To Audrey,

Whose friendship and support
in some busy times was greatly
appreciated — and who will surely
recognize an occasional patient here and there.

Donald Steinberg

September 17, 1973

CLINICAL PEDIATRIC ONCOLOGY

Clinical pediatric oncology

EDITED BY

WATARU W. SUTOW, M.D.

Pediatrician and Professor of Pediatrics, The University of
Texas M. D. Anderson Hospital and Tumor Institute at Houston,
Houston, Texas

TERESA J. VIETTI, M.D.

Professor of Pediatrics, Mallinckrodt Department of Pediatrics,
Washington University School of Medicine; Associate Pediatrician,
Barnes and Associated Hospitals; Director, Division of Hematology and
Oncology, St. Louis Children's Hospital,
St. Louis, Missouri

DONALD J. FERNBACH, M.D.

Professor of Pediatrics, Baylor College of Medicine; Chief,
Hematology and Oncology Service at Texas Children's Hospital;
Director, Research Hematology Laboratory, Texas Children's Hospital,
Houston, Texas

WITH 216 ILLUSTRATIONS

THE C. V. MOSBY COMPANY

SAINT LOUIS   1973

Contributors

Alberto G. Ayala, M.D.

Assistant Pathologist and Assistant Professor of Pathology, The University of Texas M. D. Anderson Hospital and Tumor Institute at Houston, Houston, Texas

Virginia M. Badger, M.D.

Assistant Professor of Orthopedic Surgery, Washington University School of Medicine; Assistant Surgeon, Barnes Hospital and St. Louis Children's Hospital; Assistant Surgeon, Shriners Hospital for Crippled Children; Associate, Missouri State Crippled Children's Program; Chief of Orthopedic Surgery, St. Louis City Hospital, St. Louis, Missouri

Daisilee H. Berry, M.D.

Associate Professor of Pediatrics, University of Arkansas School of Medicine; Assistant Director of Clinical Research and Attending Pediatrician, University of Arkansas Medical Center; Attending Pediatrician, Arkansas Children's Hospital, Little Rock, Arkansas

James J. Butler, M.D.

Associate Pathologist and Associate Professor of Pathology, The University of Texas M. D. Anderson Hospital and Tumor Institute at Houston, Houston, Texas

George W. Clayton, M.D.

Professor of Pediatrics and Chief, Endocrine Section, Department of Pediatrics, Baylor College of Medicine; Chief, Endocrine Service, Texas Children's Hospital, Houston, Texas

Milton H. Donaldson, M.D.

Associate Professor of Pediatrics, University of Pennsylvania School of Medicine; Senior Physician and Associate Director of Oncology, Children's Hospital of Philadelphia, Philadelphia, Pennsylvania

John W. Duckett, M.D.

Assistant Professor of Urology, University of Pennsylvania School of Medicine; Senior Surgeon, Children's Hospital of Philadelphia, Philadelphia, Pennsylvania

Donald J. Fernbach, M.D.

Professor of Pediatrics, Baylor College of Medicine; Chief, Hematology and Oncology Service at Texas Children's Hospital; Director, Research Hematology Laboratory, Texas Children's Hospital, Houston, Texas

Lillian M. Fuller, M.D.

Radiotherapist and Associate Professor of Radiotherapy, The University of Texas M. D. Anderson Hospital and Tumor Institute at Houston, Houston, Texas

Mary Ellen Haggard, M.D.

Professor of Pediatrics and Director, Division of Pediatric Hematology and Oncology, The University of Texas Medical Branch, Galveston, Texas

Martin Hrgovcic, M.D., D.Sc.(Med.)

Formerly Faculty Associate in Medicine, The University of Texas M. D. Anderson Hospital and Tumor Institute at Houston, and the Diagnostic Clinic of Houston, Houston, Texas

David H. Hussey, M.D.

Associate Radiotherapist and Associate Professor of Radiotherapy, The University of Texas M. D. Anderson Hospital and Tumor Institute at Houston, Houston, Texas

Oscar Y. King, M.D.

Project Investigator in Pediatrics, The University of Texas M. D. Anderson Hospital and Tumor Institute at Houston, Houston, Texas

Vita J. Land, M.D.

Assistant Professor of Pediatrics, Washington University School of Medicine; Assistant Pediatrician, St. Louis Children's Hospital, St. Louis, Missouri

Daniel M. Lane, M.D., M.S.(Peds.), Ph.D.

Associate Professor of Pediatrics, Tulane University School of Medicine, New Orleans, Louisiana

Derrick Lonsdale, M.B., B.S.(London)

Staff Pediatrician, Cleveland Clinic, Cleveland, Ohio

Richard G. Martin, M.D.

Surgeon and Professor of Surgery and Chief, Section of General Surgery, The M. D. Anderson Hospital and Tumor Institute at Houston, Houston, Texas

Robert W. Miller, M.D.

Chief, Epidemiology Branch, National Cancer Institute, Bethesda, Maryland; Clinical Professor of Pediatrics, Georgetown University, Washington, D. C.

S. Grant Mulholland, M.D.

Assistant Professor of Urology, University of Pennsylvania School of Medicine; Urologist, Graduate Hospital of the University of Pennsylvania; Chief, Department of Urology, Philadelphia General Hospital, Philadelphia, Pennsylvania

Carlos A. Perez, M.D.

Professor of Radiology and Chief, Clinical Section, Division of Radiation Oncology, Mallinckrodt Institute of Radiology, Washington University School of Medicine, St. Louis, Missouri

Abdelsalam H. Ragab, M.D.

Assistant Professor of Pediatrics, Washington University School of Medicine; Assistant Pediatrician, St. Louis Children's Hospital, St. Louis, Missouri

Felix Rutledge, M.D.

Gynecologist-in-Chief and Professor of Gynecology, The University of Texas M. D. Anderson Hospital and Tumor Institute at Houston, Houston, Texas

Julian P. Smith, M.D.

Gynecologist and Associate Professor of Gynecology, The University of Texas M. D. Anderson Hospital and Tumor Institute at Houston, Houston, Texas

James B. Snow, Jr., M.D.

Professor and Chairman, Department of Otorhinolaryngology, University of Pennsylvania Medical Center, Philadelphia, Pennsylvania

Kenneth A. Starling, M.D.

Assistant Professor of Pediatrics, Baylor College of Medicine; Associate Hematologist and Oncologist, Texas Children's Hospital and Research Hematology Laboratory, Houston, Texas

Herman D. Suit, M.D.

Chief, Department of Radiation Medicine, Massachusetts General Hospital; Professor of Radiation Therapy, Harvard Medical School, Boston, Massachusetts

Margaret P. Sullivan, M.D.

Associate Pediatrician and Associate Professor of Pediatrics, The University of Texas M. D. Anderson Hospital and Tumor Institute at Houston, Houston, Texas

Wataru W. Sutow, M.D.

Pediatrician and Professor of Pediatrics, The University of Texas M. D. Anderson Hospital and Tumor Institute at Houston, Houston, Texas

Jerry J. Swaney, M.D.

Associate in Pediatrics, Northwestern University; Director, Pediatric Oncology, Children's Memorial Hospital, Chicago, Illinois

Norah duV. Tapley, M.D.

Radiotherapist and Professor of Radiotherapy, The University of Texas M. D. Anderson Hospital and Tumor Institute at Houston, Houston, Texas

Jessie L. Ternberg, M.D., Ph.D.

Head, Division of Pediatric Surgery, St. Louis Children's Hospital; Professor of Surgery, Washington University School of Medicine; Associate Surgeon, Barnes Hospital and St. Louis County Hospital, St. Louis, Missouri

Patricia Tretter, M.D.

Associate Attending Radiologist and Associate Clinical Professor of Radiology, The Presbyterian Hospital in the City of New York at the Columbia-Presbyterian Medical Center, New York, New York

Frederick Valeriote, Ph.D.

Associate Professor of Radiology and Head, Section of Cancer Biology, Mallinckrodt Institute of Radiology, Washington University School of Medicine, St. Louis, Missouri

Teresa J. Vietti, M.D.

Professor of Pediatrics, Mallinckrodt Department of Pediatrics, Washington University School of Medicine; Associate Pediatrician, Barnes and Associated Hospitals; Director, Division of Hematology and Oncology, St. Louis Children's Hospital, St. Louis, Missouri

Jordan R. Wilbur, M.D.

Director, Children's Oncology Program, Children's Hospital at Stanford, Palo Alto, California

Thomas E. Williams, M.D.

Associate Professor of Pediatrics and Pathology, The University of Texas Medical School at San Antonio, San Antonio, Texas

Preface

This book represents the composite synthesis of the interest and experience of the many investigators and consultants who comprise the Pediatric Division of the Southwest Cancer Chemotherapy Study Group. The text was designed and written primarily for the clinician; correspondingly there has been less emphasis on the histopathology except as it relates to the recognition, behavior, and management of each disease entity.

Advances in the treatment of malignant neoplastic diseases are being reported with increasing regularity in all age groups, but especially in children. There has been a significant reversal of the mortality rate in some instances, a significant prolongation of the survival time in others, and effective palliation in general.

The order of the chapters was arbitrarily determined to present first the general aspects of the care of the child with cancer and to follow this with detailed discussions of the major disease entities. No attempt has been made to be all-inclusive or to provide specific modes of therapy. Our major objective was to review the status of cancer in children and to acquaint the reader with the current progress in each area.

The steady improvement in the overall survival rate of children with cancer has done much to dispel pessimism and has spawned a new era of cautious optimism. This improvement exceeds the concept of any single "wonder" drug and is, for the most part, the result of a dogged multidisciplinary approach that integrates the talents of the clinical oncologist, radiotherapist, and surgeon. By functioning in well-equipped centers they are able to extend the capability of the practicing clinician, whose increased awareness and prompt attention are still ultimately critical to the successful management of these complex problems.

As a result of the years of experience provided within the atmosphere of a collaborative group, it is obvious that the era of empirical therapy is dissipating as knowledge of the natural history of tumors, mechanisms of drug action, cellular kinetics, molecular biology, cell differentiation, and immunology continues to accumulate. The pediatric oncologist is now deeply committed in a dynamic period of experimental and investigational therapy that promises even greater benefits within the foreseeable future.

Throughout the text the reader will detect areas of overlapping material. Because of the nature of this book and an awareness of the many existing controversies, we allowed the contributing authors the freedom to express individual opinions wherever this seemed to be appropriate and desirable.

The manuscripts for many of the chapters were generously reviewed and criticized, favorably or otherwise, by our colleagues at a number of institutions.

Their assistance, as well as that of the clerks, secretaries, and others whose efforts have made this book possible, is gratefully acknowledged. We regret that all of the referring physicians, staff, and others who participated in the care of the patients involved cannot be listed here, but it is hoped that our sincere expression of appreciation will be acceptable to all. Those to whom special thanks are due include Drs. R. Cumley, D. DeVivo, C. Griffin, J. Grisham, F. Harberg, M. Ibanez, A. Kaplan, J. Kissane, G. LePage, E. Montague, and M. Smith, and especially our families.

Wataru W. Sutow
Teresa J. Vietti
Donald J. Fernbach

Contents

CLINICAL PEDIATRIC ONCOLOGY

CHAPTER 1

General aspects of childhood cancer*

WATARU W. SUTOW

CHILDHOOD CANCER

The nature and incidence of cancer in the childhood population can be estimated from several sources such as death certificates, tabulations from cancer
centers, and reports of tumor registries. Although each of these bodies of data
contains serious inherent biases, tabulations of the figures from the total group
provide information on the relative incidence of specific types of cancer in children. Age/sex/race predilections of different types of tumors will be discussed
separately in the chapter devoted to each type.

Incidence

Table 1-1 shows the combined incidence of specific types of cancer in children
as reported by two cancer centers: the Memorial Hospital for Cancer and Allied
Diseases in New York City[4] and The University of Texas M. D. Anderson Hospital and Tumor Institute in Houston.[18] Also shown in Table 1-1 is the report of
the Manchester (England) Children's Tumour Registry,[17] covering a 10-year
period (1953-1963) in a general childhood population of approximately 1 million.

Data obtained from hospital sources may reflect specialized interests of the
hospital. Thus the relative infrequency of tumors of the brain and retinoblastomas
in the two cancer hospitals shown in Table 1-1 suggests that many patients with
these tumors were referred to other centers concentrating on the care of such
patients.

The incidence rates of childhood cancer are more difficult to determine than
the mortality rates. A report based on the New York state registry data, covering
all of New York State exclusive of New York City (about 2,769,000 children
in 1960), showed an overall rate of 11.33 per 100,000 children under 15 years
of age for 1941-1943, 12.05 for 1949-1951, and 11.67 for 1958-1960.[12]

The incidence of childhood cancer within a geographically limited region
(Harris County, Texas, which includes Houston) has been determined from
a study of hospital records between 1958 and 1970.[13] During this period, 672
cases were recorded. Based on the 1960 and 1970 census reports, rates for the
0- to 15-year age group per 100,000 population per year have been calculated
for a number of childhood malignant diseases (Table 1-2).

---

*Supported in part by U. S. Public Health Service Research Career Award CA-2501.

Table 1-1. Relative incidence of specific types of cancer in children under 15 years of age

Type of cancer	Relative frequency (%)	
	Cancer center data*	Manchester (England) Tumour Registry data†
Leukemia	31	29
Lymphoma—Hodgkin's disease	10	9
Soft tissue sarcoma	14	12
Bone sarcoma	13	2 (Ewing's sarcoma)
Neuroblastoma	9	8
Wilms' tumor	7	5
Brain tumors—retinoblastoma	6	20
Miscellaneous	10	15
Total	100	100
Total number of cases	(2248)	(994)

*Data from Dargeon[4] and Sutow.[18]
†Data from Marsden and Steward.[17]

Table 1-2. Incidence of specific malignant diseases in children (0 through 14), Harris County, Texas, 1958-1970*

Type of neoplasm	Rate per 100,000 per year
Leukemia	3.72
Lymphoma	1.25
Central nervous system	1.85
Neuroblastoma	0.90
Wilms' tumor	0.85
Bone sarcoma	0.48
Rhabdomyosarcoma	0.27
Retinoblastoma	0.24
All others	1.23
Total	10.79

*Data from Texas Center for Disease Control.[13]

Table 1-3. Mortality rates in the United States for malignant tumors in children

	Mortality rate (per 100,000 population)*		
	Age under 1 yr	Ages 1-4 yr	Ages 5-14 yr
1940	4.4	4.8	3.0
1950	8.7	11.7	6.7
1960	7.2	10.9	6.4
1966†	5.6	8.3	6.4
White	5.9	8.8	6.7
Nonwhite	3.9	5.5	5.0
Male	5.2	8.8	7.3
Female	6.0	7.7	5.5

*Data from Grove and Hetzel.[11]
†Data from Public Health Service.[19]

Mortality

Cancer kills more children at the present time than does any other disease in the age group of 1 through 14 years, ranking second to accidents as a major cause of death.[19] The American Cancer Society estimates that in 1972 cancer will take the lives of approximately 4000 children under the age of 15.[1] Mortality figures extracted from U. S. Vital Statistics for the past three decades have been tabulated in Table 1-3.

Miller[15] has analyzed all (29,457) death certificates in the United States for children under the age of 15 years who died during the period 1960-1966, as well as the death certificates (2487) for those 15 to 19 years of age who died in 1965 and 1966. The relative incidence of specific types of cancer and their respective mortality rates have been summarized from Miller's report in Table 1-4.

Table 1-4. Mortality from childhood cancer*

| Type of cancer | Ages under 15 yr (1960-1966) | | Ages 15-19 yr (1965-1966) | |
	Total deaths (%)	Rate*	Total deaths (%)	Rate*
Leukemia	48	3.45	30	2.63
Brain tumor	16	1.13	11	1.01
Lymphoma	8	0.54	17	1.54
Neuroblastoma	7	0.50	1	0.10
Wilms' tumor	5	0.38	1	0.07
Bone cancer	4	0.28	13	1.19
Rhabdomyosarcoma	2	0.15	3	0.25
Liver	1	0.08	1	0.10
Retinoblastoma	1	0.05	–	0.004
Teratoma	1	0.05	2	0.17
Miscellaneous	7	0.53	21	1.81

*Per 100,000 per year, based on data from Miller.[15]

Table 1-5. Relative incidence of specific types of cancer in children and adults

| Tumor types | Children 0-14 yr* | All types of cancer (%) all ages | |
		Dorn and Cutler†	Griswold and associates‡
Leukemia/lymphoma	41	6	7
Sarcomas	27	3	3
Embryonal tumors	16	1	1
Neural tumors	6	2	1
Carcinomas and adenocarcinomas	5	85	86
All others	5	3	2
Number of cases	2248	45,311	29,260
Number of children included	2248	594	425

*Data from Dargeon[4] and Sutow.[18]
†Data from Dorn and Cutler.[5]
‡Data from Griswold, Wilder, Cutler, and Pollack.[9]

Data from death certificates are subject to variations in completeness of reporting and accuracy of diagnosis. Moreover, mortality figures cannot provide a precise estimate of the actual incidence of specific types of cancer having significant cure rates.

Comparison of childhood cancer with cancer in adults

The spectrum of types of cancer in children differs strikingly from that in adults. The types that most often affect children are the leukemias, embryonal tumors, and sarcomas. Adenocarcinomas and carcinomas, which constitute the majority of cancers in adults, are rare in children. Data from several reports have been tabulated to provide a comparison between childhood and adult cancers (Table 1-5). Although these data were obtained by various means from several tumor populations, the vast differences in the types of cancer prevalent among children as compared to those in the general population (predominantly adult) are immediately apparent.

TEAM APPROACH AND TOTAL CARE

The optimum care of children with cancer now includes the application of all known modes of therapy, particularly the multimodal and interdisciplinary approach. This is the total care concept so effectively developed by Farber.[8] Such collaboration among specialists should involve every aspect of patient care, from the diagnostic procedures through definitive therapy and family support.

That this type of organized and coordinated treatment program carried out by experienced physicians in well-staffed and well-equipped medical centers is effective has been demonstrated in published statistics. The survival rate of 89% among 53 children who were treated entirely by Farber and his group for nonmetastatic Wilms' tumor was significantly better than the survival rate of 39% among 54 children whose treatment was started elsewhere and was continued at Farber's institution.[7]

The survival times of 220 children with acute leukemia who were treated in England and Wales from 1963 through 1967 by physicians specializing in childhood leukemia (study group) were compared with those of 1025 children who were treated for this disease by other physicians (comparison group). In a report to the Medical Research Council, the Committee on Leukaemia and the Working Party on Leukaemia in Childhood concluded that the children in the study group had a considerably longer life expectancy than did the children in the comparison group.[6] It is suggested that during the period covered by the study, the "improvement in survival is due not so much to the details of the therapeutic regimens as to the availability of special facilities and expertise."[6]

The use of sensitive and sophisticated diagnostic procedures increases the likelihood, not only of establishing the proper diagnosis, but also of delineating more precisely the extent of the disease. The latter aspect may be vital in the application of effective therapy such as surgery and irradiation. Diagnostic procedures developed in recent years include lymphangiography, angiography, xerography, isotope scanning, electron microscopy, and tissue culture techniques.

Every helpful approach should be considered and used, if appropriate, in the diagnosis and treatment. If adequate facilities and personnel are not available, the patient should be referred promptly to a university clinic or cancer center wherein such help can be obtained. Surely, a child with cancer and his parents should expect and receive no less.

PERIOD OF RISK AND CURE

After diagnosis and definite therapy, when can a child with a given type of cancer be presumed to be cured? Consideration in this section will be limited to solid tumors. The reader is referred to the chapters on acute leukemia, Hodgkin's disease, lymphomas, and histiocytosis for discussions of long-term survival and cure of those diseases.

Utilizing data from published cases of Wilms' tumor and other sources, Collins[2] introduced the concept of a *period of risk* in the prognosis of solid tumors in 1955. Since a tumor in a given patient could have been present (and growing) no longer than the patient's chronologic age at the time of diagnosis plus the 9 months of gestation, it was postulated that any occult residual tumor present at the time of definitive treatment (assuming an unchanged growth rate) should reach the same size as the primary tumor in the same length of time (that is, the patient's age plus 9 months). Collins concluded that if no evidence of recurrence or metastases became apparent during this time, called the *period of risk*, the patient could be considered cured.[3] Subsequently, other independent reports appeared to substantiate the validity of this concept.[14] In fact, observations based originally on data from patients with Wilms' tumor seemed to hold also for patients with neuroblastoma and rhabdomyosarcoma.[14]

Gross[10] had commented that in children with Wilms' tumor, a fixed post-therapy period of 1 to 1½ years seemed to distinguish those who would remain free of the disease. Platt and Linden,[16] using the California Tumor Registry, compared the two criteria for survival: the period of risk as proposed by Collins and the fixed interval of 2 years. They concluded that the survival rates for the variable interval (Collins) and the fixed interval of 2 years were almost identical.

Although exceptions are uncommon, the application of any rule of this type to a single case carries a risk of being unreliable; nevertheless, these concepts are useful in discussing the prognosis with the parents. Such guidelines are also necessary for the planning and evaluation of long-term continuation therapy.

The recent development of newer antineoplastic drugs has resulted in a more prolonged control of several types of tumor, even though the patient is not cured. An example of this is the significant increase in the duration of remissions in children with acute leukemia following currently employed chemotherapeutic regimens (Chapters 9 and 10). Similar improvements in the results of chemo-therapy could well be anticipated in children with some types of solid tumors.[18] If, however, the growth rate of the tumor is appreciably retarded by these agents, modifications in the concept of the risk period will become necessary.

REFERENCES

1. American Cancer Society: '72 cancer facts and figures, 1972, The Society.
2. Collins, V. P.: Wilms' tumor, its behavior and prognosis, J. Louisiana Med. Soc. **107**:474-480, 1955.
3. Collins, V. P., Loeffler, R. K., and Tivey, H.: Observations on growth rates of human tumors, Am. J. Roentgenol. Radium Ther. Nucl. Med. **76**:988-1000, 1956.

4. Dargeon, H. W.: Tumors of childhood: a clinical treatise, New York, 1960, Paul B. Hoeber, Inc., p. 28.
5. Dorn, H. F., and Cutler, S. J.: Morbidity from cancer in the United States, Public Health Monograph No. 56 (Public Health Service Publication No. 590), 1959.
6. Duration of survival of children with acute leukaemia, Br. Med. J. 4:7-9, Oct. 2, 1971.
7. Farber, S.: Chemotherapy in the treatment of leukemia and Wilms' tumor, J.A.M.A. 198:826-836, 1966.
8. Farber, S.: The control of cancer in children. In Neoplasia in childhood, presented at the Twelfth Annual Clinical Conference on Cancer, 1967, at the University of Texas M. D. Anderson Hospital and Tumor Institute at Houston, Chicago, 1969, Year Book Medical Publishers, Inc. pp. 321-327.
9. Griswold, M. H., Wilder, C. S., Cutler, S. J., and Pollack, E. S.: Cancer in Connecticut, 1935-1951, Hartford, Conn., 1955, Connecticut State Department of Health.
10. Gross, R. E.: The surgery of infancy and childhood, Philadelphia, 1953, W. B. Saunders Co.
11. Grove, R. D., and Hetzel, A. M.: Vital statistics rates in the United States, 1940-1960, Washington, D. C., 1968, National Center for Health Statistics.
12. Handy, V. H.: Malignancies in children, Am. J. Dis. Child. 106:54-64, 1963.
13. Incidence of childhood cancer in Harris County, Texas, 1958-1970, Leukemia Section, Center for Disease Control, Feb., 1972.
14. Knox, W. E., and Pillers, E. M. K.: Time of recurrence or cure of tumors in childhood, Lancet 1:188-191, 1958.
15. Miller, R. W.: Fifty-two forms of childhood cancer: United States mortality experience, 1960-1966, J. Pediatr. 75:685-689, 1969.
16. Platt, B. B., and Linden, G.: Wilms's tumor—a comparison of 2 criteria for survival, Cancer 17:1573-1578, 1964.
17. Problems of children's tumours in Britain. In Marsden, H. B., and Steward, J. K.: Tumours in children, New York, 1968, Springer-Verlag New York, Inc., pp. 1-12.
18. Sutow, W. W.: Drug therapy and curability of childhood cancer, Postgrad. Med. 48:173-177, Nov., 1970.
19. Vital statistics of the United States, 1966, Washington, D. C., 1968, Public Health Service.

CHAPTER 2

Etiology of childhood cancer

ROBERT W. MILLER

It is understandable that in the bustle of medical practice physicians will focus their attention on diagnosis and treatment rather than exploring clues to etiology. In consequence, new clinical observations of possible research value go unnoticed or unrecorded. Such observations may concern environmental exposures, therapy, preexistent diseases in the patient, or familial disorders—any of which may portend an increased risk of certain cancers. Recognition of high-risk factors is of value in the prevention and early detection of certain neoplasms.

ENVIRONMENTAL FACTORS

A variety of environmental exposures have been described that are oncogenic in man,[10] but only one of these—ionizing radiation—has induced cancer in children.[44] In part, this difference is due to the much smaller exposure of children to oncogenic agents, which adults encounter at work or by habit.

Drugs during childhood. There is no doubt that (1) drugs containing radioisotopes and (2) immunosuppressive therapy after renal transplantation are related to an increased frequency of cancer in man.[7, 54, 58] Cancer in adults may be induced by a few other drugs, as indicated by case reports (e.g., leukemia after the use of chloramphenicol[57] or melphalan[27, 32]). There is much better evidence of chemical carcinogenesis in man caused by occupational exposures than by drug therapy.

Drugs during fetal life. A monumental finding in human oncology was announced in April, 1971: heavy doses of stilbestrol given to pregnant women to prevent abortion were implicated as the cause of adenocarcinoma of the vagina in their daughters 14 to 22 years later.[26] The initial report describing 7 cases in Boston was quickly confirmed by a search of the New York State Tumor Registry, which revealed 5 more.[23] Adenocarcinoma of the vagina is extremely rare so early in life, and these clusters of cases could not be attributed to chance. Had a more common neoplasm such as lymphoma or neuroblastoma been involved, the excess of cases would probably have gone undetected. Studies are now in progress to determine if stilbestrol during pregnancy induces other cancers or disorders in the offspring and to determine if other drugs may do the same. Sensitivity may be greater in the fetus than in later life. Indeed, there is better evidence for oncogenicity after fetal exposure to stilbestrol than there is for any drug taken later in life.

Viruses. An important development in cancer research has been the invention of statistical techniques for determining dispassionately whether the frequency with which a rare event clusters in time and space exceeds normal expectation.[41] There is no doubt that after examining the distribution of cases on a scatter map, one can identify individual clusters of rare diseases by inspection and can draw tight boundaries around them. The question is not "Do rare events cluster?" but "Do they cluster excessively?" To date, the application of these new statistical procedures in studies of leukemia has provided no solid evidence of an excess suggesting an infectious mode of spread.[20, 21] In contrast, the application of one of these techniques to data for Burkitt's lymphoma in the West Nile District of Uganda has shown considerable evidence of clustering.[56] For this reason among others, an infectious origin is far more likely for African lymphoma than for leukemia.

Tests of various hypotheses concerning the infectious transmission of leukemia have been made, and the findings were negative. For example, if there is an infectious transmission, it might be detectable among persons having the closest contact with the neoplasm. Leukemia has not been found, however, to occur excessively among marital partners of leukemic persons[43] or in children born of women with leukemia during pregnancy.[13]

Leukemia in mice can be experimentally transmitted to the young by viruses in breast milk.[24, 33] Is there a human counterpart to this laboratory observation? The answer is no. The histories of breast-feeding among 541 children with leukemia under 15 years of age were compared with those for a similar number of neighborhood control children. No significant differences in the frequency or duration of breast-feeding were found.[49]

The hypothesis that the leukemia virus may be widely prevalent in blood but of low pathogenicity is not supported by observations in man. In the series of children just described, there was no significant difference between cases and controls in the frequency of exchange transfusion for blood type incompatibility in the newborn period, when immunologic defenses are low.[44] The claim that a slow virus may be responsible for human leukemia, as is presumed to be true for kuru (cerebellar ataxia in New Guinea), meets difficulty when comparison is made of the epidemiology for the two diseases. Deaths from kuru cluster in villages and in time, but deaths from leukemia do not. Evidence for vertical transmission from mother to child is substantial for kuru, but absent for leukemia. Overall, epidemiologic studies support the belief that kuru is infectious and that leukemia is not.[49]

These observations do not exclude the possibility of a viral role in leukemogenesis. They do indicate that if viruses are involved, their mode of transmission is too subtle to be detected by methods available at present.

HOST FACTORS

Mortality rates in children with specific forms of cancer exhibit dynamic changes by single year of age. These variations must reflect important etiologic influences. Among white children in the United States, the mortality rate for acute lymphocytic leukemia exhibits a huge peak at 4 years of age that is absent among nonwhite children.[48] There is no such peak for children with acute myelogenous leukemia. Thus there must be racial differences in exposure or susceptibility to some agent that induces acute lymphocytic leukemia but not acute myelogenous leukemia.

In children about 4 years of age, there are also peaks in mortality from Wilms' tumor[34] and neuroblastoma[53]—cancers whose intrauterine origins are suggested by their occurrence in very young patients and by the high frequency with which they are found in situ (microscopically) at autopsy in patients younger than 3 months of age, but not thereafter.[59] The same age pattern is exhibited for primary liver cancers,[17] retinoblastoma,[30] ependymoma,[52] and presacral teratoma.[52] These tumors may be linked with or distinguished from one another by the specific congenital malformations with which they are associated.

Leukemia. Leukemia is at times determined prezygotically. It occurs excessively in Down's syndrome,[50] which in 95% of all cases is due to trisomy 21, in consequence of meiotic nondisjunction.[38] The probability that a child with Down's syndrome will develop leukemia is about 1 in 200—about fifteen times the normal rate.[50] The risk of developing leukemia is substantially higher in two genetically transmitted diseases, Bloom's syndrome and Fanconi's aplastic anemia.[46] The numbers of persons with these syndromes *and* leukemia, although small, indicate that the neoplasm occurs in adolescence or early adulthood and in Fanconi's anemia is limited to the acute myelomonocytic type.[11] The magnitude of the risk of leukemia in these syndromes appears to be almost 1 in 10. Both syndromes are characterized by chromosomal fragility in cell culture.

In addition, there is a high rate of leukemia among atomic bomb survivors in Japan,[29] persons occupationally exposed to benzene,[22] and patients with multiple myeloma treated with melphalan (L-phenylalanine mustard) or cyclophosphamide.[27, 32] Groups at high risk of leukemia have in common a chromosomal abnormality, although not of a single type—congenital aneuploidy in Down's syndrome, chromosomal fragility in Bloom's and Fanconi's syndromes, and long-lasting complex chromosomal aberrations after exposure to ionizing radiation, benzene, melphalan, or cyclophosphamide.[9, 46, 60]

Persons with high probability of developing leukemia do not carry a similar risk of lymphoma, a neoplasm that is associated instead with inborn, immunologic, cell-mediated deficiencies (congenital thymic alymphoplasia, Wiskott-Aldrich syndrome, and ataxia-telangiectasia).[18] Thus the constellation of diseases associated with leukemia is different from that associated with lymphoma.

Wilms' tumor. In an entirely different orbit is Wilms' tumor, adrenocortical neoplasia, and primary liver cancer, which are associated with several congenital growth excesses.[48] Each of the three neoplasms occurs excessively with congenital hemihypertrophy; the neoplasms and hemihypertrophy are independently associated with large pigmented or vascular nevi, among other hamartomas, and with the visceral cytomegaly syndrome to which Beckwith has recently called attention (Fig. 2-1). The syndrome consists of omphalocele, macroglossia, and cytomegaly of visceral organs, including the three in which neoplasia has been observed in association with hemihypertrophy.[5, 28]

Wilms' tumor also occurs excessively with congenital aniridia. This ocular defect, bilateral absence of the iris, is ordinarily extremely rare. Its frequency in children with Wilms' tumor is about a thousand times greater than normal.[46] Ordinarily aniridia is due to an autosomal dominant gene, and two thirds of the cases have a familial history of the defect. When present with Wilms' tumor, aniridia has been nonfamilial, with the exception of 1 case out of 30, indicating that the eye defect and the tumor are due to a new genetic mutation or to an environmental agent that mimics the action of a gene.

It should be noted that the malformations associated with the three categories

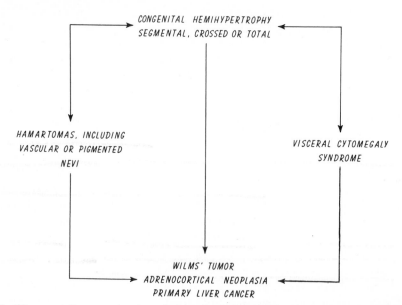

Fig. 2-1. Diagrammatic representation of the relationship among four forms of growth excess. Arrows point away from preexistent disease. (From Miller, R. W.: J. Natl. Cancer Inst. 40:1079-1085, 1968.)

of childhood cancer just described are quite different, with little overlap among them. Leukemia is associated with preexistent chromosomal abnormality, lymphoma with immunodeficiency (inborn or iatrogenic), and Wilms' tumor with various manifestations of growth abnormality. These observations can be useful in identifying circumstances of the host or the environment that carry high risk of these neoplasms. Thus they are not only of value in prevention but also can be used by laboratory scientists to further the understanding of the relationship between oncogenesis and teratogenesis.

Neuroblastomas. The vast majority of neuroblastomas are diagnosed in children under 5 years of age. Study of 504 hospital charts for children with this tumor has revealed no excessive occurrence with specific congenital anomalies.[53] This is in marked contrast to the three separate constellations of anomalies associated with leukemia, lymphoma, and Wilms' tumor.

Retinoblastomas. Nationwide study of death certificates for children in the United States who died of cancer (1960-1967) revealed that 269 deaths were due to retinoblastoma.[30] There was a peak in mortality at 2 to 3 years of age that was two and one-half times greater in Negroes than in whites. Study of 1623 hospital records of children with retinoblastoma revealed a threefold excess of mental retardation as compared with normal expectation. Associated malformations in several cases suggested D-deletion syndrome, which had previously been described in 6 case reports concerning children with retinoblastoma.

Until recently, retinoblastoma was thought to be primarily due to the action of autosomal dominant genes, with nonfamilial (sporadic) cases attributable to new germinal mutation. Current evidence indicates that only a relatively small portion of sporadic cases can be so explained.[31] It is now thought that when both eyes are affected, a germinal mutation is the cause. Thus bilaterality signifies hereditary transmission. Sporadic unilateral cases originate postzygotically.[31] Statistical study of age at diagnosis has revealed that in a semilogarithmic plot a straight line was obtained for bilateral cases and a curved line for unilateral cases, These results suggest a one-hit event in the genesis of bilateral cases and two hits in the genesis of unilateral cases.[31] Thus retinoblastoma appears to develop in two steps: in hereditary cases one step occurs prezygotically (germinal mutation) and the other postzygotically; in sporadic cases both steps are believed to involve postzygotic events.

Teratomas. Study has not yet been made of a sufficiently large series of teratoma to determine its occurrence with congenital malformations. Review of 63 cases of sacrococcygeal teratoma suggests, however, an association with maldevelopment of the hind gut and "cloacal" region.[6] It was thought that these defects may be related to pressure from the tumor during organogenesis.

Brain tumors. The only brain tumor with a well-defined peak under 5 years of age is ependymoma.[52] Study has not yet been made of its association with congenital malformations.

Medulloblastoma is diagnosed at a relatively constant rate until 8 years of age, after which there is a progressive fall in rates for both diagnosis and mortality throughout adolescence.[52] Diagnosis of glioma rises to a peak frequency in children 3 to 5 years of age. The peak in mortality from these tumors occurs at 6 years of age, with a slow decline thereafter.

The risk of glioma is very much increased in tuberous sclerosis and multiple neurofibromatosis.[55] There is a possibility that, even in subclinical form, these genetically induced hamartomatous syndromes may predispose to glioma and thus account for excessive family aggregation of the neoplasm.[35]

Apparently in the same category is the basal cell nevus syndrome. Recently this disease has been reported in several families in which young children have been observed with medulloblastoma with or without signs of the syndrome.[2] In two instances the brain tumor was the first manifestation of the syndrome, a circumstance that indicates the importance of the family history not only with regard to brain tumors but also to characteristics of syndromes in which such neoplasms may be found. Van der Wiel,[64] in a large study of relatives of persons with glioma, found 29 with major congenital defects of the spine or skull (anencephaly, spina bifida, or hydrocephalus), as compared with only 1 among the control group. His study, in effect, generates the hypothesis that these malformations are associated with glioma. It would be of interest to test this idea in a study more sharply focused on these particular anomalies.

Rhabdomyosarcomas. A peak under 5 years of age is exhibited by rhabdomyosarcoma with regard both to diagnosis and mortality.[36] Although this neoplasm exhibited familial occurrence with regard to tumors of the same cell type and specific rare tumors of other cell types, no association with congenital anomalies was detected among 280 children in a multihospital series.

In perspective, neoplasms with peaks in occurrence under 5 years of age presumably have their origins during intrauterine development. An association with congenital anomalies, however, is variable. It is most marked in Wilms' tumor and leukemia, whereas no association has yet been demonstrated with regard to neuroblastoma.

Neoplasms that do not have a peak in occurrence under 5 years of age will now be considered.

Gonadal tumors. At present, gonadoblastoma is the only neoplasm for which a congenital defect—gonadal dysgenesis—is known to be a prerequisite.[42] In Poland, the occurrence of gonadal tumors was studied in 25 patients with Turner's syndrome and in 26 other patients whose legal sex was female and who had gonadal dysgenesis with primary amenorrhea.[61] Exploratory laparotomy, mostly elective, revealed the presence of 7 unsuspected gonadal tumors in addition to 3 that were diagnosed preoperatively. The 4 classes of tumor described were gonadoblastoma, interstitial hilar cell tumor, seminoma, and Brenner tumor.

Lymphomas. Mortality patterns for children with Hodgkin's disease display several peculiarities that are presumably of etiologic significance.[45] First, there are very few deaths from this disease in patients under 5 years of age—only 22 in the entire United States between 1960 an 1964. This scarcity of cases may indicate a delay in exposure or susceptibility to oncogenic influences. Second, the sex ratio (M/F) is a static 3.0 in children from 5 to 11 years of age and then falls steadily to the level of 1.5 found in adults. The fall in sex ratio occurs in conjunction with a climb in mortality rates, which begins at 11 years of age (Fig. 2-2). Since the average survival time among children with Hodgkin's disease is about 2.7 years,[12] the rise in rates at 11 years must reflect an increase in exposure or susceptibility before 8 years of age. There is no reason to suspect one environmental agent rather than another at present. As to susceptibility, perhaps the largest physiologic change at about 8 years of age is a tremendous involution of

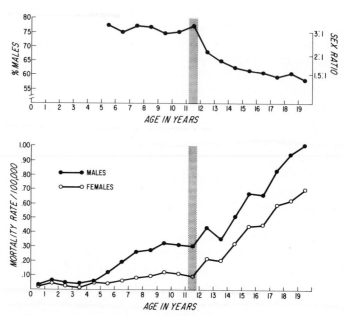

Fig. 2-2. Mortality from Hodgkin's disease among white children in the United States, 1950-1959; sex ratio (M/F) as related to death rate by single year of age and sex. (From Miller, R. W.: J.A.M.A. **198:**1216-1217, 1966.)

the lymphatic tissue (e.g., tonsils and adenoids). This involution, if faulty, might predispose to Hodgkin's disease, an ailment in which a substantial number of immunologic abnormalities have been found.[1]

Another epidemiologic characteristic that provides an etiologic clue to Hodgkin's disease is a bimodal distribution of age at death, found in all countries studied except Japan.[40] Mortality rates begin to rise at 11 years of age, reach a peak at 25 to 29 years, and then drop before another climb to a second peak late in life. In Japan the mortality patterns clearly reveal the absence of the first peak. Thus the usual bimodality represents the presence of two age distributions, an epidemiologic feature that suggests two different sets of etiologic factors are operative.

The age distribution of reticulum cell sarcoma and lymphosarcoma in children has not yet been reported. Burkitt's lymphoma exhibits a peak at about 8 years of age and, as already noted, shows evidence by its epidemic patterns of occurrence in Africa of being environmentally induced.

Although various forms of lymphoma in the United States do not show a peak occurrence under 5 years of age, they do occur excessively with heritable disorders characterized by cell-mediated immunologic deficiency.[18] There is no specificity as to cell type in the lymphomas that occur with these diseases. After immunosuppressive therapy for organ transplantation, however, a marked excess has been observed in the occurrence of reticulum cell sarcoma, especially of the brain, an organ in which this form of neoplasia is extremely uncommon.[58]

Bone sarcomas. Study of bone sarcoma in dogs strongly suggests that the occurrence of this neoplasm is closely related to bone growth. The relative risk among giant breeds of dogs, such as the Saint Bernard and Great Dane, is about two hundred times that for small- or medium-sized breeds.[62] This observation is consistent with the similarity in man between patterns of growth (stature) and mortality rates from bone cancer.[48] The average height by single year of age for boys and girls rises progressively and is virtually identical until 13 years of age when boys grow taller than girls. Mortality rates from bone cancer are virtually identical for both sexes until precisely the same age, 13 years, when the rates for boys first exceed those for girls (Fig. 2-3). It is to be expected, then, that children with bone cancer will be taller than average. Finding data collected in the past to test this hypothesis is difficult. In the one study that has been made of stature after tumor development, the affected children were significantly taller than average.[14] The absolute differences in height, however, were small.

From studies of radium-dial painters, there is no doubt that radioisotopes in sufficient dosage can induce osteogenic sarcoma in man.[4] The neoplasm also can be induced by doses of external radiation in excess of 3000 r.[63]

Recently, the study of the occurrence of bone sarcoma in Negroes vs whites revealed a very low rate of Ewing's sarcoma in Negroes, whereas the rate for osteosarcoma was similar to that for whites.[19] This finding is of clinical value in the differential diagnosis of bone lesions affecting Negroes and is of research value in considering the origins of Ewing's tumor in regard to osteosarcoma.

Study of almost 400 hospital records for children with bone cancer in the United States revealed an association with several preexistent skeletal defects such as bone cysts or multiple hereditary exostoses.[19]

Thyroid cancer. Although thyroid cancer is a rare cause of death in childhood,

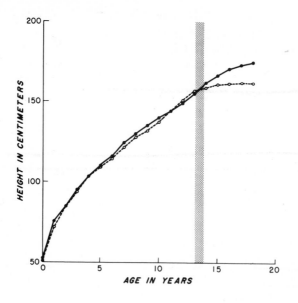

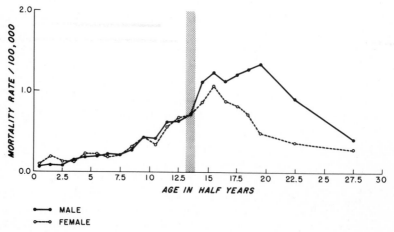

●——● MALE
○——○ FEMALE

Fig. 2-3. Comparison of stature with bone cancer mortality (1950-1959) by single year of age and sex among white children in the United States. (From Miller, R. W.: J. Natl. Cancer Inst. 40:1079-1085, 1968.)

there is no doubt that it was induced relatively easily in the past by therapeutic irradiation of the thymus in infancy.[25] Benign tumors of the thyroid have been induced by the same treatment procedure, by the ^{131}I in the fallout to which children on the Marshall Islands were exposed,[25] and by the atomic bomb exposure in Japan.[65]

Familial cancer. There is a wide array of cancers that are either heritable in themselves, such as retinoblastoma, or are manifestations of hereditary syndromes, such as astrocytomas that occur in tuberous sclerosis. Detailed reviews of these disorders have been published by Lynch,[39] Anderson,[3] and Fraumeni.[15]

Certain other childhood cancers also aggregate in families more often than can be expected by chance. When death certificates for all children who died of cancer in the United States between 1960 and 1967 were alphabetized according to mother's name, deaths involving sibs could be recognized by the repeated listing of the same mother's name, along with the same surname for more than one child. Fifty-four pairs of sibs were thus identified. Their family relationship was confirmed by reference to the death certificates, which showed that each pair had the same father and the same home address.[51]

Seven pairs were twins of like sex, who were presumably identical and had died of leukemia. The probability was very low that more than 1 pair would occur in the series by chance. For individual pairs the age at death differed by as little as 24 days, and in all but one instance the intervals between the deaths were less than 7 months. Although the ages studied ranged up to 19 years, none of the twin pairs with leukemia was over 6 years of age at death. Zuelzer and Cox[66] have shown that concordance for leukemia is virtually 100% when the first twin develops the neoplasm before 1 year of age. With increasing age at diagnosis of the first twin, there is a diminishing probability that the co-twin will develop leukemia, until a near normal value is reached at about 6 years of age. Clarkson and Boyse[8] have pointed out that this sharp fall in concordance with age is what one would expect if leukemic cells were transplanted from one identical twin to the other during intrauterine life, while they share the same placental circulation.

In the death certificate study, there were 8 pairs of sibs other than twins with brain tumor as compared with 0.9 expected. These occurrences may be due to genetic disorders, perhaps subclinical, which carry a high risk of brain tumor (e.g., neurocutaneous syndromes). The same explanation has previously been offered to account for eight brain cancers in 17 members of one family that perhaps had subclinical multiple neurofibromatosis.[35]

The death certificate study also revealed that in eight families, 1 child had died of brain cancer and another of cancer that was primary in muscle or bone. Review of the hospital records for these cases revealed tuberous sclerosis in 1 pair, but no heritable disease in the other 7.

Childhood cancer, when observed in individual pairs of sibs, will naturally be attributed to chance. Only when data for a country as large as the United States are accumulated for 5 to 10 years can an excessive occurrence be demonstrated.

Other sib pairs in the death certificate series are known to be from "cancer families"—families that had been ascertained by other means and that contained many members who developed cancers, generally at an early age. One such familial cancer syndrome included soft tissue sarcomas in 2 children and breast cancer often in the mother, but also in other female relatives. Five families with this syndrome have been described by Li and Fraumeni.[36, 37]

It is noteworthy that familial cancer may be of the same cell type or of dissimilar cell types, often rare in the general population. The recurrence of the pattern and the rarity of some of the cell types strongly suggest that these family aggregates are not due to chance, although formal statistical proof of the excess in families may be difficult to achieve.

CONCLUSION

Insight into the etiology of childhood cancer often comes from clinical observations involving small series of cases. The opportunities for such observations would be greatly enhanced if, in the hospital examination of each child with cancer, the physician would use a checklist of malformations for the child and other family members. Thus, for example, acute myelomonocytic leukemia in a phenotypically normal child may possibly be related to Fanconi's anemia in a first cousin. A self-administered questionnaire completed by parents concerning cancer in the family would also be of benefit. Parents are often willing, and even anxious, to contribute to an exploration into factors that may have influenced the development of cancer in their child. The histories they contribute may be more complete than those that the physician can obtain and record on the hospital chart.

Through the use of these devices, review of hospital cases would be greatly simplified, and potentially valuable observations could be quickly tabulated. Furthermore, the information so obtained may well contribute to recognition of individual cases of particular interest at the time of admission, allowing opportunity for special laboratory studies (e.g., cytogenetics, virology, or immunology) concerning features possibly involved in the development of the disease. The potential importance of individual family studies may thus be appreciated at a time when the index case and family are still available for study.

REFERENCES

1. Aisenberg, A. C.: Manifestations of immunologic unresponsiveness in Hodgkin's disease, Cancer Res. **26**:1152-1160, 1966.
2. Aita, J. A.: Genetic aspects of tumors in the nervous system. In Lynch, H. T., editor: Hereditary factors in carcinoma, vol. 12 in Recent results in cancer research, New York, 1967, Springer-Verlag New York, Inc., pp. 86-110.
3. Anderson, D. E.: Genetic varieties of neoplasia. In Genetic concepts and neoplasia, Twenty-Third Annual Symposium on Fundamental Cancer Research, Baltimore, 1970, Williams & Wilkins Co., pp. 85-104.
4. Aub, J. C., Evans, R. D., Hempelmann, L. H., and Martland, H. S.: The late effects of internally-deposited radioactive materials in man, Medicine **31**:221-329, 1952.
5. Beckwith, J. B.: Macroglossia, omphalocele, adrenal cytomegaly, gigantism, and hyperplastic visceromegaly, Birth Defects: Original Article Series **5**:188-196, 1969.
6. Berry, C. L., Keeling, J., and Hilton, C.: Coincidence of congenital malformation and embryonic tumours of childhood, Arch. Dis. Child **45**:229-231, 1970.
7. Boyd, J. T., Langlands, A. O., and Maccabe, J. J.: Long-term hazards of thorotrast, Br. Med. J. **2**:517-521, 1968.
8. Clarkson, B. D., and Boyse, E. A.: Possible explanation of the high concordance for acute leukaemia in monozygotic twins, Lancet **1**:699-701, 1971.
9. Cohen, M. M.: Drugs and chromosomes, Ann. N. Y. Acad. Sci. **171**:467-477, 1970.
10. Doll, R.: Prevention of cancer: pointers from epidemiology, London, 1967, Whitefriars Press, Ltd.
11. Dosik, H., Hsu, L. Y., Todaro, G. J., Lee, S. L., Hirschhorn, K., Selirio, E. S., and Alter, A. A.: Leukemia in Fanconi's anemia: Cytogenetic and tumor virus susceptibility studies, Blood **36**:341-352, 1970.
12. Evans, H. E., and Nyhan, W. L.: Hodgkin's disease in children, Bull Johns Hopkins Hosp. **114**:237-248, 1964.
13. Fraumeni, J. F., Jr.: Sex ratio of children born of leukemic mothers, Pediatrics **33**:587-589, 1964.
14. Fraumeni, J. F., Jr.: Stature and malignant tumors of bone in childhood and adolescence, Cancer **20**:967-973, 1967.

15. Fraumeni, J. F., Jr.: Genetic factors in the etiology of cancer. In Holland, J. F., and Frei, E., III: Cancer medicine, Philadelphia, Lea & Febiger (in press).
16. Fraumeni, J. F., Jr., and Glass, A. G.: Wilms' tumor and congenital aniridia, J.A.M.A. **206:**825-828, 1968.
17. Fraumeni, J. F., Jr., Miller, R. W., and Hill, J. A.: Primary carcinoma of the liver in childhood: An epidemiologic study, J. Natl. Cancer Inst. **40:**1087-1099, 1968.
18. Gatti, R. A., and Good, R. A.: Occurrence of malignancy in immunodeficiency diseases. A literature review, Cancer **28:**89-98, 1971.
19. Glass, A. G., and Fraumeni, J. F., Jr.: Epidemiology of bone cancer in children, J. Natl. Cancer Inst. **44:**187-199, 1970.
20. Glass, A. G., and Mantel, N.: Lack of time space clustering of childhood leukemia, Los Angeles County, 1960-64, Cancer Res. **29:**1995-2001, 1969.
21. Glass, A. G., Mantel, N., Gunz, F. W., and Spears, G. F. S.: Time space clustering of childhood leukemia in New Zealand, J. Natl. Cancer Inst. **47:**329-336, 1971.
22. Goguel, A., Cavigneau, A., and Bernard, J.: Les leucémies benzéniques de la région parisienne entre 1950 (etude de 50 observations), Nouv. Rev. Fr. Hematol. **7:**465-480, 1967.
23. Greenwald, P., Barlow, J. J., Nasca, P. C., and Burnett, W. S.: Vaginal cancer after maternal treatment with synthetic estrogen, N. Engl. J. Med. **285:**390-392, 1971.
24. Gross, L.: Transmission of mouse leukemia virus through milk of virus-injected C3H female mice, Proc. Soc. Exp. Biol. Med. **109:**830-836, 1962.
25. Hempelmann, L. H.: Risk of thyroid neoplasms after irradiation in childhood, Science **160:**159-163, 1968.
26. Herbst, A. L., Ulfelder, H., and Poskanzer, D. C.: Adenocarcinoma of the vagina: association of maternal stilbestrol therapy with tumor appearance in young women, N. Engl. J. Med. **284:**878-881, 1971.
27. Holland, J. F.: Epidemic acute leukemia, N. Engl. J. Med. **283:**1165-1166, 1970.
28. Irving, I. M.: The "E. M. G." syndrome (exomphalos, macroglossia, gigantism), Progr. Pediatr. Surg. **1:**1-61, 1970.
29. Ishimaru, T., Hoshino, T., Ichimaru, M., Okada, H., Tomiyasu, T., Tsuchimoto, T., and Yamamoto, T.: Leukemia in atomic bomb survivors, Hiroshima and Nagasaki, 1 October 1950-30 September 1966, Radiat. Res. **45:**216-233, 1971.
30. Jensen, R. D., and Miller, R. W.: Retinoblastoma: epidemiologic characteristics, N Engl. J. Med. **285:**307-311, 1971.
31. Knudson, A. G., Jr.: Mutation and cancer: statistical study of retinoblastoma, Proc. Natl. Acad. Sci. U.S.A. **68:**820-823, 1971.
32. Kyle, R. A., Pierre, R. V., and Bayrd, E. D.: Multiple myeloma and acute myelomonocytic leukemia, N. Engl. J. Med. **283:**1121-1125, 1970.
33. Law, L. W., and Moloney, J. B.: Study of congenital transmission of a leukemia virus in mice, Proc. Soc. Exp. Biol. Med. **108:**715-723, 1961.
34. Ledlie, E. M., Mynors, L. S., Draper, G. J., and Gorbach, P. D.: Natural history and treatment of Wilms' tumour: An analysis of 335 cases occurring in England and Wales 1962-6, Br. Med. J. **4:**195-200, 1970.
35. Lee, D. K., and Abbott, N. L.: Familial central nervous system neoplasia. Case report of a family with von Recklinghausen's neurofibromatosis, Arch. Neurol. **20:**154-160, 1969.
36. Li, F. P., and Fraumeni, J. F., Jr.: Rhabdomyosarcoma in children: Epidemiologic study and identification of a familial cancer syndrome, J. Natl. Cancer Inst. **43:**1365-1373, 1969.
37. Li, F. P., and Fraumeni, J. F., Jr.: Soft-tissue sarcomas, breast cancer, and other neoplasms. A familial syndrome? Ann. Intern. Med. **71:**747-752, 1969.
38. Lilienfeld, A. M.: Epidemiology of mongolism, Baltimore, 1969, Johns Hopkins Press, p. 26.
39. Lynch, H. T.: Hereditary factors in carcinoma, vol. 12 in Recent results in cancer research, New York, 1967, Springer-Verlag New York, Inc.
40. MacMahon, B.: Epidemiology of Hodgkin's disease, Cancer Res. **26:**1189-1200, 1966.
41. Mantel, N.: The detection of disease clustering and a generalized regression approach, Cancer Res. **27:**209-220, 1967.
42. Melicow, M. M.: Tumors of dysgenetic gonads in intersexes: Case reports and discussion regarding their place in gonadal oncology, Bull. N. Y. Acad. Med. **42:**3-20, 1966.

43. Milham, S.: Leukemia in husbands and wives, Science **148**:98-100, 1964.
44. Miller, R. W.: Radiation, chromosomes and viruses in the etiology of leukemia: Evidence from epidemiologic research, N. Engl. J. Med. **271**:30-36, 1964.
45. Miller, R. W.: Mortality in childhood Hodgkin's disease, J.A.M.A. **198**:1216-1217, 1966.
46. Miller, R. W.: Persons at exceptionally high risk of leukemia, Cancer Res. **27**(part I): 2420-2423, 1967.
47. Miller, R. W.: Effects of ionizing radiation from the atomic bomb on Japanese children, Pediatrics **41**:257-263, 1968.
48. Miller, R. W.: Relation between cancer and congenital defects: An epidemiologic evaluation, J. Natl. Cancer Inst. **40**:1079-1085, 1968.
49. Miller, R. W.: The viral etiology of leukemia: An epidemiologic evaluation. In Zarafonetis, C. J. D.: Proceedings of the International Conference on Leukemia-Lymphoma, Philadelphia, 1968, Lea & Febiger.
50. Miller, R. W.: Neoplasia and Down's syndrome, Ann. N. Y. Acad. Sci. **171**:637-644, 1970.
51. Miller, R. W.: Deaths from childhood leukemia and solid tumors among twins and other sibs in the United States, 1960-67, J. Natl. Cancer Inst. **46**:203-209, 1971.
52. Miller, R. W.: Unpublished data.
53. Miller, R. W., Fraumeni, J. F., Jr., and Hill, J. A.: Neuroblastoma: Epidemiologic approach to its origins, Am. J. Dis. Child. **115**:253-261, 1968.
54. Modan, B., and Lilienfeld, A. M.: Polycythemia vera and leukemia—the role of radiation treatment. A study of 1222 patients, Medicine **44**:305-344, 1965.
55. Paulson, G. W., and Lyle, C. B.: Tuberous sclerosis, Dev. Med. Child Neurol. **8**:571-586, 1966.
56. Pike, M. C., Williams, E. H., and Wright, B.: Burkitt's tumour in the West Nile District of Uganda 1961-5, Br. Med. J.**2**:395-399, 1967.
57. Pisciotta, A. V.: Drug-induced leukopenia and aplastic anemia, Clin. Pharmacol. Ther. **12**:13-43, 1971.
58. Schneck, S. A., and Penn, I.: De-novo brain tumours in renal-transplant recipients, Lancet **1**:983-986, 1971.
59. Shanklin, D. R., and Sotelo-Avila, C.: In situ tumors in fetuses, newborns and young infants, Biol. Neonate **14**:286-316, 1969.
60. Shaw, M. W.: Human chromosome damage by chemical agents, Ann. Rev. Med. **21**:409-432, 1970.
61. Teter, J., and Boczkowski, K.: Occurrence of tumors in dysgenetic gonads, Cancer **20**: 1301-1310, 1967.
62. Tjalma, R. A.: Canine bone sarcoma: Estimation of relative risks as a function of body size, J. Natl. Cancer Inst. **36**:1137-1150, 1966.
63. United Nations: Report of the United Nations Scientific Commitee on the effects of atomic radiation, General Assembly, official records, nineteenth session, supp. no. 14 (a/5814), New York, 1964, United Nations.
64. Van der Wiel, H. J.: Inheritance of glioma. The genetic aspects of cerebral glioma and its relation to status dysraphicus, Amsterdam, 1960, Elsevier Publishing Co.
65. Wood, J. W., Tamagaki, H., Neriishi, S., Sato, T., Sheldon, W. F., Archer, P. G. Hamilton, H. B., and Johnson, K. G.: Thyroid carcinoma in atomic bomb survivors, Hiroshima and Nagasaki, Am. J. Epidemiol. **89**:4-14, 1969.
66. Zuelzer, W. W., and Cox, D. E.: Genetic aspects of leukemia, Semin. Hematol. **6**:228-249, 1969.

CHAPTER 3

General surgical considerations

JESSIE L. TERNBERG
VIRGINIA M. BADGER

The surgeon has a central role in the modern multidiscipline treatment of malignant childhood tumors. This role includes (1) *treatment*, (2) *diagnosis*, (3) *staging of disease*, and (4) *palliation*. If surgical treatment is to be effective, technical skill must be coupled with judgment. The surgeon who operates on a child with cancer must have a thorough knowledge of not only the existence of age-dependent physiologic differences but also the unique differences encountered in childhood tumors. Even the prognosis for the same tumor type (e.g., neuroblastoma) may differ from one age to another. The treatment of a malignant tumor will be dictated by its pathologic behavior, location, size, the involvement of adjacent structures, and the knowledge of past results using various therapeutic modalities.

When the pediatric cancer surgeon undertakes an operation, he must understand its limitations and its risks. This implies a careful preoperative assessment of the patient. Extensive surgery is now possible because of improvement in anesthetic and surgical techniques and better preoperative and postoperative support and care. In contrast to adult malignancies, many pediatric tumors are very responsive to chemotherapy and may be converted from inoperable to operable tumors by preoperative treatment to decrease tumor size. Similarly, metastatic disease associated with childhood tumors can be treated more aggressively with excision of isolated metastases to the brain, lung, and liver. It is important that the first operation be an adequate cancer operation whenever possible. Multiple operations reduce the chance of a successful outcome. If a surgeon encounters a more complex problem than he is prepared to handle during a routine procedure, he should close the wound and refer the child to a center where optimal management of the tumor can be provided.

It is extremely important to maintain good communication among the specialists involved in treating the child with a malignant tumor. Ideally, the surgeon, chemotherapist, radiologist, and radiotherapist should each consult at the beginning of the diagnostic evaluation. The availability of a well-trained pathologist is essential. When it is decided that an operative procedure is indicated, the surgeon should assume the primary role to ensure that the necessary diagnostic procedures and preoperative arrangements are efficiently coordinated. Once the child is returned to a nonsurgical status, surgical service may resume a consultative role.

PREOPERATIVE CARE
Preparation of parents

The parents must clearly understand the indications for surgery; parents who are adequately informed will cope with the rest of the problems related to the

19

surgery more easily. The necessity for counseling and preparation of the parents of a child who is about to be operated on for tumor will vary. After a brief descriptive explanation as to what the operation entails, the parents should be encouraged to ask questions to allay specific fears. The emphasis should be on residual function and plans for rehabilitation. The problems and alternatives that may result if the operation is not done should be detailed to avoid misunderstanding and to support the parents, who must give their informed consent. Possible discomfort the child may experience postoperatively should be explained, as well as how long it might last and what will be done to minimize it.

The parents should be prepared for the actual mechanics of the procedure: premedication, transportation to surgery, use of blood and intravenous fluids, and the use of a recovery area. The parents are also prepared for possible variations in the time spent in the operating room and in the recovery room so that any unexpected delay will not take on the significance of a disaster. The use of supportive measures and various nursing routines should be explained. Occasionally, families are upset by the sheer number of personnel involved in caring for their children and should be prepared for this, with particular emphasis on the importance of the continuous care provided by the house staff. The necessity for laboratory tests should also be explained in advance.

The ability of the child to cope with a given procedure and its consequences will often depend on the manner in which the parents react to the child before and after the operation.

Preparation of child

The preparation of the child for an operation is a more difficult problem and will vary with the age and background of the child. Under most circumstances the preparation is the same as for any surgical procedure; the child should be informed in simple terms about the mechanics of the surgical process and the resulting sequelae. In general, simple explanations are inadequate, particularly with the older child, who should be given an opportunity to ask questions and express his doubts. As with the parents, the emphasis should be less on what is to be done and more on how he will be afterward. It is important that this be a matter-of-fact approach without withdrawal on part of the professional people or the parents and that the child never receive cold impersonal treament along the way. Hospital units designed to care for children should be warm (in the personal sense) bright places geared to a normal child's environment. Accordingly, they often appear to be areas of rampant confusion to individuals accustomed to the quiet, sedate environment of adult hospitals.

Preoperative evaluation

A detailed preoperative evaluation of the child's condition is essential so that proper measures can be taken before operation (1) to decrease the risk of surgery, (2) to ensure an adequate operation, and (3) to decrease complications. Evaluation of the patient for surgery can appropriately be started by considering the tumor: location, size, systemic effects, and involvement of adjacent organs. In certain clinical situations, angiography may be helpful in defining the extent of the tumor and the blood supply. The potential hazards of this procedure in infants and small children should be kept in mind.

The child should be evaluated next from a general point of view. Unlike the adult, the child has a changing physiologic status conferred by growth. If the child appears to have developed normally, chances are his *nutritional* status is satisfactory. History, physical examination, and radiologic examinations combine to provide a satisfactory evaluation of the *respiratory* and *cardiovascular* systems. Hypertension has been noted in some of the patients with Wilms' tumor and in some with neuroblastoma. No specific treatment for the hypertension is usually required in these patients; it should, however, be noted and followed up in case a problem arises. After surgery the blood pressure frequently returns to normal levels. On the other hand, the child with a pheochromocytoma presents a serious problem requiring rigorous control of the blood pressure through the preoperative, intraoperative, and postoperative periods.

Renal function is assessed by a routine urinalysis and blood urea nitrogen. Most of the children will have had an intravenous pyelogram as part of their diagnostic workup, and, although this will not supply reliable quantitative information about renal function, it will furnish the important information of location of functioning renal tissue. It is advisable to do the intravenous pyelogram by injecting the dye into a leg vein. This provides an inferior venacavogram, which may give additional information about tumor site and extent. When bilateral renal involvement is present or suspected, arteriography is useful to indicate extent of involvement, plus the location and number of vessels supplying the tumor.

The hemodynamic status of the child is an important preoperative consideration, especially when a major surgical procedure is contemplated. Although a minimum hemoglobin level of 10 grams/100 ml is a widely established prerequisite for elective surgery, it is the blood volume and red blood cell mass of the patient that are more directly related to anesthesia complications. When transfusion is indicated because of chronic blood losses, packed cells are given preoperatively. If immediate surgery is indicated in the presence of a severe chronic anemia, a modified exchange transfusion with packed red blood cells can be done to increase the red cell mass without increasing the total blood volume. The intravascular component of body fluid can be decreased in certain tumors, notably pheochromocytoma and probably in all catecholamine secretors. Preoperative detection of a blood volume abnormality and appropriate treatment ensures a safer operation.

Electrolyte imbalance may be present, especially if there is any history of diarrhea or vomiting. Imbalances should be corrected preoperatively, but correction may be almost impossible if losses are continuing. For example, tumors arising from the sympathetic nervous system may be associated with severe uncontrolled diarrhea. Generally, removal of the tumor will result in an abrupt cessation of the diarrhea. In a situation such as this, prolonged preparation is not indicated.

Possible problems caused by *bleeding* or *clotting errors* must also be considered. For example, a low platelet count may result from the preoperative use of chemotherapy, and platelet transfusions may be indicated.

Preoperative orders

There are no specifically different preoperative orders for the child who is to be operated on for a tumor. The surgeon must be informed about possible drug allergies and present and past drug history. The past or present use of steroids in particular may require use of an additional amount of steroid preoperatively and intraoperatively.

OPERATIVE CARE
Anesthesia

When an intravenous route is to be established, two important factors must be considered: (1) the potential blood loss and (2) the length of time an intravenous infusion will be required. A large-bore, secure, intravenous catheter route must be available if sudden large blood loss is possible. Placement of the intravenous catheter may also depend on the sites of potential blood loss; for example, major losses from the inferior vena cava cannot be replaced through an infusion in a lower extremity. A Silastic catheter is introduced via a tunneling technique when it appears that prolonged intravenous treatment will be necessary.

Physiologic monitoring

The measurement of the *central venous pressure (CVP)* is a valuable aid, particularly if large amounts of blood or intravenous fluids or both are administered. Correct central venous pressure monitoring requires the catheter tip to be in the superior vena cava or right atrium. The location of the catheter tip at the time of insertion is established by x-ray examination. CVP measurements must be made serially to be of significance as an indicator of hypervolemia. If a central venous catheter is inserted, proper precautions must be taken to avoid the complications of air embolism.

A running estimate of blood loss is kept. This requires the use of small calibrated suction traps and dry laparotomy pads or sponges that are weighed to provide a gravimetric method of determining loss.

Blood pressure is also monitored. The Doppler technique is advocated for blood pressure measurements in young infants. In special situations it may be important to monitor arterial pressure directly. This can be done by direct percutaneous puncture of the radial artery in older children, but a cutdown may be required in smaller children and infants. Use of the ulnar artery is contraindicated because of the close proximity of the ulnar nerve, which may be traumatized. The needle or catheter is connected to a transducer for pressure monitoring. Periodic heparinized saline irrigations are required to keep the system patent. Arterial blood gases can be followed more frequently in this situation than if a separate arterial puncture is required for each determination.

Electrocardiograph (ECG) monitoring is recommended as a routine procedure. It provides a visual pulse rate plus quick identification of cardiac irregularity.

Urinary output can be followed up and will indicate whether adequate perfusion of the kidneys is being maintained.

Temperature regulation in small children and infants can be a serious problem, and it is necessary to be prepared to warm or cool the patients.

Positioning and draping of patients

Positioning of the patient and draping of the operation site are all important. On the chest, abdomen, or back, the use of a Steri-drape or a similar device allows exposure of a much larger operative field without extensive surface skin exposure. These drapes also aid in decreasing excessive heat loss in the infant.

During draping, consideration must be given to the possible need to extend the operative incision. For example, if a sacrococcygeal teratoma has a large pelvic and intra-abdominal extension, the preparation and draping of the infant should allow repositioning to permit both a sacral and an intra-abdominal approach. The entire operation can then be completed in a single stage. Similarly, possible thoracic extensions should be allowed by appropriate skin preparation and draping. The abdomen and perineum can be handled as a single field in combined abdominoperineal procedures. In all situations in which an intra-abdominal procedure is to be combined with an extra-abdominal procedure, care is taken to use separate instrument setups and to change the gowns and gloves of the operating team.

When amputation of an extremity is to be done, the extremity should be draped freely to allow movement of the next proximal joint. A double tourniquet technique may be used in treating tumors of the leg or forearm if it is probable that the surgical pathologist will be able to make a diagnosis from frozen sections. The distal tourniquet is inflated during the biopsy procedure. If the decision for amputation is made, the extremity can then be amputated between the two tourniquets (after inflation of the most proximal one) without the potential spread of tumor cells in the general circulation from the original biopsy site. Obviously the extremity should not be exsanguinated with a rubberized bandage before distal tourniquet inflation. If a hip disarticulation or hemipelvectomy procedure is anticipated, then catheter drainage for the bladder is mandatory, as is also purse-string suturing of the anal sphincter.

Intravenous fluids

Intraoperative intravenous fluids will vary with the problem presented by the patient. The administration of Ringer's lactate at 5 ml/kg/hr is used when minimal translocation or loss of extracellular fluid is assumed. The amount may be increased, depending on the kind and extent of surgery. Whole blood is replaced after an estimated 10% loss of blood volume if further significant loss is anticipated; otherwise replacement is withheld until losses are estimated to be 15% of the blood volume.

SURGERY—GENERAL PRINCIPLES

The surgical approach depends on why the operation is to be done: (1) to establish a definitive diagnosis, (2) as a curative resection, (3) for staging of disease, (4) as a palliative procedure, or (5) as a combination of two or more of these. Specific details of various surgical approaches are beyond the scope of this chapter; however, certain general principles are pertinent to tumor operations.

Curative surgery is based on the rationale of total removal of the tumor without breaking its continuity. Although biopsy of the tumor may compromise a curative operative procedure, an operation that imposes risk and possible physiologic impairment cannot be recommended without a pathologic diagnosis. Judgment is based to a considerable extent on knowledge of tumor pathology and behavior and the consequences of the proposed surgical procedure. For example, it is difficult to biopsy an intra-abdominal mass and avoid potential contamination by tumor cells. In the instance of a probable Wilms' tumor, biopsy would not be indicated if the intravenous pyelogram was considered diagnostic and the intraoperative appearance was that of Wilms' tumor. Errors in diagnosis may be made (e.g., most commonly dysplastic kidney), but impairment of function is not a consequence, since nephrectomy would be indicated anyway.

In general, if the operation that will satisfactorily remove a tumor or lesion masquerading as a tumor can be done without physiologic impairment or undue risk, the procedure can be done as an excisional biopsy. Incisional biopsy is mandatory for definitive tumor therapy when (1) the tumor location or extent prevents its complete removal, (2) the tumor removal will result in serious physiologic or functional impairment (e.g., amputations, urinary tract diversions), (3) tumor removal may be accompanied by high mortality risk, or (4) radiotherapy or chemotherapy or both may be as effective and less mutilating then attempted surgical excision. The importance of an adequate biopsy must be stressed, and extensive surgery may be necessary to obtain this. Superficial biopsies in the presence of inflammatory, fibrovascular reaction around a tumor are frequently nondiagnostic. Tumor necrosis may also be the basis for diagnostic problems. The pathologist should be consulted before the biopsy procedure is completed. A frozen section will frequently indicate if the tissue obtained will be adequate for diagnosis. If there is a question about the adequacy of the specimen obtained, further biopsies can be obtained before the procedure is terminated. Diagnostic difficulties may also be associated with the use of cutting or cauterizing current secondary to charring and dehydration of tissue. Care should be exercised during biopsy to protect normal tissue from contamination by tumor cells, especially if future surgical resection of the tumor is a probability.

Lymph nodes should be biopsied by excising the entire node; this may avoid a draining fistula if the lesion is infectious instead of neoplastic. In the presence of neoplastic adenopathy, biopsy of superficial nondiagnostic nodes may result in delayed treatment. It is important that node biopsies be done carefully and that the most suspicious nodes are obtained. When generalized adenopathy is present, the inguinal nodes are best avoided in children over 1 year of age because of the high frequency of an overlying inflammatory process, which makes tissue diagnosis difficult. Lymph node imprints and cultures should be obtained before the node is placed in fixative. In undertaking staging operations, the principle of adequate lymph node biopsy must be followed or the procedure has no value.

A careful and complete exploration with adequate documentation is mandatory in staging, diagnostic, and therapeutic operative procedures. It should be emphasized that familiarity with tumor behavior is important, for example, the potential bilaterality of Wilms' tumors and likely sites of and the appearance of metastatic disease. Whether biopsying, staging, or undertaking an extirpative operation, a surgical incision should be made that will give optimal exposure. It is well to remember the surgical adage that a wound heals from side to side and not from end to end. Knowledge of the regional distribution of lymphatics is important for en bloc tumor and regional node dissection. Whenever possible, the vascular supply to a tumor should be isolated and clamped before the tumor is manipulated to prevent vascular dissemination of tumor cells. The diagnosis of metastatic disease should be confirmed by biopsy. Silver clips should be placed to mark biopsy and tumor removal sites as an aid to subsequent evaluation and possible future radiotherapy.

The palliative role of surgery may be extremely useful, for example, in resections for pain, obstruction, infected ulcerations, or hemorrhage. The surgeon's goal in undertaking a palliative procedure is the relief of symptoms or the lessening of a child's illness. The expected relief should be balanced against the morbidity of the operative procedure. Prolongation of life may result from the palliative operation, but the surgeon should be careful not to do an operation that prolongs life without the relief of symptoms.

POSTOPERATIVE CARE

Dressings

Subcuticular skin closure allows operative incisions to be dressed with Steri-strips that can be removed in 2 to 3 days. The advantages of this dressing include almost full visualization of the operative site and absence of tape burns. Radiation therapy fields can be easily located and marked, and therapy can be begun without removing dressings. When body secretions or excretions may be a problem, wounds can be left completely undressed so that they can be constantly visualized and cleaned. Cotton balls and soap are used to clean the soiled area, followed by a saline rinse and gentle drying.

In the case of an extremity amputation for a tumor, the wound is closed primarily, drained (Penrose drain or Hemovac suction), and then dressed with a rigid elastic or plaster dressing. At the second cast change (approximately 10 days), if a leg wound is sufficiently healed, a plaster pylon may be applied to allow the patient to begin early ambulation.

Intravenous fluids

The general assumption is made that intraoperative fluid losses have been replaced during surgery; therefore orders are written for maintenance fluids only. If there is any concern about renal function (e.g., any procedure involving both kidneys), potassium should be omitted from the postoperative fluids until there is practical information available that adequate urinary output is established. In addition to maintenance fluids, provision must be made for continuing losses (e.g., through the nasogastric drainage). It is important that the patient be reevaluated frequently and fluid orders changed as necessary if clinically indicated. Plasma or albumin is rarely used unless a specific problem such as protein-losing enteropathy or extensive liver resection exists. If low serum proteins are present on a nutritional basis and restoration of normal alimentation will be delayed, a program of parenteral hyperalimentation will be instituted in preference to plasma or albumin supplementation.

Medications

Antibiotics are rarely used routinely in clean operations. If it is anticipated that the biliary system, the bowel, or the urinary tract will be opened, systemic antibiotics are started just before the operation and continued for 2 days postoperatively. If unanticipated peritoneal contamination occurs, antibiotics are started during surgery.

Pain medication orders will vary, depending on the age and condition of the child and the operation done. Children are generally hesitant to request injections so that a PRN order for pain medication may not be satisfactory unless the nursing service accepts the responsibility of giving the medication when it appears indicated.

Special provision should be made for the child who has had an amputation. Immediately postoperatively he may experience phantom sensations described as pain or abnormal position. It should be explained that this is a normal phenomenon that will become less and less noticeable, although it may never go away completely. A mild sedative may relieve the discomfort associated with phantom sensations, but for the first 36 to 48 hours it may be necessary to supplement this with a mild analgesic as well. By 72 hours, it is usually possible to start wheelchair or ambulation activities or both, which definitely decreases this complaint. Phantom limb sensations must also be explained to the parents so that they too will appreciate this phenomenon.

Care must be taken to be sure that preoperative medications have renewal orders if indicated. A child who has been on steroids preoperatively will require higher doses immediately after the operation, but the customary dose should be resumed as soon as possible.

Chemotherapy can be resumed or started immediately postoperatively if indicated. Ordinarily, postoperative recovery is smoother if these agents can be delayed until the patient is taking liquids orally without difficulty, especially those agents that are associated with nausea, vomiting, and obstipation.

Physiologic monitoring

The postoperative monitoring of patients consists of routine recording of their pulse, blood pressure, respiration, temperature, and urine output and accurate measurements of drainage tube contents, coupled with comments about the patient's general appearance and state of consciousness. When intra-arterial or central venous pressure monitoring has been established during the operation, it can be continued postoperatively. ECG monitoring, respiratory monitoring, and automatic blood pressure monitoring are available in many intensive care units. These are not generally necessary but can be extremely valuable under specific circumstances such as postoperative pheochromocytoma patients. Of equal importance are the skills of an adequate number of competent, enthusiastic, and sympathetic nurses.

Respiratory problems

Endotracheal tubes are occasionally left in place for several hours up to 1 to 2 days postoperatively if the patient needs the support of a respirator or an airway problem exists. The following special care will be required: (1) adequate humidification of the air, (2) careful aseptic suctioning of the tube, and (3) close observation for mechanical problems related to the tube or the respirator. When a tracheostomy has been done, the same care must be given.

Activity

The infant or younger child who is left unrestrained will usually become active almost immediately postoperatively. Although a child is not forced to sit up on the day of surgery, he may if he wants—he may also go to the bathroom, etc. If no voluntary activity has been undertaken, the patient is placed in a chair during the first postoperative day, and he is encouraged to be up and about increasing his activity daily. After brief instructions to the mother by the nurses, we allow the mother to hold the patient shortly after an operation if he is an infant or toddler. This removes some of her apprehension and provides activity and security for the patient.

The child who has had an amputation is encouraged to sit up within the first 24 to 36 hours and then is encouraged to move about in a wheelchair or is started on crutches by the physical therapy staff. Active motion exercises are started by the second postoperative day, and the lower extremity amputee is encouraged to lie prone part of the day to prevent hip flexion contracture. The use of pillows under an amputated stump is discouraged unless there is a need for postoperative elevation.

Every effort is made to fit the child amputee with a permanent prosthesis as soon as the circumference measurements of the stump are stabilized and his weight is stabilized. This general philosophy is followed even though the long-term prognosis is entirely unpredictable. A child is usually ready for prosthetic fitting between 10 and 12 weeks postoperatively.

Feeding

One of the early problems postoperatively is to obtain adequate fluid intake orally. If there is no gastrointestinal problem or other reason for ileus, the child is offered clear liquid when he is fully alert. Carbonated beverages are frequently used, since they are generally more acceptable to the patient and intake is therefore better. Once clear liquids are tolerated well, the diet is advanced to a general diet modified only according to the age of the patient.

When the gastrointestinal tract is involved (e.g., an anastomotic site or ileus), gastrointestinal decompression is continued until functional intestinal activity is demonstrated. Clear liquids are then started and, if tolerated, are followed by a full liquid diet. In turn this progresses to a regular diet. Soft diets are similar to regular diets, but generally they are less palatable and serve no real purpose.

CHAPTER 4

Basic concepts and clinical implications of radiation therapy

CARLOS A. PEREZ

Since the discovery of x rays by Roentgen in 1896 and radium by Curie and Becquerel in 1898, ionizing radiations have been widely used in the treatment of malignant tumors, alone or in combination with surgical procedures or cytotoxic agents. A significant improvement has been demonstrated in treatment results when these different modalities are combined. It is critical that specialists in all areas concerned with the treatment of cancer patients be familiar with the basic concepts of radiation therapy so that a coordinated interdisciplinary strategy of management will be fully understood and carried out.

PRACTICAL ASPECTS OF RADIATION THERAPY

Irradiation is frequently used in the treatment of pediatric neoplasias, usually in conjunction with an operation or chemotherapy or both.[117, 118] Also, palliation can be accomplished with relief of symptoms or shrinkage of masses.[116] The attitude of the parents toward the distressful experience of taking care of a child with cancer who is to be treated by irradiation and their interrelationship with the child are important to the adjustment of the young patient to this new environment. The radiotherapist must discuss in detail not only what he hopes to accomplish with radiation therapy but also the probable transient as well as late undesirable side effects. Since these sequelae may be frightening to the parents, it is helpful to have the referring pediatrician reassure them that radiation therapy is the most optimal approach of the treatment modalities available and discuss with them the effects of other alternative therapy or the prognosis of the child if he does not receive treatment. Sometimes it is necessary to have a second interview with the parents before consent for radiation therapy is obtained. Complete and informed consent with a signed permit by the parents or legal guardian is necessary before radiation therapy is administered to a child.

Adequately trained technical personnel with experience in the handling of children will be required. It is very important that they have the proper psychologic attitude to inspire confidence in their little patients, since this is the single most important principle in immobilization during the treatment. An apprehensive child is restless and will not lie still. Sometimes, in special circumstances, heavy sedation or even a light general anesthetic is needed to ensure satisfactory immobilization.

Devices can be used to facilitate the treatment setup and make the patient more comfortable. Head holders, restraining bands, and foam pillows are very helpful.[22, 108] A vacuum-operated head holder has been particularly useful in the

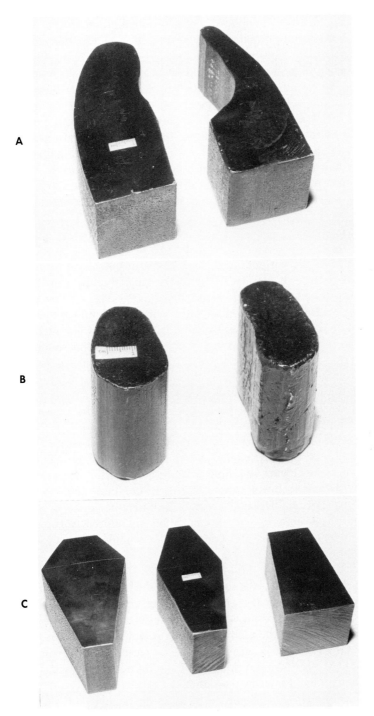

Fig. 4-1. Examples of lead shielding blocks used during external beam radiation therapy. **A**, For the lungs. **B**, For the kidneys. **C**, For the gonads.

treatment of children with head and neck neoplasias. Immobilizing plastic molds can be worn during treatment to reduce inaccuracy in positioning. In patients with angled beams, a back pointer and a pin and arc will allow accurate alignment of the beams. A simple way of reproducing this type of complex treatment setup can be accomplished with a cardboard cutout as described by Fletcher in his textbook.[57]

Properly designed protective lead or tungsten blocks are imperative to provide maximum shielding of normal uninvolved organs[122, 123] such as the eyes, ears, spinal cord, lungs, heart, kidneys, and gonads (Fig. 4-1). If personnel and adequate facilities are available, tailored individual shielding blocks for each patient are ideal. Likewise, special compensating filters may be required to correct the distribution of radiation in a patient with an irregular external surface such as the thoracic inlet or to compensate for density inhomogeneity of the tissues treated. To achieve optimal results, accurate treatment techniques are mandatory so that the dose received by the patient is the one plotted on the treatment computations.

Supportive care

Because of the various side effects that can be caused by irradiation, optimal supportive care is necessary. If this is lacking, therapy may have to be discontinued or protracted over a long period of time.

Acute reactions such as nausea and vomiting should be promptly controlled. This usually can be done with phenothiazine derivatives such as Compazine or Thorazine. If persistent vomiting is present, medication should be given parenterally (IM) or in suppositories until normal oral intake is reinstated. Diarrhea, which usually appears when the abdomen or the pelvis is irradiated, can be controlled with antispasmodics and preparations with kaolin pectine. In more severe cases of vomiting and diarrhea, oral intake should be discontinued and intravenous fluid administration instituted. Careful monitoring of fluid and electrolyte balance with repeated laboratory determinations is necessary.

Mucositis of the oral cavity and the pharynx can be significantly decreased with continuous mouth washing with salt water or commercial mouthwashes mixed with water. Local care of the lips and oral cavity is mandatory, using topical glycerin on ulcerated areas. Administration of local anesthetics such as lidocaine (Xylocaine) is not recommended in children. Soft or liquid diet with a high content of proteins and carbohydrates should be given, unless the patient is unable to swallow.

Dental care is very important during and after radiotherapy.[107] Removal of metallic dental prostheses is recommended during the period of irradiation. When irradiation of the salivary glands is necessary, the composition of the saliva changes, which may result in a significant increase in caries.[58, 61] At this time, fluorine treatment of the teeth, as well as periodic visits to the dentist, is in order. If a dental extraction is necessary, special care should be applied to make it as atraumatic as possible, and the patient should be treated with antibiotics prior to, at the time of, and for a few days after the extraction.

The irradiated skin should be kept clean during and after therapy, washed daily with a mild soap and without scrubbing. As soon as erythema or dry desquamation appears, continuous use of a lubricating agent such as petrolatum or, better, hydrous lanolin, applied two or three times daily will help prevent further damage to the skin and will keep it moist and pliable.

In those patients in whom moist desquamation develops, the direct application of these ointments on the skin is difficult and painful. In this situation it is better to smear the lanolin on a thin piece of gauze and gently apply it over the denuded skin. If there is crusting or hemorrhage, the area should be cleaned with hydrogen peroxide (half-strength) and soap at least once daily.

Occasionally, ointments containing 0.25% to 0.5% hydrocortisone are helpful in controlling more severe skin reactions. If any infection is present, steroids should not be used. Instead, increasing use of the hydrogen peroxide is recommended, as well as topical application of 1% zinc oxide ointments. Varying degrees of skin care should be continued for 4 to 6 weeks after completion of therapy until complete reepithelization occurs.

Treatment planning

Since a tumor is not isolated in space, but situated within a patient who has structures sensitive to radiation, adequate treatment planning is crucial (Fig. 4-2). This is a complex equation with multiple functions,[115] which include the following:

1. Characteristics of the patient (age, sex, general condition)
2. Pathologic and biologic features of the tumor, including accurate localization and consideration of routes of spread[101]
3. Anatomic and physiologic characteristics of the normal tissues and their tolerance to irradiation[93, 143]
4. Aim of radiation therapy, that is, curative or palliative
5. Distribution of ionizing radiation in the treated volume
6. Dose-time relationship of irradiation

It is very important to approach the patient with a malignant tumor in an interdisciplinary fashion, with the pediatrician, chemotherapist, surgeon, and radiation therapist participating in the overall treatment planning. From the radiation therapist's viewpoint, it is imperative to determine whether the patient is going to be treated solely by radiation or in combination with one or more of the other techniques, namely, chemotherapy or surgery. This may determine not only the treated volume but also the dose that will be given to the patient and whether irradiation will be done preoperatively or in the postoperative period.[117, 118] A thorough knowledge of the biologic and pathologic characteristics of the tumor is basic to successful therapy. If a lesion is amenable to surgical extirpation, with high cure rates, surgery should be the treatment of choice, since ionizing radiation or chemotherapy may produce some undesirable side effects, particularly in growing children. However, in lesions that are not completely resectable or have a tendency toward dissemination, combination therapy should be preferred. This is the case in many pediatric malignant neoplasms such as rhabdomyosarcoma, Ewing's tumor, neuroblastoma, and Wilms' tumor. Leukemias are primarily treated by chemotherapy. Lymphomas, when localized to the lymph nodal system, are managed by irradiation; in more advanced stages, they are treated with a combination of irradiation and chemotherapeutic agents.

In addition to simple dose calculations, hand or computerized representa-

RADIATION THERAPY

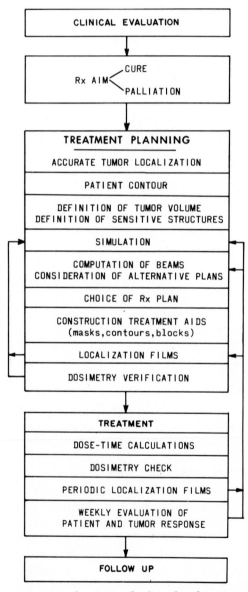

Fig. 4-2. Schematic representation of steps involved in the planning and delivery of radiation therapy.

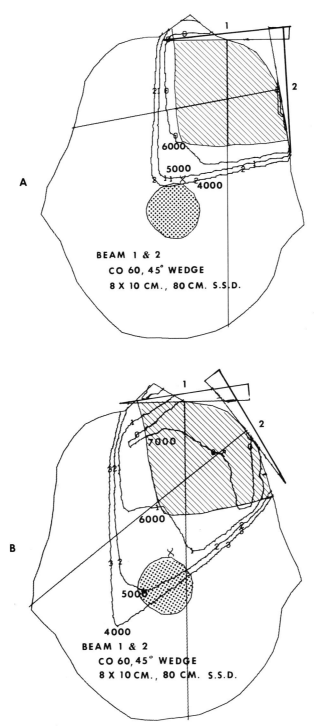

Fig. 4-3. Alternative treatment plans for an orbital tumor. Plan **A** delivers a minimum of 6000 rads to the tumor and less than 4000 rads to the brainstem (dotted area). Plan **B**, although treating the tumor adequately, delivers an excessive amount of irradiation to the brainstem, which may cause radiation myelitis.

tions of external beams are done to obtain a graphic image of the optimal dose distribution of radiation.[36, 94] Fig. 4-3 shows the alternative distributions for an orbital tumor, one of them giving an excessive dose to the brainstem. At the present time, the available computer techniques give mostly planar computations, but it is expected that in the near future three-dimensional representations such as illustrated by Mansfield and associates[109] and Laughlin[94] can be obtained routinely. In addition to the dose computations, several other important steps are an integral part of the treatment planning in radiation therapy:

1. *Simulation* of treatment areas to relate the external landmarks on the patient to the internal structures. The localization of the tumor volume must be done in many instances by means of fluoroscopy and films, before the patient is taken to the therapy room.

2. Additional *localization* films should be obtained using the therapy unit, with the patient in the treatment position.

3. In some cases, verification of the treatment plan is necessary, either with in vivo thermoluminescent dosimeters when feasible, or by direct measurements on a phantom loaded with suitable dosimeters.

Since the degree of precision required to cure a tumor by radiation is highly critical if large doses are applied and at the same time a low incidence of complications is sought,[74] particularly in long-surviving pediatric patients, the importance of adequate treatment planning cannot be overemphasized.

BIOLOGIC EFFECTS OF IONIZING RADIATIONS

In the ionization process, when a radioactive particle interacts with an atom, an electron is ejected, leaving a positive ion. The free electron is eventually either captured by an atom or molecule to produce a negative ion or recaptured by the same or another positive ion. Since tissue contains a significant proportion of water, many of the ionizations will occur primarily in the water, the effect being called *indirect*. This is in contrast to the interaction in which the molecules or atoms under study are primarily excited or ionized by the incident radioactive particles, this effect being called *direct*. When ionization occurs, a significant proportion of the energy released will be absorbed by the water in the cell, which in turn will generate a number of interactions with other ions in solution, forming several free radicals (H^+ and OH^- among them) and H_2O^+, H_2O_2, etc.[131] The critical target in cell death is the nucleus.[86, 189] DNA and RNA may be damaged by ionizing radiation in at least three different ways:

1. Base damage that is mainly to the pyrimidine bases cytosine, thymine, and uracil

2. Single strand breaks

3. Double helical strand breaks

A number of nuclear and cytoplasmic molecular changes follow,[2, 79, 85] which result in varied biologic effects (Fig. 4-4).

Lethal and sublethal damage

When a cell is hit by an ionizing particle, several types of damage may be observed:

1. If the cell is killed by the radiation, this is referred to as *lethal damage*.[47]

2. If the cell is severely affected and any modification in its environment will cause it to die, the damage is considered *potentially lethal*.[128]

3. In other instances, if the cell undergoes some damage that is subsequently repaired, this type of injury is classified as *sublethal damage.*[46]

Cell-survival curves

Biologically speaking, cell killing by radiation is defined as the loss of unlimited proliferative capacity.[136] Several studies have shown that nonviable cells may survive with intact metabolic functions and even undergo several divisions before lysis.[35, 179] In mathematical terms, the loss of cell viability in-

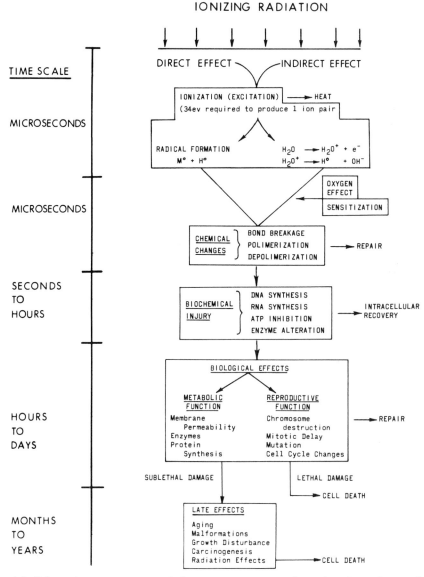

Fig. 4-4. Schematic representation of the various processes that take place after irradiation of an organism.

duced by radiation follows a complex exponential function, so that a specified dose of radiation kills a constant fraction of irradiated cells.[76, 136] This means that the fraction of cells killed is independent of the number of cells that are irradiated, but by the same token, the absolute number of cells killed by a given dose of radiation will vary with the initial number of cells. Fowler[58] and Elkind and Whitmore[48] have comprehensively reviewed the survival curve theory and defined the different types that can be encountered in mathematical models and in some experimental systems.

An exponential curve of cell survival indicates that cell killing is a random event, in which a single hit must affect a single target to kill the cell (Fig. 4-5, curve A). A number of cell-survival curves have an initial "shoulder," which suggests that more than one target must be hit by an ionizing event several times before the cell is inactivated (Fig. 4-5, curve B). The "shoulder" seen in the initial portion of the survival curve has been interpreted as due to (1) repair of sublethal damage, (2) progression of some cells through the cell cycle, or (3) repopulation from surviving cells.[46]

The extrapolation number of mammalian cells usually is in the range of two to ten and has been interpreted as the number of targets that should be hit for the cell to be killed.[48, 82]

Two doses are frequently referred to in biologic and sometimes in clinical papers. One is the D_0 (mean lethal dose), which is the dose of radiation that

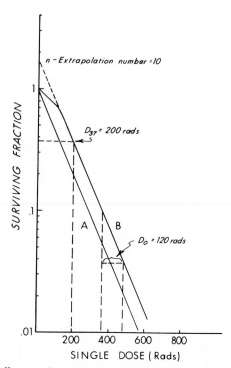

Fig. 4-5. Theoretical cell-survival curve. **A,** Single-hit curve represented by the equation SF $= 1-e^{D/D_0}$. **B,** Multihit survival curve with an initial shoulder, represented by the equation SF $= 1-(1-e^{D/D_0})$n. (See above for further explanation.)

is required to destroy 63% of the cells as shown on the survival curve. The other is the D_{37}, which is the single dose of radiation that kills 63% of the cells, leaving 37% survival fraction taken in the exponential portion of the survival curve.[82] If the survival curve is strictly exponential (Fig. 4-5, curve A), D_0 and D_{37} are the same.[82]

Chromosomal damage and genetic effects of radiation

The appearance of chromosomal aberrations in interphase is a well-known visible manifestation of cellular radiation damage.[51, 103] Radiation may cause either single or double strand breaks on the DNA molecule.[2, 85] The chromosome structure itself is resistant, and aberrations in cells irradiated during metaphase are not seen until subsequent mitosis.[103] The frequency of aberrations depends not only on the initial production of chromosome breaks but also on the repair mechanisms (reunion or restitution).[189]

The genetic effect of radiation is different from the somatic in that there is probably no threshold for the mutational effects, so that even a small dose of radiation may cause chromosomal aberrations.[113] However, a continuous repair process is in progress, so that a number of mutations are eliminated.[145] Excellent treatises discussing the effect of radiation on human heredity are available.[120, 200]

Carcinogenesis

Ionizing radiation can induce skin cancer, leukemia, thyroid cancer, some bone tumors, and some mesenchymal tumors.[24, 25, 43, 70, 170] To date, the published cases of leukemia that are correlated with prior exposure to radiation have been acute leukemia of all types and chronic granulocytic leukemia.[37] The appearance of malignant tumors after irradiation has been reported in children treated for retinoblastoma,[170] adenoid lymphoid tissue (osteosarcoma, soft tissue sarcoma), or thymic enlargement (thyroid carcinoma) and after irradiation of the long bones (osteochondroma or chondrosarcoma).*

Although the adult thyroid gland may tolerate as much as 4000 rads without significant effects, this gland in children is particularly sensitive to radiation. About 3% of children who received doses between 200 and 800 rads to the neck for thymic enlargement have developed thyroid carcinoma.[43, 130, 154, 155]

Sensitivity to radiation and cell generation cycle

Several investigators have demonstrated experimentally that the sensitivity of cells to radiation and to most of the chemotherapeutic agents varies, depending on the phase of reproductive capacity in which the cell is at the time it is exposed to the physical or chemical event.[21, 64, 155, 174, 193] Terasima and Tolmach[174] showed that synchronized Hela cells in culture irradiated with a single dose of 300 rads were more sensitive to radiation during late G_1 and late G_2 phases and more resistant during G_1 and the late S. Sinclair[155] reported that Chinese hamster cells are more sensitive during mitosis and particularly resistant during the latter part of the S period. Although this differential sensitivity could

---

*References 26, 56, 72, 146, 173, 180.

be useful to the treatment of patients, the lack of knowledge about these parameters of the cell cycle in man at the present time makes this impractical.

Cell sensitivity, response to irradiation, and tumor curability

Years ago Bergonie and Tribondeau[10] formulated the classic law that in essence states that cells are more sensitive to radiation, the greater their mitotic activity. The cells need not be in mitosis at the time of irradiation. Experimentally or in clinical practice, a straightforward correlation between cellular sensitivity and tumor curability is not constant, suggesting that other factors play a role in tumor control.[75, 133] In clinical practice, a distinction must be made between sensitivity and response to radiation. In some tumors such as seminoma, dysgerminoma, and some lymphoproliferative or hemoproliferative disorders (lymphoma, leukemia, multiple myeloma) the tumor may be very sensitive and disappear after a few doses of radiation. However, the patient may or may not be cured because he may eventually die of distant metastases. On the other hand, it was a long-held classic misconception that adenocarcinoma of the breast or the prostate was resistant to radiation. Recent clinical trials have shown that a significant number of these tumors may be sterilized by high doses of radiation and although the mass may take a long time to regress completely the patient may be cured.

FACTORS AFFECTING THE BIOLOGIC EFFECTS OF IONIZING RADIATIONS
Linear energy transfer (LET)

When an ionizing particle traverses a medium, the energy is released along the particle's track and is described by the rate of ionizations per unit of pathway. The LET of an ionizing particle depends in a complicated way on the energy and charge possessed by the particle[82]; the greater the charge and the smaller the velocity, the higher its LET (Fig. 4-6). This varying rate of energy released in an absorber will be expressed in different biologic effects in living cells. Because of this, the term *relative biologic effect* (RBE) is used to compare the biologic effectiveness of a given ionizing radiation with a standard: the effect produced by 250 kvp x rays. For instance, cobalt 60 has a *relative biologic effect* (RBE) of about .95,[67] neutrons have an RBE of approximately

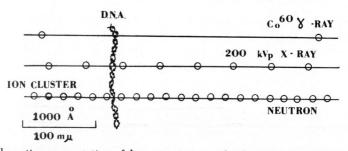

Fig. 4-6. Schematic representation of linear energy transfer for various ionizing particles and x rays. Neutrons have a large number of ionizations and are recognized as high LET particles. (Modified from Young, M. E. J.: Radiological physics, ed. 2, London, 1967, H. K. Lewis & Co., Ltd.)

2.3.[59] This means that a comparatively large or smaller dose of these radiations is necessary to produce the same biologic effect as a given dose of 250 kvp x rays.

Oxygen enhancement effect

Growing tumors rapidly develop a hypoxic population of cells[134] because of inadequate capillary circulation and oxygen diffusion in the tissues.[176, 184] The dose of radiation required to produce a given effect is, in general, two to three times as great in the absence of oxygen as under normal oxygen tension (Fig. 4-7). Experimental observations with high LET particles such as neutrons have shown less dependence of biologic effect of irradiation on oxygen concentration.[3, 24, 59, 119] Gray[66] was the first to postulate that the oxygen effect might be important in radiation therapy because malignant tumors are frequently avascular and therefore have a significant population of hypoxic cells that is irradiated at a low oxygen tension. It has been postulated that if patients are treated by breathing oxygen, preferably under pressure in a sealed chamber (3 to 4 atmospheres), an increased response would be obtained in the hypoxic cells.[176, 184] Assuming that normal tissue is well oxygenated, the in-

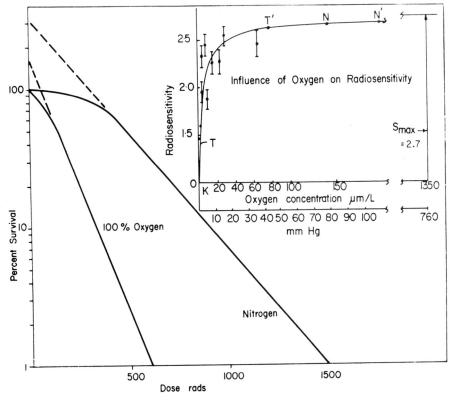

Fig. 4-7. Influence of oxygen tension on radiosensitivity according to Deschner and Gray. Survival curve for human embryo liver cells in tissue culture, irradiated with and without oxygen. (From Johns, H., and Cunningham, J.: The physics of radiology, ed. 3, Springfield, Ill., 1971, Charles C Thomas, Publisher.)

crease in radiosensitivity would be minimal, so that a given dose of radiation would have a greater relative effect on the tumor than on normal cells.[31, 184, 185, 196]

Several clinical trials dealing with tumors of the head and neck, cervix, bladder, etc. have been reported by Churchill-Davidson,[28] van den Brenk,[184] Wildermuth,[197] and others, sometimes with encouraging, sometimes with inconclusive, results. Although the incidence of complications may be greater, appropriate adjustment in dose and fractionation has shown no significant enhancement of skin or mucosal reactions or permanent damage to other normal tissues.[185, 196] To our knowledge, no clinical trials of hyperbaric oxygen have been carried out in pediatric patients.

Dose fractionation and dose-time relationship

In general, radiation therapy is given to patients in fractionated doses, usually daily (4 to 5 fractions per week). The rationale for fractionation is based on the observations that multiple doses spread several hours apart will result in some repair of sublethal damage and that, in general, normal cells have a greater and faster capacity than tumor cells to repair this damage.[30, 49, 199] Therefore after each treatment the normal tissue cells will recover from the effects of radiation, whereas the tumor cells cannot, so that eventually a complete

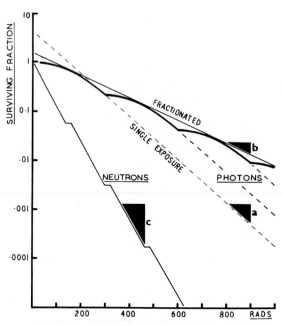

Fig. 4-8. Theoretical cell-survival curve showing the effects of fractionation compared with a single exposure dose with photons and neutrons. A larger dose of radiation is required with a fractionated dose of photons, but due to the lack of repair, no significant difference exists between the single or fractionated doses with neutrons. (From Cohen, L. In Schwartz, E. M., editor: The biological basis of radiation therapy, Philadelphia, 1966, J. B. Lippincott Co.)

sterilization of the tumor will be obtained without causing significant injury to the surrounding normal tissues. Furthermore, experimental observations in animal tumors have demonstrated that during fractionated irradiation there is a reoxygenation process with transfer of hypoxic cells into the more sensitive well-oxygenated compartment.[162, 163, 177, 186] Larger doses of fractionated irradiation are necessary to produce the same effect as a single dose, high LET particles being an exception (Fig. 4-8).

It is essential for the radiation therapist to specify not only the total dose and the total period of time during which the therapy is given but also the number of fractions. This dose-time relationship has been expressed mathematically by Ellis[50] as the Nominal Standard Dose. The first isoeffect curve to be derived was that for carcinoma of the skin by Strandqvist[161] in 1944. Subsequently, similar dose-time curves have been constructed for squamous cell carcinoma of the skin,[124, 190] recurrent carcinoma of the breast, testicular tumors, Hodgkin's disease, other lymphomas, Kaposi's sarcoma, and other lesions. Some time-dose relationships have been derived for a number of normal tissues (Fig. 4-9).

Split course radiation therapy

In addition to protraction and fractionation, the time-dose factor can be further applied to clinical radiotherapy by dividing the total doses that are given

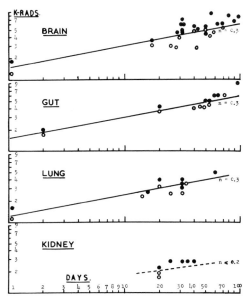

Fig. 4-9. Tolerance limits for various tissues. ● = high-dose effects; ○ = maximum safe level. Data for brain and cord by Jones (1964), Wachowski (1945), Greenfield (1948), Boden (1948), Friedman (1952), Lampe (1958), Pallis (1961), Lindgren (1958), and Dynes (1962); for gut by Amory (1951), Friedman (1952), and Gray (1957); for lung by Whitfield (1956), Ross (1956), and Gish (1957); and for kidney by Kunkler (1952), Ledingham (1959), Luxton (1964), and Paterson (1952). Although data are somewhat scanty, the kidney appears to have a recovery function lower than average, which is about $n = 0.3$ for most normal tissues. (From Cohen, L. In Schwartz, E. M., editor: The biological basis of radiation therapy, Philadelphia, 1966, J. B. Lippincott Co.)

to a patient in two or three series of fractions that are spaced 1 or 2 weeks apart.[147] The increased effectiveness of split course radiotherapy could be explained by (1) partial regression of the tumor with increased vascularization and improved oxygenation of hypoxic cells or (2) a greater therapeutic ratio between the lethal effect on the tumor and the effect on the normal cells, which presumably will have a greater reparative capacity.[147, 148]

Combination therapy

In an effort to increase the control of a radioresistant tumor cell population, which may be found in some lesions, combined therapeutic approaches have been used. These may include the combination of radiation therapy and surgery,[132, 151] with the irradiation administered prior to or after the surgical procedure, or the combination of radiation therapy with chemotherapy.*

Combination chemotherapy with radiotherapy is discussed further in Chapters 10 to 26.

Chemical protection to radiation

The current status of chemical radiation protection was reviewed by Bacq[8] in 1965. Although a number of substances such as histamine, cyanides, catecholamines, p-aminopropiophenone, thiols, and disulfide compounds have been shown to possess radioprotective properties, none at the present time are used in clinical work because of the toxicity of these compounds at doses affording radioprotection.

High LET particle therapy

Because of the differential sensitivity to radiation of well-oxygenated and hypoxic cells, one of the possibilities to eliminate this difference is the use of high LET particles such as fast neutrons[3, 4] or pi-mesons.[16] A considerable amount of experimental research on the effects of neutrons on in vitro and in vivo biologic systems,[24, 59, 119] as well as exploration of possible sources of neutrons or pi-mesons applicable to clinical therapy, has been carried out in recent years.† Protons and alpha particle beams have been used in clinical trials in the past.[95, 178]

EFFECTS OF RADIATION ON NORMAL TISSUES

Excellent reviews of the effects of high doses of radiation on man were published after the atomic bomb explosions over Nagasaki and Hiroshima,[114] radiation accidents with nuclear reactors,[71, 77] and fallout exposure of some Marshall Islands inhabitants.[32]

Chronic exposure to low doses of radiation in a young organism will cause slow growth and shortening of the life-span (premature aging). In several animal experiments, doses as small as 0.1 rad per day produced some reduction in life-span.[1, 37] Concern has been expressed that low doses of radiation from diagnostic or therapeutic procedures[14, 113, 158] or fallout,[31] in addition to the possibility of carcinogenesis, may have significant genetic effects in future genera-

---

*References 12, 13, 41, 42, 45, 150, 152, 164, 171, 188.
†References 6, 20, 60, 149, 160, 202.

tions.[102] This would be due to damage either to the germ cell chromosomes[35, 51] before fertilization (genetic damage) or from exposure of the embryo in utero.[78] The embryo is very sensitive to irradiation,[1] particularly during the first 8 to 12 weeks. Since this is a period of cellular and organ differentiation, exposure to ionizing radiation may induce a variety of malformations.[39]

Although most of the information concerning the effects of radiation in normal tissues is fragmentary and, in general, incomplete, several reviews have been published,[11, 93] the most comprehensive by Rubin and Casarett.[143] Significant changes in those organs commonly irradiated in the treatment of pediatric tumors will be briefly discussed in the following paragraphs. A graphic representation of known tolerance doses of radiation is shown in Fig. 4-10.

Nervous system

Acute changes of the brain and spinal cord are due to edema and are not of great clinical significance. Chronic changes may include necrosis of the brain, which is rarely seen, sometimes after retreatment of a lesion in the cerebrum.[18, 141]

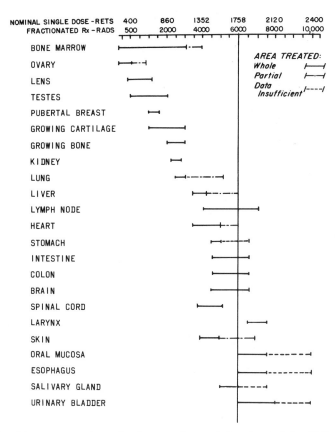

Fig. 4-10. Graphic representation of tolerance doses of fractionated irradiation for various organs. (Modified from Rubin, P., and Casarett, G. In Vaeth, J. M., editor: Frontiers of radiation therapy and oncology, vol. 6, Baltimore, 1972, University Park Press.)

A transient form of reaction of the spinal cord to irradiation, known as *Lhermitte's syndrome,* may occur a few weeks after completion of therapy and is characterized by some electric shock–like sensations that radiate along the spinal cord into the extremities.[84] In most cases, the situation is reversible, and it does not seem to be correlated with subsequent permanent radiation myelopathy. A more severe form of brainstem or spinal cord injury may appear after 6 months and as late as several years after irradiation.[15, 54, 104, 183] This myelitis is manifested by motor and sensory changes referable to the segment of the cord irradiated. If the entire width is included, there will be complete paraplegia and anesthesia similar to a total transection of the spinal cord. However, if only half the spinal cord has been irradiated, the neurologic picture is that of a Brown-Séquard syndrome.

Although a small segment of brainstem or spinal cord may tolerate higher doses of radiation, doses over 3750 to 4500 rads given in weekly increments of more than 800 rads may have a significant probability of inducing radiation myelopathy.[183] However, if adequate fractionation is observed, this complication is rare.

The permanent changes in the brain and the spinal cord are due to severe capillary degeneration, fibrinoid necrosis of the small arterioles, and necrosis of neurons and other oligodendrocytes, accompanied by marked demyelination of the white matter.[143]

In my experience, no cases of brain necrosis in children have been observed with the following dose schedules:

Under 2 years of age: 3000 rads tumor dose
2 to 5 years of age: 3750 rads tumor dose
5 to 12 years of age: 4500 rads tumor dose
Over 12 years of age: 5000 rads tumor dose

In special circumstances a small volume of the cerebrum can be given an additional 500 to 1000 rads.

The eye

The eye is a complex organ with a variety of tissues that exhibit different sensitivity to ionizing radiation. With doses in the range of 1500 to 2000 rads, the conjunctiva and cornea may show an acute inflammatory reaction manifested by pain and photophobia.[106] Doses in the range of 5000 to 6000 rads may cause severe inflammatory changes in the cornea and conjunctiva, which may be painful or may be complicated by necrosis or perforation requiring an operation. Suppression of the secretions of the lacrimal gland appears. With this relatively large dose of radiation, iridocyclitis may develop, and secondary glaucoma occurs in some patients.[62, 106, 143]

Among the chronic changes, the most frequent is cataract formation, which occurs in the posterior capsule of the lens. Other minor lenticular opacities may be observed, but they rarely produce visual loss, and they tend to be stationary.[143] The doses of radiation necessary to induce cataracts have been thoroughly studied by Merriam and Focht, [111, 112] ranging from 200 rads in a single dose to 1100 rads in fractionated doses.

Although the choroid and the retina have been considered rather resistant to irradiation, severe degeneration, hemorrhage, and capillary obliteration have been described with doses over 3500 rads.[40, 62, 127] The optic nerve is relatively radioresistant.[40]

The ear

Radiation-induced otitis media due to the hyperemia and swelling of the membranes and the eustachian tube is a relatively frequent complication. Dizziness and Meniere's syndrome may occur, probably because of increased perilymphatic and endolymphatic pressure secondary to the acute edema and vasculitis. With higher doses of radiation between 4000 and 6000 rads, progressive or delayed sclerosis of the auditory ossicles, as well as degenerative changes in the cochlea, may result in loss of hearing.[63]

The skin

Depending on the type of radiation and energy used, different exposure doses of radiation will be necessary to produce skin changes. These effects range from erythema and dry desquamation to moist desquamation and ulceration with

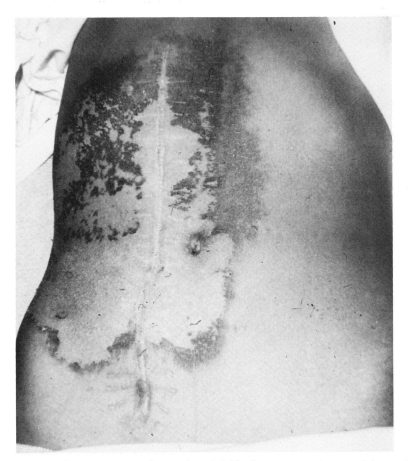

Fig. 4-11. Moist desquamation in the irradiated field of a young patient receiving postoperative actinomycin D and radiation therapy for Wilms' tumor.

necrosis and are seen with lower energy and orthovoltage equipment. With cobalt 60, high-energy x rays, neutrons, and high-energy electrons, subcutaneous fibrosis is more frequently observed.

In general, single doses ranging from 300 rads (superficial machine) to 750 rads (orthovoltage machines) are necessary to produce erythema. With fractionated doses, this is usually noted after 2000 rads and with cobalt 60, after higher doses. Dry desquamation appears with doses over 3000 rads with supervoltage equipment. At this dose level, depending on the field size, moist desquamation will begin to appear with orthovoltage equipment. Severe ulceration and necrosis of the skin should never be seen with therapeutic exposures, but sometimes they are observed after the injudicious use of radiation therapy equipment.

With moderate doses of radiation (2000 to 4000 rads), there is transient depilation, from which the patient usually recovers in 3 to 6 months. The other skin appendages, as well as the fingernails, follow the same recovery pattern. It has been shown that these effects may be enhanced by the combination of irradiation and some chemotherapeutic agents, particularly actinomycin D[99] (Fig. 4-11). With larger doses of radiation (over 5000 rads), permanent epilation, as well as depopulation of sebaceous and sweat glands, may be observed. Chronic and late effects are characterized by atrophy of the epidermis, epilation with loss of hair follicles and sebaceous and sweat glands, telangiectasis, sometimes hyperpigmentation, and even areas of hyperkeratosis. Large doses of radiation may produce necrosis and ulceration with complete denudation of the skin, vascular degeneration, fibrosis, and associated inflammation. Prolonged exposure to low doses of radiation may produce chronic dermatitis, which is associated with an increasing incidence of skin carcinoma.

Mucosas of oral cavity and pharynx

As in the skin, the reactions in the oral cavity and the pharynx are related to damage of the germinal cell layers of the epithelium and to vascular changes of the underlying tissues. During the first 2 weeks, erythema is observed, which is followed by studded mucositis and increasing vascular injection. After 2000 rads, a patchy fibrinous exudate is observed throughout these cavities, which will become more confluent with doses over 3000 rads. Usually these changes are reversible, although sometimes some atrophy of the irradiated mucosa is observed with telangiectasis and fibrosis of the underlying tissues.

Gastrointestinal tract

The esophagus. The appearance of mucositis in the esophagus is similar to that of the pharynx. However, in the chronic phase there is a tendency for the esophagus to show some mild reduction in caliber or sometimes demonstrable strictures. Such strictures are due to fibrosis of the muscular layers and are frequently associated with atrophic changes in the overlying mucosa, sometimes with ulcerations.[153] These changes are more likely to be seen after doses of 5000 rads.[143]

The stomach. A total fractionated dose of 2000 rads or less generally is well tolerated by the stomach and results only in some temporary suppression of gastric acidity.[143] Increasing doses of radiation will cause nausea, vomiting, and epigastric distress. The gastroscopic and radiographic picture is similar to acute gastritis. Higher doses of radiation (4000 rads) may produce atrophic changes in the mucosa with long-term decrease in the activity of the chief and parietal cells. Doses over 5000 rads may cause gastric ulceration, which may bleed and occasionally be complicated by a perforation.

The small and large intestine. It is not uncommon to observe watery diarrhea with intermittent abdominal cramping during the second or third week of abdominal irradiation. There is increased peristalsis, disturbance of the absorption mechanisms, and a decreased transit time.[44, 137, 140, 187] When the rectum is included in the irradiated volume, there is rectal discomfort, tenesmus, and mucus, sometimes admixed with blood on the stools.

Despite a rapid cell turnover,[98, 194] the small bowel mucosal changes have been associated with necrosis of proliferating epithelial cells in the crypts of Lieberkühn, degeneration of endothelial cells, edema of the submucosal connective tissues, inflammatory cell infiltration, and sometimes leakage of erythrocytes.[194, 195] If the dose of radiation is large enough, it may cause a temporary or permanent ulceration.[126] This type of lesion may be associated with either stenosis or perforation with fistula formation.[68, 126] In general, doses of 6000 rads are necessary to produce this more advanced radiation damage to the bowel.[92] Severe injuries to the bowel are uncommon in pediatric patients, except for occasional small bowel obstruction.

Concannon and co-workers[33] experimentally showed that in dogs the combination of irradiation and actinomycin D significantly increased the effects of irradiation in the small intestine, when compared to animals treated with similar doses of radiation alone.

Salivary glands

The salivary glands are frequently irradiated during the treatment of head and neck tumors. In the first 12 to 24 hours after the initial exposure, there might be some swelling of the glands with pain. Kashima and associates[88] showed a sharp rise in the serum amylase level, which reached a peak between 9 and 36 hours after exposure. With fractionated doses, after 3 to 4 weeks the saliva becomes less abundant and more viscous. After moderate doses of radiation (3000 to 4000 rads), there is a transient dryness of the mouth that lasts for 3 to 6 months. With higher doses (in the range of 5000 to 6000 rads) the effects of radiation on the salivary glands tend to be more permanent and are characterized by atrophy and destruction of the glandular acini, degeneration of the small vessels, epithelial degeneration, obliteration of the ducts, and diffuse interstitial fibrosis. Sometimes the fibrosis and deformity of the salivary glands is such that they are confused with metastatic lymph nodes.[52] Another sequela of radiation effects on the salivary gland is the development of caries and trophic changes in the teeth, which are secondary to abnormalities in the chemical composition of the saliva.[58, 61, 107]

The liver

Recent clinical and pathologic studies have shown that the liver is not a radioresistant organ. Ogata and co-workers[121] described postradiation changes in hepatic vessels, particularly in the centrolobular vein branches of three patients in whom part of the liver was irradiated when lung tumors were treated. Ingold and associates[80] reported similar findings on a group of 40 patients receiving irradiation to the entire liver during the treatment of disseminated ovarian carcinoma of malignant lymphoma.

Hepatic cell necrosis and connective tissue proliferation within the lumen of small efferent veins, without preexisting thrombosis, have been described.[139]

The clinical course and liver changes depend on the dose of irradiation and are characterized by weight gain, liver enlargement, and varying amounts of ascites.[80] Laboratory studies frequently show abnormal liver function tests, but the alkaline phosphatase test has been the most reliable single laboratory study.[80] No damage is generally observed with doses below 3000 rads. After doses of between 3500 and 4000 rads, almost half the patients will show radiation damage, and with doses of over 4000 rads, 75% of the patients may develop radiation hepatitis.[80] Tefft[172] has reported radiation hepatitis in children treated with a combination of chemotherapeutic agents and irradiation with doses as low as 2000 rads.

The lung

Acute radiation pneumonitis may be asymptomatic, or the patient may complain of cough or minimal chest discomfort. When more than 75% of the pulmonary bed is irradiated, after doses of 2000 rads, the patient may develop a severe respiratory distress, spiking temperature, and shortness of breath and even die of acute respiratory insufficiency and cor pulmonale.[191] Sputum cultures are negative unless there is a superimposed bacterial infection, which is common and may be life threatening. The chest x-ray film shows diffuse pulmonary infiltrates that may become coalescent and be associated with pleural or interlobar effusions. Pathologic features of radiation pneumonitis have been thoroughly described both in experimental animals and patients.[9, 34] The underlying pathologic damage is alveolar degeneration and hyaline membrane formation, followed by fibrosis of the alveolar wall and interlobar septa, as well as capillary thrombosis and fibrinoid degeneration of the small arterioles.[9, 191] With moderate doses of radiation, many of these acute changes are reversible after 3 to 4 weeks, or the patients may have subclinical subacute changes characterized by some interstitial pulmonary fibrosis. However, with larger doses, late chronic changes become permanent and can be seen after 3 months following irradiation. Functional impairment may appear.[19] If the fibrotic process is localized to less than 50% of one lung, it is generally asymptomatic and detected only on x-ray films.

Cardiovascular system

Depending on the volume irradiated and the dose and the fractions given, a transient, subacute, or chronic pericarditis may appear accompanied or unaccompanied by endocardial and myocardial damage.[96, 159, 192] The symptomatology is that of a pericardial effusion or in the late phase a constrictive pericarditis. Some of these patients developed endocardial or myocardial fibrosis, and in some young patients, myocardial infarctions have been reported.[159]

Although a few cases of cardiac complications have been seen with doses less than 3000 rads, most of the patients reported by Stewart and Cohn[159] received doses of over 4000 rads to almost the entire volume of the heart. This complication may be more frequent in patients who are retreated to volumes including most of the heart. Adequate treatment planning and special shielding of some portions of the heart, if possible, may prevent a significant number of these complications.[159]

The kidney

Functional changes have been described after exposure of the kidney to irradiation. The symptoms of acute radiation nephritis, which usually appear within 6 months of irradiation to doses in the range of 2000 rads in 3 to 5 weeks,[105] are lassitude, headaches, shortness of breath, vomiting, nocturia, and edema of the legs. Both systolic and diastolic pressures are elevated and, if the hypertension is severe, abnormal changes in the retina are seen on fundoscopic examination. Urinary output is adequate, and urinalysis shows albuminuria and low specific gravity. Gross hematuria never occurs, although epithelial and hyaline casts are seen and red blood cells may be observed on microscopic examination. A normocytic, normochromic anemia may appear. Renal function studies are abnormal, and the BUN is elevated. Grave prognostic signs are generalized edema and a blood urea nitrogen level over 100 mg/100 ml. The blood pressure alone is not a reliable prognostic sign, but increasing hypertension associated with progressive anemia and a rising BUN is ominous.[105]

Chronic nephritis usually appears about 18 months or later after exposure to radiation. The clinical course is slow, with progressive anemia, arterial hypertension, and impairment of renal function. Some patients may not have manifestations of the acute form of nephritis, and the first manifestation of renal damage is decreased specific gravity of the urine and albuminuria. The BUN may be elevated. Anemia is always present. Renal function studies show decreased blood flow and filtration rates. Intravenous pyelograms may show good excretion of contrast material, but the kidneys are small.

Rather uncommon is the development of malignant hypertension, which is manifested by severe hypertensive encephalopathy, throbbing headaches, papilledema, and retinitis with hemorrhages. This usually appears after a latent period of 18 to 24 months, and the absence of acute renal failure or severe renal impairment suggests a different pathophysiologic mechanism.[105] Albuminuria may be present, but the urine is otherwise normal. Renal function is preserved until the terminal phase.

Patients with chronic radiation nephritis may die in chronic uremia or renal failure or because of malignant hypertension, a cerebral vascular accident, or congestive heart failure secondary to the increased blood pressure.

Urinary bladder

As in other organs, increasing doses of radiation produce mucosal degeneration, edema, and increased capillary permeability in the acute phase during irradiation. These findings may be more severe in patients receiving cyclophosphamide, a drug that by itself is known to produce severe hypertrophic cystitis. More severe changes such as mucosal atrophy, ulceration, telangiectasis, or fibrosis are rare with the doses of radiation given to children.

The gonads

The testicles. In a number of patients treated with radiation to the pelvis, as high as 5% to 10% of the exposure dose may be given to the testicles because of scattered radiation. The germinal cells in the gonads are very sensitive to irradiation, and either prolonged periods of azoospermia or oligospermia are noted even with small doses of radiation; permanent sterility will probably occur after doses of 1200 to 1500 rads.[204]

This injury is practically asymptomatic, and eventually the testes may become smaller and softer. The epididymis retains its normal size. Because of a lesser sensitivity of the interstitial Leydig cells in the adult, the internal secretions (testosterone) are not affected, and the secondary sexual characteristics and social behavior of the individual do not change.

The ovaries. Small doses of radiation (as low as 200 rads) may produce appreciable cellular killing[204]; with larger doses, menopausal symptoms and sterility may be produced. Ovarian irradiation was shown to reduce significantly the urinary excretion of estrogens.[38] In women treated with low doses of irradiation in the range of 100 to 200 rads, which may be equivalent to the scattered dose that some patients could receive during the treatment of a thoracic or abdominal malignancy, some transient effects on the granulosa cells have been observed. With larger doses causing greater injury to the granulosa cells, there may be no recovery. The oocyte degenerates, and the follicle becomes atrophic. Since there are no stem cells in the ovary analogous to the type A spermatogonia of the male, the radiation damage of the follicles may result in permanent sterility.

The dose necessary to castrate a woman depends on her age; a larger dose is required during the period of more active follicular proliferation. A single dose of 650 to 750 rads or fractionated doses in the range of 1500 to 2500 rads are known to produce permanent castration and sterility in most patients.

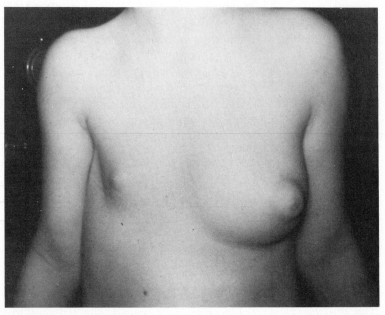

Fig. 4-12. Hypoplasia of the right breast and thorax, 14 years after irradiation for a malignant sympathetic tumor (2500 rads in 3 weeks, 250 kvp x rays).

After small doses of radiation in both the testes and ovaries, numerous chromosomal abnormalities are observed in the germ cells, even for prolonged periods of time.[14]

The breasts

The atrophy or underdevelopment of a breast in a patient irradiated for a thoracic tumor is not uncommon (Fig. 4-12). Although in general, the adult breast is resistant to irradiation, this is not true in young girls. The hypoplastic changes are irreversible and do not respond to hormones.[29, 182]

Bone and cartilage

The growing cartilage is a radiosensitive organ, and the clinical sequelae appear somewhat later, some becoming more apparent as the child grows. Rubin

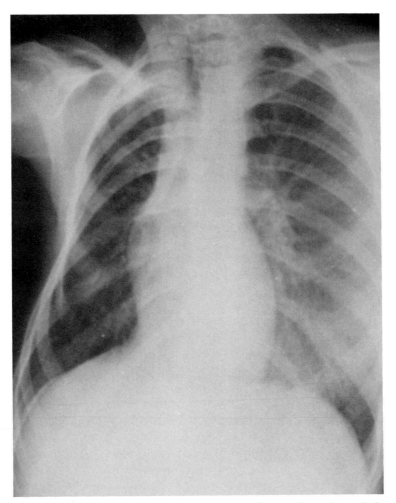

Fig. 4-13. Chest x-ray film of the patient in Fig. 4-12, showing hypoplasia of the thoracic cage and hyperradiolucency of the lung, probably secondary to underdevelopment.

and Casarett[143] and others have shown experimentally that depending on what portion of the growing bone or cartilage is irradiated and the dose levels, a different type of deformity may be induced in long bones.

If minimal injury is produced in the long bones, a series of transverse growth arrest lines is noted in the metaphysis that progresses into the diaphysis and may eventually disappear. Irradiation of the epiphyseal plate may result in stunting of the long bones because of damage to the proliferating cartilage cells in the zones of endochondral ossification.[89]

In the skull, changes may involve underdevelopment of the calvarium or the facial bones, including the nasal bone as well as the mandible. Injury to secondary tooth buds and delay in the appearance of teeth may also be observed. Hypoplasia of the ribs and asymmetry of the chest may occur (Fig. 4-13).

About 25% to 30% of the surviving patients irradiated for neuroblastoma or Wilms' tumor will have a significant degree of vertebral column deformity, which includes kyphosis, scoliosis, or lordosis (Fig. 4-14), secondary to varying degrees of osteochondrodystrophy.[125, 143] Pelvic tilt may compensate the scoliosis, and pronounced limping is infrequently seen. In contrast to idiopathic scoliosis, radiation-induced spine deformities are not progressive.[143, 144]

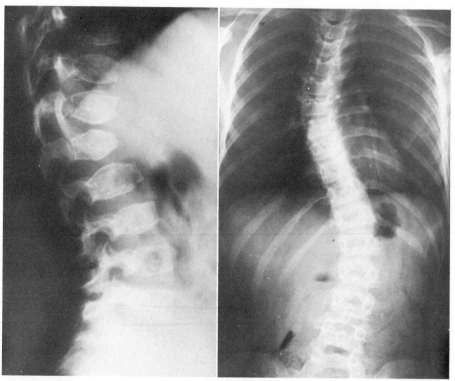

Fig. 4-14. Varying degrees of postirradiation changes of the spine in children irradiated for malignant sympathetic tumors.

Recovery may occur, and after a variable time of growth retardation normal bone growth may resume following exposure to doses in the range of 600 to 1500 rads. Permanent damage is produced with doses over 2000 rads.

The induction of cartilaginous benign tumors (osteochondroma) or sometimes chondrosarcomas or fibrosarcomas is not infrequent[125, 129] (Fig. 4-15). The ingestion of radium salts by watch dial painters some years ago resulted in a high incidence of osteosarcomas.[25, 70, 73]

Mature bone and cartilage when heavily irradiated may undergo necrosis. Fractures of some flat bones, particularly the pelvis, femoral neck, or ribs may be noted after high doses of radiation.[55, 57]

Bone marrow

The acute effects of radiation on the bone marrow are usually observed after whole body irradiation, and they are mostly due to direct cell killing.[1] Within a few hours after a large dose of radiation, there is prompt reduction in the number of lymphocytes and, consequently, the white blood count. A significant drop in lymphocytes has been found in man after a single dose as little as 25 rads total body irradiation. This is due to the marked sensitivity of circulating lympho-

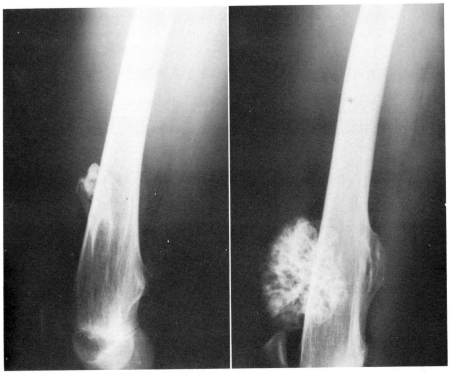

Fig. 4-15. Benign osteochondroma of the left distal femur and a low-grade chondrosarcoma of the right distal femur on a child surviving 15 years after irradiation of a mediastinal neuroblastoma with multiple skeletal metastases. Only 800 rads over a period of 2 weeks were given to the femurs.

cytes to interphase death. The lymphocyte count will remain low for a week, and if the dose of radiation is not lethal, slow repopulation may be seen after this period of time. The granulocyte decrease is noted a day after radiation, and the lowest value is reached after about a week. This is due to the killing of stem cells and lack of repopulation.[1] After sublethal doses of radiation, the granulocytes do not return to normal for at least 2 to 3 weeks, and it is at this period of time that death due to bone marrow depression during acute radiation sickness occurs. Thrombocytopenia due to radiation effect on the platelets leads to hemorrhages in these patients, with ecchymosis, hematemesis, and melena, which complicate the fluid and electrolyte imbalance during the first and second week after exposure. The circulating red cells are extremely radioresistant. Chronic irradiation, however, may give rise to protracted anemia because erythropoietic tissue seems to have less ability to recover from radiation damage than the granulopoietic tissue has.[1]

More permanent chronic changes are noted even when small segments of the bone marrow are irradiated to doses over 3000 rads,[97] and recovery may take up to 18 months or longer in a small proportion of the patients, with good reparative capacity. Vascular degeneration and fibrosis is noted,[91, 167] preventing repopulation.

These changes are more prominent in patients who have received bone marrow–depressing chemotherapeutic agents or in patients treated with these drugs after radiation therapy.[83] Special care should be exercised for patients receiving combination therapy or retreatment after irradiation or chemotherapy; frequent white blood cell and platelet counts are necessary. This is particularly true if the bone marrow is infiltrated with malignant cells.

Endocrine glands

The pituitary. Occasionally, clinical evidence of hypopituitarism may be observed after high doses of radiation,[169] but this is rarely seen in children.

The thyroid. It is well known that the administration of therapeutic doses of ^{131}I causes marked glandular degeneration, perivascular fibrosis, and damage to the fine vasculature of the thyroid with resulting hypothyroidism.[143] With the increasing treatment of the neck for malignant lymphomas to relatively high doses, mild to severe cases of hypothyroidism are being reported.[110]

Patients with usual thyroid studies within normal ranges may have elevated TSH levels. Patients who have a lymphangiogram prior to irradiation have been reported to develop hypothyroidism more frequently than those who did not have a lymphangiogram.[142] It is postulated that the prolonged high iodine level after the injection of ethiodol induces thyroid hyperplasia, which increases the radiosensitivity of the gland.

External radiation to the neck and thorax in children* has been implicated as a cause of thyroid carcinoma. A significant number of these patients received moderate doses of radiation in the range of 500 to 1500 rads for benign disease such as thymus enlargement,[180] lymphoid tissue in the Waldeyer ring, or cervical adenitis. The average latent period is 10 to 15 years,[138] and most of the lesions

---

*References 43, 53, 72, 130, 154, 198.

histologically are papillary adenocarcinomas.[17] In addition to malignant tumors, Conard and associates[32] described a large number of adenomatous nodules in the thyroid in a group of children accidentally exposed to radioactive fallout 6 to 10 years previously, at ages less than 10 years. Similar experimental observation in rats was reported by Lindsay and co-workers.[100]

Adrenal and parathyroid glands. Soanes and co-workers[156] have described a variable response of the adrenals to irradiation, with functional stimulation at low doses (2000 to 3000 rads) and some impairment under stress following 3500 rads. There are no reports in the literature describing the effects of external irradiation on the human parathyroid glands.[143]

BASIC PHYSICS OF IONIZING RADIATIONS

Only a few fundamental concepts of physical aspects of radiation will be reviewed here. The reader is referred to more comprehensive treatises for further information.[82, 203]

Sources of ionizing radiations

Some substances are radioactive, such as polonium and radium, and are called *natural isotopes.* The great majority of the isotopes used in medicine are man produced, usually by bombardment of a stable compound with fast neutrons, either on a nuclear reactor or a cyclotron. *Radioisotopes* are elements with different atomic weights or masses (excess of neutrons) and identical atomic numbers as the stable elements. They have the same chemical properties but give off energy, emitting ionizing radiation. Other sources of external irradiation (x rays, electrons) will be discussed later.

The *physical half-life* of a radioactive isotope is the period of time required for half its radioactivity to disappear.

Types of ionizing particles

Depending on their electromagnetic charge and penetration, ionizing radiations are classified into four types (Fig. 4-16).

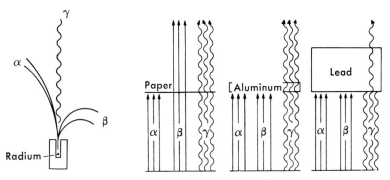

Fig. 4-16. Deflection of ionizing particles emitted from a radium source in a magnetic field, alpha particles being attracted by the negative and beta particles by the positive fields. Schematic representation of the penetrating power of alpha, beta, and gamma radiation. (From Young, M. E. J.: Radiological physics, ed. 2, London, 1967, H. K. Lewis & Co., Ltd.)

1. *Alpha rays* are equivalent to the nucleus of helium, which has two protons and two neutrons. They have a large mass, are positively charged, and are stopped by a few sheets of paper or a few centimeters of air.
2. *Beta particles* are similar to electrons, are negatively charged, and are more penetrating than the alpha rays, but they are stopped by a few millimeters of aluminum. These particles can traverse a few millimeters in tissues (about 4 mm/1 mev maximum energy).
3. *Gamma rays*, which have the same diffusion characteristics as light, are not deflected by electric or magnetic fields and are considered to be electromagnetic radiation, similar to x rays.
4. *X rays* are artificially produced by bombardment of a target with high-speed electrons in a vacuum.

In external beam therapy, usually only gamma rays and x rays are of significance, beta rays being filtered out. However, in the internal administration of radioactive isotopes, such as iodine 131, gold 198, or phosphorus 32, the beta particles are very important, since the main contribution to the tissue dose is derived from these particles. External electron beams are used in the treatment of relatively superficial lesions.

Measurement of ionizing radiations

Measurement of ionizing radiations is thoroughly discussed in Handbook 87 of the National Bureau of Standards.[69]

The aim of measuring the radiation is to be able to assess the physical and biologic effects observed. Several types of dosimeters are available.[26, 82, 87, 201]

Exposure or *given dose* is that amount of radiation to which a particular object or a region of a patient has been exposed, without reference to the nature of the particular material in which the radiation is absorbed.[203] This measurement is usually determined in air or, in the case of high energy beams, at the point of maximum ionization.

Absorbed dose is the dose of radiation that is delivered to a particular material at the point of interest.

Units of radiation[69, 81]

The *roentgen* is the unit of exposure and can be abbreviated by the letter "R." "Roentgen is that amount of x or gamma radiation such that the associated corpuscular emission per 0.001293 gram of air produces in air ions carrying one electrostatic unit or quantity of electricity of either sign."[*]

The *rad* is the unit of absorbed dose and is equal to that amount of ionizing radiation that delivers 100 erg/gram of absorber.

Another unit of radiation that has been used in the past is the *curie*, which is equal to 3.7×10^{10} disintegrations/second. The curie may be used to describe the activity of any radioactive isotope and is approximately the equivalent of the number of disintegrations per second undergone by 1 gm of radium.[82]

---

[*]From International Commission on Radiological Units and Measurements (ICRU): Report 10B, Handbook 85, Washington, D. C., 1962, U. S. National Bureau of Standards.

Dosimetry in radiation therapy (Fig. 4-17)

The dose of radiation given to a patient is expressed in several ways, as follows:

1. *Air dose.* This is used for energies below 400 kvp and denotes the number of roentgens per minute at a given distance for a specified area.
2. *Back scatter dose.* These are secondary electrons produced in the absorber and ejected to the surface.
3. *Surface dose.* This is the amount of radiation received by the more superficial layers of the skin. The surface dose is used only for orthovoltage equipment, in which the maximum effect is at the skin level. It is equal to the summation of the air dose, plus the back scattering dose.
4. *Maximum dose or given dose.* Because of the higher energy of the incident photons and the secondary electrons produced by the interaction of higher energy x rays or gamma rays, there is a point of maximum electronic equilibrium usually several millimeters below the skin, depending on the effective energy of the beam. The dose for this type of radiation is expressed in rads, as the maximum dose or in some institutions as the given dose. The point of maximum ionization (electronic equilibrium) for cesium 137 is about 2 mm below the skin, for cobalt 60, 5 mm, for 4 mev x rays, 8 mm, and for 22 mev x rays, 4 cm.[82, 175, 203]
5. *Central axis percent depth dose.* The distribution of radiation in an absorber can be expressed as a percentage of the surface or maximum electronic equilibrium dose at a reference point that is at a given distance below the surface. The best compendium of these tables is published in Supplement No. 11 of the *British Journal of Radiology.*[166]
6. *Tumor air ratios.* This concept is defined as the ratio of the absorbed dose that would be measured at the same point in free air.[82] It is particularly

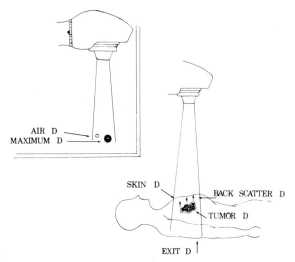

AIR D
MAXIMUM D

SKIN D

BACK SCATTER D

TUMOR D

EXIT D

Fig. 4-17. Various types of doses commonly used in radiation therapy. (See above for detailed explanation.)

useful in the dose calculations for isocentric techniques as well as in rotational therapy.

7. *Tumor dose.* In general, this is defined as the minimal amount of radiation that is given at a point within or around the tumor.[165]

8. *Integral dose.* This can be defined as the total absorbed dose integrated over the entire body or, in other words, as the total energy absorbed by the entire volume of the patient during irradiation.[27] The unit of integral dose is the rad-gram or megarad gram.

Isodose curves

Isodose curves are two-dimensional representations in a plane of the distribution of radiation (Fig. 4-18). They can be obtained by direct measurements, irradiating water phantoms, or by complex mathematical calculations.[157]

Filters

With low- and medium-energy x-ray beams, various types of filters have been used to eliminate soft radiations and improve the quality of the beam. Usually, these consist of 1 to 2 mm of aluminum, sometimes combined with 0.25 mm of copper for 100 to 120 kvp x rays, and at higher energies such as 250 kvp a Thoreaus III filter (combination of tin, copper, and aluminum) is employed. With megavoltage x rays, compensating filters are used to flatten the beam and make it more homogeneous.

Half-value layer

Half-value layer is that thickness of absorber (Al, Cu, Pb) that reduces by 50% the intensity of an incident beam of radiation.[82, 203]

Table 4-1. Characteristics of radiation therapy equipment

	Superficial X rays	Orthovoltage	Van de Graaf generator
Basic components	X-ray tube	X-ray tube	High-voltage electron source, x-ray tube, accelerating electrodes
Energy	50-140 kvp	200-400 kvp	2 mev
Radiation produced	X rays (photons)	X rays (photons)	X rays (photons)
Size of source or target	5-7 mm	5-7 mm	3 mm
Penumbra	+++	+++	+
Dose rates (rads/min)	At 20 cm, depending on filter, varies from 50-300	At 80 cm, 50-75, depending on filter	
Depth maximum ionization	Skin	Skin	About 0.5 cm. below skin
Clinical use	Skin lesions	Superficial lesions	Deep-seated lesions, moderate doses

EQUIPMENT

Table 4-1 illustrates the basic characteristics of radiation therapy equipment; the only mention of the different therapy machines in this text follows. More detailed information can be found in physics textbooks.[82, 181, 203]

Orthovoltage x-ray machines

This unit basically consists of a therapy vacuum tube made out of glass, with a cathode that when headed, emits electrons that are accelerated and hit a fixed tungsten target (anode), resulting in the production of x rays.

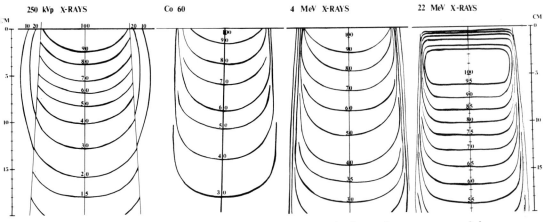

Fig. 4-18. Comparative isodose curves showing the depth dose of various external beam energies.

^{137}Cs	^{60}Co	Betatron	Linear accelerator
Radioactive source	Radioactive source	Circular accelerating tube and magnets	Electron gun, klystron wave guide
.66 mev	1-2 mev	Variable 18-40 mev	Variable 4-35 mev
Gamma rays	Gamma rays	Photons electrons	Photons electrons
-3 cm	1.5-2.5 cm	1-2 mm	1-2 mm
++	++	—	—
0-200, depending on strength of source	50-200, depending on strength of source	50 at 1 meter	200 to 1000
.2 cm below skin	0.5 cm below skin	4 cm or more below skin	Variable with energy 0.8 to 5 cm. below skin
Deep-seated lesions, moderate doses (5000-6000 rads)	Deep-seated lesions, moderate doses (5000-6000 rads)	Deep-seated lesions, high doses (6000-7000 rads)	Deep-seated lesions, high doses (6000-7000 rads)
			Electrons used for lesions at known depths

Although superficial units in the range of 80 to 100 kvp with aluminum or very thin copper filters are used for superficial lesions, most of the pediatric patients with deeper-seated tumors have been treated with energies in the range of 200 to 400 kvp.

The main disadvantage of this type of equipment is the relative lack of penetration with low-depth doses and the maximum ionization occurring at the skin, so that erythema and either dry or moist desquamation will appear even with moderate doses of radiation.

Cesium 137 and cobalt 60 units (Fig. 4-19, A)

The two radioisotopes most frequently used for teletherapy units are cobalt 60 and cesium 137. These therapy machines have the advantage of some skin sparing effect and better depth doses.

The Van de Graaf generator

These megavoltage x-ray units, designed at the Massachusetts Institute of Technology, are used in a few institutions and usually operate at 2 mev. Johns and Cunningham[82] offer a summarized basic description of the machine in their textbook.

Linear accelerators

The linear accelerators are high-energy electron accelerators that can be used as either electron or x-ray sources (Fig. 4-19, B). Linear accelerators

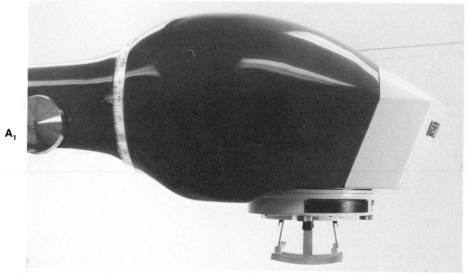

A₁

Fig. 4-19. Photograph (A₁) and schematic representation (A₂) of the head of a cobalt 60 unit. **B,** Schematic diagram of a linear accelerator showing the electronic circuitry on the left and the head, with deflecting magnets, collimator, and flattening filter on the right. **C,** Diagrammatic representation of a Betatron tube and position in magnetic systems. (A₁ and A₂ courtesy of Atomic Energy Commission of Canada, Ltd.; **B** from Johns, H. E., and Cunningham, J. R.: The physics of radiology, Springfield, Ill., 1971, Charles C Thomas, Publisher; **C** from Young, M. E. J.: Radiological physics, ed. 2, London, 1967, H. K. Lewis & Co., Ltd.)

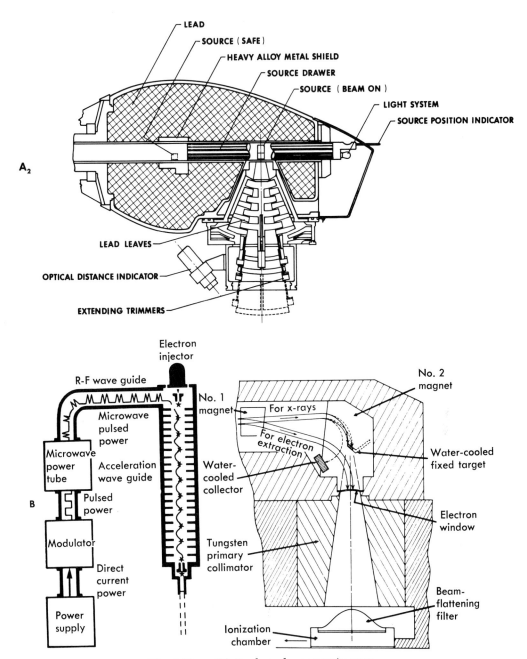

Fig. 4-19, cont'd. For legend see opposite page.

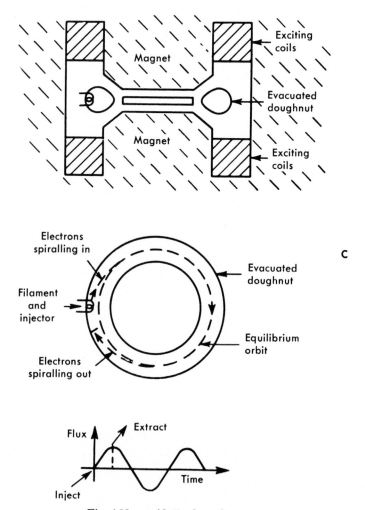

Fig. 4-19, cont'd. For legend see p. 60.

have a high output (200 to 1000 rads at the center of rotation, depending on the type of units). The beam is more homogenous than cobalt 60 and there is little penumbra because of the small focal spot.

Betatrons (Fig. 4-19, *C*)

The Betatron is a machine designed for acceleration of electrons; the only difference is that this is done in a circular tube. Betatrons generate high energy, relatively homogenous x-ray beams with sharp edges, and no penumbra. The maximum electronic equilibrium is at 4 cm below the skin; thus this machine is excellent for deep-seated lesions.

The Betatron can also be used as an electron source. The main advantage of the electrons is that they have a definite range in tissues, which is dependent on their energy.

Most pediatric patients have no need for these high energies. However, in some areas such as in the face, where protection of normal structures and minimal scattering are desired, as in the treatment of retinoblastoma or orbital rhabdomyosarcoma, linear accelerators or Betatrons are particularly useful.

Other radioactive sources and internally administered isotopes

Sometimes it is advantageous to treat a tumor with radiation sources that are directly implanted in the tumor (interstitial therapy) or in cavities that contain the tumor or that are adjacent to it (intracavitary therapy). However, this is not frequently done in children. Likewise, the systemic administration of radioisotopes is extremely rare in children.[5, 65, 168] Several years ago, instillation of ^{198}Au in the spinal subarachnoid space was used in children with medulloblastoma.[90]

REFERENCES

1. Alexander, P.: Atomic radiation and life, rev. ed., Baltimore, 1965, Penguin Books, Inc.
2. Alexander, P., Dean, C. J., Hamilton, L. D. G. ,Lett, J. T., and Parkins, G.: Critical structures other than DNA as sites for primary lesions of cell death induced by ionizing radiations. In Cellular radiation biology: a symposium considering radiation effects in the cell and possible implications, Baltimore, 1965, The Williams & Wilkins Co.
3. Alper, T., and Moore, J. L.: The interdependence of oxygen enhancement ratios for 250 KVP x-rays and fast neutrons, Br. J. Radiol. 40:843-848, 1967.
4. Andrews, J. R., and Hollister, H.: Fast neutron beam radiotherapy, Am. J. Roentgenol. 99:954-961, 1967.
5. Arthur, K.: Radioactive phosphorus in the treatment of polycythemia, a review of ten years' experience, Clin. Radiol. 18:287-291, 1967.
6. Atkins, H. L.: The medical use of 252 CF, Californium-252 proceedings of a symposium sponsored by the New York Metropolitan Section of the American Nuclear Society, New York, 1968, Brookhaven National Laboratory.
7. Avioli, L. V., Lazor, M. Z., Cotlove, E., Brace, K. C., and Andrews, J. R.: Early effects of radiation on renal function in man, Am. J. Med. 34:329-337, 1963.
8. Bacq, Z. M.: Chemical protection against ionizing radiation, American lectures in living chemistry, Springfield, Ill., 1965, Charles C Thomas, Publisher.
9. Bennett, D. E., Million, R. R., and Ackerman, L. V.: Bilateral radiation pneumonitis, a complication of the radiotherapy of bronchogenic carcinoma, Cancer 5:1001-1018, 1969.
10. Bergonie, J., and Tribondeau, L.: De quesques resultats de la radiotherapie et essai de fixation d'une technique rationelle, C. R. Acad. Sci. 143:983-985, 1906.
11. Berkjis, C. C.: Pathology of irradiation, Baltimore, 1971, The Williams & Wilkins Co.
12. Berry, R. J.: Modification of radiation effects, Radiol. Clin. North Am. 3:249-258, 1965.
13. Berry, R. J.: Effects of some metabolic inhibitors on x-ray dose response curves for survival of mammalian cells in vitro and an early recovery between fractionated x-ray doses, Br. J. Radiol. 39:458-463, 1966.
14. Blood, A. D., and Tijo, J. H.: In vivo effects of diagnostic x-irradiation on human chromosomes, N. Engl. J. Med. 270:1341-1344, 1964.
15. Boden, G.: Radiation myelitis of the cervical spinal cord, Br. J. Radiol. 21:464-469, 1948.
16. Bond, V. P.: Negative pions: their possible use in radiotherapy, Am. J. Roentgenol. 111:9-26, 1971.
17. Bonte, F. J.: Radioiodine and the child with thyroid cancer, Am. J. Roentgenol. 95:1-24, 1965.
18. Bouchard, J., and Pera, J.: Radiation therapy in the management of neoplasms of the central nervous system with a special note in regard to children: twenty years' experience, 1939-1958, Am. J. Roentgenol. 84:610-628, 1960.
19. Brady, L. W., Germon, P. A., and Cander, L.: The effects of radiation therapy on pulmonary function in carcinoma of the lung, Radiology 85:130-135, 1965.

20. Brennan, J. T.: Fast neutrons for radiation therapy, Radiol. Clin. North Am. 7:365-374, 1969.

21. Bruce, W. R., Meeker, B. E., and Valeriote, F. A.: Comparison of the sensitivity of normal hematopoietic and transplanted lymphoma colony-forming cells to chemotherapeutic agents administered in vivo, J. Natl. Cancer Inst. 37:233-245, 1966.

22. Bunting, J. S.: A head and neck immobilization unit for use with megavoltage or teletherapy units, Br. J. Radiol. 39:151-152, 1966.

23. Burch, P. R. J.: Radiation carcinogenesis: a new hypothesis, Nature (Lond.) 182:135-142, 1960.

24. Bweley, D. K.: Radiobiological research with fast neutrons and the implications for radiotherapy, Radiology 86:251-257, 1966.

25. Cade, S.: Radiation induced cancer in man, Br. J. Radiol. 30:393-402, 1957.

26. Cameron, J. R., Suntheralingam, N., and Kenny, G. N.: Thermoluminescence dosimetry, Madison, Wis., 1968, University of Wisconsin Press.

27. Carlsson, C.: Determination of integral absorbed dose from exposure measurements, Acta Radiol. (Ther.) 1:433-458, 1963.

28. Churchill-Davidson, I., Foster, C. A., Wiernik, G., Collins, C. D., Pizui, N. C. D., Skeggs, D. B. L., and Purser, P. R.: The place of oxygen in radiotherapy, Br. J. Radiol. 39:321-331, 1966.

29. Cluzet, J., and Soulie, A.: De l'action des rayons x sur l'evolution de la glande mammaire du cobaye pendant la grossesse, C. R. Soc. Biol. 62:145-147, 1907.

30. Cohen, L.: Radiation response and recovery: radiobiological principles and their relation to clinical practice. In Schwartz, E., editor: The biological basis of radiation therapy, Philadelphia, 1968, J. B. Lippincott Co.

31. Comar, C. L.: Fallout from nuclear tests, rev. ed., 1966, United States Atomic Energy Commission.

32. Conard, A., Dobyns, B., and Sutow, W.: Thyroid neoplasia as late effect of exposure to radioactive iodine in fallout, J.A.M.A. 214:316-324, 1970.

33. Concannon, J. P., Summers, R. E., King, J., Tcherkow, G., Cole, C., and Rogow, E.: Enhancement of x-ray effects on the small intestinal epithelium of dogs by actinomycin D, Am. J. Roentgenol. 105:126-136, 1969.

34. Cooper, G., Jr., Guerrant, J. L., Harden, A. G., and Teates, D.: Some consequences of pulmonary irradiation, Am. J. Roentgenol. 85:865-874, 1961.

35. Court Brown, W. M., Buckton, K. E., and McLean, A. S.: Quantitative studies of chromosome aberrations in man following acute and chronic exposure to x-rays and gamma rays, Lancet 1:1239-1241, 1965.

36. Cox, J. R., Gallagher, T. L., Holmes, W. F., and Powers, W. E.: Programmed console: an aid to radiation treatment planning, IBM Medical Symposium 8:179-188, 1967.

37. Cronkite, E. P.: Radiation injury in man. In Schwartz, E. J., editor: The biological basis of radiation therapy, Philadelphia, 1966, J. B. Lippincott Co., pp. 163-207.

38. Dealy, J. B., Jr., and Jessiman, A. G.: Personal communications. In Rubin, P., and Casarett, G. W., editors: Clinical radiation pathology, Philadelphia, 1968, W. B. Saunders Co., p. 399.

39. Dekaban, A. S.: Abnormalities in children exposed to x-irradiation during various stages of gestation. Tentative time table of radiation injury to the human fetus, Int. J. Nucl. Med. 9:471-477, 1968.

40. de Schryver, A., Wachtmeister, L., and Baryd, I.: Ophthalmologic observations on long-term survivors after radiotherapy for nasopharyngeal tumours, Acta Radiol. (Ther.) 10:193-209, 1971.

41. Di Angio, G. J., Farber, S., and Maddock, C. L.: Potentiation of x-rays effected by actinomycin-D, Radiology 73:175-177, 1959.

42. Doggett, R. L. S., Bagshaw, M., and Kaplan, H. S.: Combined therapy using chemotherapeutic agents and radiotherapy, Mod. Trends Radiotherapy 1:107-131, 1967.

43. Duffy, B. J., and Fitzgerald, P. J.: Cancer of the thyroid in children, A report of 28 cases, J. Clin. Endocrinol. 10:1296, 1950.

44. Duncan, W., and Leonard, J. C.: Malabsorption syndrome following radiotherapy, Q. J. Med. 34:319-329, 1965.

45. Eldjarn, L., and Pihl, A.: Mechanisms of protective and sensitizing action. In Errera, M.,

and Forssberg, A. G., editors: Mechanisms in radiobiology, vol. 2, Multicellular organisms, New York, 1961, Academic Press, Inc., pp. 231-296.

46. Elkind, M. M., and Sutton, H.: Radiation response of mammalian cells grown in cuture. I. Repair of x-ray damage in surviving Chinese hamster cells, Radiat. Res. **13**:556-593, 1960.

47. Elkind, M. M., Sutton, G., Moses, W. B., and Kamper, C.: Sub-lethal and lethal radiation damage, Nature (Lond.) **214**:1088-1092, 1967.

48. Elkind, M. M., and Whitmore, G. F.: The radiobiology of cultural mammalian cells, New York, 1967, Gordon & Breach, Science Publishers, Inc., pp. 7-143.

49. Ellis, F.: Fractionation in radiotherapy, Mod. Trends Radiotherapy **1**:34-51, 1967.

50. Ellis, F.: Dose-time and fractionation: a clinical hypothesis, Clin. Radiol. **20**:1-7, 1969.

51. Evans, H. J.: Chromosome aberrations induced by ionizing radiations, Int. Rev. Cytol. **13**:221-321, 1962.

52. Evans, J. C., and Ackerman, L. V.: Irradiated and obstructed submaxillary salivary glands simulating cervical lymph node metastasis, Radiology **62**:550-555, 1954.

53. Exelby, P. E., and Frazel, E. L.: Carcinoma of the thyroid in children, Surg. Clin. North Am. **49**:249-259, 1969.

54. Eyster, E. F., and Wilson, C. B.: Radiation myelopathy, J. Neurosurg. **32**:414-420, 1970.

55. Falchi, L., and Pierotti, P.: Bilateral fracture of the neck of the femur following telecobalt therapy of the pelvis, Radiol. Med. **49**:847-863, 1963.

56. Fendel, H., and Feine, U.: Late sequelae of therapeutic irradiation for benign conditions in childhood, Ann. Radiol. **13**:291-296, 1970.

57. Fletcher, G. H.: Textbook of radiotherapy, Philadelphia, 1966, Lea & Febiger, p. 21.

58. Fowler, J. F.: Differences in survival curve shapes for formal multi-target and multi-hit morals, Phys, Med. Biol. **9**:177-188, 1964.

59. Fowler, J. F., and Margan, R. L.: Symposium on pretherapeutic experiments with fast neutrons and x-rays on tumour and normal tissue in the rat, Br. J. Radiol. **36**:115-121, 1963.

60. Fowler, P. H., and Perkins, D. H.: The possibility of therapeutic applications of beams of negative Pi-mesons, Nature **189**:524-528, 1961.

61. Frank, R. M., Herdly, J., and Philippe, E.: Acquired dental defects and salivary gland lesions after irradiation for carcinoma, J.A.D.A. **70**:868-883, 1965.

62. Fry, W. E.: Secondary glaucoma, cataract and retinal regeneration following radiation, Trans. Am. Acad. Ophthalmol. Otolaryngol. **56**:888-889, 1952.

63. Gamble, J. E., Peterson, E. A., and Chandler, J. R.: Radiation effects on the inner ear, Arch. Otolaryngol. **88**:156-161, 1968.

64. Gillette, E. L., Withers, H. R., and Tannock, I. F.: The age sensitivity of epithelial cells of mouse small intestine, Radiology **96**:639-643, 1970.

65. Goolden, A. W. G., and Szur, L.: Therapeutic uses of radioactive iodine and radioactive phosphorus, Mod. Trends Radiotherapy **1**:317-348, 1967.

66. Gray, L. H.: Radiobiologic basis of oxygen as modifying factor in radiation therapy, Am. J. Roentgenol. **85**:803-815, 1961.

67. Hall, E. J.: The relative biological efficiency of x-rays generated at 220 KVP and gamma radiation from a cobalt 60 therapy unit, Br. J. Radiol. **34**:313-322, 1961.

68. Halls, J. M.: Radiation damage of the small intestine, Clin. Radiol. **16**:173-176, 1965.

69. Handbook 87, National Bureau of Standards, Washington, D. C.

70. Hatcher, C. H.: Development of sarcoma in bone subjected to roentgen or radium irradiation, J. Bone Joint Surg. **27**:179-195, 1945.

71. Hempelmann, L. H., Lisco, H., and Hoffman, J. G.: The acute radiation syndrome: A study of nine cases and a review of the problem, Ann. Intern. Med. **36**:279-510, 1952.

72. Hempelmann, L. H., Pifer, J. W., Burke, G. H., Terry, R., and Ames, W. R.: Neoplasms in persons treated with x-rays in infancy for thymic enlargement, J. Natl. Cancer Inst. **38**:317-341, 1967.

73. Hems, G.: The risk of bone cancer in man from internally deposited radium, Br. J. Radiol. **40**:506-511, 1966.

74. Herring, D. F., and Compton, D. M. J.: The degree of precision required in the radiation dose delivered in cancer radiotherapy, Enviro-Med Report, EMI-216, 1970.

75. Hewitt, H. B.: Fundamental aspects of the radiotherapy of cancer, Sci. Basis Med. Annu. Rev. **1962**:305-326, 1962.
76. Hewitt, H. B., and Wilson, C. W.: Survival curve for mammalian leukemia cells irradiated in vivo, Br. J. Cancer **13**:69-75, 1959.
77. Howland, J. W., Ingram, M., Mermagen, H., and Hansen, C. L., Jr.: The Lockport incident: Accidental partial body exposure of humans to large doses of x-irradiation, In Diagnosis and treatment of acute radiation injury, Proceedings of the International Atomic Energy Commission 1961, WHO International Document Service, pp. 11-16.
78. Hulse, E. V.: The effects of ionizing radiation in the embryo and foetus, a review of experimental data, Clin. Radiol. **15**:312-319, 1964.
79. Hutchinson, F.: Molecular basis for radiation effects on cells, Science **134**:533-538, 1961.
80. Ingold, J. A., Reed, G. B., Kaplan, H. S., and Bagshaw, M. A.: Radiation hepatitis, Am. J. Roentgenol. **93**:200-208, 1965.
81. International Commission on Radiological Units and Measurements (ICRU): Report 10B, Handbook 85, Washington, D. C., 1962, U. S. National Bureau of Standards.
82. Johns, H. E., and Cunningham, J. R.: The physics of radiology, ed. 3, Springfield, Ill., 1969, Charles C Thomas, Publisher.
83. Johnson, R. E., Kagan, A., Hafermann, M. D., and Keyes, J. W., Jr.: Patient tolerance to extended irradiation in Hodgkin's disease, Ann. Intern. Med. **70**:1-6, 1969.
84. Jones, A.: Transient radiation myelopathy (with reference to Chermitte's syndrome of electrical paresthesia), Br. J. Radiol. **37**:727-744, 1964.
85. Kaplan, H. S.: Biochemical basis of reproductive death in irradiated cell, Am. J. Roentgenol. **90**:907-916, 1963.
86. Kaplan, H. S.: Proceedings of Eleventh International Congress, Biologic Foundations of Radiotherapy, Rome, Sept., 1965.
87. Kartha, M.: A ferrous sulfate mini-dosimeter, Radiat. Res. **42**:220-231, 1970.
88. Kashima, H. K., Kirkham, W. R., and Andrews, J. R.: A study of the clinical features, histopathologic changes and serum enzyme variations following irradiation of human salivary glands, Am. J. Roentgenol. **94**:271-291, 1965.
89. Kember, N. F.: Cell survival and radiation damage in growth cartilage, Br. J. Radiol. **40**:496-505, 1967.
90. Kerr, F. W. L., Schwartz, H. G., and Seaman, W. B.: Experimental effects of radioactive colloidal gold in the subarachnoid space, Arch. Surg. **69**:694-706, 1954.
91. Knospe, W. H., Blom, J., and Crosby, W. H.: Regeneration of locally irradiated bone marrow. I. Dose dependent long-term changes in the rat, with particular emphasis upon vascular and stromal reaction, Blood **28**:398-415, 1966.
92. Kottmeier, H. L.: Complications following radiation therapy in carcinoma of the cervix and their treatment, Am. J. Obstet. Gynecol. **88**:854-866, 1964.
93. Lacassagne, A., and Gricouroff, G.: Action of radiation on tissues: an introduction to radiotherapy, New York, 1958, Grune & Stratton, Inc.
94. Laughlin, J. S.: Realistic treatment planning, Cancer **22**:716-729, 1968.
95. Lawrence, J. H., Tobias, C. A., Born, J. L., Gottschalk, A., Linfoot, J. A., and Kling, R. P.: Alpha particle and proton beams in therapy, J.A.M.A. **186**:236-245, 1963.
96. Leach, J. E.: Some of the effects of roentgen irradiation on cardiovascular system, Am. J. Roentgenol. **50**:616-628, 1943.
97. Lehar, T. J., Kiely, J. M., Pease, G., and Scanlon, P. W.: Effect of focal irradiation on human bone marrow, Am. J. Roentgenol. **96**:183-190, 1966.
98. Lesher, S. W., and Bauman, J.: Cell proliferation in the intestinal epithelium. In Fry; Griem, and Kirsten, editors: Recent results in cancer research, normal and malignant cell growth, New York, 1969, Springer-Verlag New York, Inc., pp. 49-56.
99. Liebner, E. J.: Actinomycin D and radiation therapy, Am. J. Roentgenol. Radium Ther. Nucl. Med. **87**:94-105, 1962.
100. Lindsay, S., Nichols, C. W., Jr., and Chaikoff, I. L.: Carcinogenic effect of irradiation, Arch. Pathol. **85**:487-492, 1968.
101. Lingran, M.: Techniques for tumor localization, Cancer **22**:735-744, 1968.
102. Little, J. B.: Environmental hazards: ionizing radiation, N. Engl. J. Med. **275**:929-938, 1966.

103. Little, J. B.: Cellular effects of ionizing radiation, N. Engl. J. Med. **278**:308-315, 369-376, 1968.
104. Locksmith, J., and Powers, W. E.: Permanent radiation myelopathy, Am. J. Roentgenol. **102**:916-926, 1968.
105. Luxton, R. W., and Kunkler, P. B.: Radiation nephritis, Acta Radiol. **2**:169-178, 1962.
106. MacFaul, P. A., and Bedford, M. A.: Ocular complications after therapeutic irradiation, Br. J. Ophthal. **54**:237-247, 1970.
107. Maintenance of oral and general health in the management of the oral cancer patient, 1968-1969, American Cancer Society, Inc.
108. Mallion, W. E., and White, D. R.: Immobilization of the head in radiotherapy, Br. J. Radiol. **41**:236, 1968.
109. Mansfield, C. M., Galkin, B. M., Suntharalingam, N., et al.: Three-dimensional dose distribution in cobalt 60 teletherapy of the head and neck, Radiology **93**:401-404, 1969.
110. Markson, J. L., and Flatman, G. E.: Myxoedema after deep x-ray therapy to the neck, Br. Med. J. **1**:1228-1230, 1965.
111. Merriam, G. R., Jr., and Focht, E. F.: A clinical study of radiation cataracts and the relationship to dose, Am. J. Roentgenol. **77**:759-785, 1957.
112. Merriam, G. R., Jr., and Focht, E. F.: Radiation dose to the lens in treatment of tumors of the eye and adjacent structures, Radiology **71**:357-369, 1958.
113. Millard, R. E.: Abnormalities of human chromosomes following therapeutic irradiation, Cytogenetics **4**:277-294, 1965.
114. Miller, R. W.: Delayed effects occurring within the first decade after exposure of young individuals to the Hiroshima atomic bomb, Pediatrics **18**:1-17, 1956.
115. Montague, C.: The organization of clinical dosimetry. I. The four stages of clinical dosimetry, Acta Radiol. **4**:233-235, 1966.
116. Montague, E. D.: Palliative irradiation for the cancers of infancy and childhood. In Hickey, R. D., editor: Palliative care of the cancer patient, Boston, 1967, Little, Brown & Co. pp. 188-193.
117. Moss, W., and Brand, W.: Therapeutic radiology, St. Louis, 1969, The C. V. Mosby Co.
118. Murphy, W. T.: Radiation therapy, ed. 2, Philadelphia, 1967, W. B. Saunders Co.
119. Neary, G. J.: Oxygen effect with 14 MEV neutrons, Nature (Lond.) **204**:197, 1964.
120. Neel, J. V., and Schull, W. J.: Human heredity, Chicago, 1954, University of Chicago Press.
121. Ogata, K., Hozawa, K., Yoshika, M., Kitamuro, T., Akagi, G., Kagawa, K., and Fukuda, F.: Hepatic injury following irradiation—a morphologic study, Tokushima, J. Exp. Med. **9**:240-251, 1963.
122. Page, V., Gardner, A., and Karzmark, C. J.: Physical and dosimetric aspects of the radiotherapy of malignant lymphomas. I. The mantle technique, Radiology **96**:609-618, 1970.
123. Page, V., Gardner, A., and Karzmark, C. J.: Physical and dosimetric aspects of the radiotherapy of malignant lymphomas. II. The inverted-Y technique, Radiology **96**:619-626, 1970.
124. Paterson, R.: The treatment of malignant disease by radiotherapy, ed. 2, Baltimore, 1963, The Williams & Wilkins Co.
125. Perez, C. A., Vietti, T., Ackerman, L. V., Eagleton, M. D., and Powers, W. E.: Tumors of the sympathetic nervous system in children, Radiology **88**:750-760, 1967.
126. Perkins, D. E., and Spjut, H. J.: Intestinal stenosis following radiation therapy, Am. J. Roentgenol. **88**:953-966, 1962.
127. Perrers-Taylor, M., Brinkley, D., and Reynolds, T.: Choroidoretinal damage as a complication of radiotherapy, Acta Radiol. **3**:431-440, 1965.
128. Phillips, R. A., and Tolmach, L. J.: Repair of potentially lethal damage in x-irradiated Hela cells, Radiat. Res. **29**:413-432, 1966.
129. Phillips, T. L., and Sheline, G. E.: Bone sarcomas following radiation therapy, Radiology **81**:992-996, 1963.
130. Pifer, J. W., Toyooka, E. T., Murray, R. W., Ames, W. A., and Hempelmann, L. H.: Neoplasms in children treated with x-rays for thymic enlargement. I. Neoplasms and mortality, J. Natl. Cancer Inst. **31**:1333-1356, 1963.
131. Pollard, E. C.: Physical considerations influencing radiation response. In Schwartz, E.,

editor: The biological basis of radiation therapy, Philadelphia, 1966, J. B. Lippincott Co., pp. 10-12.

132. Powers, W. E., and Palmer, L. A.: Biological basis of preoperative radiation treatment, Am. J. Roentgenol. **102**:176-192, 1968.

133. Powers, W. E., Palmer, L. A., and Tolmach, L. J.: Cellular radiosensitivity and tumor curability, Conference on Radiology and Radiotherapy, Natl. Cancer Inst. Monogr. **24**:169-185, 1967.

134. Powers, W. E., and Tolmach, L. J.: A multicomponent x-ray survival curve for mouse lymphosarcoma cells irradiated in vivo, Nature **197**:710-711, 1963.

135. Puck, T. T., and Marcus, P. I.: Action of x-rays on mammalian cells, J. Exp. Med. **103**: 653-668, 1956.

136. Puck, T. T., Marcus, P. I., and Cieciura, S. J.: Clonal growth of mammalian cells in vitro, J. Exp. Med. **103**:273-284, 1956.

137. Ratzkowski, E., and Hochman, A.: Gastro-intestinal function after abdominal cobalt irradiation, Acta Radiol. (Ther.) **7**:417-432, 1968.

138. Raventos, A., Horn, R. C., and Ravdin, I. S.: Carcinoma of the thyroid gland in youth, a second look ten years later, J. Clin. Endocrinol. **22**:886-891, 1962.

139. Reed, G. B., and Cox, A. J.: The human liver after radiation injury, Am. J. Pathol. **48**: 597-611, 1966.

140. Reeves, R. J., Sanders, A. P., Isley, J. K., Sharpe, K. W., and Baylin, G. J.: Fat absorption studies and small bowel x-ray studies in patients undergoing Co 60 teletherapy and or radium application, Am. J. Roentgenol. **94**:848-851, 1965.

141. Rider, W. D.: Radiation damage to the brain—a new syndrome, J. Canad. Assoc. Radiol. **14**:67-69, 1963.

142. Rogoway, W. M., Finkelstein, S., Rosenberg, S. A., and Kriss, J. P.: Myxedema developing after lymphangiography and neck irradiation, Clin. Res. **14**:133-134, 1966.

143. Rubin, P., and Casarett, G. W.: Clinical radiation pathology, Philadelphia, 1968, W. B. Saunders Co.

144. Rubin, P., Duthie, R. B., and Young, L. W.: The significance of scoliosis in postirradiated Wilms' tumor and neuroblastoma, Radiology **79**:539-559, 1962.

145. Russell, W. L., Russell, L. B., and Kelly, E. M.: Radiation dose rate and mutation frequency, Science **128**:1546-1550, 1958.

146. Saenger, E. L., Silverman, E. N., Sterling, T. D., and Turner, M. D.: Neoplasia following therapeutic irradiation for benign conditions in childhood, Radiology **74**:889-904, 1960.

147. Sambrook, D. K.: Split course radiation therapy in malignant tumors, Am. J. Roentgenol. **91**:37-45, 1964.

148. Scanlon, P. W.: Initial experience with split-dose periodic radiation therapy, Am. J. Roentgenol. **84**:632-644, 1960.

149. Schlea, C. S., and Stoddard, D. H.: Californium isotopes proposed for intracavity and interstitial radiation therapy with neutrons, Nature **206**:1058-1059, 1965.

150. Schneider, D. O., and Johns, R. M.: Enhancement of radiation-induced mitotic inhibition by BUdR incorporation in L-cells, Radiat. Res. **28**:657-667, 1966.

151. Schroeder, A. F., Crews, Q., Jr., and Rotner, M. B.: Combined treatment of non-seminoma testicular cancer. In Vaeth, J. M., editor: Frontiers of radiation therapy oncology, vol. 5, San Francisco, 1970, University Park Press.

152. Schwartz, E. E.: The modification of radiation response, the biological basis of radiation therapy, Philadelphia, 1968, J. B. Lippincott Co.

153. Seaman, W. B., and Ackerman, L. V.: The effect of radiation on the esophagus; a clinical and histological study of the effects produced by the Betatron, Radiology **68**: 534-541, 1957.

154. Simpson, C. L., and Hempelmann, L. H.: The association of tumors and roentgen ray treatment of the thorax in infancy, Cancer **10**:42-56, 1957.

155. Sinclair, W. K.: Cyclic x-ray responses in mammalian cells in vitro, Radiat. Res. **33**:620-643, 1968.

156. Soanes, W. A., Cox, R. S., Jr., and Maher, J. R.: The effects of roentgen irradiation on adrenal cortical function in man, Am. J. Roentgenol. **85**:133-144, 1961.

157. Sterling, T. D., Perry, H., and Katz, L.: Derivation of mathematical expression for the percent depth dose surface of Cobalt 60 beams and visualization of multiple field dose distributions, Br. J. Radiol. 37:544-550, 1964.

158. Stewart, A., and Kneale, G. W.: Radiation dose effects in relation to obstetric x-rays and childhood cancers, Lancet 1:1185-1188, 1970.

159. Stewart, J. R., Cohn, K. E., Fajardo, L. F., Hancock, E. W., and Kaplan, H. S.: Radiation induced heart disease, a study of twenty-five patients, Radiology 89:302-310, 1967.

160. Stone, R. S.: Neutron therapy and specific ionization, Am. J. Roentgenol. 59:771-785, 1948.

161. Strandqvist, M.: Studien uber Die Kumulative Wirkung der Rontgenstrahlen bei Fraktionierung, Acta Radiol. (supp.) 55:1-300, 1944.

162. Suit, H. D., and Maeda, M.: Hyperbaric oxygen and radiobiology of a C3H mouse mammary carcinoma, J. Natl. Cancer Inst. 39:639-652, 1967.

163. Suit, H. D., and Shalek, R. J.: Response of anoxic C3H mouse mammary carcinoma isotransplants (1-25 MM3) to x-irradiation, J. Natl. Cancer Inst. 31:479-495, 1963.

164. Sullivan, M. P., Vietti, T. J., Fernbach, D. J., Griffith, K. M., Haddy, T. B., and Watkins, W. L.: Clinical investigations in the treatment of meningeal leukemia: radiation therapy regimens vs. conventional intrathecal methotrexate, Blood 34:301-319, 1969.

165. Sundbom, L., and Asard, P. E.: Tumor dose concept, Acta Radiol. 3:135-142, 1965.

166. Supplement No. 11 Depth dose tables for use in radiotherapy, Br. J. Radiol., 1971.

167. Sykes, M. P., Savel, H., Chu, F. C. H., Bonadonna, G., Farrow, J., and Mathis, H.: Long-term effects of therapeutic irradiation upon bone marrow, Cancer 17:1144-1148, 1964.

168. Szur, L., and Lewis, S. M.: The haematological complications of polycythaemia vera and treatment with radioactive phosphorus, Br. J. Radiol. 39:122-130, 1966.

169. Tan, B. C., and Kunaratnam, N.: Hypopituitary dwarfism following radiotherapy for nasopharyngeal carcinoma, Clin. Radiol. 17:302-304, 1966.

170. Tapley, N. D.: The treatment of bilateral retinoblastoma with radiation and chemotherapy. In Boniuk, M., editor: Ocular and adnexal tumors, St. Louis, 1964, The C. V. Mosby Co., pp. 158-170.

171. Tapley, N. D.: Bilateral retinoblastoma, combined treatment with irradiation and chemotherapy. In Vaeth, J. M., editor: Frontiers of radiation therapy and oncology, vol. 4, Baltimore, 1969, University Park Press.

172. Tefft, M., Traggis, D., and Filler, R. M.: Liver irradiation in children: acute changes with transient leukopenia and thrombocytopenia, Am. J. Roentgenol. 106:750-765, 1969.

173. Tefft, M., Vawter, G. F., and Mitus, A.: Second primary neoplasms in children, Am. J. Roentgenol. 103:800-822, 1968.

174. Terasima, T., and Tolmach, L. J.: Variations in several responses of Hela cells to x-irradiation during division cycle, Biophys. J. 3:11-33, 1963.

175. Ter-Poggosian, M.: The physical aspects of radiation therapy of carcinoma of the cervix uteri, Clin. Obstet. Gynecol. 4:466-503, 1961.

176. Thomlinson, R. H.: Oxygen therapy-biological considerations, Mod. Trends Radiotherapy 1:52-72, 1967.

177. Thomlinson, R. H.: Reoxygenation as a function of tumor size and histopathological type. In Time and dose relationships in radiation biology as applied to radiotherapy, Upton, N. Y., 1970, Brookhaven National Laboratory, Associated Universities, Inc., pp. 242-259.

178. Tobias, C. A., and Todd, P. W.: Heavy charged particles in cancer therapy. In Conference on radiobiology and radiotherapy, Natl. Cancer Inst. Monogr. 24:1-21, 1967.

179. Tolmach, L. J.: Growth patterns in x-irradiated Hela cells, Ann. N. Y. Acad. Sci. 95: 743-757, 1961.

180. Toyooka, E., Pifer, J. W., Dutton, A. M., Crump, L., and Hempelmann, L. H.: Neoplasms in children treated with x-rays for thymic enlargement. II. Tumor incidence as function of radiation factors, J. Natl. Cancer Inst. 31:1357-1377, 1963.

181. Tubiana, M., and Lalanne, C. M.: Treatment by supervoltage machines—Telecurie apparatus, Mod. Trends Radiotherapy 1:232-249, 1967.

182. Turner, C. W., and Gomex, E. T.: The radiosensitivity of the cells of the mammary gland, Am. J. Roentgenol. 36:79-93, 1936.

183. Vaeth, J.: Radiation-induced myelitis. In Buschke, F., editor: Progress in radiation therapy, New York, 1965, Grune & Stratton, Inc.

184. van den Brenk, H. A. S.: Hyperbaric oxygen in radiation therapy, Am. J. Roentgenol. **102**:8-26, 1968.

185. van den Brenk, H. A. S., Madigan, J. P., and Kerr, R. C.: Experience with megavoltage irradiation of advanced malignant disease using high pressure oxygen. In Boerema, I., editor: Clinical application of hyperbaric oxygen, Amsterdam, 1964, Elsevier Publishing Co., p. 144.

186. Van Putten, L. M., and Kallman, R. F.: Oxygenation status of a transplantable tumor during fractionated radiation therapy, J. Natl. Cancer Inst. **40**:441-451, 1968.

187. Vatistas, S., and Hornsey, S.: Radiation induced protein loss into the gastrointestinal tract, Br. J. Radiol. **39**:547-550, 1966.

188. Vermund, H., and Gollin, F. F.: Mechanisms of action of radiotherapy and chemotherapeutic adjuvants, Cancer **21**:58-76, 1968.

189. Von Borstel, R. C.: Effects of radiation on cells. In Schwartz, F., editor: The biological basis of radiation therapy, Philadelphia, 1966, J. B. Lippincott Co., pp. 60-125.

190. Von Essen, C. F.: A spatial model of time dose-area relationships in radiation therapy, Radiology **81**:881-883, 1963.

191. Whitfield, A. G. W., and Bond, W. H., and Arnott, W. M.: Radiation reactions in the lung, Q. J. Med. **25**:67-86, 1956.

192. Whitfield, A. G. W., and Kunkler, P. B.: Radiation reactions in the heart, Br. Heart J. **19**:53-58, 1957.

193. Whitmore, G. J., Gulgas, S., and Botond, J.: Radiation sensitivity throughout the cell cycle and its relationship to recovery. In Cellular radiation biology, Baltimore, 1965, The Williams & Wilkins Co., pp. 423-441.

194. Wiernik, G. In Sullivan M. F., editor: Mucosal cell kinetics in patients exposed to abdominal irradiation, gastrointestinal radiation injury, New York, 1968, Excerpta Medica Foundation.

195. Wiernik, G., and Plant, M.: Radiation effects on the human intestinal mucosa, Curr. Top. Radiat. Res. **6**:325, 368, 1970.

196. Wildermuth, O.: Hybaroxic radiation therapy in cancer management, Radiology **82**:767-777, 1964.

197. Wildermuth, O.: The present status of hybaroxic radiotherapy: A perspective view from five years' clinical experience, Radiol. Clin. North Am. **7**:345-351, 1969.

198. Wilson, S. M., Platz, C., and Block, G. M.: Thyroid carcinoma aafter irradiation, characteristics and treatment, Arch. Surg. **100**:330-337, 1970.

199. Withers, H. R.: Capacity for repair in cells of normal and malignant tissues. In Time and dose relationships in radiation biology as applied to radiotherapy, Upton, N. Y., 1970, Brookhaven National Laboratory, Associated Universities, Inc., pp. 54-69.

200. World Health Organization, International Documents Service: Effect of radiation on human heredity, New York, 1957, Columbia University Press.

201. Worton, R. G., and Holloway, A. F.: Lithium fluoride thermoluminescence dosimetry, Radiology **87**:938-943, 1966.

202. Wright, C. N., Boulogne, A. R., Reinig, W. C., and Evans, A. G.: Implantable Californium-252 neutron sources for radiotherapy, Radiology **89**:337-339, 1967.

203. Young, M. E. J.: Radiological physics, ed. 2, London, 1967, H. K. Lewis & Co., Ltd.

204. Zuckerman, S.: The sensitivity of the gonads to radiation, Clin. Radiol. **16**:1-15, 1965.

CHAPTER 5

Cellular kinetics and conceptual basis of chemotherapy[*]

FREDERICK VALERIOTE
TERESA J. VIETTI

Cancer can be considered the result of a failure of those cellular regulatory mechanisms that maintain cell populations at "homeostatic," or optimal, numbers. This malfunction results in a continuous proliferation of the aberrant cell population that, if not successfully controlled, leads to the death of the host. Because the therapist has been frustrated so often by the trial-and-error approach to the cancer patient, a clearer understanding of both the cellular basis of tumor growth and the factors involved in the response of tumor cells to therapy should provide a basis for the development of successful treatment regimens. In this chapter we have attempted to provide such a basis for the development of rational therapeutic regimens. Comprehensive referencing for each concept is not developed here, but appropriate documentation may be found in the references.

NORMAL CELL GROWTH AND DIFFERENTIATION

Some concept of normal cell proliferation is essential before discussing the proliferative kinetics of abnormal cells. In the adult, most of the cell populations are static (i.e., nonproliferating). Many of the cells are irreversibly differentiated (e.g., muscle cells and neurons), whereas some can undergo active proliferation after stress, such as hepatocytes after partial hepatectomy. The cells of the fetus, infant, and child represent an expanding cell population in which proliferation is controlled by feedback mechanisms with cessation of tissue growth as the child attains various developmental stages.

In the adult, as well as the child, some of the body tissues continuously renew their cell populations. Myelopoiesis is an example of a cell renewal population for which a graphic representation is shown in Fig. 5-1. While the different cell types in the myelopoietic series are intermingled in hematopoietic tissues, the various maturation stages can be compartmentalized. The stem cell compartment comprises less than 1% of the marrow population, and under normal conditions, few of these cells are actively proliferating. Depending on the demands of the body, the stem cell will undergo cell division and either differentiate into two granulocytic precursors (myeloblasts) or remain as two stem cells to maintain the size of this compartment. Once differentiation into a myeloblast is initiated, this process is irreversible, with commitment to continued active proliferation

---

[*]The research for this chapter was supported by United States Public Health Service Grant CA-10435 from the National Cancer Institute, N.I.H.

and progressive maturation and ultimate differentiation to a mature neutrophilic polymorphonuclear cell. In the proliferative or amplification compartment the myeloblasts undergo cell division and give rise to the promyelocytes, which subsequently differentiate into the granulocytic precursors, the myelocytes. After the next division, the cell enters the nonproliferative compartment and without further cell division matures to a metamyelocyte, to a band or stab cell, and finally to a fully mature polymorphonuclear granulocyte. The cells in the nonproliferative compartment are insensitive to chemotherapeutic agents, whereas those in the proliferative compartment are sensitive and, as will be discussed later, the cells in the stem cell compartment are relatively insensitive to most agents even though it is the effect on this cell population that is most important with regard to therapy.

Other blood cells, cells of the gastrointestinal tract, epithelial cells of skin and skin appendages, and germinal cells contain similar drug-sensitive renewal cell populations. Furthermore, the cells of the young infant and child that are undergoing active proliferation until optimal organ size is attained are susceptible to the toxic effects of anticancer agents. Although the following discussions consider the effects of anticancer agents in terms of their lethal effect on proliferating cellular systems, one should be aware that some of the drugs affect cellular processes separate from proliferation, which can cause pathologic changes in tissues.

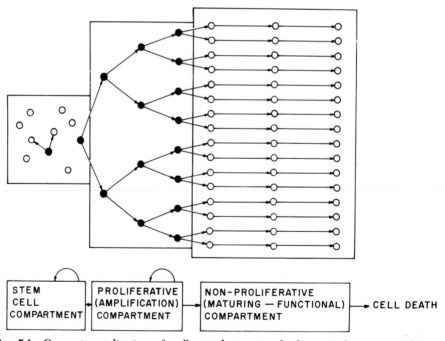

Fig. 5-1. Compartmentalization of cell populations involved in myelopoiesis. Proliferating cells are represented by solid circles and nonproliferating cells by open circles. The type of compartment is indicated in the lower half of the illustration. The arrows indicate passage of cells from one compartment to the next or proliferation within a given compartment.

BIOLOGY OF TUMOR GROWTH

The study of viral and chemical carcinogenesis of mammalian cells and the biochemistry of this transformation holds promise for the future in diagnosis as well as treatment; however, current knowledge is too premature to meaningfully modify the present management of patients. In contrast to this, accumulating knowledge of normal and tumor cell populations is now being used to help the clinician understand and thereby devise more effective therapeutic regimens. Because of this, we have restricted our discussion to a cellular approach to tumor biology in which we will (1) define the functionally different cell populations that might compose a tumor during its growth, (2) provide a clearer understanding of the proliferative (kinetic) processes that are taking place among the different cell populations of the tumor, (3) synthesize this information into a model for a "typical" tumor, and (4) present some therapeutic implications of the model.

The presumed starting point of all tumors is the development of a single malignant cell. For this discussion, let us assume that the one property that characterizes this malignant cell is an inability to respond to the mechanisms regulating cell growth so that it continues to proliferate.

Constant proliferation

A constantly proliferating cell continuously repeats a cycle of biochemical events that terminates with cell division as shown in Fig. 5-2.

Since each proliferating cell gives rise to two daughter cells that continue the proliferative process, the cell population increases geometrically in number as shown schematically in Fig. 5-3.

The model of cellular proliferation shown in Fig. 5-3 would exist for a perfectly synchronized population. Such synchrony implies that all cells in the popu-

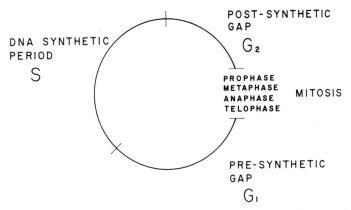

Fig. 5-2. Schematic representation of the cell cycle. The time of replication of the genetic material is termed the DNA synthetic period (S); cell division or cytokinesis occurs at mitosis (M). The periods between these two events are known as the presynthetic gap (G_1) and the postsynthetic gap (G_2). The length of time for a cell to progress from one mitosis to the next is termed the generation time (T_G). Classically, the life history of a proliferating cell was divided only into mitosis and interphase.

lation carry out mitosis at exactly the same time, thereby increasing the population number in a stepwise manner,* as illustrated in Fig. 5-4.

Since the underlying biochemical events involved in the progression of a cell through the cell cycle are statistically distributed in nature, there are considerable variations in the time different cells take to pass through the cell cycle. This results in a distribution of generation times for cells in a population of proliferating mammalian cells; such a frequency distribution is shown in Fig. 5-5.

There is a certain minimum period of time required for a cell to pass through the cell cycle, since it requires some finite period of time to accomplish both the synthesis of total cellular DNA and the process of cytokinesis. This minimum period is probably on the order of 5 to 10 hours. Furthermore, the distribution shown is neither symmetrical nor normal, but rather it is log-normal, for example, if one were to plot the logarithm of generation times, the distribution would be normal. Thus some cells have relatively long generation times that could last for days. This type of distribution of generation times has been demonstrated often for proliferating cells. As a consequence, the cell population proliferates asynchronously, so that at any given time cells can be found in all phases of the cell cycle.† Such a cell population increases exponentially in numbers with time as shown in Fig. 5-6.

At the present time, considerable study is being directed toward determining some of the parameters that define a growing population of tumor cells. The techniques involving labeled mitosis and double labeling (in which radioactive DNA precursors are incorporated into proliferating cells and are observed autoradiographically) have provided estimates not only for the generation times of cell populations but also for the lengths of the different phases of the cell cycle.

Since most of the generation times so far measured for both animal and human tumor cells are around 10 to 30 hours, such tumors should grow rapidly. For example, if it requires 10^{12} tumor cells (approximately 1 kg) to kill a man and all are the progeny of one cell, then

$$10^0 \rightarrow 10^{12} \simeq 2^{40}$$

---

*Mathematically, this geometric increase can be expressed as

$$N(t) = 2^x \qquad (1)$$

where "N(t)" is the number of cells in the population at time "t" and "x" is the number of divisions that the population has carried out in time "t" starting from a single cell. A base of 2 is used, since the process of mitosis that leads to the increase in the population is one of binary fission.

†The increase in the cell population (dN) in any increment of time (dt) is due solely to passage of cells through mitosis. Since we are concerned with an asynchronous population containing N cells, a constant fraction (K) will always be passing through mitosis during dt. Thus:

$$\frac{dN}{dt} = KN$$

The solution of this equation is $N(t) = N_o \cdot e^{Kt}$, where N_o is the number of cells at time "O." To put this equation in a form similar to that shown in (1), the base "e" can be changed to base "2":

$$N(t) = N_o \cdot 2^{t/TG} \qquad (2)$$

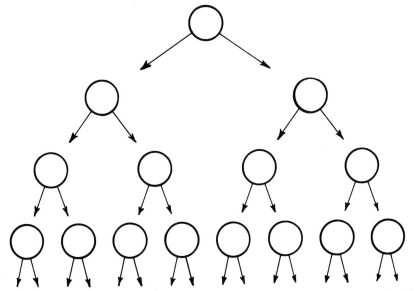

Fig. 5-3. Progressive increase in cellularity for a continuously proliferating population of cells.

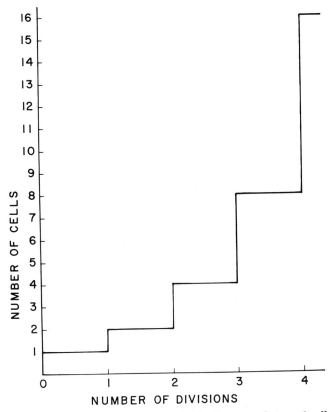

Fig. 5-4. Change in cellularity of a synchronously dividing population of cells as a function of the number of divisions it has carried out.

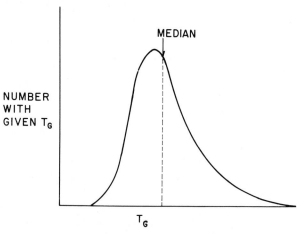

Fig. 5-5. Idealized distribution of generation times (T_G) for a population of mammalian cells.

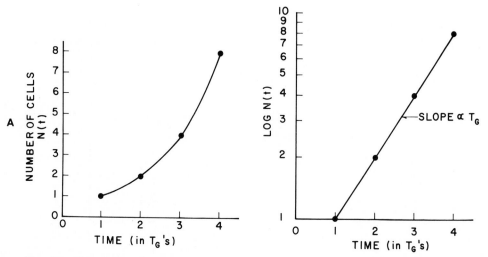

Fig. 5-6. Change in cellularity of an asynchronous population of cells as a function of time plotted either linearly (**A**) or semilogarithmically (**B**).

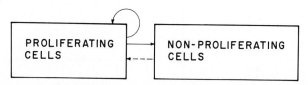

Fig. 5-7. Compartmental relationship between proliferating and nonproliferating cells in a tumor. The solid arrows indicate movement of cells, whereas the dotted arrow indicates the possibility of movement of cells from the nonproliferating to the proliferating compartment.

or 40 cell doublings, are required. If clinical diagnosis occurred at 10^9 cells (1 gram), the time required from diagnosis to death would be that required for 10 cell doublings. If the generation time was 24 hours, death would occur in 10 days, which is rarely encountered. This is likely because there are few, if any, human malignancies in which *all* tumor cells are in the proliferative state, even though this is observed for a number of the transplantable leukemias and lymphomas in experimental animals. Since the model developed to this point does not reflect the growth kinetics observed for most (human) tumors, there must exist modifying factors of tumor growth that have to be considered because of their importance in the design of therapy.

Growth fraction

The fact that tumors often grow at rates less than that expected on the basis of the generation times of their constituent cells can be explained partially by the existence of a fraction of cells in the tumor that are not proliferating. The fraction of cells that are proliferating is defined as the growth fraction (GF) of the tumor, illustrated in Fig. 5-7 in terms of cell compartments. Postulating the existence of nonproliferating cells in a tumor does not preclude the possibility that these cells can become proliferative at some later time. This possibility will be discussed in more detail later.

The addition of a nonproliferating fraction of cells leads to a decrease in the rate of tumor growth* from that that would exist without this restraint. Provided

---

*The equation describing the tumor population growth is
$$N(t) = N_o \cdot 2^{t/T_D} \tag{3}$$

where T_D, the doubling time of the tumor cell population, is that time required for the tumor cell number (or tumor volume) to double. This parameter is greater than the generation time except when all cells in the population are proliferating, that is

$$T_D \geq T_G$$

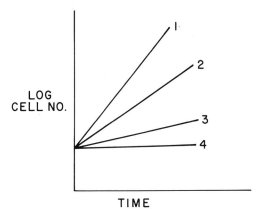

LOG CELL NO.

TIME

Fig. 5-8. Relative growth curves for hypothetical tumor populations. The slope of the curve depends on the fraction of cells that are proliferating. Assume curve 1 represents a tumor in which all cells are proliferating (GF = 1.0), whereas for curve 4 none of the cells proliferate (GF = 0). Curves 2 and 3 represent tumors with values between these extremes.

the rate of movement of cells from the proliferating to the nonproliferating compartment remains constant, the population will increase exponentially with time. Fig. 5-8 shows a number of relative growth curves one might observe for a tumor with different growth fractions.

In an attempt to comprehend the biology of tumor growth it is essential to analyze factors that might influence tumor growth rate. Separate categories of nonproliferating cells discussed here are shown in Fig. 5-9 as cell compartments.

Differentiated cells. Many of the cell populations in the body are characterized by the production of a final functional cell population that does not proliferate such as columnar cells in intestinal mucosa, metamyelocytes and segmented cells in the marrow, and spermatids in testes. In many tumors, morphologically and functionally differentiated cells that do not incorporate tritiated thymidine can be identified. Small lymphocytes in acute lymphocytic leukemia, mature ganglion cells in ganglioneuroblastoma, and keratin-producing squamous carcinoma cells all have functional properties characteristic of differentiated cells. Although it seems reasonable to assume that these differentiated cells cannot again become proliferative, the possibility of dedifferentiation cannot be excluded.

Nutritionally limited, or hypoxic, cells. Nutritionally limited, or hypoxic, cells can arise in areas of a tumor as a result of a deprivation of oxygen or other required substrates, thereby yielding a nonproliferating or dying cell population or both. The limitation of essential metabolites in vitro will cause cells to cease proliferating. Although this condition is generally reversible, if the deprivation continues, cell death will occur. In untreated tumors this category of cells is usually related to its vascularization; for solid tumors, as the size increases, the blood supply to the central area becomes insufficient, with consequent cell death and lysis in the depleted area. Fig. 5-10 illustrates this point.

G_0 cells. G_0 cells refer to those cells that, although not proliferating, do have the capacity to proliferate. This cellular concept was proposed to explain the large number of cells moving into cell cycle after partial hepatectomy. Experimental demonstration of this population is very difficult, and some investi-

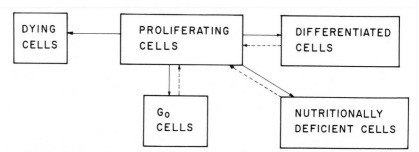

Fig. 5-9. Representation of a tumor containing a proliferating cell compartment and different categories of nonproliferating cell compartments. Solid arrows indicate movement of cells between compartments, whereas dotted arrows indicate a potential for movement between compartments.

gators consider it indistinguishable from cells with a long G_1; however, these two populations can be considered distinct, at least theoretically. Although cells with a long G_1 may exist under conditions of nutritional deprivation, the G₀ cell is outside the cell cycle. Normal cells in the body that are in a G_0 state may be fully differentiated and functionally active, such as the hepatocyte, or exist as primordial stem cells that, if called on, will give rise to functionally active cells such as the hematopoietic stem cell.

Dead cells. Dead cells constitute a separate category. Although these cells will eventually lyse, while they are still intact they will contribute to the size of the nonproliferating population. The fact that these cells exist is attested to by the occurrence of necrotic areas in many tumors. Natural senescence or limitation of nutrients by population pressures or both are often reasons for the death of tumor cells. This latter situation can result if the intervening population becomes so large that nutrients are utilized by intervening cells, or the pressure of the intervening cells leads to the constriction of a capillary, thereby obstructing the normal movement of substrates through the vessel.

It is at this point that present biologic knowledge has not been matched by an adequate mathematical description of tumor growth.* At present the techniques are not available to quantitate the cells in the different compartments that have been discussed or to determine the parameters that define their kinetic

---

*To date, the most useful definition of tumor growth is by the Gompertz equation

$$N(t) = N_o \cdot \exp \left[\frac{Ao(1 - e^{-\alpha t})}{\alpha} \right]$$

where Ao is the initial growth rate, which decreases exponentially with time proportional to α. Although most tumors fit this mode of growth, the biologic basis for it has not been determined.

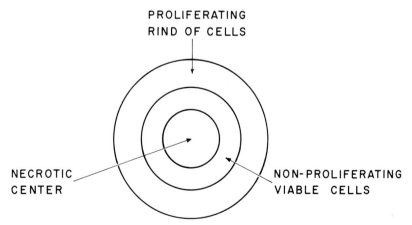

PROLIFERATING RIND OF CELLS

NECROTIC CENTER

NON-PROLIFERATING VIABLE CELLS

Fig. 5-10. Idealized representation of a tumor subunit. It has been demonstrated in experimental tumors that as cells become further removed from the vascular supply that exists at the periphery of the tumor, the growth fraction decreases. This results in a rind of proliferating cells close to the vascular supply of the tumor, nutritionally limited cells at distances greater than about 100 μ from the vascular supply, and a necrotic area of dead and lysing cells when this distance becomes greater than approximately 150 μ.

interrelationships. Because of this, empiricism has been relied on to define the kinetics of tumor growth. However, even though the description of the kinetics of tumor cell population is already complex at this stage, there is yet another important concept to be discussed, that of cell loss.

Cell loss

If the cells die or leave the tumor, then any estimate of the growth rate must take this cell loss into consideration. Cells may be lost in the following ways:

1. *Cell death*. This may be due to a number of factors, some of which have already been discussed, such as natural senescence, nutritional deficiencies, and anoxia. These cells will eventually lyse, and the debris will either be removed from the tumor or remain as areas of necrosis (Fig. 5-9 and p. 79).

2. *Immune response*. The existence of acquired immunity against tumor cells has been demonstrated for a wide variety of experimental tumors and seems likely to be of major importance in human tumors as well. The presence of cell-mediated immunity could lead to the direct killing of tumor cells and their lysis.

3. *Migration*. This process by which cells leave the tumor can be further subdivided:

    a. *Exfoliation*. Cells are removed to the outside of the organism.

    b. *Metastasis*. Cells leaving the tumor subsequently settle and grow in another area of the host to produce secondary "metastatic" tumors.

    c. *Nonproliferative or nonviable cells*. The cells that migrate may be either nonproliferative or nonviable before or after reaching the lymphatic and circulatory system. They may be removed by immune mechanisms or settle into an area that is not amenable to their survival.

Cell loss is extremely difficult to measure directly and thus must be approximated. The approximation is based on the rate of cell loss (the difference between the measured rate of cell production in the tumor and the measured rate of growth of the tumor).

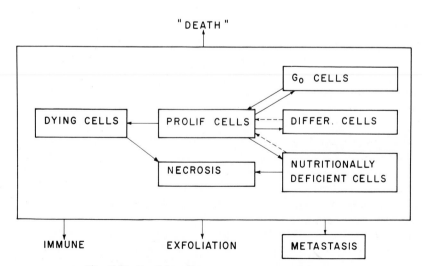

Fig. 5-11. Possible cell compartments in a solid tumor.

Finally, a population model for tumor growth can be developed that takes into consideration all these categories. This model is shown in Fig. 5-11.

From this model, some of the dynamic interrelationships among cell populations within a tumor should be clearer. It should be noted that these interrelationships may be modified continuously during tumor growth. For example, in the very early stages of tumor growth, compartments such as necrosis, G_0 cells, or nutritionally deficient cells probably do not exist. These subpopulations as well as an active immune response probably arise as the tumor grows. Unfortunately for most human tumors, essentially nothing is known about the rate constants between these different compartments; indeed, even the existence of many of these compartments in most tumors has not yet been demonstrated.

RELATIONSHIPS BETWEEN CELL COMPARTMENTS AND THERAPY

Having defined a number of distinct cell populations in a tumor, it is possible to explore their individual importance with respect to therapeutic measures designed to destroy the tumor.

Proliferating cells

The proliferating cell population represents the central point of attack in therapy. In fact, most agents presently used in cancer therapy preferentially kill proliferating cells. Proliferating malignant cells can be separated into those with limited proliferative capacity and those with unlimited proliferative capacity. It is these latter cells that therapy is specifically designed to eliminate. Although those cells with limited proliferative capacity could become important therapeutically if the number of divisions they carried out were large enough, the definition implies only a "few" divisions; therefore such cells are self-limiting in population size. Since it is likely that the survival of a single proliferating cell could reinitiate a tumor, the present rationale of therapy is that every single proliferating tumor cell must be destroyed to cure the host.

Nonproliferating cells

G_0 cells. G_0 cells possibly present the major limitation to eradication of many tumors by chemotherapy as present administered. These cells are not in cycle and are therefore relatively insensitive to the majority of the agents employed. Those agents that have some lethal effect on these cells most likely do so at a very low efficiency when compared to the proliferating cells. It is possible, however, that ionizing radiation may be as effective in killing these nonproliferating cells as it is in destroying proliferating cells, but there are other factors that modify the effectiveness of radiotherapy. The limitation imposed by this population on therapeutic effectiveness results from such cells reentering the proliferating cell pool after therapy so that tumor growth continues. Unfortunately, the kinetics of such movement is unknown but is of paramount importance in the design of effective therapy.

Nutritionally deficient cells. Nutritionally deficient cells are also known to influence successful therapy. Hypoxic cells are relatively radiation resistant and in most tumors would survive host-limiting doses of radiation were it not for the fact that radiation is given in a fractionated schedule. During the intervals between the fractions, population changes occur, and previously hypoxic cells become oxygenated. This is termed _reoxygenation_ and involves concomitant sensitization of these cells during therapy. Since hypoxic cells are in locations where there is an inadequate perfusion of substrates, it is likely that chemotherapeutic agents would be similarly limited in their penetration so that cytoxic levels of the agents may not be reached. An additional complication is suggested by in vitro studies that show that nutritionally deficient cells are arrested in certain phases of the cell cycle; thus they might be in a phase insensitive to the administered agent should it have an age response.* A possible consequence of therapy might then result from the destruction of substrate-utilizing, sensitive cells in that the previously nutritionally deficient cells can now obtain sufficient substrates to commence proliferation and consequently become sensitive to further therapy.

Differentiated cells. Differentiated cells presumably are "end-stage" cells and thus need not be taken into consideration from a therapeutic point of view. However, if dedifferentiation occurs, these cells might again become proliferative. In this event, they could be treated like the two prior cell populations in which a fractionated therapy would be warranted.

Dying cells. Dying cells are of little therapeutic consequence, since this is the category into which we are attempting to put all tumor cells. However, in the process of dying, they might yield metabolites and catabolites that accumulate locally and are potentially able to reverse the lethal action of a given anticancer agent; for example, the liberation of thymidine or its phosphorylated derivatives might lead to the reversal of the action of methotrexate.

Cell loss from primary tumor

The existence of metastases is frequently the major reason why present therapy fails; therefore metastases are of extreme importance in planning therapy. Although surgical excision alone or in combination with x-radiation is the main modality used to control cancer, both surgical excision and x-radiation are forms of local therapy and therefore of little value in the treatment of disseminated disease. This also applies to chemotherapy when the malignant cells metastasize to "protected" areas in the body into which the drug penetrates with difficulty. An example of this is the failure of most antileukemic drugs to pass the "blood-brain" barrier.

Immune mechanisms have intrinsically important functions in the host, both as a surveillance mechanism directed against neoplasms and perhaps also as an active participant against established tumors. In these reactions, cell-mediated immunity plays the most important role. Present evidence suggests that immunoglobulins have little or no positive role in moderating tumor growth and may actually enhance it. Since chemotherapeutic agents and x-radiation are potent immunosuppressants, the immunoreactivity of the host against the neoplasm may be severely compromised during therapy.

As for exfoliation, necrosis, or other modes of cell death, these need not be considered in the design of therapy.

---

*Age response is a term used to denote the sensitivity of cells in different parts of the cell cycle to a given agent. The existence of a differential sensitivity about the cell cycle was first shown for radiation and recently for many of the anticancer drugs now in clinical use.

EXPERIMENTAL CHEMOTHERAPY MODELS IN ANIMALS

A number of animal tumors have been used to evaluate the effectiveness of chemotherapeutic agents, with the mouse-transplantable lymphocytic leukemia L1210 currently being used as the chief tumor screen of the National Cancer Institute. One approach to experimental chemotherapy involving the use of this tumor is illustrated by the work of Goldin and his collaborators. Generally, about 10^5 leukemic cells are injected intraperitoneally into susceptible host mice. After a 2-day period during which the leukemic cells establish exponential growth in their new host, the animals are treated with different doses of an experimental agent. An antileukemic effect is evidenced by a prolongation of the mean survival time as compared to a control group. Active compounds then

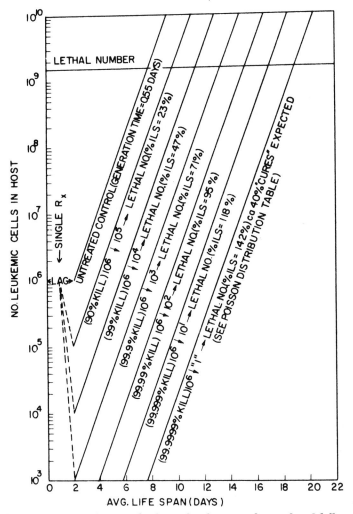

Fig. 5-12. Illustration of the theoretical relationship between drug-induced killing of leukemic cells and the increase in host life-span after single dose therapy. (From Skipper, H. E., Schabel, F. M., Jr., and Wilcox, W. S.: Cancer Chemother. Rep. **35**:1-111, 1964.)

enter a second phase of study in which dose schedules are varied to obtain the maximal antileukemic effect. Because this test system is essentially dealing with an "early leukemia," some of the more powerful agents do cure the mice of their disease. However, if the interval between the injection of the cells and the treatment is prolonged and the mice are allowed to develop "advanced" leukemia, it is at present impossible to cure them with single agents alone. In fact, only with the combination of several effective agents such as 1,3-bis(2-chloroethyl)-1-nitrosourea (BCNU) and cyclophosphamide or cytosine arabinoside and cyclophosphamide is it possible to cure mice with advanced transplanted leukemia.

Skipper and his colleagues have attempted to quantitate this model system by comparing the surviving time of treated mice with that of hosts given known numbers of leukemic cells so that an estimate of the number of leukemic cells killed in the host after therapy is obtained (Fig. 5-12).

One day after injecting 10^6 leukemic cells into susceptible syngenic hosts, a cytotoxic agent is administered and the mice observed for survival. The duration of survival is then compared with the survival time of animals who received varying numbers of leukemic cells to determine the number of leukemic cells surviving after therapy. The extent of the prolongation of the survival time when compared to the untreated control group gives some indication of the magnitude of the destruction of the leukemic cells. This is shown in Fig. 5-12 in terms of both the percentage survival of leukemic cells and the increase in life-span. Quantitation has been further improved by Bruce's group by employing a spleen colony assay in which the exact cell kill could be determined. The effect of anticancer agents on the survival of both a rapidly proliferating malignant cell population (a transplantable AKR mouse leukemia) and a normal nonproliferating population (mouse hematopoietic stem cells) could be compared with respect both to drug dose and time after drug administration. These

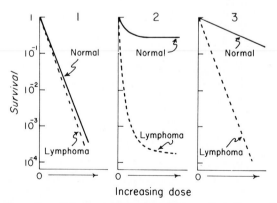

Fig. 5-13. Classification of anticancer agents according to the shape of their dose-survival curves. Different classes are indicated by the numbers 1, 2, and 3. All curves are normalized for comparison. (From Bruce, W. R., and Valeriote, F. A.: The proliferation and spread of neoplastic cells, Baltimore, 1968, The Williams & Wilkins Co.)

studies enabled the investigators to classify agents as illustrated in Fig. 5-13 and diagrammatically presented in Fig. 5-14.

Class 1 consists of *nonspecific agents* in which there is little or no difference in the destruction of leukemic cells as compared to normal stem cells. The lethal effect of the agent occurs independent of the proliferative state of the cell population. This class includes ionizing radiation as well as many of the alkylating agents such as nitrogen mustard. Since an animal with advanced leukemia has a leukemic cell population much larger than that of the hematopoietic stem cells (10^4-fold or more), a nonspecific agent such as x-radiation administered systemically would be of little value because doses lethal to the host would have to be administered to eradicate the malignant cell population. Obviously, if the disease was localized or if the leukemia was very early (i.e., less than a thousand malignant cells), this form of therapy might be effective.

Class 2 consists of *phase-specific agents* such as vincristine or cytosine arabinoside, which destroy cells only during a specific interval in the cell cycle. Most of the antimetabolites effective against tumor cells act in this manner. For this transplantable leukemia, all the cells are presumably in cycle, whereas most of the hematopoietic stem cells are not; thus a degree of selectivity in killing is obtained. Most of the agents in this class kill cells during DNA synthesis (the S phase of the cell cycle). In reference to the schematic representation of the cell cycle in Fig. 5-2, it should be apparent that if S occupies 35% of the cycle, then 35% of the cells would be killed with one exposure to a class 2 agent, assuming that the agent is given at a cytotoxic dose. To obtain optimal therapy with the class 2 agents, they should be administered repeatedly at defined time intervals until all the proliferating malignant cells have entered the sensitive phase and are exposed to lethal concentrations of the drug.

Class 3 consists of *cycle-specific agents* believed to be lethal for proliferating (leukemia) cells, irrespective of the phase of the cell cycle, but relatively in-

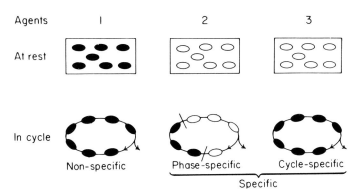

Fig. 5-14. Schematic representation of the assumed cellular action of the three different classes of anticancer agents. The cells that are sensitive to the lethal action of the drugs are indicated in black. (From Bruce, W. R., and Valeriote, F. A.: The proliferation and spread of neoplastic cells, Baltimore, 1968, The Williams & Wilkins Co.)

effective for cells that are out of cycle such as hematopoietic stem cells. Thus a drug in this class, such as cyclophosphamide or 5-fluorouracil, is best administered as a single maximum-tolerated dose. Repeated drug doses can be administered at intervals sufficient to allow the host to recover from any toxicity of the drug to normal tissues.

One of the difficulties that arises with the use of class 2 and class 3 agents is that after their administration, normal stem cells proliferate. This recruitment into cell cycle is apparently due to killing of both the small fraction of the stem cells that are normally undergoing active proliferation and any descendants of the stem cells that are in proliferative compartments (Fig. 5-1). The stem cells then proliferate and differentiate in an attempt to replace the loss in these compartments. A subsequent drug administration during stem cell proliferation destroys them to the same degree as the constantly proliferating leukemic cells, and the differential sensitivity is lost. Therefore in designing appropriate therapeutic regimens, one must be cognizant of the deleterious effects on normal tissues and attempt to minimize toxicity to these cell populations while obtaining maximum destruction of malignant cells.

APPLICATION OF EXPERIMENTAL RESULTS TO THERAPY OF HUMAN TUMORS

In this discussion we have attempted to provide a rationale for the use of anticancer agents in the treatment of disseminated leukemia in mice. It is unlikely that any human tumor has growth properties similar to this model system but rather, as illustrated in Fig. 5-11, consists of a number of functionally distinct cell populations. Therefore in designing therapy for human tumors, the possibility of G_0 or other nonproliferating cells becoming proliferative after therapy must be considered. Other complications such as the development of

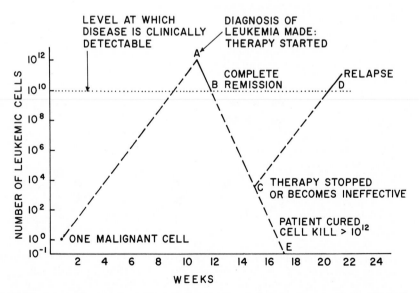

Fig. 5-15. Schematic representation of the results of therapy in a patient with leukemia.

drug resistance, the existence of cells in sites not penetrated by the drug, the interaction of the drugs when given in combination, the physical and mental status of the patient, as well as other factors, including the possible persistence of the tumor-inducing agent, must enter the therapeutic design.

Because of the present inability to define a given human tumor in quantitative, compartmental cellular terms, the clinician is restricted to a presentation of the results of therapy in qualitative terms such as partial remission, complete remission, duration of remission, duration of survival, and cure. The biologist, on the other hand, has at his disposal accurate laboratory assays and thus talks in quantitative terms such as the fraction of cells killed. Fig. 5-15 is presented in an attempt to correlate the terminology of the clinician with that of the biologist, using childhood leukemia as the example.

Since 10^{12} malignant cells weigh about 1 kg, it is not unreasonable to postulate that a child weighing 25 kg with massive hepatosplenomegaly, adenopathy, 50,000 lymphoblasts/mm³ in his peripheral blood, and a packed marrow with 99% blasts would have about 1 kg of tumor cells distributed throughout the tissues of his body at the time of diagnosis as indicated in Fig. 5-15, A. With the start of therapy, a remission is induced that progresses until the liver, spleen, and lymph nodes return to normal size and the percent of blast cells in the marrow decreases to less than 5%. At the point when the patient is considered clinically to be in complete remission (Fig. 5-15, B), the tumor population has been reduced by 99%, leaving 10 grams of tumor tissue still present in the patient. The tumor biologist would say that the tumor population has been reduced by a factor of 10^{-2} or to 10^{10} cells. If therapy is stopped at this point, relapse rapidly ensues, and without further therapy the patient will die of the disease, whereas if therapy is continued, a further reduction in the leukemic cell population is possible. Although the clinician can only guess at the number of leukemic cells that have been destroyed by noting the duration of remission, the biologist can measure this by assaying for the remaining leukemic cells. Obviously, if the patient is cured of his disease, then all malignant cells would have been eradicated, indicating a cell kill of 10^{12} as shown in Fig. 5-15, E. Even if total cell kill is not achieved but can be closely approximated, it is possible that the normal immune mechanisms of the host might help eradicate the last vestiges of malignant cells. This possibility is supported by the finding that in the surgical excision of tumors such as basal cell carcinoma, even though tumor tissue can be presumably left in the patient, complete remission in such patients is usual.

Difficulty in the interpretation of clinical results is frequently observed after radiation therapy and chemotherapy. Consider the hypothetical case of a large tumor seen in the lungs and treated with radiation therapy. Initially there is a poor response, but on long-term follow-up it is observed that the tumor gradually disappears, leaving the patient cured of his disease. Although this might appear puzzling to the clinician, a number of explanations for this result are possible:

1. The tumor growth fraction (proliferating cells) was small, and this cellular fraction was completely destroyed by the therapy; however, sufficient time was required for the large fraction of irreversible differentiated cells to finally die off.

2. The blood supply to the tumor cells was permanently damaged by the treatment, resulting in eventual death of the tumor cells by starvation.

3. Antigenic changes were induced in the cells, and the host's immune mechanism rid the body of these malignant cells.

These two clinical examples illustrate the problems presently experienced in attempting to devise rational approaches to the therapy of human tumors. The major difficulty in the attempt to achieve curative therapy in humans lies in the necessary reliance of the clinician on an empirical approach because of the lack of appropriate techniques to quantitate the cellular effects of therapy.

There are still too many unknown factors to devise optimal therapeutic regimens. Although the experimental studies do provide some basis for a more rational therapy, much more investigation is required to (1) separate tumor cell populations into their respective compartments, (2) define the kinetic interrelationship between these compartments during tumor growth, (3) predict the kinetics of any changes produced by therapy in the cell compartment size as well as the rates of movement of cells between the compartments, and (4) explain the action of the therapeutic agents at the molecular, cellular, and somatic levels.

The tools and knowledge to define some of these factors in animal tumors are now available, and hopefully the obstacles to their application to human tumors will be overcome soon. When this transition (animal-to-human) is successfully accomplished, it should be possible to organize therapeutic schedules with greater confidence of success.

REFERENCES

1. Baserga, R., editor: The cell cycle and cancer, New York, 1971, Marcel Dekker, Inc.
2. Cameron, I. L., and Thrasher, J. D., editors: Cellular and molecular renewal in the mammalian body, New York, 1971, Academic Press, Inc.
3. Field, E. O., editor: Cell and tissue Kinetics, a bimonthly journal, Oxford, Blackwell Scientific Publications, Ltd.
4. Fry, R. J. M., Griem, M. L., and Kirsten, W. H., editors: Recent results in cancer research: Normal and malignant cell growth, New York, 1969, Springer-Verlag New York, Inc.
5. Harris, J. E., and Sinkovics, J. G.: The immunology of malignant disease, St. Louis, 1970, The C. V. Mosby Co.
6. Human tumor cell kinetics, Natl. Cancer Inst. Monogr. **30**, 1969.
7. Lamerton, L. F., and Fry, R. J. M., editors: Cell proliferation, Oxford, 1963, Blackwell Scientific Publications, Ltd.
8. M. D. Anderson Tumor Institute: The proliferation and spread of neoplastic cells, Baltimore, 1968, The Williams & Wilkins Co.
9. Mihich, E., editor: Immunity, cancer, and chemotherapy, New York, 1967, Academic Press, Inc.

CHAPTER 6

General aspects of chemotherapy[*]

WATARU W. SUTOW
FREDERICK VALERIOTE

The immense volume of literature covering each aspect of chemotherapy, from the biochemical and cellular mechanisms of action of the agents to their antitumor activity and effects on the host, precludes a comprehensive review of the subject in this chapter. This chapter has been clinically oriented so that the scope and direction of the discussion are limited to that which, in our opinion, may be of concern to physicians who deal with practical chemotherapy at the patient level. The experimental and conceptual bases for chemotherapy as derived from in vivo and in vitro models have been presented in the previous chapter. Although a number of considerations related to the application of chemotherapy in the clinic will be discussed in some detail, current information concerning the biochemical and pharmacologic aspects of drug activity has been condensed.

GENERAL CONSIDERATIONS
Objectives of chemotherapy

From the clinical viewpoint, the objectives of chemotherapy for cancer might be outlined as follows[50]:

A. Cure
  1. Complete eradication of tumor
  2. Complete eradication of residual tumor
  3. Complete eradication of metastatic tumor (occult or apparent)
  4. Synergism or additive effect with other treatment modalities
B. Palliation
  1. Partial eradication or temporary control of tumor
  2. Symptomatic relief
C. Prevention
  1. Prevention of metastases
  2. Prevention of cancer in populations at increased risk of developing specific malignant diseases (theoretical)
  3. Prevention of reinduction of tumor (theoretical)

Cure of cancer by the use of drugs alone has been reported in patients with Burkitt's lymphoma[16] and those with metastatic gestational trophoblastic tu-

---

*This work was supported in part by Research Career Award CA-2501 (to W. W. S.) and by Grants CA-03713 and CA-13053 from the National Cancer Institute, USPHS.

mors.[35] The fact that some children with acute leukemia are now living more than 10 years without any evidence of disease suggests that cures may be occurring.[16] Among other tumors that respond regularly to chemotherapeutic regimens are Wilms' tumor[22] and rhabdomyosarcoma[40, 52]; in both these conditions the duration of survival or cure rate or both has been dramatically improved by adjuvant chemotherapy. Occasionally, chemotherapy has produced impressive responses in patients with neuroblastoma and some testicular and ovarian cancers. Although the disease may be controlled in varying degree by combination of drugs, curative treatment by drugs alone in Hodgkin's disease and other malignant lymphomas with the exception of Burkitt's tumor remains to be established.[25]

It seems likely that curative schedules of anticancer agents in the future will be those that employ combinations of chemotherapeutic agents or chemotherapeutic agents as adjuvants with surgery or radiotherapy. Inability to predict curative schedules at present lies in our deficiency of knowledge concerning the biochemical and cellular action of anticancer agents, the cell population kinetics of different tumors, and the interaction of the drugs with the host as well as with themselves or with radiation therapy.

Details concerning the use of drugs are given in Chapters 10 to 26. The spectrum of childhood cancers sensitive to each of the most frequently used antineoplastic drugs is outlined in Table 6-2.

The recurrence of tumor or the development of metastases long after the treatment for the primary tumor (e.g., 5 years or longer) evokes consideration of the possibility of "reinduction" of the primary cancer. If some cancers are induced by a virus, it might be postulated that the delayed manifestations of tumor activity represent new "transformation" by the same oncogenic agent. If this is a fact, then cytologic cure must be complemented by the destruction or elimination of the carcinogenic agents.

Finally, the potential effectiveness of chemotherapy as a true prophylactic measure requires investigation. The risk of leukemia is higher than normal in children with Down's syndrome.[36] Children exposed to large doses of ionizing radiation and identical twins of leukemic children are often examples of those with increased risk of leukemogenesis.[15, 36] This increased risk of cancer is also present in those with congenital anomalies such as aniridia (Wilms' tumor), and in those who have received therapeutic irradiation (bone sarcoma and other malignant tumors). No systematic study of the potential benefits of prophylactic chemotherapy in these groups has been reported. Skin cancers invariably develop in children with xeroderma pigmentosum.[47] Exposure of the thyroid gland of children to ionizing irradiation has resulted, years later, in the development of malignant tumors in the gland.[18] Efforts to prevent such types of carcinogenesis have not been rewarding; nevertheless, the necessity for continued efforts in this direction remains.

Factors influencing effectiveness of chemotherapy

The factors that may influence the response of tumors to treatment with cytotoxic drugs can be separated into three categories based on a consideration of the drug, the host, and the tumor. In Fig. 6-1 a representation of these three categories is shown, together with the specific factors that must be taken into consideration. A number of the factors are not specific for a single category but exist in areas in which the categories overlap.

Antitumor activity. The choice of the agent depends on the predicted sensitivity of the tumor from previous animal and human studies. Usually an agent that has demonstrated activity against the tumor to be treated will be chosen.

Drug combination. Many of the present and likely most of the future therapy protocols for cancer will encompass the use of chemotherapeutic agents in combination. Because of its major importance, the strategy of combination therapy is discussed separately in a later section of this chapter.

Sensitivity. The sensitivity of a given tumor to a chemotherapeutic agent is obviously one of the first considerations in the design of therapy. A major problem in present-day chemotherapy is the restricted ability of the chemotherapist to measure meaningfully and quantitatively the response of a population of malignant cells, as well as of normal cells, to anticancer agents.

The recognition of the need for uniform, objective criteria[33] has not been matched by the formulation and agreement on the nature of such criteria except in acute leukemia (Chapters 9 and 10). Yet the evaluation of tumor sensitivity or therapeutic efficacy is critically pertinent to decisions regarding the continuance, discontinuance, or modification of therapy. The parameters most

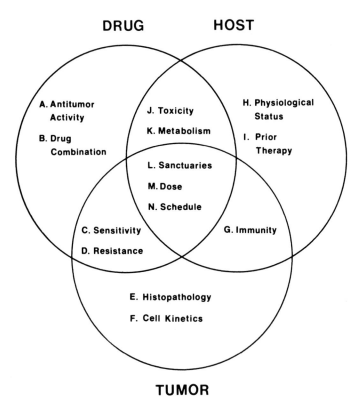

Fig. 6-1. Schema indicating drug, tumor, and host factors and their interactions that influence effectiveness of chemotherapy.

frequently used at present for evaluation of results of chemotherapy include the following:

1. Estimation of the probability of cure or permanent control of the disease as projected from survival (in disease-free state) beyond an arbitrary fixed duration of time (e.g., 2 years, 5 years, or a calculated "period of risk")[17, 39]
2. Actual duration of remission or of tumor regression
3. Measurement of the change in growth rate of the tumor
4. Assessment of change in the performance status of the patient
5. Serial determination of specific biochemical substances, for example, gonadotropins in choriocarcinoma, VMA patterns in neuroblastoma, alkaline phosphatase in osteogenic sarcoma, and copper in Hodgkin's disease
6. Serial determination of routine peripheral blood counts and other pertinent laboratory tests

The development of some quantitative measurement of residual disease or of the "depth of therapeutic response" would aid immensely in the comparison of the effectiveness of different treatment protocols. When in vitro systems become available for the quantitation of the proliferative capacity of human malignant cells, the assessment of drug effects on both specific types of tumors and individual tumors in the patient undergoing therapy will be possible. Similarly, a test for the cytocidal activity of anticancer agents in the sera of patients undergoing therapy would be helpful.

Resistance.[29] A major problem in clinical cancer chemotherapy is the development of drug-resistant tumor cells. At the cellular level there are a number of possible mechanisms for the development of this resistance[51]:

1. Modification of the plasma membrane such that the drug is either no longer transported or able to move across it. This is probably the major mechanism through which resistance to many drugs develops.[28, 34]

2. Decreased activity or loss of the enzyme that converts the parent drug into an active form such as uridine phosphorylase, which converts 5-FU to 5-FUR.

3. An increased production or decreased turnover of target macromolecules. Although the drug still inactivates those targets with which it binds, the ratio of drug to target molecules becomes low so that a number of active target macromolecules persist and are sufficient for survival of the cell. This phenomenon is known to occur in the development of resistance to methotrexate, during which levels of folate reductase increase substantially.

4. An increased activity of the repair system for the inactivated target such that the cell is more able to recover from the drug-induced lesion. An increased activity of DNA polymerase I in cells selected through exposure to some alkylating agents would be an example.

5. An increased activity of the enzyme or enzyme system that metabolizes the anticancer agent so that cytotoxic concentrations are no longer reached. This may be true for a number of the antimetabolites.

6. The synthesis of a number of macromolecules with which the drug can bind. The binding to a second "target" would act to reduce the intracellular concentration of the drug. Also, the second target might be less important to the survival of the cell than was the inactivation of the first target. The produc-

tion or accumulation of electron-rich substances to "discharge" alkylating agents would be such a mechanism.[31]

7. A modification of the structure of the target so that it is no longer able to bind the drug but can still carry out its required function.

8. An increase in the activity or de novo synthesis of another macromolecule that can carry out the function of the target macromolecule but is not affected by the drug. Since there are often a number of biochemical pathways through which a product can be produced, the selection of cells utilizing an alternate pathway might occur. The combination of agents in effective chemotherapy schedules has as one of its rationales the ability of a second agent to destroy those cells resistant to the first agent and vice versa.

Histopathology. Histologic considerations involve the diagnosis, the possible mixture of morphologically different cancer types (e.g., in malignant teratoma), and the possible coexistence of sensitive and resistant cell populations in the same tumor. One important aspect of present-day histopathology of malignant tumors is its use to predict those chemotherapeutic agents to which the tumor will respond. It is also important in defining those tumors for which other modes of therapy would be most effective or for which experimental chemotherapy protocols might be worthwhile.

Kinetics.[37, 42, 48, 49, 53] The different types of cell populations that exist in a tumor as well as the interrelationships among these populations are most important in designing a rational schedule of chemotherapy. For example, clinical experience indicates that "early disease" responds to chemotherapy better than "advanced disease." Such a difference might well be due to the existence in the late tumor of a large fraction of cells in a G_0 state (nonproliferative state), in which phase-specific and cycle-specific agents have little effect. In such tumors with low growth fractions, administration of phase-specific agents would be far from optimal, since they would have little effect on the tumor cell population but would have their normal toxic effect on the host. Furthermore, if one knew the rate of recruitment of cells during therapy from the G_0 compartment, more effective therapy could be designed. A similar situation probably exists with regard to the lack of response exhibited by populations of tumor cells in poorly vascularized areas of the tumor (these would be hypoxic and thus fairly insensitive to radiation therapy). If information concerning the rate of revascularization or reoxygenation of these cells were available, more optimal therapeutic regimens could be employed, thereby decreasing the total dose of therapy required, as well as increasing cure rates. Much of this analysis of cell population kinetics is discussed in Chapter 5. Although considerably more knowledge is needed for a competent understanding of cell population kinetics of tumors in the intact human host, these various concepts are being utilized in the strategic programming of clinical chemotherapy for patients with acute leukemia and solid tumors.

Immunity. It has been found that in a wide variety of human tumors the host initiates an immune response against the tumor during its development. This immune response can be both effective in terms of a cell-mediated immune system resulting in sensitized lymphocytes specifically against the tumor cells or it can be detrimental in terms of the production of a blocking antibody by a humoral-mediated immune system. In any event, it is necessary to consider that most of the anticancer agents currently employed are immunosuppressive and might be expected to modify this interaction between the tumor and host. At present, little quantitative information on the effects of different schedules or different agents on the immune responses in tumor-bearing hosts is available on which to base any such considerations.

Physiologic status.[41] The age, nutrition, and metabolic status of the patient may require modification of the course of chemotherapy. Factors such as the presence of a bacterial or viral infection, bone marrow failure, electrolyte imbalance, hepatic and renal functions, and the psychologic condition of the patient must be taken into consideration. It has been emphasized that the physiologic state of the patient may alter drug interactions.

Prior therapy. The type, intensity, and recency of prior treatment determine the choice and timing of subsequent therapy. If the patient has had radiation therapy to a large fraction of the bone marrow, sufficient time must be allowed after irradiation to permit repopulation of the hematopoietic cells (especially the stem cells). Any newly proposed chemotherapy schedule should preclude the administration of those agents that could show cross resistance or aggravate residual toxicity.

Toxicity. Toxicity to the host limits the single and total dose of a chemotherapeutic agent. Toxicity is a function not only of the dose of the agent used but also of the schedule employed. Depending on the route of administration as well as the specific agent, toxicity may be more manifest in one organ system than in another. Since most anticancer agents have been selected because of their lethal effects on proliferating cells, normal host cell populations undergoing rapid renewal are usually the most affected by these chemotherapeutic agents. This is especially true of the hematopoietic tissues, intestinal mucosa, hair, and gonadal tissue. However, the toxicity of a number of agents is expressed on nonproliferating systems such as the *Vinca* alkaloids on nervous tissue and daunorubicin on cardiac tissue. By combining agents with completely different toxic effects, an additive (increased) killing of the tumor cell population may be obtained while maintaining a tolerable host toxicity.

Metabolism. Since drugs such as cyclophosphamide are activated in vivo,[57, 61] whereas others such as cytosine arabinoside are inactivated, the ability of the host to carry out metabolic functions at the time of therapy will determine the amount of drug to which the malignant cells are exposed. It is known that many factors affect the rates of metabolism of anticancer agents, such as the action of phenobarbital on microsomal enzymes to increase the rate of activation of cyclophosphamide or of steroids that compete for these enzymes to decrease drug activation. Since many agents are metabolized by the liver, impairment of liver function is of importance in determining dosage levels. Similarly, any impairment of kidney function must also be considered, since this might lead to an increased half-life of the drug in the patient and hence a more lethal effect on tumor cells but also greater toxicity.

Sanctuaries. A major limitation of curative chemotherapy is the persistence of malignant cells at the completion of therapy in anatomic sites to which the drugs did not penetrate. For example, most of the anticancer agents do not cross the "blood-brain barrier" and thus are not effective when leukemic cells penetrate this barrier and proliferate in the meninges. A similar situation might exist for brain metastases of other tumors. One might then consider the use of agents that do penetrate the barrier, such as BCNU, employ ionizing radiation to the cerebrospinal axis, or administer anticancer agents such as methotrexate intrathecally. Sanctuaries may also exist within a tumor and be a function of its vascularization, that is, there might be areas within the tumor in which viable tumor cells exist; however, the capillaries are at such a distance from these cells that minimally required levels of nutrients can reach them, but effective levels of anticancer agents cannot.[23]

Dose. The dose of the drug(s) depends not only on the host tolerance but also on tumor sensitivity. The optimum drug dosage is that sufficient to achieve cytotoxic concentration for all malignant cells. Pinkel[38] suggested the use of body surface area as the base instead of body weight alone for dosage calculations of antineoplastic agents.[20] Gehan and George[27] recently reviewed the

Table 6-1. Body surface area (m^2) as a function of height and weight*

Height (cm)	Weight (kg)				Height (cm)	Weight (kg)					Height (cm)	Weight (kg)				
	4	6	8	10		12	14	16	18	20		22	24	26	28	30
50	0.25	0.31	0.36		50						75					
55	0.26	0.32	0.37		55						80					
60	0.27	0.33	0.39	0.43	60						85					
65	0.28	0.34	0.40	0.45	65						90					
70		0.36	0.41	0.46	70	0.51					95					
75			0.42	0.48	75	0.52	0.57				75					
80			0.44	0.49	80	0.54	0.58				80					
85				0.50	85	0.55	0.60	0.64			85					
90				0.51	90	0.56	0.61	0.65			90					
95				0.53	95	0.58	0.63	0.67			95					
100					100	0.59	0.64	0.68	0.73	0.77	100	0.81				
105					105	0.60	0.65	0.70	0.74	0.78	105	0.82				
110					110			0.71	0.76	0.80	110	0.84	0.88			
115					115			0.73	0.77	0.81	115	0.86	0.89			
120					120				0.79	0.83	120	0.87	0.91	0.95		
125					125					0.84	125	0.89	0.93	0.97	1.00	
130					130						130	0.90	0.94	0.98	1.02	1.06

Height (cm)	24	26	28	30		32	34	36	38	40		42	44	46	48	50
135	0.96	1.00	1.04	1.07	135	1.11	1.15	1.18			135					
140		1.01	1.05	1.09	140	1.13	1.16	1.20	1.23	1.26	140					
145			1.07	1.11	145	1.14	1.18	1.22	1.25	1.28	145	1.32				
150				1.12	150	1.16	1.20	1.23	1.27	1.30	150	1.34	1.37	1.40	1.43	1.46
155				1.14	155	1.18	1.21	1.25	1.29	1.32	155	1.35	1.39	1.42	1.45	1.48

Height (cm)	42	46	50	54		58	62	66	70	74		78	82	86	90	94
160	1.37	1.44	1.50	1.56	160	1.62					160					
165		1.46	1.52	1.58	165	1.64	1.70	1.75			165					
170		1.48	1.54	1.60	170	1.66	1.72	1.78	1.83		170					
175				1.62	175	1.68	1.74	1.80	1.85	1.91	175					
180					180	1.70	1.76	1.82	1.88	1.93	180					
185					185			1.84	1.90	1.95	185	2.01	2.06	2.11	2.16	2.21
190					190			1.86	1.92	1.97	190	2.03	2.08	2.13	2.18	2.23
195					195					2.00	195	2.05	2.11	2.16	2.21	2.26

*Based on data furnished by E. A. Gehan and I. L. George, Department of Biomathematics, The University of Texas M.D. Anderson Hospital and Tumor Institute at Houston, Houston, Texas.

methodology of surface area determinations and prepared a table showing surface areas for height and weight categories (Table 6-1). It has been claimed that the use of body surface area calculations simplifies the application of animal data to human drug trials and permits better evaluation of the dose to toxicity relationships for a comparison of different body sizes such as adults versus children.[26] Shirkey[46] has reveiwed the clinical experience utilizing body surface area as the basis for drug dosage in pediatric patients and has concluded that such dosage innovations are "reliable for all age groups except the premature and full term newborn human." A number of nomograms have been published for estimation of body surface area from stature and weight determinations.[20, 44, 45]

   Schedule. All these factors just mentioned and available information are then synthesized into the construction of the schedule of anticancer agents for a particular tumor.[24, 29] The schedule considers the timing, sequence, route, and frequency of administration. "Reversing agents" that will counteract the prolonged action of a drug may be indicated when very large doses of anticancer agents are administered. In this case, a large dose of the reversing agent(s) is administered at the specified time. An example of this is the administration of methotrexate with folinic acid as the reversing agent.[21, 30, 43] The schedule of chemotherapy may also depend on the concomitant or sequential use of other treatment modalities.

   From this brief description of the many factors involved in establishing therapeutic regimens, it should be obvious that to rely on empiricism alone in the development of the optimal regimens for specific tumors would be futile. More information concerning the three interacting categories—drug, host, and tumor—is required to develop a scientific rationale for cancer chemotherapy. In any event, experienced clinical judgment must be constantly exercised to anticipate the course of the disease and the possible impact of the therapy itself on the patient.

SITES OF ACTION OF ANTICANCER AGENTS

   The screening systems generally employed for anticancer agents select out those that are particularly lethal to proliferating cells.[19] Two of the most important and characteristic features of proliferating cells are the biochemical sequences during the chromosome duplication phase and the subsequent cytokinesis during mitosis. It is not surprising then that the biochemical mode of cell lethality of most anticancer agents is an interference with the synthesis of deoxyribonucleic acid (DNA) or cell division.

   For the following discussion of various anticancer agents, the sites of action have been illustrated (Fig. 6-2) in terms of DNA synthesis (replication), the synthesis of ribonucleic acid (RNA) from the DNA (transcription), and the synthesis of proteins from the messenger RNA (translation).

   The agents have been classified into the several conventional categories: alkylating agents, antimetabolites, antibiotics, steroid hormones, plant extracts, and miscellaneous compounds.

Alkylating agents

   War-oriented investigations of poison gases led to studies that resulted in the development of a group of cytotoxic chemicals classified as alkylating agents.

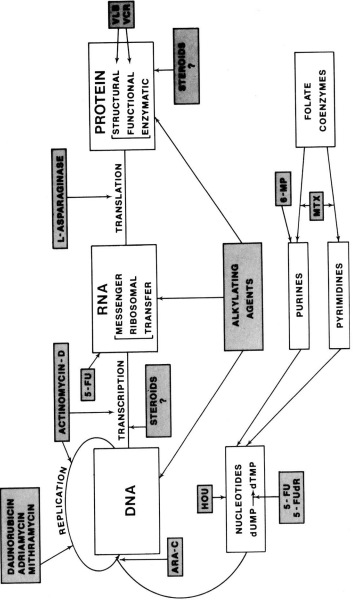

Fig. 6-2. Sites of action of antineoplastic agents in relation to synthesis of DNA, RNA, and protein. DNA, deoxyribonucleic acid; RNA, ribonucleic acid; ara-C, cytosine arabinoside; HOU, hydroxyurea; 5-FU, 5-fluorouracil; 5-FUdR, 5-fluorodeoxyuridine; 6-MP, 6-mercaptopurine; MTX, methotrexate; VLB, vinblastine; VCR, vincristine; dUMP, deoxyuridine monophosphate; dTMP, deoxythymidine monophosphate.

The clinical trials of these agents were begun in 1942[62]; subsequently a number of monographs, reviews, and symposia provided condensed perspectives on the ever-expanding literature.*

The chemical reaction of alkylation is the replacement of a hydrogen atom in the molecule to be alkylated with an alkyl group ($R \cdot CH_2-$). Since the active part of the alkylating agent is electrophilic, it will react at sites in molecules where there is high electron density.

In the structure of nitrogen mustard, the parent alkylating agent in cancer chemotherapy, two chloroethyl groups are attached to a nitrogen atom. Each of the chloroethyl groups can alkylate a nucleophilic structure; for this reason, nitrogen mustard is called a *bifunctional* alkylating agent. The alkylating agents are classified into several categories: the nitrogen mustards such as mechlorethamine, chlorambucil, and cyclophosphamide; the methane sulfonates such as busulfan (Myleran); the ethylene imines such as thio-TEPA and triethylenemelamine (TEM); and the epoxides such as benzoquinone.

In their intracellular interaction in mammalian cells, these chemicals will react with the following groups preferentially: phosphate, guanine, carboxyl, imidazole, sulfhydryl, and amino. Therefore the major loci of action in the cell are the proteins and polynucleotides. Although many investigators have indicated that the site of action for *all* alkylating agents is the same, that being the alkylation of DNA,[71, 75] other investigators have provided evidence that indicates that RNA and protein are also targets in the cell whose alkylation would lead to cell death.[56, 64, 69] For example, it has been proposed that nitrogen mustard produces death of the target cells by alkylating the macromolecules in the cytoplasm of the cell. Although DNA in vitro is sensitive to alkylating agents, it is protected from alkylation in vivo as a consequence of its complexing with proteins.[72] It is likely, however, that many alkylating agents do lead to cell death through reaction with DNA.

In the interaction of the alkylating agents with DNA, the N-7 atom of guanine reacts preferentially, after which several outcomes are possible: alkylation and cross-linking with a second guanine on the opposite strand of the double helix may occur, thereby preventing strand separation and resulting in inhibition of DNA replication[65-67]; depurination might occur, resulting in breakage of the DNA chain; a reaction with a second guanine residue on the same strand might occur, thereby interfering with DNA synthesis[68]; ring cleavage might result; an abnormal base pair with thymine might be formed; and finally, cross-linking may occur between DNA and its associated proteins.[63, 74]

Another consideration in assessing lethal damage resulting from the reaction of alkylating agents with DNA is the existence of a repair mechanism through which part of the damage is repaired.[60, 75] Alexander[54] hypothesized that "lethal lesions arise from injuries produced during enzymatic removal of the cross-links introduced by the alkylating agents." Ochoa and Hirschberg's[70] conclusion in their extensive review that "it does not appear possible to identify in an unequivocal way a single mechanism of action for the alkylating agent" appears more true than ever at the present time.

---

*References 55, 58, 59, 70, 71, 73, 74, and 75.

Antimetabolites

A second group of anticancer agents are structurally similar to normal metabolites of the cell and thereby act as substrates for the enzymes of the metabolites they resemble. These antimetabolites then either bind strongly to the enzyme, thereby decreasing or blocking its activity, or the antimetabolite is converted to a product that is incorporated into a macromolecule that, because of its difference, produces a nonfunctional macromolecule.

Because this is the largest and most commonly used category of anticancer agents in clinical practice, we have discussed a number of them in some detail here.

Methotrexate. Studies of the antileukemic activities of folic acid analogs were begun in 1947 with the use of aminopterin.[90] The most common antifolate presently used in therapy is methotrexate, which binds strongly to and stoichiometrically inhibits folic acid reductase, thus interfering with reduction of folic acid to tetrahydrofolic acid.[78, 106, 111] Tetrahydrofolic acid is converted to a number of cofactors that take part in important reactions requiring the transfer of 1-carbon units.[78] Consequently, antifolates inhibit a number of biochemical pathways, the most important of which are de novo synthesis of both purines and pyrimidines and specifically the synthesis of thymidylate. The final result is inhibition of DNA synthesis, leading to cell death.[79, 101] Since RNA and protein synthesis are not concomitantly inhibited with DNA synthesis, the cell is said to be in a state of "unbalanced growth," which leads to the lethal outcome. The administration of a number of cell metabolites together with methotrexate is known to modify the degree of cytotoxicity. The cytotoxic action of methotrexate can be reversed by folinic acid, which is an end product of the enzyme that methotrexate inhibits, or by the use of thymidine or other deoxynucleosides.

6-Mercaptopurine. Many purine analogs have been studied as potential antineoplastic agents.[105, 107] To date, the most successful of these analogs has been 6-mercaptopurine (6-MP), which was synthesized as a hypoxanthine analog and was first tested as an antitumor agent in 1951.[99] It is converted in vivo to the active form, 6-MP ribonucleotide (6-MPRP),[98, 100] which interferes at one or more steps in the metabolic pathway of inosinic acid to xanthylic acid.[88]

6-MPRP acts as an analog of inosinic acid, thereby feedback inhibiting the first enzymatic step in the de novo synthesis of purines. Also, by competing for the enzymes that convert inosinic acid to both adenylsuccinic acid and xanthylic acid, it inhibits the synthesis of both deoxyadenosine diphosphate and deoxyguanosine diphosphate, thereby inhibiting DNA synthesis.* There are a number of other purine analogs such as azathioprine (Imuran), 6-methylthiopurine ribonucleoside, and 2-amino-6-mercaptopurine (6-thioguanine).

Another purine analog, 4-hydroxy pyrazolo[3,4-d]pyrimidine (allopurinol), has little if any antineoplastic activity but greatly increases the activity of 6-mercaptopurine when combined with it. Allopurinol is preferentially bound to xanthine oxidase, which is the enzyme responsible for the oxidation and degradation of 6-mercaptourine in vivo. Thus when these agents are given together, a significant increase in the amount of 6-mercaptopurine in the serum occurs as a function of time after administration, and the antitumor activity is increased.

---

*References 77, 80, 88, 89, 98, 104.

Pyrimidine analogs.[81, 82, 87, 95-97] A large number of pyramidine analogs have been synthesized, the first being 6-azauracil. At the present time, the two most utilized of the pyrimidine analogs are 5-fluorouracil (5-FU) and cystosine arabinoside (ara-C).

5-Fluorouracil (5-FU). 5-FU is a fluorinated uracil analog synthesized in 1957 by Heidelberger and his colleagues.[97] Intracellularly, there are probably two active forms of this analog: the riboside, 5-FUR, and the deoxynucleotide, 5-fluoro-2′-deoxyuridine (FUdR). Although the production of 5-FUR and its eventual incorporation through its triphosphate FUTP into RNA is not generally considered to lead to death of mammalian cells, recent evidence does implicate this as a mechanism of a cell death in leukemic cells. The mechanism of cytotoxicity is generally considered to be through the production of 5-FUdR, which is a substrate for the enzyme thymidylate synthetase. This enzyme normally converts deoxyuridine to thymidylate but binds FUdR, thereby becoming unavailable for thymidylate synthesis. In this way, one of the substrates required for the biosynthesis of DNA is not available, leading to an inhibition of DNA synthesis, resulting in unbalanced growth and cell death.

1-β-D-Arabinofuranosylcytosine (ara-C).[*] Ara-C was synthesized in 1959 as the analog of the nucleoside deoxycytidine. Ara-C must be phosphorylated in vivo to the active form ara-CTP. The drug probably has several sites of action such as indirect inhibition in the reduction of CDP, thereby inhibiting the formation of DNA. The drug may be incorporated directly into DNA, thereby preventing its replication. Finally, ara-C competes with dCTP for DNA polymerase, resulting in suppression of DNA synthesis; this is believed to be its major locus of action.[91] Incorporation of ara-C into RNA has been noted but is not believed to be the cause of subsequent cell death. Chromosome abnormalities have been reported, and the genesis of the chromatid breaks is believed to be intimately related to interruption of DNA synthesis; however, such an effect is not specific for ara-C but is observed for most of the anticancer agents.[102]

An important effect often observed with ara-C is inhibition in the progression of cells through the cell cycle. Although the mechanism responsible for this effect is unclear, its magnitude is extremely important in the optimal design of combination chemotherapy.

Antibiotics

The discovery of the anticancer antibiotics resulted from a comprehensive screening program for isolating antimicrobial substances from soil-inhabiting microorganisms, especially the actinomycetes. Because of their toxicity and rapid excretion from the blood, they afforded little protection against bacterial infections; however, concomitant studies on their antineoplastic activity were fruitful. Of the large number of antibiotics examined, a few have been found to be effective in cancer therapy.[123]

Actinomycin D.[117, 119-127, 130-132, 138, 142] Actinomycin D, one of a group of polypeptide antibiotics produced by several *Streptomyces* species, was first described in 1940. Investigations concerning its cytotoxic effects, however, did not begin until 1952.[141]

---

*References 76, 83-86, 92-94, 103, 109, 110.

This agent forms a tight reversible complex with DNA but not with RNA and shows an absolute base specificity for the guanine residues in DNA. Although it was initially thought that actinomycin D was bound to the DNA and projected along the minor groove of the DNA helix, increasing evidence indicates that the antibiotic intercalates between the base pairs of the DNA and binds to two deoxyguanosine residues.[136] Because of this binding, it interferes with the transcription function of DNA, thereby blocking DNA-directed synthesis of RNA. The inhibition of species of RNA seems to be dose dependent, with ribosomal RNA synthesis most sensitive. However, the synthesis of all species of RNA can be inhibited at concentrations of the antibiotic at which DNA replication is relatively unaffected.

Mitomycin C. The isolation of mitomycin C from *Streptomyces caespitosus* was reported in 1958.[140] It belongs to a group of antibiotics with a common structural pattern that includes porfiromycin. These agents are activated by enzymatic reduction to become effective bifunctional alkylating agents and likely exert their lethal effect through the formation of covalent cross-links in DNA.[137] This results in a steric hindrance leading to a prompt and selective inhibition of DNA synthesis.[133, 134]

Daunorubicin and adriamycin.[*] The anthracycline class of antibiotics includes daunorubicin and adriamycin as anticancer agents. In 1962, Italian investigators obtained daunomycin from *Streptomyces peucetius*. An identical antibiotic, rubidomycin, was isolated independently in France from *Streptomyces coerulorubidus*. The antibiotic has been studied in Russia as the "C fraction of rubomycin."[112] Adriamycin or 14-hydroxydaunomycin was isolated in 1967 from the same bacterial strain, *Streptomyces peucetus caesius*. Both agents probably exert their cytotoxic action through their intercalation with DNA, thereby inhibiting the polymerases. These agents have a near immediate effect on inhibition of mitosis, as well as fragmentation of chromosomes in exposed cells.

Mithramycin. Mithramycin is an antibiotic that was isolated from a *Streptomyces* species in 1960.[129] This drug forms a complex with DNA and Mg^{++}; the DNA-antibiotic complex is thought to be different from that formed by actinomycin D.[118, 126] This interferes with the separation of DNA and inhibits DNA-directed RNA synthesis at concentrations that have little effect on DNA replication.

Bleomycin. Bleomycin was isolated from a strain of *Streptomyces verticillus*[139] and has shown significant antineoplastic activity against some tumors. Although its mechanism of action is not presently known, it probably interferes with transcription. Its main lethal effect is on cells in late G_2 and mitosis; it has therefore been postulated as interfering with the synthesis of proteins known to be required for cell division.

Vinca alkaloids

Two active anticancer alkaloids, vinblastine and vincristine, were extracted from the periwinkle plant (*Vinca rosea Linnaeus*) in 1958.

Vincristine inhibits the synthesis and processing of nuclear RNA precursors

---

[*]References 112, 113-116, 119, 126, 127, 135, 137, 143.

of ribosomal RNA through an effect on the DNA-dependent RNA polymerase system.

Both compounds probably act in a manner similar to colchicine by binding the subunit protein of microtubules. The microtubules are presently believed to be important with regard to nerve conduction (the site of toxicity of these agents), spindle formation for cytokinesis, and chromosome replication. For these last two reasons, it is likely that the agents selectively kill cells in DNA synthesis or mitosis.[152] As such, these agents are powerful inhibitors of mitosis, specifically inhibiting the passage of cells through metaphase.

Steroids[155-162]

Adrenocortical steroids have well-known and profound physiologic effects in man. In cells of lymphoid origin and in leukemic and lymphomatous cells, the hormones inhibit mitosis, produce pyknosis of cells, and induce lymphocytorrhexis. Prednisone (1-dehydrocortisone), a synthetic analog of cortisone, has been widely used as an anticancer agent since 1955 for remission induction in acute leukemia.

The exact mechanism of action of corticosteroids remains unclear. Available data suggest that one mechanism is a direct cytolytic effect of the steroid, which could be a reflection of the property of steroids to bind to cell membranes and affect their permeability. Furthermore, from the treatment of breast cancer with androgens and estrogens, it appears that a growth-regulating effect is involved, in which case the cell is not killed but rather its rate of growth is modified.[161] Inhibition of thymidine kinase has been reported.[160]

Miscellaneous agents

Ortho, para'-DDD (o,p'-DDD). This drug, fractionated in 1958 from the commercial insecticide DDD,[174] acts specifically on the mitochondria of adrenal cortical cells,[181] producing focal degeneration of the fascicular and reticular zones.[186, 192] Hormone production of glucocorticoids and 17-ketosteroids is diminished, aldosterone secretory capacity remaining unchanged.[169, 179, 191, 192] The peripheral metabolism and conjugation of the hormones are altered.[164]

Hydroxyurea. Hydroxyurea is a hydroxylamine derivative first synthesized in 1869.[197] The inhibition of DNA synthesis by the drug has been attributed to the suppression of the enzymatic activity of ribonucleoside diphosphate reductase thereby blocking the reduction of ribonucleotides to deoxyribonucleotides.[183, 197] DNA synthesis is inhibited, but protein and RNA synthesis is less affected, and unbalanced growth with concomitant cell death ensues.[198] In some experimental systems, other sites of action appear to be implicated,[187] since low levels of DNA synthesis may proceed in the presence of hydroxyurea. The resulting DNA remains as small fragments that are not joined together, which might then account not only for cell death but also for the large number of chromosome aberrations seen in treated cells.[173] The drug is known to strongly inhibit the movement of cells from G_1 phase (drug-insensitive) into S phase (sensitive), an important point in the consideration of combination therapy.[190]

Nitrosoureas. A large number of N-substituted nitrosoureas have been synthesized, the most active ones to date of clinical significance being 1,3-bis (2-chloroethyl)-1-nitrosourea (BCNU),[189] 1-(2-chloroethyl)-3-cyclohexyl-1-nitrosourea (CCNU), and a methyl derivative of CCNU. The compounds are generally believed to act as alkylating agents with their conversion to appropriate carbonium ions and reaction with DNA[175, 189, 194, 196]; however, there is an indication that reaction of derived isocyanates with cellular proteins might be a significant component of the cytotoxicity.[170, 193]

The importance of these compounds derives from their proved effectiveness in mice inoculated intracerebrally with L1210 leukemic cells; that is, the agents cross the blood-brain barrier in cytotoxic quantities.

L-*Asparaginase.* In 1953 it was observed that normal guinea pig serum produced regression of 6C3HED lymphoma in mice.[182] The active antitumor component in the guinea pig serum was later identified as L-asparaginase.[166] L-Asparaginase was extracted from *Escherichia coli* in 1964, thus providing a source of the enzyme for clinical investigations.[172, 177]

L-Asparaginase is an enzyme that catalyzes the hydrolysis of L-asparagine (a nutritionally nonessential amino acid) to L-aspartic acid, thereby producing a depletion of L-asparagine in the body fluids.[161] This leads to the inhibition of certain neoplastic cells such as those in acute lymphoblastic leukemia that require L-asparagine, since they are not capable of synthesizing the amino acid in adequate amounts.[178] Protein synthesis is first suppressed, followed later by the inhibition of DNA and RNA synthesis.[168] Normal cells synthesize L-asparagine and therefore are unaffected by a deficiency of it.[168, 171, 172] Some inhibitory effect on RNA polymerase activity has been noted.[163]

Procarbazine. Procarbazine was synthesized in 1962 after observations that a related monoamine oxidase inhibitor possessed some antitumor activity.[180] Although some of the biologic reactions of procarbazine resemble those of alkylating agents,[165] the mechanism of action of methylhydrazines is still uncertain.[176] Chromatid breaks and suppression of mitosis have been reported.[188] Degradation products appear to be the active forms.[176] Synthesis of DNA, RNA, and protein are inhibited.[176] Interference with normal transmethylation of methyl groups of methionine to transfer RNA has been reported.[60, 184]

DRUGS AND DOSAGE REGIMENS

The current trend toward the use of increasingly more complex combination chemotherapy regimens makes difficult any simple tabular presentation of dose and toxicity data. A full knowledge of the various patterns and significance of acute and chronic toxicity of each drug used is required of the clinician who undertakes the chemotherapy of the child with cancer. Some pertinent data in this regard has been compiled in Table 6-2.

The first column lists the names of the chemotherapeutic agents employed at present. The second column shows the dosage forms available. The third column indicates the routes of administration of the drugs. The fourth and fifth columns give data on formulation, solution, and stability.

The sixth column shows some dosage regimens that have been followed in clinical studies by different investigators. Almost all these doses are based on trials of a single agent.

The seventh and eighth columns indicate the toxic manifestations that have been observed with each agent. Major toxicity includes those manifestations that usually require cessation of therapy or alteration in dose or schedule of admin-

Text continued on p. 110.

Table 6-2. Anticancer agents: dose, toxicity, and indications

Drug	Dosage forms	Route of administration	Storage	Solution and stab‖
Alkylating agents				
Mechlorethamine (nitrogen mustard, HN₂, Mustargen)	10 mg vial	Intravenously; intracavitary	Room temperature	Add 10 ml sterile water or norm saline; unstable solution; use as as possible; dis‖ unused portion‖
Chlorambucil (CB-1348, Leukeran)	2 mg tablets	Orally	Room temperature	
Cyclophosphamide (Cytoxan, Endoxan)	50 mg and 25 mg tablets; 100 mg, 200 mg, and 500 mg vials	Orally; intravenously; intramuscularly	Room temperature	Add 5 or 10 ml st‖ water; use with‖ hours; discard unused portion‖
Busulfan (Myleran)	2 mg tablets	Orally	Room temperature	
Antimetabolites				
Methotrexate (amethopterin)	2.5 mg tablets; 5 or 50 mg/2 ml vials (in solution)	Orally; intravenously; intramuscularly; intrathecally	Room temperature; solutions have expiration date; keep at room temperature	

Dosage regimens	Clinical toxicity, major	Clinical toxicity, minor	Target tumors
g/kg × 1 IV q̄ 3 wk as tolerated	Marrow depression	Nausea and vomiting; anorexia; intense local reaction on extravasation; acute contact vesicant; phlebitis; thrombosis; alopecia; rash Immunosuppression	Hodgkin's disease (++)* Lymphosarcoma (++) Reticulum cell sarcoma (++) Chronic leukemia (+) Testicular tumors (+) Neuroblastoma (+) Retinoblastoma (±) Wilms' tumor (±)
.2 mg/kg/day × 3-6 , PO (often given in urses)	Marrow depression; hepatotoxicity	Nausea and vomiting; diarrhea; dermatitis	Hodgkin's disease (++) Lymphosarcoma (++) Reticulum cell sarcoma (++) Testicular tumor (++) Chronic leukemia (++) Histiocytosis X (+) Ovarian cancer (+) Soft tissue sarcoma (±) Neuroblastoma (±)
.0 mg/kg/day, PO g/kg/day IV or PO til WBC drops below 00/mm³ or for 7-10 ys; repeated q̄ 3-6 k as courses	Marrow depression; hemorrhagic cystitis	Nausea and vomiting; stomatitis; diarrhea; epigastric pain; alopecia (common); skin rash; skin pigmentation; transverse ridging of nails Immunosuppression	Hodgkin's disease (++) Lymphosarcoma (++) Reticulum cell sarcoma (++) Burkitt's tumor (++) Acute leukemia (++) Neuroblastoma (++) Rhabdomyosarcoma (++) Ewing's tumor (+) Retinoblastoma (+) Wilms' tumor (±) Osteogenic sarcoma (±)
mg/day to WBC of ,000-20,000; then se titrated to main- in this WBC level	Marrow depression; "busulfan lungs" (interstitial pulmonary fibrosis); "wasting syndrome"	Alopecia; melanoderma; nausea and vomiting; glossitis; gynecomastia	Chronic myelogenous leukemia (++)
.0 mg/day orally;) mg/m² twice week- , IV, IM, or PO; 0-15 mg/m² q 5-7 ays intrathecally maximum dose of 5 mg)	Oral ulcers and stomatitis; intestinal ulcers; diarrhea; hemorrhagic enteritis; liver damage; osteoporosis (after prolonged usage); marrow depression (caution in patients with impaired renal function)	Nausea and vomiting; abdominal pain; skin rash; alopecia; hyperpigmentation; megaloblastosis Immunosuppression	Acute leukemia (++) Gestational trophoblastic tumors (++) CNS leukemia (++) Epithelial cancer (+) Lymphoma (+) Testicular tumors (+)

timation of degree of effectiveness: ++ = marked; + = definite; ± = variable.

Continued.

Table 6-2. Anticancer agents: dose, toxicity, and indications—cont'd

Drug	Dosage forms	Route of administration	Storage	Solution and sta
Mercaptopurine (6-mercaptopurine, Purinethol, 6-MP)	50 mg tablet; 500 mg vial (lyophilized powder) (investigational)	Orally; intravenously (investigational at present)	Room temperature	
Fluorouracil (5-fluorouracil, 5-FU)	500 mg ampule (in solution, 10 ml)	Orally; intravenously	Room temperature (protect from light)	
Cytarabine (cytosine arabinoside, arabinosyl cytosine, ara-C, Cytosar)	100 and 500 mg vial (lyophilized powder)	Intravenously; intramuscularly; subcutaneously; intracavitary; intrathecally	Refrigerate until reconstituted	Dissolve in 5-10 ▮ diluent (suppli◀ solution stable room temperat for 48 hours (d card if haze appears)
Antibiotics				
Dactinomycin (actinomycin D, Cosmegen)	500 mcg vial (lyophilized powder)	Intravenously	Room temperature	Add 1.1 ml steril◀ water for injec◀ discard unused portion
Mithramycin (Mithracin)	2500 mcg (lyophilized powder)	Intravenously	Refrigerated	Add 4.9 ml steril◀ water for injec◀ discard unused portion
Vinca alkaloids				
Vincristine (Oncovin)	1 and 5 mg vial (lyophilized powder)	Intravenously	Refrigerated	Add 10 ml of dilu◀ solution (suppli◀ solution stable 14 days if refrigerated
Vinblastine (vincaleukoblastine, Velban)	10 mg vial (lyophilized powder)	Intravenously	Refrigerated	Add 10 ml of nor▮ saline; solution stable for 30 da◀ if refrigerated

osage regimens	Clinical toxicity, major	Clinical toxicity, minor	Target tumors
g/kg/day, PO	Marrow depression; liver dysfunction	Abdominal pain; nausea and vomiting; diarrhea; fever; alopecia; dermatitis; stomatitis Immunosuppression	Acute leukemia (++)
g/kg/day IV for 4-5 s followed by 6 /kg qod to mild icity (monthly rses)	Glossitis; stomatitis; pharyngitis; intestinal ulceration; enteritis; marrow depression	Nausea and vomiting; alopecia; skin eruptions; megaloblastosis; cerebellar signs	Carcinomas (+) Neuroblastoma (±) Ewing's sarcoma (±) Hepatoma (±) Lymphoma (±) Osteogenic sarcoma (±)
us dose schedules 1 combinations with er drugs are under ensive study	Marrow depression; hepatitis (usually reversible and subclinical); oral ulceration	Nausea and vomiting; oral ulceration; megaloblastosis Immunosuppression	Acute leukemia (+) Lymphoma (+) CNS leukemia (+)
amma/kg/course ven in 5-7 days); rses repeated every mo	Bone marrow depression (especially thrombocytopenia); mucositis; stomatitis	"Flare reaction" of previously irradiated tissues; nausea and vomiting; abdominal pain; enteritis; <u>severe local tissue reaction on extravasation;</u> acne; alopecia Immunosuppression	Wilms' tumor (++) Gestational trophoblastic tumors (++) Testicular cancer (++) Soft tissue sarcoma (+) Ewing's sarcoma (±) Neuroblastoma (±)
cg/kg dose qod IV; to 8 doses/course	Hemorrhagic syndrome; hepatic damage; renal damage; marrow depression	Nausea and vomiting; hypocalcemia; GI tract toxicity; skin necrosis; fever	Embryonal carcinoma of testis (+) Hypercalcemia (+)
/m² weekly; ravenously	Severe abdominal pain; peripheral neuropathy; obstipation	<u>Cellulitis on extravasa</u>tion; muscle pain; numbness and tingling; alopecia; marrow depression (mild to moderate); jaw pain Immunosuppression	Acute leukemia (++) Wilms' tumor (++) Rhabdomyosarcoma (++) Hodgkin's disease (+) Other lymphomas (+) Neuroblastoma (+) Ewing's sarcoma (+) Retinoblastoma (+) Brain tumors (+) Histiocytosis X (+)
.15 mg/kg IV weekly every 2 wk	Marrow depression	Nausea and vomiting; stomatitis; alopecia; peripheral neuropathy; <u>cellulitis on extravasa</u>tion	Hodgkin's disease (++) Choriocarcinoma (++) Lymphosarcoma (+) Reticulum cell sarcoma (+) Histiocytosis X (+)

Continued.

Table 6-2. Anticancer agents: dose, toxicity, and indications—cont'd

Drug	Dosage forms	Route of administration	Storage	Solution and sta
Glucocorticoids				
Prednisone (Meticorten, Deltasone, Paracort, many other proprietary names)	2.5 mg, 5 mg, or 20 mg tablets	Orally	Room temperature	
Hydrocortisone sodium succinate (Solu-Cortef)	100 mg plain; 100 mg, 250 mg, 500 mg, or 1000 mg "Mix-O-Vials"	Intravenously; intramuscularly; intrathecally	Room temperature	Two compartmer "Mix-O-Vials"; discard unused portion after 3 Add 2 ml sterile for injection to mg "plain" via
Miscellaneous agents				
Mitotane (O, p¹-DDD, Lysodren)	500 mg tablets	Orally	Room temperature	
Hydroxyurea (Hydrea)	500 mg capsules	Orally	Room temperature	
Procarbazine (methylhydrazine, Matulane)	50 mg capsules	Orally	Room temperature	
Investigational agents				
Daunorubicin (daunomycin, rubidomycin)	20 mg vial (red crystals)	Intravenously	Room temperature	Add 10 ml sterile water; use imm diately (*Note:* animal studies indicate stabilit for 3 wk in refrigerated solut
Adriamycin	10 mg vial (red crystals)	Intravenously	Room temperature	Add 10 ml norma saline; use immediately

Dosage regimens	Clinical toxicity, major	Clinical toxicity, minor	Target tumors
g/M²/day for 28-35 /s	Diabetes mellitus; psychoses; GI tract ulceration; osteoporosis	Cushing syndrome; water retention; muscle wasting; hypertension; hyperphagia; electrolyte disturbances Immunosuppression	Acute leukemia (++) Lymphomas (+) Histiocytosis X (+)
	See under prednisone	See under prednisone	See under prednisone
Gm daily PO trated individually patient)	Hypoadrenalism; severe nausea and vomiting	Vertigo; mental depression; diarrhea; somnolence; skin eruption; muscle tremors	Metastatic functional carcinoma of adrenal gland (++)
mg/kg/day PO; -80 mg/kg PO q̄ days	Marrow depression	Nausea and vomiting; stomatitis; diarrhea; rash; mucosal ulceration; alopecia	Melanoma (+) Hypernephroma (±) Sarcomas (±) Carcinomas (±) Adenocarcinomas (±)
0 mg/M²/ day × 7), then 125-150 mg/ ²/day PO, as erated	Bone marrow depression; severe nausea and vomiting; lethargy; CNS depression; drug dermatitis	Stomatitis (uncommon); myalgia; arthralgia; alopecia (uncommon); neuropathy (uncommon); diarrhea (uncommon)	Hodgkin's disease (+) Lymphomas (+) Melanoma (±) Neuroblastoma (±) Embryonal cell carcinoma (±)
er study	Bone marrow depression; cardiac toxicity (especially at total cumulative doses—around 500 mg/m² or higher)	Skin rash; nausea and vomiting; alopecia; "red" urine; local phlebitis; fever	Acute leukemia (++) Neuroblastoma (+) Lymphomas (±) Rhabdomyosarcomas (±)
er study	Bone marrow depression; cardiac toxicity	Nausea and vomiting; stomatitis (severe); alopecia; "red" urine; local phlebitis; skin rash	Acute leukemia (++) Neuroblastoma (+) Osteogenic sarcoma (+) Wilms' tumor (±) Rhabdomyosarcoma (±)

Continued.

Table 6-2. Anticancer agents: dose, toxicity, and indications—cont'd

Drug	Dosage forms	Route of administration	Storage	Solution and sta
BCNU (1,3-bis (2-chloroethyl)-1-nitrosourea)	100 mg vial (lyophilized powder)	Intravenously	Refrigerated	Add 3 ml absolut ethanol (suppli then add 7 ml sterile water; u immediately; c card unused pe
L-Asparaginase	10,000 or 50,000 IU vial (lyophilized powder)	Intravenously; intramuscularly	Refrigerated	Add 5 ml sterile water without preservative; u immediately

istration. The minor toxic manifestations are those that generally require no modification of drug administration. Potentially serious problems must be anticipated when combination chemotherapy regimens involve the use of drugs having overlapping types or times of major toxicity.

The final column lists as "target tumors" those neoplasms in which a given drug has produced variable degrees of antitumor effect, objectively measured as improved survival or tumor regression. Some measure of the response is indicated in brackets beside each tumor listed.

COMBINATION CHEMOTHERAPY

Henderson and Samaha[204] recently reviewed the evidence that drugs in multiple combinations have materially advanced the treatment of malignant diseases in human beings. The successful achievement of remission in almost every child with acute lymphocytic or unclassified leukemia is based on the use of combination chemotherapy[205] (Chapter 10). Improved survival among children with acute leukemia has been similarly accredited to the increased application of multidrug programs. Improved results after combination chemotherapy have also been observed in patients with Hodgkin's disease, malignant lymphoma (in adults), Wilms' tumor, and testicular tumors. To this list might be added Ewing's sarcoma, rhabdomyosarcoma, and some gynecologic tumors (see specific chapters). From such data, one might conclude that tumors in general respond in various degrees to each of several drugs, that tumors do not respond consistently to any drug or combination of drugs, and that the response to each drug differs according to the clinical stage of the tumor.

The biologic basis for combination chemotherapy can be divided into at least five categories. The first is termed *sequential blockade*. This is illustrated in purine biosynthesis, in which a number of enzymatic steps are sensitive to inhibition by a variety of agents. This pathway may be affected in at least two different sites by azaserine and by methotrexate. The administration of the two agents together would be expected to put two separate blocks sequentially in this metabolic pathway. A second combination is termed *concurrent blockage*, in which two different pathways, both leading to a common end product, are

osage regimens	Clinical toxicity, major	Clinical toxicity, minor	Target tumors
r study	Leukopenia (delayed 4-6 wk); thrombocytopenia (delayed 4-6 wk)	Nausea and vomiting; local venous pain; flushing of face; jaundice	Hodgkin's disease (+) Brain tumor (+) CNS leukemia (+) Ewing's tumor (±) Lymphoma (±)
r study	Hypersensitivity reaction; pancreatitis; hypergly-cemia; convulsions	Inhibition of protein synthesis; fever; ano-rexia; nausea and vomiting; weight loss; abnormal liver function tests; abnormal EEG	Acute leukemia (++) Lymphoma (±)

inhibited. For example, a drug such as azaserine, which blocks purine formation, could be combined with some purine analog that is incorporated into poly-nucleotides, thereby making nonfunctional DNA or RNA. A third type of inhi-bition is *complementary inhibition,* in which a second agent acts to prevent the repair of the damage done by the first agent. An example of this is found clinical-ly in the case of Wilms' tumor, for which treatment radiation and actinomycin D is given; in this circumstance, the actinomycin D is thought to interfere with the cellular repair processes after radiation damage to tumor cells. A fourth type of combination may produce *metabolic sensitization.* In this case, one agent acts to increase the sensitivity of the cell to the damaging effects of a second agent. For example, the administration of an agent such as BUdR, which is incorporated into cells at nonlethal concentrations, will enhance the sensitivity of these cells and when a subsequent dose of radiation is administered, there will be an in-creased cell kill. Finally, a combination called *relapse prevention* exists, in which both agents have lethal effects on the cell population. The combination of the two agents circumvents the emergence of resistant populations. Although many of these biochemical concepts have been used to explain the synergistic effects of drug combinations, it is difficult, if not impossible, at the present time to predict which drugs will be synergistic, additive, or even inhibitory when used in combi-nation.

Empirically, the strategy of combination chemotherapy has been to increase the overall antitumor effect without increasing correspondingly the toxic effect. This has been approached by selection for combination of those drugs that, when used alone, show definite antineoplastic activity, have different biochemical mechanisms of action, and produce different types of major toxicities. The in-creasing knowledge concerning cell population kinetics and the development of quantitative cellular methods (Chapter 5) are expected to provide a more rational basis for application of data from animal model systems and other laboratory studies to clinical regimens. As one example, it would not seem appropriate to administer simultaneously maximal doses of two phase-specific agents that destroy cells in the same phase of the cell cycle. The administration of the two drugs might better be separated by a sufficient interval, so that all cells in the sensitive phase would be exposed to the first drug and the cells in the insensitive phase would have time to move into the sensitive phase to be affected by the second agent.

MULTIMODAL THERAPY

Multimodal therapy implies the concurrent or sequential use of more than one major method of treatment. At present, four forms of treatment are clinically utilized: surgery, radiotherapy, chemotherapy, and, to a limited extent, immunotherapy. This approach to cancer therapy requires that each modality utilized be at least partially effective in the given clinical situation. The objective of any multimodal program should be the strategic combination of measures to obtain the maximum therapeutic effect. The obvious reason for combined therapy derives from the fact that a single method fails to rid the host of all malignant cells. This might be due to one or more of the following reasons: tumor, dose, metastasis, or resistance.

Tumor. The location or size of the tumor makes it inoperable or unamenable to complete eradication by a single mode of therapy. In this case, one might reduce the tumor to an operable size by the administration of preoperative radiation. In some situations, as in children with Wilms' tumor, preoperative chemotherapy can be administered to achieve a similar result.

Dose. The dose of radiation or chemotherapy that can be given without severe toxicity or the extent of surgery possible is insufficient to eradicate the entire malignant cell population. After surgical removal of a tumor, radiation or chemotherapy may subsequently be administered to destroy any malignant cells remaining at the site of the primary tumor. The rationale for the use of combination chemotherapy was discussed on pp. 110 and 111.

Metastasis. After surgery or irradiation, which are "target-limited" forms of therapy, malignant cells may remain outside the field of treatment or as distant metastases. Postoperative radiation therapy is directed to such cells not removed by the surgical procedure. Similarly, chemotherapy has been administered after either or both of the physical modalities to eradicate malignant cells disseminated outside the limited field of treatment.

Resistance. Although it may have been possible to administer theoretically sufficient doses of radiation or drugs, a population of cells might remain that is resistant to further administration of the given agent. The resistance might be physiologic, as in the case of hypoxic cells with regard to radiation, or genetic, which is the usual situation with chemotherapy. The use of combinations of chemotherapeutic agents is intended to decrease the likelihood of the emergence of a resistant cell population. Cells that are unresponsive to one of the drugs may be destroyed by the second agent.

VARIATIONS OF DOSAGES AND SCHEDULES

Mathé,[207] working with L1210 murine leukemia, summarized his findings by stating that "the same total dose does not give the same results according to whether the drug is given continuously, divided into small daily doses, or intermittently in a massive dose. Goldin's and co-workers' observation[29] that methotrexate given every 4 days was more effective than daily doses in the treatment of early L1210 leukemia has been utilized clinically in an extensive study of remission maintenance in children with acute leukemia.[199] Intermittent infusions of large doses of methotrexate have been administered in the treatment of children with acute leukemia.[201]

In early studies with cyclophosphamide, Lane[206] reported that intermittent doses (e.g., once weekly) produced significantly greater increases in survival than daily (or three times weekly) doses given to mice with L1210 leukemia. Cyclophosphamide is now being administered clinically in intermittent "pulses" (Chapter 21) as a treatment for solid tumors[52, 203] and acute leukemia.[202] The use of extremely high doses of methotrexate in conjunction with "Leucovorin rescue" has been mentioned earlier.[21, 29, 30, 43]

Conceptually, the data now being derived from studies of cell population kinetics and cell cycle sensitivity can be expected to provide rational guidelines for the definition and application of optimum doses and schedules in clinical cancer chemotherapy.[200, 208, 209, 211]

REFERENCES
General references

1. Brodsky, I., Kahn, S. B., and Moyer, J. H., III, editors: Cancer chemotherapy: Basic and clinical applications, New York 1967, Grune & Stratton.
2. Calabresi, P., and Welch, A. D.: Chemotherapy of neoplastic diseases, Annu. Rev. Med. 13:147-202, 1962.
3. Cole, W. H., editor: Chemotherapy of cancer, Philadelphia, 1970, Lea & Febiger.
4. Goldin, A., Kaziwara, K., Kinosita, R., and Yamamura, Y., editors: Cancer chemotherapy (Japanese Cancer Association, Gann Monograph 2), Tokyo, 1967, Maruzen Co., Ltd.
5. Greenwald, E. S.: Cancer chemotherapy, Flushing, N. Y., 1967, Medical Examination Publishing Co., Inc.
6. Hall, T. C.: Principles of chemotherapy. In Rubin, P., and Bakemeier, R. F., editors: Clinical oncology for medical students and physicians: A multidisciplinary approach, ed. 3, Rochester, N. Y., 1970-1971, American Cancer Society, pp. 60-75.
7. Karnofsky, D. A., and Clarkson, B. D.: Cellular effects of anticancer drugs, Annu. Rev. Pharmacol. 3:357-428, 1963.
8. Livingston, R. B., and Carter, S. K.: Single agents in cancer chemotherapy, New York, 1970, Plenum Publishing Corp.
9. Mathé, G., editor: Scientific basis of cancer chemotherapy, New York, 1969, Springer-Verlag, New York Inc.
10. Montgomery, J. A.: On the chemotherapy of cancer, Progr. Drug Res. 8:431-507, 1965.
11. Olivero, V. T., and Zubrod, C. G.: Clinical pharmacology of effective antitumor drugs, Annu. Rev. Pharmacol. 5:335-356, 1965.
12. Schnitzer, R. J., and Hawking, F., editors: Experimental chemotherapy, vol. 4, Chemotherapy of neoplastic diseases, part I and vol. 5, Chemotherapy of neoplastic diseases, part II, New York, 1966-1967, Academic Press, Inc.
13. Sullivan, R. D., editor: Clinical cancer chemotherapy, including ambulatory infusion, Springfield, Ill., 1970, Charles C Thomas, Publisher.
14. Symposium: A critical evaluation of cancer chemotherapy, Cancer Res. **29:**2255-2485, 1969.

General considerations

15. Arlen, M., Higinbotham, N. L., Huvos, A. G., Marcove, R. C., Miller, T., and Shah, I. C.: Radiation-induced sarcoma of bone, Cancer **28:**1087-1099, 1971.
16. Burchenal, J. H.: Analysis of long-term survival in acute leukemia and Burkitt's tumor —effects to be expected from intensive therapy and asparaginase. In Sixth National Cancer Conference Proceedings, Philadelphia, 1970, J. B. Lippincott Co., pp. 127-132.
17. Collins, V. P., Loeffler, R. K., and Tivey, H.: Observations on growth rates of human tumors, Am. J. Roentgenol. Radium Ther. Nucl. Med. **76:**988-1000, 1956.

18. Conard, R. A., Dobyns, B. M., and Sutow, W. W.: Thyroid neoplasia as a late effect of acute exposure to radioiodines in fallout, J.A.M.A. **214**:316-324, 1970.
19. Connors, T. A.: Anti-cancer agents. Their detection by screening tests and their mechanism of action, Recent Results Cancer Res. **21**:1-17, 1969.
20. Crawford, J. D., Terry, M. E., and Rourke, G. M.: Simplification of drug dosage calculation by application of the surface area principle, Pediatrics **5**:783-790, 1950.
21. Djerassi, I., Rominger, C. J., Kim, J., Turchi, J., and Meyer, E.: Methotrexate-citrovorum in patients with lung cancer, Proc. Am. Assoc. Cancer Res. **11**:21, March, 1970.
22. Farber, S.: Chemotherapy in the Treatment of leukemia and Wilms' tumor, J.A.M.A. **198**:826-836, 1966.
23. Folkman, J.: Tumor angiogenesis: therapeutic implications, N. Engl. J. Med. **285**:1182-1186, 1971.
24. Frei, E., III, Bickers, J. N., Hewlett, J. S., Lane, M., Leary, W. V., and Talley, R. W.: Dose schedule and antitumor studies of arabinosyl cytosine (NSC 63878), Cancer Res. **29**:1325-1332, 1969.
25. Frei, E., III, and Gehan, E. A.: Definition of cure for Hodgkin's disease, Cancer Res. **31**:1828-1833, 1971.
26. Freireich, E. J., Gehan, E. A., Rall, D. P., Schmidt, L. H., and Skipper, H. E.: Quantitative comparison of toxicity of anticancer agents in mouse, rat, hamster, dog, monkey, and man, Cancer Chemother. Rep. **50**:219-244, May, 1964.
27. Gehan, E. A., and George, S. L.: Estimation of human body surface area from height and weight, Cancer Chemother. Rep. **54**:225-235, Aug., 1970.
28. Goldenberg, G. J., Vanstone, C. L., Israels, L. G., Ilse, D., and Bihler, I.: Evidence for a transport carrier of nitrogen mustard in nitrogen mustard-sensitive and resistant L5178Y lymphoblasts, cancer Res. **30**:2285-2291, 1970.
29. Goldin, A., Venditti, J. M., Humphreys, S. R., and Mantel, N.: Modification of treatment schedules in the management of advanced mouse leukemia with amethopterin, J. Natl. Cancer Inst. **17**:203-212, 1956.
30. Goldin, A., Venditti, J. M., Kline, I., and Mantel, N.: Eradication of leukaemic cells (L 1210) by methotrexate and methotrexate plus citrovorum factor, Nature (Lond) **212**:1548-1550, 1966.
31. Hirono, I.: Non-protein sulphydryl groups in the original strain and sub-line of the ascites tumour resistant to alkylating reageants, Nature (Lond) **186**:1059-1060, 1960.
32. Hutchison, D. J.: Studies on cross-resistance and collateral sensitivity (1962-1964), Cancer Res. **25**:1581-1595, 1965.
33. Karnofsky, D. A.: Problems and pitfalls in the evaluation of anticancer drugs, Cancer **18**:1517-1528, 1965.
34. Kessel, D., and Bosmann, H. B.: On the characteristics of actinomycin D resistance in L5178 Y cells, Cancer Res. **30**:2695-2701, 1970.
35. Lewis, J., Jr.: Chemotherapy for metastatic gestational trophoblastic neoplasms, Clin. Obstet. Gynecol. **10**:330-341, June, 1967.
36. Miller, R. W.: Epidemiology of childhood neoplasia. In Neoplasia in childhood. Chicago, 1969, Year Book Medical Publishers, Inc., pp. 13-24.
37. Perry, S., editor: Human tumor cell kinetics introduction, Natl. Cancer Inst. Monogr. **30**:vi-ix, 1969.
38. Pinkel, D.: The use of body surface area as a criterion of drug usage in cancer chemotherapy, Cancer Res. **18**:853-856, 1958.
39. Platt, B. B., and Linden, G.: Wilms' tumor—A comparison of criteria for survival, Cancer **17**:1573-1578, 1964.
40. Pratt, C. B., Hustu, H. O., Fleming, I. D., and Pinkel, D.: Coordinated treatment of childhood rhabdomyosarcoma with surgery, radiotherapy, and combination chemotherapy, Cancer Res. **32**:606-610, 1972.
41. Rall, D. V.: New approaches in administration of anticancer drugs, Cancer Res. **29**:2471-2474, 1969.
42. Schabel, F. M., Jr.: The use of tumor growth kinetics in planning "curative" chemotherapy of advanced solid tumors, Cancer Res. **29**:2384-2389, 1969.
43. Selawry, O. S.: Tolerance to sequential use of methotrexate and leucovorin in cancer patients, Proc. Am. Assoc. Cancer Res. **11**:72, March, 1970.

44. Sendroy, J., Jr., and Cecchini, L. P.: Determination of human body surface area from height and weight, J. Appl. Physiol. **7**:1-12, 1954.
45. Sendroy, J., Jr., and Collison, H. A.: Nomogram for determination of human body surface area from height and weight, J. App. Physiol. **15**:958-959, 1960.
46. Shirkey, H. C.: Drug dosage for infants and children, J.A.M.A. **193**:443-446, 1965.
47. Siegelman, M. H., and Sutow, W. W.: Xeroderma pigmentosum—report of three cases, J. Pediatr. **67**:658-673, 1965.
48. Skipper, H. E., Schabel, F. M., Jr., Mellett, L. B., Montgomery, J. A., Wilkoff, L. J., Lloyd, H. H, and Brockman, W.: Implications of biochemical, cytokinetic, pharmacologic, and toxicologic relationships in the desgin of optimum therapeutic schedules, Cancer Chemother. Rep. **54**:431-450, Dec., 1970.
49. Skipper, H. E., Schabel, F. M., Jr., and Wilcox, W. S.: Experimental evaluation of potential anticancer agents. XIII. On the criteria and kinetics associated with "curability" of experimental leukemia, Cancer Chemother. Rep. **35**:1-111, Feb., 1964.
50. Sutow, W. W.: Chemotherapy in childhood cancer (except leukemia)—an appraisal, Cancer **18**:1585-1589, 1965.
51. Wheeler, G. P.: Studies related to mechanisms of resistance to biological alkylating agents, Cancer Res. **23**:1334-1349, 1963.
52. Wilbur, J. R., Sutow, W. W., Sullivan, M. P., Castro, J. R., and Taylor, H. G.: Successful treatment of rhabdomyosarcoma with combination chemotherapy and radiotherapy (Abstract No. 56), American Society of Clinical Oncology Proceedings, 1971.
53. Wilcox, W. S., Griswold, D. P., Laster, W. R., Jr., Schabel, F. M., Jr., and Skipper, H. E.: Experimental evaluation of potential anticancer agents. XVII. Kinetics of growth and regression after treatment of certain solid tumors, Cancer Chemother. Rep. **47**:27-39, Aug., 1965.

Alkylating agents

54. Alexander, P.: Comparison of the mode of action by which some alkylating agents and ionizing radiations kill mammalian cells, Ann. N.Y. Acad. Sci. **163**:652-674, 1969.
55. Biological effects of alkylating agents, Ann. N.Y. Acad. Sci. **163**:589-1029, 1969.
56. Brewer, H. B., and Aronow, L.: Effects of nitrogen mustard on the physicochemical properties of mouse fibroblast deoxyribonucleic acid, Cancer Res. **23**:285-290, 1963.
57. Brock, N.: Pharmacologic characterization of cyclophosphamide (NSC—26271) and cyclophosphamide metabolites, Cancer Chemother. Rep. **51**:315-325, Oct., 1967.
58. Brown, S. S.: Nitrogen mustards and related alkylating agents, Adv. Pharmacol. **2**:243-295, 1963.
59. Comparative clinical and biological effects of alkylating agents, Ann. N.Y. Acad. Sci. **68**:657-1266, 1958.
60. Dowling, M. D., Jr., Krakoff, I. H., and Karnofsky, D. A.: Mechanism of action of anti-cancer drugs. In Cole, W. H., editor: Chemotherapy of cancer, Philadelphia, 1970, Lea & Febiger.
61. Foley, G. E., Friedman, O. M., and Drolet, B. P.: Studies on the mechanism of action of cytoxan. Evidence of activation *in vivo* and *in vitro*, Cancer Res. **21**:57-63, 1961.
62. Gilman, A., and Philips, F. S.: The biological actions and therapeutic applications of the B-chloroethyl amines and sulfides, Science **103**:409-415, 1946.
63. Golder, R. H., Martin-Guzman, G., Jones, J., Goldstein, N. O., Rotenberg, S., and Rutman, R. J.: Experimental chemotherapy studies. III. Properties of DNA from ascites cells treated *in vivo* with nitrogen mustard, Cancer Res. **24**:964-968, 1964.
64. Goldstein, N. O., and Rutman, R. J.: Experimental chemotherapy studies. VII. The effect of alkylation on the *in vitro* thymidine-incorporating system of Lettré-Ehrlich cells, Cancer Res. **24**:1363-1367, 1964.
65. Lawley, P. D.: Effects of some chemical mutagens and carcinogens on nucleic acids, Progr. Nucleic Acid Res. Mol. Biol. **5**:89-131, 1966.
66. Lawley, P. D., and Brookes, P.: Molecular mechanism of the cytotoxic action of difunctional alkylating agents and of resistance to this action, Nature (Lond) **206**:480-483, 1965.
67. Lawley, P. D., and Brookes, P.: Interstrand cross-linking of DNA by difunctional alkylating agents, J. Mol. Biol. **25**:143-160, April 14, 1967.

68. Lawley, P. D., Lethbridge, J. H., Edwards, P. A., and Shooter, K. V.: Inactivation of bacteriophage T7 by mono- and difunctional sulphur mustards in relation to cross-linking and depurination of bacteriophage DNA, J. Mol. Biol. **39:**181-198, Jan. 14, 1969.

69. Milner, A. N., Klatt, O., Young, S. E., and Stehlin, J. S., Jr.: The biochemical mechanism of action of L-phenylalanine mustard. I. Distribution of L-phenylalanine mustard-H[3] in tumor bearing rats, Cancer Res. **25:**259-264, 1965.

70. Ochoa, M., Jr., and Hirschberg, E.: Alkylating agents. In Schnitzer, R. J., and Hawking, F., editors: Experimental chemotherapy vol. 5, New York, 1967, Academic Press, Inc. pp. 1-132.

71. Ross, W. C. J.: Biological alkylating agents, London, 1962, Butterworth and Co., Ltd.

72. Ruddon, R. W., and Johnson, J. M.: The effects of nitrogen mustard on DNA template activity in purified DNA and RNA polymerase systems, Mol. Pharmacol. **4:**258-273, May, 1968.

73. Schmidt, L. H., Fradkin, R., Sullivan, R., and Flowers, R.: Comparative pharmacology of alkylating agents, Cancer Chemother. Rep. supp **2:**1-1528, 1965.

74. Warwick, G. P.: The mechanism of action of alkylating agents, Cancer Res. **23:**1315-1333, 1963.

75. Wheeler, G. P.: Studies related to the mechanisms of action of cytotoxic alkylating agents: A review, Cancer Res. **22:**651-688, 1962.

Antimetabolites

76. Benedict, W. F., Harris, N., and Karon, M.: Kinetics of 1-β-D-Arabinofuranosylcytosine-induced chromosome breaks, Cancer Res. **30:**2477-2483, 1970.

77. Bennett, L. L., Jr., and Allan, P. W.: Formation and significance of 6-methylthiopurine ribonucleotide as a metabolite of mercaptopurine, Cancer Res. **31:**152-158, 1971.

78. Bertino, J.: The mechanism of action of the folate antagonists in man, Cancer Res. **23:**1286-1306, 1963.

79. Bertino, J. R., and Johns, D. G.: Folate antagonists, Annu. Rev. Med. **18:**27-34, 1967.

80. Brockman, R. W.: Biochemical aspects of mercaptopurine inhibition and resistance, Cancer Res. **23:**1191-1201, 1963.

81. Chaudhuri, N. K., Montag, B. J., and Heidelberger, C.: Studies on fluorinated pyrimidines. III. The metabolism of 5-fluorouracil-2-C[14] and 5-fluoroorotic-2-C[14] acid *in vivo*, Cancer Res. **18:**318-328, 1958.

82. Chaudhuri, N. K., Mukherjee, K. L., and Heidelberger, C.: Studies on fluorinated pyrimidines. VII. The degradative pathway, Biochem. Pharmacol. **1:**328-341, 1958.

83. Chu, M. Y., and Fischer, G. A.: A proposed mechanism of action of 1-β-D-arabino-furanosyl-cytosine as an inhibitor of the growth of leukemic cells, Biochem. Pharmacol. **11:**423-430, 1962.

84. Chu, M. Y., and Fischer, G. A.: Comparative studies of leukemic cells sensitive and resistant to cytosine arabinoside, Biochem. Pharmacol. **14:**333-341, 1965.

85. Chu, M. Y., and Fischer, G. A.: The incorporation of ^{3}H-cytosine arabinoside and its effect on murine leukemic cells, Biochem. Pharmacol. **17:**753-767, 1968.

86. Cohen, S. S.: Introduction to the biochemistry of D-arabinosyl nucleosides, Progr. Nucleic Acid Res. Mol. Biol. **5:**1-88, 1966.

87. Cohen, S. S., Flaks, J. G., Barner, H. D., Loeb, M. R., and Lichtenstein, J.: The mode of action of 5-fluorouracil and its derivatives. Proc. Natl. Acad. Sci. **44:**1004-1012, 1958.

88. Elion, G. B.: Biochemistry and pharmacology of purine analogues, Fed. Proc. **26:**898-904, 1967.

89. Elion, G. B., and Hitchings, G. H.: Metabolic basis for the actions of analogs of purines and pyrimidines, Adv. Chemother. **2:**91-177, 1965.

90. Farber, S., Diamond, L. K., Mercer, R. D., Sylvester, R. F., Jr., and Wolff, J. A.: Temporary remissions in acute leukemia in children produced by folic acid antagonist, 4-amino-pteroyl-glutamic acid (aminopterin), N. Engl. J. Med. **238:**787-793, 1948.

91. Furlong, N. B., and Gresham, C.: Inhibition of DNA synthesis but not of Poly-dAT synthesis by the arabinoside analogue of cytidine *in vitro*, Nature New Biol. **233:**212-214, Oct. 13, 1971.

92. Furth, J. J., and Cohen, S. S.: Inhibition of mammalian DNA polymerase by the 5'-triphosphate of 1-β-D-arabinofuranosylcytosine and the 5'-phosphate of 9-β-D-arabino-furanosyladenine, Cancer Res. **28**:2061-2067, 1968.
93. Graham, F. L., and Whitmore, G. F.: The effect of 1-β-D-arabino furanosylcytosine on growth, viability, and DNA synthesis of mouse L-cells, Cancer Res. **30**:2627-2635, 1970.
94. Graham, F. L., and Whitmore, G. F.: Studies in mouse L-cells on the incorporation of 1-β-D arabinosylcytosine into DNA and on inhibition of DNA polymerase by 1-β-D arabino-furanosylcytosine 5'-triphosphate, Cancer Res. **30**:2636-2644, 1970.
95. Heidelberger, C.: Fluorinated pyrimidines. Progr. Nucleic Acid Res. Mol. Biol. **4**:2-50, 1965.
96. Heidelberger, C.: Cancer chemotherapy with purine and pyrimidine analogues, Annu. Rev. Pharmacol. **7**:101-124, 1967.
97. Heidelberger, C., Chaudhuri, N., and Danneburg, P.: Fluorinated pyrimidines, a new class of tumour-inhibitory compounds, Nature (Lond) **179**:663-666, 1957.
98. Hitchings, G. H.: Chemotherapy and comparative biochemistry. G.H.A. Clowes Memorial Lecture, Cancer Res. **29**:1895-1903, 1969.
99. Hitchings, G. H., and Elion, G. B.: The chemistry and biochemistry of purine analogs, Ann. N.Y. Acad. Sci. **60**:195-199, 1954.
100. Hitchings, G. H., and Elion, G. B.: Mechanisms of action of purine and pyrimidine analogs. In Brodsky, I., Kahn, S. B., and Moyer, J. H., III, editors: Cancer chemotherapy: basic and clinical applications, New York, 1967, Grune & Stratton, pp. 26-36.
101. Holland, J. F.: Folic acid antagonists. Clin. Pharmacol. Ther. **2**:374-409, May-June, 1961.
102. Kihlman, B. A.: Actions of chemicals on dividing cells, Englewood Cliffs, N. J., 1966, Prentice-Hall, Inc.
103. Kihlman, B. A., Nichols, W. W., and Levan, A.: The effect of deoxyadenosine and cytosine arabinoside on the chromosomes of human leukocytes *in vitro*, Hereditas Genetiskt Ark. **50**:139-143, 1963.
104. LePage, G. A., and Jones, M.: Purinethol as feedback inhibitors of purine synthesis in ascites tumor cells, Cancer Res. **21**:642-649, 1961.
105. 6-Mercaptopurine, Ann. N.Y. Acad. Sci. **60**:185-507, 1954.
106. Nichol, C. A., and Welch, A. D.: On the mechanism of action of aminopterin, Proc. Soc. Exp. Biol. Med. **74**:403-411, June, 1950.
107. Roy-Burman, P.: Analogues of nucleic acid components, Recent Results Cancer Res. **25**:1-111, 1970.
108. Scannell, J. P., and Hitchings, G. H.: Thioguanine in deoxyribonucleic acid from tumors of 6-mercaptopurine treated mice, Proc. Soc. Exp. Biol. Med. **122**:627-629, 1966.
109. Silagi, S.: Metabolism of 1-β-D arabino-furanosylcytosine in L cells, Cancer Res. **25**:1446-1453, 1965.
110. Walwick, E. R., Roberts, W. K., and Dekker, C. A.: Cyclisation during the phosphorylation of uridine and cytidine by polyphosphoric acid: a new route to the 0^2, 2'-cyclonucleosides, Proc. Chem. Soc. 84, March, 1959.
111. Werkheiser, W. C.: The biochemical, cellular and pharmacological action and effects of the folic acid antagonists, Cancer Res. **23**:1277-1285, 1963.

Antibiotics

112. Bernard, J., Paul, R., Boiron, M., Jacquillat, C., and Maral, R.: Rubidomycin, New York, 1969, Springer-Verlag New York, Inc.
113. Bonadonna, G., Monfardini, S., De Lena, M., Fossati-Bellani, F., and Beretta, G.: Phase I and preliminary phase II evaluation of adriamycin (NSC-123127), Cancer Res. **30**:2572-2582, 1970.
114. Calendi, E., DiMarco, A., Reggiani, M., Scarpinato, B., and Valentini, L.: On physico-chemical interactions between daunomycin and nucleic acids, Biochim. Biophys. Acta **103**:25-49, 1965.
115. DiMarco, A.: Daunomycin-pharmacological activity at the cellular level, Pathol. Biol. **15**:897-902, 1967.

116. DiMarco, A., Gaetani, M., Dorigotti, L., Soldati, M., and Bellini, O.: Daunomycin: A new antibiotic with antitumor activity, Cancer Chemother. Rep. **38**:31-38, May, 1964.

117. Franklin, R. M.: The inhibition of ribonucleic acid synthesis in mammalian cells by actinomycin D, Biochim. Biophys. Acta **72**:555-565, 1963.

118. Gause, G. F.: Olivomycin, mithramycin, chromomycin: three related cancerostatic antibiotics, Adv. Chemother. **2**:179-195, 1965.

119. Goldberg, I. H.: Mode of action of antibiotics. II. Drugs affecting nucleic acid and protein synthesis, Am. J. Med. **39**:722-752, 1965.

120. Goldberg, I. H., and Rabinowitz, M.: Actinomycin D inhibition of deoxyribonucleic acid-dependent synthesis of ribonucleic acid, Science **136**:315-316, 1962.

121. Goldberg, I. H., Rabinowitz, M., and Reich, H.:Basis of actinomycin action. I. DNA binding and inhibition of RNA—polymerase synthetic reaction by actinomycin, Proc. Natl. Acad. Sci. **48**:2094-2101, 1962.

122. Goldberg, I. H., and Reich, E.: Actinomycin inhibition of RNA synthesis directed by DNA, Fed. Proc. **23**:958-964, 1964.

123. Gottlieb, D., and Shaw, P. D., editors: Antibiotics. I. Mechanism of action, New York, 1967, Springer-Verlag New York, Inc.

124. Hamilton, L. D., Fuller, W., and Reich, E.: X-ray diffraction and molecular model building studies of the interaction of actinomycin with nucleic acids, Nature (Lond) **198**:538-540, 1963.

125. Hurwitz, J., Furth, J. J., Malamy, M., and Alexander, M.: The role of deoxyribonucleic acid in ribonucleic synthesis. III. The inhibition of the enzymatic synthesis of ribonucleic acid and deoxyribonucleic acid by actinomycin D and proflavin, Proc. Natl. Acad. Sci. **48**:1222-1230, 1962.

126. Kersten, W., Kersten, H., and Szybalski, W.: Physicochemical properties of complexes between deoxyribonucleic acid and antibiotics which affect ribonucleic acid synthesis (actinomycin, daunomycin, cinerubin, nogalomycin, chromomycin, mithramycin, and olivomycin), Biochemistry **5**:236-244, 1966.

127. Newton, B. A.: Chemotherapeutic compounds affecting DNA structure and function, Adv. Pharmacol. Chemother. **8**:149-184, 1970.

128. Northrop, G., Taylor, S. G., III, and Northrop, R. L.: Biochemical effects of mithramycin on cultured cells, Cancer Res. **29**:1916-1919, 1969.

129. Rao, K. V., Cullen, W. P., and Sobin, B. A.: A new antibiotic with antitumor properties, Antibiot. Chemother. **12**:182-186, March, 1962.

130. Reich, E.: Biochemistry of actinomycin, Cancer Res. **23**:1428-1441, 1963.

131. Reich, E.: Actinomycin: Correlation of structure and function of its complexes with purines and DNA, Science **143**:684-689, 1964.

132. Reich, E., and Goldberg, I. H.: Actinomycin and nucleic acid function, Progr. Nucleic Acid Res. Mol. Biol. **3**:183-234, 1964.

133. Schwartz, H. S., Sternberg, S. S., and Philips, F. S.: Pharmacology of mitomycin C. IV. Effects *in vivo* on nucleic acid synthesis; comparison with actinomycin D, Cancer Res. **23**:1125-1136, 1963.

134. Shiba, S., Terawaki, A., Taguchi, T., and Kawamata, J.: Selective inhibition of formation of DNA in *Escherichia coli* by Mitomycin C, Nature (Lond) **183**:1056-1057, 1959.

135. Silvestrini, R., DiMarco, A., and Dasdia, T.: Interference of daunomycin with metabolic events of the cell cycle in synchronized cultures of rat fibroblasts, Cancer Res. **30**:966-973, 1970.

136. Sobell, H. M., Jain S. C., Sakore, T. D., and Nordman, C. E.: Stereochemistry of actinomycin-DNA binding, Nature New Biol. **231**:200-205, June 16, 1971.

137. Szybalski, W., and Iyer, V. N.: Crosslinking of DNA by enzymatically or chemically activated mitomycins and porfiromycins, bifunctionally "alkylating" antibiotics, Fed. Proc. **23**:946-957, 1964.

138. The actinomycins and their importance in the treatment of tumors in animals and man, Ann. N. Y. Acad. Med. **89**:283-486, 1960.

139. Umezawa, H., Maeda, K., Takeuchi, T., and Okami, Y.: New antibiotics, bleomycin A and B, J. Antibiot. Series A **19**:200-209, Sept., 1966.

140. Wakaki, S., Marumo, H., Tomioka, K., Shimizu, G., Kato, E., Kamada, H., Kudo, S.,

and Fujimoto, Y.: Isolation of new fractions of antitumor mitomycins, Antibiot. Chemother. **8**:228-240, May, 1958.

141. Waksman, S. A.: Actinomycin: Nature, formation activity, New York, 1968, (Interscience) John Wiley & Sons, Inc.

142. Waksman, S. A., and Woodruff, H. B.: Bacteriostatic and bactericidal substances produced by a soil actinomyces, Proc. Soc. Exp. Biol. Med. **45**:609-614, 1940.

143. Ward, D. C., Reich, E., and Goldberg, I. H.: Base specificity in the interaction of polynucleotides with antibiotic drugs, Science **149**:1259-1263, 1965.

Vinca alkaloids

144. Armstrong, J. G.: The mechanism of action of the vinca alkaloids. In Brodsky, I., Kahn, S. B., and Moyer, J. H., III, editors: Cancer chemotherapy: Basic and clinical applications, New York, 1967, Grune & Stratton, pp. 37-45.

145. Cardinali, G., Cardinali, G., and Enein, M. A.: Studies on the antimitotic activity of leurocristine (vincristine), Blood **21**:102-110, 1963.

146. Cline, M. J.: Effect of vincristine on synthesis of ribonucleic acid and protein in leukaemic leucocytes, Br. J. Haematol. **14**:21-29, 1968.

147. Creasey, W.: Effect of the vinca alkaloids on RNA synthesis in relation to mitotic arrest, Fed. Proc. **27**:760, 1968.

148. Creasey, W. A.: Modifications in biochemical pathways produced by the vinca alkaloids, Cancer Chemother. Rep. **52**:501-507, 1968.

149. Creasey, W. A., and Markiw, M. E.: Biochemical effects of the vinca alkaloids. II. A comparison of the effects of colchicine, vinblastine and vincristine on the synthesis of ribonucleic acids in Ehrlich ascites carcinoma cells, Biochim. Biophys. Acta **87**:601-609, 1964.

150. George, P., Journey, L. J., and Goldstein, M. N.: Effect of vincristine on the fine structure of HeLa cells during mitosis, J. Natl. Cancer Inst. **35**:355-361, 1965.

151. Johnson, I. S., Armstrong, J. G., Gorman, M., and Burnet, J. P., Jr.: The vinca alkaloids: a new class of oncolytic agents, Cancer Res. **23**:1390-1427, 1963.

152. Madoc-Jones, H., and Mauro, F.: Interphase action of vinblastine and vincristine: Differences in their lethal action through the mitotic cycle of cultured mammalian cells, J. Cell. Physiol. **72**:185-196, Dec., 1968.

153. Neuss, N., Johnson, I. S., Armstrong, J. G. and Jansen, C. J.: The vinca alkaloids, Adv. Chemother. **1**:133-174, 1964.

154. Wagner, E. K., and Roizman, B.: Effect of vinca alkaloids on RNA synthesis in human cells *in vitro*, Science **162**:569-570, 1968.

Glucocorticoids

155. Bush, I. E.: Chemical and biological factors in the activity of adrenocortical steroids, Pharmacol. Rev. **14**:317-445, 1962.

156. Bush, I. E.: Structure and mechanism of action of steroid hormones and analogues. In, Martini, L., Fraschini, F., and Motta, M., editors: Proceedings of the Second International Congress on Hormonal Steroids, International Congress Series No. 132, Amsterdam, 1967, Excerpta Medica Foundation, pp. 60-67.

157. Dougherty, T. F., and White, A.: Influence of hormones on lymphoid tissue structure and function. The role of the pituitary adrenotrophic hormone in the regulation of the lymphocytes and other cellular elements of the blood, Endocrinology **35**:1-14, July, 1944.

158. Gabourel, J. D., and Fox, K. E.: On the site of cortisol inhibition of thymus ribonucleic synthesis, Biochem. Pharmacol. **20**:885-895, 1971.

159. Herzog, H. L., Payne, C. C., Jevnik, M. A., Gould, D., Shapiro, E. L., Oliveto, E. P., and Hershberg, E. B.: 11-oxygenated steroids. XIII. Synthesis and proof of structure of $\Delta^{1,4}$-pregnadiene-17α, 21-diol, 11, 20-trione and $\Delta^{1,4}$-pregnadiene-11β, 17α, 21-triol-3, 20-dione, J. Am. Chem. Soc. **77**:4781-4784, 1955.

160. Kaneko, T., and LePage, G. A.: Inhibition of thymidine kinase by cortisone, Proc. Soc. Exp. Biol. Med. **133**:229-233, 1970.

161. Kollmorgen, G. M., and Griffin, M. J.: The effect of hydrocortisone on HeLa cell growth, Cell and Tissue Kinetics **2**:111-122, 1969.

162. Makman, M. H., Nakagawa, S., and White, A.: Studies of the mode of action of adrenal steroids on lymphocytes, Recent Progr. Horm. Res. **23**:195-227, 1967.

Miscellaneous drugs

163. Becker, F. F., and Broome, J. D.: L-Asparaginase; inhibition of endogenous RNA polymerase activity in regenerating liver, Arch. Biochem. Biophys. **130**:332-336, 1969.
164. Bradlow, H. L., Fukushima, D. K., Zumoff, B., Helman, L., and Gallagher, T. F.: A peripheral action of o,p'-DDD on steroid biotransformation, J. Clin. Endocrinol. Metab. **23**:918-922, 1963.
165. Brookes, P.: Studies on the mode of action of ibenzmethyzin. In Jellife, A. M., and Mark, J., editors: Natulan (Ibenzmethyzin), Bristol, England, 1965, John Wright & Sons, Ltd., pp. 9-12.
166. Broome, J. D.: Evidence that L-asparaginase activity of guinea pig serum is responsible for its antilymphoma effects, Nature (Lond) **191**:1114-1115, 1961.
167. Broome, J. D.: Studies on the mechanism of tumor inhibition by L-asparaginase. Effects of the enzyme on asparagine levels in the blood, normal tissues, and 6C3HED lymphomas of mice: Differences in asparagine formation and utilization in asparaginase-sensitive and -resistant lymphoma cells, J. Exp. Med. **127**:1055-1072, 1968.
168. Capizzi, R. L., Bertino, J. R., and Handschumacher, R. E.: L-Asparaginase, Annu. Rev. Med. **21**:433-444, 1970.
169. Cazorla, A., and Moncloa, F.: Action of 1,1, dichloro-2-p-chlorophenyl-2-0-chloro-phenylethane on dog adrenal cortex, Science **136**:47, 1962.
170. Cheng, C. J., Fujimura, S., Grunberger, D., and Weinstein, I. B.: Interaction of 1-(2-chloroethyl)-3-cyclohexyl-1-nitrosourea (NSC79037) with nucleic acids and proteins *in vivo* and *in vitro*, Cancer Res. **32**:22-27, 1972.
171. Cooney, D. A., and Handschumacher, R. E.: Investigation of L-asparagine metabolism in animals and human subjects, Proc. Am. Assoc. Cancer Res. **9**:15, March, 1968.
172. Cooney, D. A., and Handschumacher, R. E.: L-Asparaginase and L-asparaginase metabolism, Annu. Rev. Pharmacol. **10**:421-440, 1970.
173. Coyle, M. B., and Strauss, B.: Cell killing and the accumulation of breaks in the DNA of HEp-2 cells incubated in the presence of hydroxyurea, Cancer Res. **30**:2314-2319, 1970.
174. Cueto, C., and Brown, J. H. U.: The chemical fractionation of an adrenocorticolytic drug, Endocrinology **62**:326-333, March, 1958.
175. Gale, G. R.: Effect of 1,3-bis-(2-chloroethyl)-1-nitrosourea on Ehrlich ascites tumor cells, Biochem. Pharmacol. **14**:1705-1710, 1965.
176. Gale, G. R., Simpson, J. G., and Smith, A. B.: Studies of the mode of action of N-isopropyl-α-(2-methlhydrazino)-p-toluamide, Cancer Res. **27**:1186-1191, 1967.
177. Grundmann, E., and Oettgen, H. F., editors: Experimental and clinical effects of L-asparaginase, New York, 1970, Springer-Verlag New York, Inc.
178. Horowitz, B., Madras, B. K., Meister, A., Old, L. J., Boyse, E. A., and Stockert, E.: Asparagine synthetase activity of mouse leukemias, Science **160**:533-535, 1968.
179. Hutter, A. M., Jr., and Kayhoe, D. E.: Adrenal cortical carcinoma. Results of treatment with o,p'DDD in 138 patients, Am. J. Med. **41**:581-592, 1966.
180. Jelliffe, A. M., and Marks, J., editors: Natulan (Ibenzmethyzin), Bristol, England, 1965, John Wright & Sons, Ltd.
181. Kaminsky, N., Luse, S., and Hartroft, P.: Ultrastructure of adrenal cortex of the dog during treatment with DDD, J. Natl. Cancer Inst. **29**:127-159, 1962.
182. Kidd, J. G.: Regression of transplanted lymphomas induced *in vivo* by means of normal guinea pig serum. I. Course of transplanted cancers of various kinds in mice and rats given guinea pig serum, horse serum, or rabbit serum, J. Exp. Med. **98**:565-581, 1953.
183. Krakoff, I. H., Brown, N. C., and Reichard, P.: Inhibition of ribonucleoside diphosphate reductase by hydroxyurea, Cancer Res. **28**:1559-1565, 1968.
184. Kreis, W., Burchenal, J. H., and Hutchison, D. J.: Influence of a methylhydrazine derivative on the *in vivo* transmethylation of the S-methyl group of methionine onto purine and pyrimidine bases of RNA, Proc. Am. Assoc. Cancer Res. **9**:38, March, 1968.
185. Mashburn, L. T., and Wriston, J. C., Jr.: Tumor inhibitory effect of L-asparaginase from Escherichia coli, Arch. Biochem. Biophys. **105**:450-452, 1964.

186. Nelson, A. A., and Woodard, G.: Severe adrenal cortical atrophy (cytotoxic) and hepatic damage produced in dogs by feeding 2,2-bis (parachlorophenyl) -1,1-dichloro-ethane (DDD or TDE), Arch. Pathol. **48**:387-394, Oct., 1949.

187. Rosenkranz, H. S., and Carr, H. S.: Hydroxyurea and Escherichia coli nucleoside diphosphate reductase, Cancer Res. **30**:1926-1927, 1970.

188. Rutishauser, A., and Bellag, W.: Cytological investigations with a new class of cytotoxic agents: methylhydrazine derivatives, Experientia **19**:131-132, 1963.

189. Schabel, F. M., Jr., Johnston, T. P., McCaleb, G. S., Montgomery, J. A., Laster, W. R., and Skipper, H. E.: Experimental evaluation of potential anticancer agents. VIII. Effects of certain nitrosoureas on intracerebral L1210 leukemia, Cancer Res. **23**:725-733, 1963.

190. Sinclair, W. K.: Hydroxyurea: Differential lethal effects on cultured mammalian cells during the cell cycle, Science **150**:1729-1731, 1965.

191. Temple, T. E., Dexter, R. N., Liddle, G. W., and Jones, D. J.: Dissociation of cortisol and aldosterone in o,p' DDD treated Cushing's disease, Clin. Res. **17**:24, 1969.

192. Vilar, O., and Tullner, W. W.: Effects of o,p' DDD on histology and 17-hydroxycorti-costeroid output of the dog adrenal cortex, Endocrinology **65**:80-86, July, 1959.

193. Wheeler, G. P.: Mechanism of action of alkylating agents: nitrosoureas. In Sartorelli, A. C., and Johns, D. G., editors: Handbook of experimental pharmacology: Antineo-plastic and immunosuppressive agents (in press).

194. Wheeler, G. P., and Bowdon, B. J.: Some effects of 1,3-bis (2-chloroethyl)-1-nitro-sourea upon the synthesis of protein and nucleic acids *in vivo* and *in vitro*, Cancer Res. **25**:1770-1778, 1965.

195. Wheeler, G. P., and Bowdon, B. J.: Effects of 1,3-bis (2-chloroethyl)-1-nitrosourea and related compounds upon the synthesis of DNA by cell-free systems, Cancer Res. **28**:52-59, 1968.

196. Wheeler, G. P., and Chumley, S.: Alkylating activity of 1,3 bis-(2-chloroethyl)-1-nitrosourea and related compounds, J. Med. Chem. **10**:259-261, March, 1967.

197. Yarbro, J. W.: Further studies on the mechanism of action of hydroxyurea, Cancer Res. **28**:1082-1087, 1968.

198. Young, C. W., and Hodas, S.: Hydroxyurea: inhibitory effect on DNA metabolism, Science **146**:1172-1174, 1964.

Combination chemotherapy

199. Acute Leukemia Group B.: New treatment schedule with improved survival in child-hood leukemia, J.A.M.A. **194**:75-81, 1965.

200. DeVita, V. T.: Cell kinetics and the chemotherapy of cancer, part III, Cancer Chemother. Rep. **2**:23-33, Oct., 1971.

201. Djerassi, I., Abir, E., Royer, G. L., Jr., and Treat, C. L.: Long-term remissions in child-hood acute leukemia; use of infrequent infusions of methotrexate; supportive roles of platelet transfusions and citrovorum factor, Clin. Pediatr. **5**:502-509, 1966.

202. Fernbach, D. J., Starling, K. A., Olivos, B. J., and Jones, R. R.: High-dose cyclo-phosphamide therapy in children with advanced acute leukemia, Proc. Am. Assoc. Cancer Res. **12**:86, April, 1971.

203. Finkelstein, J. Z., Hittle, R. E., and Hammond, G. D.: Evaluation of a high dose cyclophosphamide regimen in childhood tumors, Cancer **23**:1239-1242, 1969.

204. Henderson, E. S., and Samaha, R. J.: Evidence that drugs in multiple combinations have materially advanced the treatment of human malignancies, Cancer Res. **29**:2272-2280, 1969.

205. Holland, J. F.: Hopes for tomorrow versus realities of today: Therapy and prognosis in acute lymphocytic leukemia of childhood, Pediatrics **45**:191-193, 1970.

206. Lane, M.: Some effects of cyclophosphamide (Cytoxan) on normal mice and mice with L 1210 leukemia, J. Natl. Cancer Inst. **23**:1347-1360, 1959.

207. Mathé, G.: Operational research in cancer chemotherapy: Chemotherapy in the strategy of cancer treatment. In Scientific basis of cancer chemotherapy, New York, 1969, Springer-Verlag New York, Inc., pp. 72-96.

208. Mendelsohn, M. L.: Cell cycle kinetics and mitotically linked chemotherapy, Cancer Res. **29**:2390-2393, 1969.

209. Mueller, G. C.: The G_1-S conversion: a target for cancer chemotherapy, Cancer Res. **29**:2394-2397, 1969.
210. Sartorelli, A. C.: Some approaches to the therapeutic exploitation of metabolic sites of vulnerability of neoplastic cells, Cancer Res. **29**:2292-2299, 1972.
211. Venditti, J. M.: Treatment schedule dependency of experimentally active (L 1210) drugs, part III, Cancer Chemother. Rep. **2**:35-59, Oct., 1971.
212. Young, C. W.: Formal discussion: Cautionary considerations of combination chemotherapy in the treatment of human malignancies, Cancer Res. **29**:2281-2283, 1969.

CHAPTER 7

Principles of total care—
physiologic support[*]

JORDAN R. WILBUR
OSCAR Y. KING
JERRY J. SWANEY

Improvement in survival time of children with malignancies can be attributed to a number of factors. An important one has been the development and utilization of new chemotherapeutic agents, both more intensively and in combination. However, perhaps equally important has been the development of improved techniques of supportive care for the prevention and treatment of infections and bleeding.

INFECTIONS

The most frequent and most serious complication of neoplastic disease in children is infection.[2, 8, 34] There has been an increase in the spectrum of infectious complications associated with intensification of chemotherapy programs and the prolongation of the patient's life. This increase in infections is also related to the patient's decreased resistance, which may be caused by both the disease process itself or the therapy utilized.

In the past, infections in children with malignancy occurred primarily in patients with leukemia. The increased utilization of radiotherapy and intensive combination chemotherapy in children with solid tumors has made this group also susceptible to a variety of infectious complications.

Several specific entities are involved in patients with decreased resistance to infection. The most familiar and obvious is a reduction in the number of circulating granulocytes[5] due to the disease or, more frequently, the therapy. Altered metabolic and phagocytic activities of the leukocytes may also occur.[55, 60] Impaired delayed cellular immune response is often a factor. It has been particularly noted in Hodgkin's disease, other lymphomas, and leukemias.[20, 61] This defect in the cell-mediated immune response is also caused, at least temporarily, by the many types of therapy, including chemotherapy, radiotherapy, and even surgery. A decrease in immunoglobulins may also occur. However, studies of the relationship of immunoglobulin levels to malignant diseases have not shown consistent results.[20, 32, 43, 47]

Physical changes in the patient also increase the risk of infection. These include the presence of necrotic tumor tissue, the collection of fluids such as pleural effusion, and the compression of bronchopulmonary segments by metastatic foci,

[*]Supported in part by USPHS Grants CA-3713, CA-8000, CA-11844, and CA-08859.

with resulting atelectasis and impaired circulation. These pathologic areas promote rapid growth of bacteria when infected. The obstruction to normal drainage may leave specific areas more susceptible to infection. The breaking of the natural barrier of the body, the skin, with surgery or needle punctures provides new avenues for invasion by infectious organisms. Ulcerations in mucous membranes throughout the gastrointestinal tract, in the upper respiratory tract, and on the perineal areas leave the patient susceptible to invasion by organisms at the site of ulceration. The use of urinary and intravascular catheters provides other potential sources for introduction of infectious agents. Inflammatory reaction and tissue damage secondary to radiotherapy may leave local tissues more susceptible to the rapid spread of infection.

Significant infections are frequently caused by enteric bacteria and frequently involve organisms that are not normally pathogens. Respiratory and enteric viral infections occur in the child with a malignancy as often as they do in a healthy individual. This type of infection usually causes no greater toxicity than that occurring in the healthy child. However, some viral infections may not be self-limited because of the breakdown of the normal immune defenses that usually limit the ultimate development of the disease. Fungal infections form an increasing number of secondary infections, frequently occurring after prolonged antibiotic therapy for bacterial infections. Certain protozol infections (*Pneumocystis carinii*[54] and toxoplasmosis[1, 17]) may cause severe problems, but intestinal protozoal infestation does not usually cause any significant additional morbidity.[3]

Bacterial infections. Enteric bacterial infections continue to cause a significant number of generalized systemic infections in children with malignancies. Although the initial site of infection may be localized as an abscess or as a pulmonary infiltrate, frequently the infection is initially noted as a septicemia. The portal of entry is often an ulceration in some part of the intestinal tract, occurring anywhere from the mouth to the anus.

A list of the frequency of occurrence of different microorganisms in blood cultures obtained from children with malignancies with fever is shown in Table 7-1. It should be particularly noted that some bacteria usually considered to be nonpathogenic are frequently cultured. Although often interpreted as contaminants from the skin, they may represent a true septicemia in the child with decreased resistance to infection. Staphylococcal infections, although less prominent than in previous years, are still seen and are usually associated with an infected puncture site—most frequently a finger-stick. Susceptibility to tuberculosis is not increased in children with malignancies and has been detected in only one pediatric patient in our institution in the past 3 years.

A number of techniques have been attempted to reduce the frequency of systemic and local bacterial infections in the patient who is at high risk. The traditional approach of reverse isolation on a general inpatient unit has not been notably effective. This is in part because the major sources of infection are gram-negative bacteria from the intestinal tract and not the gram-positive bacteria usually associated with person-to-person contacts. A major disadvantage of reverse isolation is that the patient may not get checked as readily or as frequently. This is due to the complexity of the requirements that medical personnel must follow in properly donning the protective gowns and associated paraphernalia prior to entering the room. On the pediatric inpatient unit at M. D. Anderson Hospital

Table 7-1. Blood cultures in children (M. D. Anderson Hospital, June, 1970-May, 1971)

Organism*	Positive cultures	Patients
Staphylococcus aureus	18	11
Diphtheroids, anaerobic	17	15
Klebsiella species	13	8
Staphylococcus epidermidis	13	11
Alpha streptococci	9	7
Candida species	9	5
Escherichia coli	9	7
Pseudomonas species	8	5
Gamma streptococci	2	2
Beta streptococci	2	2
Saccharomyces species	1	1
Bacteroides species	1	1
Fusobacterium fusiforme	1	1
Streptococcus faecalis	1	1
Bacillus species	1	1
Total cultures	859	
Negative	763	
Positive	96	

*Eight of the cultures grew out two organisms in one culture.

and at some other institutions, reverse isolation techniques are not utilized for patients with neutropenia. This does not appear to affect the frequency of infections. However, patients with draining abscesses or contagious viral infections are kept in strict isolation. Reverse isolation techniques may still be necessary on a general hospital ward where other patients with significant bacterial infections (e.g., cystic fibrosis with pneumonitis) are located in the same unit.

Oral antibiotics given to eradicate bacteria from the intestinal tract have been tried most effectively in protected environment programs. The potential danger of this technique is the eradication of normal bacterial flora, allowing either resistant bacteria or fungi to predominate and subsequently cause generalized infection. The prophylactic use of systemic antibiotics is generally contraindicated.

Different techniques of protected environments have been under study.[6, 36, 41, 49, 58] There is some evidence that individual patients may be able to tolerate higher doses of intensive chemotherapy when they have been "sterilized" as completely as possible while in a protected environment.[7] Neither the Life Island Unit nor the Laminar Flow Room has been utilized with many young children in this country. The psychologic and practical problems involved with the management of young children in these units do not justify their general use at this time. If studies in adults establish the value of protected environment programs, suitable modifications for use by children could be developed.

Simple techniques of examination and hygiene provide an important basis for the prevention and early detection of infections in patients with granulocytopenia. These include particular attention to skin care and care of mucous membranes. Preparation of the skin with povidone-iodine complex (Betadine) prior to puncture reduces the possibility of introducing local infection. Finger-nails should be kept clipped to reduce trauma secondary to scratching and irritation of nasal mucous membranes. The patient should be completely examined daily for skin and mucous membrane lesions. Intramuscular injections should be avoided whenever possible. Perineal abscesses are a major problem and can be minimized by good perineal hygiene, including sitz baths when indicated. Regular careful inspection for early lesions should include spreading of the buttocks and examination of the genitalia. Rectal manipulation by thermometers or enemas should be avoided whenever possible.

Oral hygiene should include daily dental hygiene with a soft brush or sponge and mouthwash. Early evidence of *Candida* infection can be treated with 1:1000 nystatin mouthwash or aqueous benzalkonium chloride (Zephiran). Particular attention must be given to patients with postirradiation or medication-induced mucositis. Salt and soda rinses will help remove debris and mucus and provide some symptomatic relief.

The presence of a foreign body such as an indwelling catheter provides a potential route of entry for infectious organisms. The use of closed urinary drainage systems helps prevent infections occurring with indwelling urinary catheters. Antibiotic solution irrigations may also be of value. Indwelling vascular catheters are a potential source of thrombophlebitis and should be removed as soon as possible in the granulocytopenic patient. Intravenous needles have not appeared to be a source of local infection and in many patients are frequently left in place for up to 5 days without difficulty.

The diagnosis of local bacterial infection in granulocytopenic patients is often difficult because of the associated decrease in, or absence of, an inflammatory response. Localized lesions may contain no pus, and incision and drainage is generally not indicated. A diagnostic aspiration of a possible soft tissue infection, after injection of a small amount of sterile saline, may be sufficient to diagnose the type of infection by direct smear or culture.

The diagnosis of meningitis or urinary tract infection may not be excluded on the basis of absent white cells in the granulocytopenic patient. Classic x-ray evidence of pneumonia may also be lacking in the patient with no granulocytes.

The diagnosis of bacterial sepsis and even localized bacterial infection is often difficult in the patient with decreased resistance to infection. The most common presenting sign is fever. Since there are frequently many other possible causes for the fever, including the malignancy itself, drug therapy, and the usual viral illnesses that occur in children, the clinical diagnosis is much more difficult. Our policy has been that after the development of significant temperature (over 101° F, oral) in the patient with granulocytopenia (less than 1000/mm³) the patient should be assumed to have a septicemia, appropriate cultures should be done, and systemic antibiotic therapy should be started promptly. Appropriate cultures include blood, throat, stool, and urine cultures. If a bone marrow examination is done to determine the status of the marrow, a marrow culture is also obtained.

The antibiotic treatment utilized has been devised as an attempt to cover as completely as possible all the usual organisms that may cause such a systemic infection. The possible presence of two infecting organisms must be recognized (Table 7-1). Our current program utilizes cephalothin[56] (Keflin), gentamycin[30, 64] (Garamycin), and carbenicillin[46, 53, 57] (Geopen) (Table 7-2). Antibiotic sensitivities are routinely tested on all cultured organisms. If the organism is not a *Pseudomonas* organism, the carbenicillin may be discontinued from the treatment program if the patient is improving.

The possibility of a combined infection should always be kept in mind. Other specific antibiotics may be added as determined by laboratory-proved sensitivity of the organism if the patient does not improve. If the blood culture is negative and the patient has improved but the granulocyte count is still inadequate, the antibiotics are continued for a week. It is frequently difficult to determine the proper length of antibiotic therapy. Ideally, it should be adequate to treat the proved or presumed bacterial infection and yet insufficient to allow the development of a superinfection due to suppression of normal bacterial flora. When a patient is suspected of having sepsis, it is most important that antibiotic treatment be promptly started. There may not be time to wait for the return of a positive blood culture before starting therapy, since overwhelming shock due to gram-negative sepsis may rapidly develop. Frequently, gram-negative septicemia is associated with septic shock. In addition to the usual supportive measures described for the treatment of septic shock, we have found the use of high-dose corticosteroids (50 mg/kg, hydrocortisone, maximum 1 Gm), intravenous push, also helpful in retrieving fallen blood pressure and providing the patient with sufficient vascular support to allow time for the antibiotic program to become effective.[15]

Our experience with *Pseudomonas* infections has indicated that carbenicillin is effective treatment when given promptly and in adequate doses (Table 7-2). During a 6-month period of study, four pediatric patients with granulocytopenia and *Pseudomonas* sepsis, although in relapse, survived after treatment with carbenicillin and subsequently also achieved remission of their leukemia. A preventive approach regarding *Pseudomonas* infections is currently under study and may be of value in the future for children with leukemia. This technique involves the use of a prophylactic vaccine.[42]

White blood cell transfusions are being studied as a technique for the treatment of granulocytopenic patients with sepsis (p. 133).

Fungus infections. The development of intensive anticancer combination chemotherapy and the successful utilization of intensive antibiotic treatment for bacterial infections have both been contributing factors to the marked increase in patients susceptible to fungal infections.[4, 33] The use of corticosteroids has been frequently associated with the devolpment of *Candida* infections; the organism most usually involved is *Candida albicans*.[2] Generalized candidiasis often develops with the prolonged use of broad-spectrum antibiotics in granulocytopenic

Table 7-2. Combination antibiotic therapy

Drug	Dosage	Administration
Cephalothin (Keflin)	100 mg/kg/day	IV, divided doses every 6 hr, infused over 1 hr in minimum of 50 ml fluid
Gentamycin (Garamycin)	3 mg /kg/24 hr	IV every 8 hr, infused over 1 hr in minimum of 50 ml fluid
Carbenicillin (Geopen)	20 Gm/M²/day	IV every 4 hr, infused over 1 hr in minimum of 50 ml fluid

patients. Broad-spectrum bacteriostatic antibiotics such as tetracycline should not be used in patients with granulocytopenia.

Less frequent fungus infections, usually occurring only in the immunosuppressed and debilitated host, may be caused by any of several different fungi. On our pediatric unit we have encountered generalized infections such as aspergillosis and histoplasmosis. Others have reported cryptococcosis, mucormycosis, coccidioimycosis, and sporotrichosis.[2]

Techniques to minimize the risk of fungus infection include (1) the use of specific antibiotics rather than broad-spectrum ones, (2) short-pulse therapy with antitumor agents rather than prolonged treatment, and (3) the prompt treatment of local fungal infections with topical therapy. Studies have been undertaken to try to prevent the development of fungal infections in the gastrointestinal tract with oral prophylactic agents, including nystatin, amphotericin B, and iodine-containing mouthwash preparations. The effectiveness of these techniques in the subsequent prevention of systemic fungal infections has not been established.

The diagnosis of local fungal infection in the oral cavity can be frequently established simply by direct examination. Suspicious areas can be smeared and examined under the microscope and cultured for further identification. The presence of *Candida* organisms in the urine culture of a child with granulocytopenia is frequently an indication of a generalized *Candida* infection. A positive blood culture clearly establishes the presence of systemic fungal infection and is an obvious indication for intensive systemic therapy. However, many patients with disseminated candidiasis do not have positive blood cultures.

Localized lesions of the oral mucosa are best treated with topical nystatin or 1% aqueous gentian violet solution. Others have used 1:1000 aqueous benzalkonium chloride.[24] *Candida* esophagitis, a frequent problem, may sometimes be prevented by the ingestion of a nystatin solution. Mucous membrane infection of the vagina may occur but is relatively rare in prepubertal girls. Skin infections can be treated with topical nystatin.

Systemic candidiasis or *Candida* infections of the urinary tract, esophagus, or lungs require treatment with systemic antifungal agents. The most effective agent is amphotericin B. This potentially toxic antibiotic is administered intravenously in a 5% dextrose solution over a 4- to 6-hour period. The initial dose is 0.1 mg/kg/24 hr. If the dose is tolerated, it is gradually increased to a maximum dose of 1 mg/kg/day. Side effects are significant, and immediate ones include chills, fever, nausea, and vomiting. Secondary toxic effects include interference with adequate renal function, with associated azotemia and potassium loss. Duration of therapy is usually long (4 to 12 weeks) if an attempt is being made to actually eradicate the fungal infection. Both granulocytopenia and immunologic incompetence seem to interfere with effective therapy for systemic fungus infection.

5-Fluorocytosine, a relatively new antifungal agent that can be given orally, has shown some effectiveness against systemic fungus infections.[22]

Viral infections. Some of the usual childhood viral infections are much more serious when they occur in the child who has a malignancy and whose immune defenses are not functioning normally. In addition, other virus infections that are usually seen only in the immunoincompetent host are also frequently seen in children with malignancy receiving intensive therapy. The usual childhood viral infections that may cause a fatal infection are varicella (chicken pox) and measles.

Varicella and herpes zoster (shingles) are caused by the same virus. Herpes zoster has been well known as a common secondary problem occurring in adults with malignancy, particularly with lymphoma or leukemia. Herpes zoster in children is becoming a more significant problem, with more frequent occurrence. This is apparently due in part to the use of intensive combination therapy, which temporarily makes the patient immunoincompetent. In the past 3 years, we have seen over 15 children with herpes zoster on the pediatric service. For most of these patients the disease was limited to a localized area. However, a few patients developed subsequent extension of the disease to a generalized herpes zoster in spite of the fact that they previously had chicken pox. Another serious problem is that patients with herpes zoster are contagious, and other children who have not had generalized varicella may readily receive this highly communicable virus from the child with herpes zoster.[11] Patients with leukemia and patients on high-dose corticosteroid therapy are at high risk when generalized varicella develops.[50]

Previously there was no effective therapy for the varicella-zoster (VZ) virus. However, the development of several agents with antiviral properties has raised the possibility of effective systemic antiviral therapy. These drugs include floxuridine (5-FUdR), idoxuridine (IUDR), and cytosine arabinoside.[51, 52] In our own experience with 6 children under treatment with chemotherapy for malignant disease who developed geenralized varicella or disseminated herpes zoster, the efficacy of cytosine arabinoside in treating this type of infection was clearly established. Cytosine arabinoside was initially given in a dose of 3 mg/kg/day intravenously for 3 days, with associated rapid control of the spreading lesions, drying of the old lesions, and recovery of the patient. A more recent study reported that smaller doses of cytosine arabinoside are effective.[35] In our treatment of two patients, equally satisfactory results were obtained using a dose of 1 mg/kg/day given as a continuous 24-hour drip for 3 days.

If possible, it is better to prevent the development of a varicella infection. It had previously been shown that massive doses of gamma globulin (0.6 ml/lb) given promptly after exposure to varicella would decrease the intensity of the disease. More recently, the development of zoster immune globulin (ZIG) has been shown to be effective in preventing the development of varicella when given within 72 hours of known exposure.[12]

In acute leukemia, measles virus infection has been frequently fatal due to the development of measles pneumonia. Fortunately, with the development of the measles vaccine, the incidence of measles has markedly decreased and is less of a threat than before. It should be noted that the live virus measles vaccine is also a threat to patients and has resulted in fatalities when given to patients with leukemia.[48] Similar problems have been reported with the use of smallpox vaccination utilizing the live vaccinia virus. In the immunoincompetent patient the vaccination is not self-contained and may become generalized and possibly fatal. Methisazone has been shown to be effective in controlling generalized vaccinia and should be considered for use in the patient with progressive or generalized vaccinia.[10]

Because of the past experience of potentially fatal complications resulting from both measles vaccination and smallpox vaccination, children with malignancy who are receiving chemotherapy or whose disease is not in control should not receive any live virus vaccine. Even oral polio vaccine has the potential to cause a generalized clinical illness in the immunodeficient child.[23] Since immuno-deficiency may occur in association with both malignancy and immunosuppressive drugs, there is a potential risk from any live viral vaccine immunization of either progressive viral disease or lack of antibody response to the immunization.

Other viral infections seen frequently in children with malignancy include herpes simplex infections and cytomegalic inclusion disease virus infections. Although usually a localized infection, herpes simplex may become generalized in the patient who has an impaired immune mechanism. A recent patient with generalized herpes simplex infection was successfully treated with cytosine arabinoside utilizing a dosage schedule similar to that for the treatment of varicella-zoster virus infection.

Cytomegalic inclusion disease pneumonia (CMID) has been a significant complication of intensive combination chemotherapy for acute leukemia.[13] The usual initial presenting signs are temperature of 102° to 104° F, tachypnea, and no abnormal findings on ausculatory examination of the lungs. The initial chest x-ray film may show a faint, diffuse haziness consistent with interstitial pneumonia.

Such films can often be mistakenly interpreted as poor quality films. As the patient becomes increasingly ill, an increase in the general haziness develops, although the disease may be clinically limited to one area of the lung. Diffuse interstitial pneumonia has also been described secondary to methotrexate therapy.[16] This type of severe pneumonia responds to treatment with cortico-steroids (2 mg/kg/day of prednisone) and withdrawal of the methotrexate.

Needle aspiration of the lung can be utilized to establish the diagnosis of a diffuse lung infiltrate if the patient's clinical condition will permit this procedure. Potential complications are pneumothorax or bleeding if the patient has severe thrombocytopenia. The presence of CMID inclusion bodies in the urine is suggestive of generalized CMID infection but not diagnostic of CMID pneumonia.

The CMID pneumonia has previously been reported as being successfully treated with the antiviral agent 5-FUdR.[14] Since the time of that report, 15 children with leukemia with clinical findings and radiographic evidence consistent with CMID pneumonia have been treated orally with 2 mg/kg/day × 5 of prednisone and 20 mg/kg/day × 5 of 5-FUdR as intravenous push. This therapy usually brought about a prompt decrease in fever and improvement in the patient's general condition within 12 hours. Improvement usually continued during the next 4½ days of therapy, with rapid improvement in the x-ray films in 1 to 2 days, and frequently complete clearing within 5 to 7 days. At the time of initial improvement in the first 1 to 2 days, the patient may look and appear better; but auscultatory examination of the chest may now reveal the presence of scattered fine rales.

Protozoal infections. The protozoal infection commonly seen in children with malignancy is *Pneumocystis carinii* pneumonia.[31, 37] This is an organism that grows actively in the lungs in the immunosuppressed host, causing severe pneumonia, usually with rapid onset. It is frequently diagnosed only at autopsy. Definitive diagnosis can only be obtained by either lung biopsy or aspiration.[9]

The x-ray picture differs significantly from that of CMID pneumonia in that there are large fluffy areas of infiltration much more dense and localized than that seen in CMID pneumonia. A frequently associated clinical sign is the presence of unexplained drowsiness. Other signs include fever, cough, tachypnea, and relative bradycardia, with rapid progression of infiltrate seen on the x-ray film. Respiration and pulse rates may be almost equal. The patient can be successfully treated with 4 mg/kg/day of pentamidine isethionate, for 14 days, given intramuscularly.[21, 25, 62]

The main problem is keeping the patient alive during the therapy, since therapeutic effectiveness is often not noted for several days. We have been able to successfully treat several patients with *Pneumocystis carinii* pneumonia, either biopsy proved or clinically suspected. In some patients intensive supportive therapy with intermittent respirator assistance was required in addition to the systemic pentamidine isethionate. Four patients were cyanotic in 100% oxygen at the time of initiation of therapy, and three of them subsequently recovered completely.

Toxoplasmosis may occur in patients with malignancy, and treatment can be attempted with pyrimethamine and sulfonamides in combination.[1] With the increased utilization of white cell transfusions, the risk of possible transmission of toxoplasmosis also increases.[59]

BLEEDING AND DEFICIENCIES OF BLOOD COMPONENTS

Bleeding and deficiencies of blood components have been a significant cause of morbidity and mortality in children with cancer. However, the development of improved techniques of blood component therapy has helped make treatment more specific, thereby reducing the frequency of this problem. Blood loss due to hemorrhage is a well-known and usually easily recognized problem. Other forms of blood loss are often more subtle. Lack of production of new blood components due to disease or to a side effect of therapy is frequent.

Current blood banking techniques allow specific therapy for specific needs. Those techniques utilized in patients with malignancy include whole blood transfusion, packed cell transfusion (including white cell–poor red blood cells), platelet transfusion, albumin transfusion, and gamma globulin for intramuscular injection. Clinical research studies of techniques for obtaining and administering granulocyte transfusions are also in progress.

Anemia. Anemia due to blood loss or lack of new red cell production is a frequent complication in children with both leukemia and solid tumors. The rate of the blood loss is an indication of how rapidly it should be replaced. Gradual reduction in hemoglobin and hematocrit to exceedingly low levels may occur without apparent symptoms. Initial treatment should be slow transfusion of packed red cells, since the biggest risk to the patient is the development of congestive heart failure due to overload of the cardiovascular system from too rapid infusion of fluid volume. In the small child split units should be utilized when possible. This allows the child to receive multiple transfusions over an extended period of time utilizing a single donor. When packed cells are difficult to infuse because of the need for a relatively small needle, the addition of physiologic saline to the transfusion will allow it to flow more readily. Patients with suspected leukemia who have a severe anemia may be transfused prior to bone marrow aspiration without interfering with the subsequent bone marrow morphologic examination.

For acute hemorrhage the prompt administration of whole blood is required to prevent the development of shock. Whole blood should be used to replace acute blood loss.

Patients with a hemoglobin level below 10 gm/100 ml who are expected to have continuing problems with production of red cells due either to disease or therapy are electively transfused to maintain their hemoglobin above that level. Through this technique the child generally feels better and stronger and has a more adequate reserve of blood should a sudden hemorrhage develop. In the patient receiving radiotherapy this provides better oxygenation of the tissues being treated. The major potential dangers of transfusion, allergic reaction, and hepatitis have been minimized by good blood bank techniques, including careful cross matching and testing for Australia antigen in the donor prior to blood administration.

Thrombocytopenia. Thrombocytopenia is a frequent complication of leukemia and of several of the solid tumors. It may be due to marrow replacement with malignant cells. With the advent of more intensive chemotherapy programs, thrombocytopenia is frequently induced by the chemotherapy. The presence of thrombocytopenia is often indicated by the development of petechiae, ecchymoses, or bleeding that does not stop as expected. This is most frequently noted at the site of skin punctures or when the patient has epistaxis.

Platelet transfusion will usually promptly provide circulating platelets to help blood coagulation and stop bleeding.[40] Traditionally, platelets were obtained by transfusion of either fresh whole blood or platelet-rich plasma. More recently, the development of techniques of platelet plasmapheresis has enabled physicians to provide multiple platelet units from the same donor to be given to the patient at one time. A platelet unit is defined as the number of platelets normally available in a unit of blood. This represents approximately 10^{11} platelets. The transfusion of 10^{11} platelets will usually result in an average increase in circulating platelet count of about 12,000 platelets/mm^3 in a 1 M^2 child.[29] The life-span of the transfused platelets is shortened by the presence of infection, fever, gross bleeding, significant splenomegaly, or the presence of platelet antibodies.

The technique of multiple unit transfusion provides several benefits. Using a platelet plasmapheresis technique, as many as 4 units may be safely obtained from a single donor at one time. Infusion of multiple units of platelets from a single donor achieves higher platelet levels. Therefore fewer transfusions are required, and the risk of exposure to multiple donors is lessened. Parent donors are frequently used, since the donor may be used as often as twice weekly, the child may frequently be maintained with adequate platelets from a single donor. Limitation of the number of different donors helps reduce the risk of transfusion hepatitis. HL-A antigen–matched donors provide the best opportunity for platelet compatibility and effectiveness.[63] Platelets may be preserved for short periods for utilization when needed. Platelet packs stored at room temperature maintain platelet effectiveness for up to 48 hours. However, the potential risk of a contaminated unit increases during storage at room temperature.

After platelet transfusion febrile reactions frequently occur, consisting of hives, skin flush, and chills. These reactions are readily controlled with diphenhydramine hydrochloride (Benadryl), usually 25 mg, given orally when the reaction is mild and intravenously when the reaction is more severe. Subsequent use of diphenhydramine hydrochloride, given prophylactically prior to platelet transfusion, significantly reduces the number and severity of reactions.

Frequent platelet counts are necessary to monitor platelet levels in thrombo-cytopenic patients if platelet transfusions are to be given to prevent significant bleeding. Bleeding is not usually seen in patients with platelet counts above 20,000/mm³, except in the presence of infection or at a site predisposed to bleed-ing. Patients with recurrent epistaxis may reactivate bleeding at counts below 50,000/mm³. It is our policy to give platelet transfusions prophylactically to patients with platelet counts of 20,000/mm³ or below to prevent the develop-ment of serious hemorrhage. A possible disadvantage of this policy is that after frequent platelet transfusion subsequent transfusions may be less effective in achieving a significant rise in platelet level. In some cases this may be due to the development of platelet antibodies. The policy of prophylactic transfusion for severe thrombocytopenia has worked effectively in our patients; it allows the children freedom to continue their usual physical activities, which would otherwise have been limited because of fear of bleeding.

Granulocytopenia. Granulocytopenia may occur secondary to marrow in-vasion by tumor cells, loss of granulocytes by trapping in the spleen or in signif-icant areas of infection, and frequently myelosuppression secondary to intensive chemotherapy. It is of particular importance that evaluation of the patient's white blood count not be limited to a total white count but that a differential count be done to determine the percentage of granulocytes present. The pres-ence of 1000/mm³ or more granulocytes has usually provided adequate pro-tection against significant or overwhelming infection. Thus a patient with a white count of 1500/mm³ with 80% granulocytes is at much less risk than the patient with a white blood count of 1500/mm³ and only 10% granulocytes. The risk of overwhelming gram-negative sepsis is much greater in patients with granulocytes counts below 100/mm³.[5]

Clinical studies with white blood cell transfusions have indicated their ef-fectiveness in helping fight infection. Transfusions with granulocytes from chronic myelogenous leukemia (CML) donors were utilized initially.[28] These CML cells and granulocytes from normal donors are now more readily obtained in larger volumes since the development of the white blood cell separator.[26, 27] Granulocytes from CML donors and both matched and unmatched parent and sibling donors have been utilized to treat patients with severe granulocytopenia and sepsis.[45] These transfusions significantly reduce morbidity and mortality from septicemia and other severe infections. Patients with *Pseudomonas* sepsis with a large localized *Pseudomonas* abscess and with no circulating granulocytes have survived after granulocyte transfusion and intensive antibiotic therapy.

Reactions to transfused granulocytes include chills, high fever, and at times urticaria. These reactions may be minimized with the use of intravenous diphen-hydramine hydrochloride and hydrocortisone. These transfused granulocytes go immediately to areas of infection. Pulmonary infiltrates may become much more apparent immediately after granulocyte transfusion. Biopsies of infected tissues after granulocyte transfusion have shown the donor granulocytes present. Significant levels of circulating granulocytes may be achieved and maintained for several days in some patients who have severe immunosuppression. The granulocytes can be found in the bone marrow as well as the peripheral blood. In some patients not achieving significant circulating levels, the granulocytes may have been utilized promptly at the site of localized infection. Further studies on increasing utilization of the white cell separator have been accomplished with the use of etiocholanolone to stimulate the flow of donor white cells into the peripheral blood and hydroxyethyl starch to more effectively separate the granulocytes in the white cell separator.[44]

Another experimental technique for white cell separation utilizing a special filter is being developed. Cells obtained in this manner also seem to have clinical effectiveness in treating infection.[19]

Coagulation disorders. Bleeding due to the vitamin K–dependent factors (II, prothrombin, VII, proconvertin, IX, Christmas, and X, Stuart-Prower) is often due to vitamin K deficiency. Deficiency may result from gut sterilization by prolonged antibiotic therapy, but, with the exception of the newborn, the most likely cause is hepatic failure, which may be relatively mild, or perhaps a combination of both factors. If prolonged broad-spectrum antibiotic therapy is given, the patient should receive supplemental water-soluble vitamin K. If the bleeding patient has a low prothrombin level and hepatic disease is suspected, then he should receive a parenteral lipid-soluble vitamin K.

Liver dysfunction resulting from chemotherapy may interfere with protein synthesis. A drug such as L-asparaginase interferes not only with the synthesis of the vitamin K–dependent factors but also with fibrinogen synthesis. This rarely causes any symptomatic bleeding despite the fact that fibrinogen levels may be startlingly low. A severely damaged liver, regardless of the cause, will fail not only to synthesize the coagulation factors but also to detoxify the fibrinolytic enzymes. Massive bleeding from this cause is generally not reversible unless some improvement in liver damage occurs. Fresh whole blood and supportive measures to decrease the liver damage are indicated.

Another serious coagulation disorder that was almost universally fatal until the pathophysiology was understood is disseminated intravascular clotting (DIC). DIC is caused by extensive and prolonged consumption of coagulation factors, usually within the arterial system.[38] It may be due to septic emboli, vasculitis and thromboses, or massive intratumoral hemorrhage. The development of DIC must be recognized and treated promptly to prevent generalized bleeding and irreversible shock. A low prothrombin associated with a low platelet count and fragmentation of the red blood cells can be regarded as presumptive evidence of DIC, and therapy should be initiated after definitive laboratory studies have been done. These should include assays of factor (I, V, and VIII) levels and determination of the presence and amount of fibrin-split products. Therapy, in addition to vigorous antishock measures, consists of 100 units/kg of heparin given every 4 hours and continued until there is no evidence of DIC, as indicated by the disappearance of fibrin-split products from the plasma.[15, 18] If bleeding is severe, immediate correction of the coagulation factors with fresh whole blood or fresh platelet-rich plasma is indicated *after* the heparin therapy has been started.

Evaluation and management of coagulation problems resulting from severe liver failure or DIC can be complex, and early consultation should be sought when indicated.

Protein loss. Blood proteins are frequently decreased in children with malignant disease. This decrease may be secondary to significant blood loss, liver dysfunction, postoperative oozing after extensive abdominal lymph node surgery, ascites, or lack of protein intake. The presence of edema should suggest this possibility. Regular laboratory determinations of serum albumin and immunoglobulin levels are helpful in the prompt diagnosis of these defects. Significantly low gamma globulin levels leave the patient more susceptible to infection.

Protein replacement can be accomplished with the use of albumin or plasma. Patients with severe hypogammaglobulinemia associated with recurrent bacterial infection may be treated with the intramuscular administration of gamma globulin if thrombocytopenia is not present. Hospitalized patients with profound protein loss and an expected prolonged defect in oral intake or intestinal absorption of protein may benefit from a deep intravenous hyperalimentation program. Pilot studies indicate that risk of infection at catheter entry sites may preclude the regular utilization of this technique in the child with a malignancy and associated granulocytopenia and immunosuppression.

INTRAVENOUS TECHNIQUE

The importance of an intravenous access for the administration of fluids, antibiotics, blood, and blood components is well recognized by all who deal with children with malignancies. The difficulty in achieving and maintaining a needle in the child's vein is also well known. Techniques for achieving and maintaining intravenous needles in children are constantly being studied. The use of the "heparin lock" technique has been a significant addition in recent years.[39] This technique involves the use of a heparinized saline solution containing 100 units of heparin/ml saline. A special butterfly needle with a rubber stopper for multiple puncture at the end of the tubing is generally utilized. However, a regular butterfly needle can be utilized with a 1 ml syringe attached to plug off the end. Once an IV needle has been placed in the vein, it may be saved for subsequent use by introducing the heparin solution into the needle and then plugging it off.

This technique is of particular value in several situations. When intravenous medications have to be given at infrequent intervals, such as every 8 hours, the IV need not be kept open but may be maintained with a "heparin lock." The patient is then free to do what he wishes without being attached to an intravenous fluid bottle. When a blood or platelet transfusion is anticipated, the blood can be withdrawn through the butterfly needle, the needle plugged off with a "heparin lock," and the transfusion plugged into the needle when it is ready. Patients who have to be sent to the x-ray department or elsewhere off the pediatric unit can have the "heparin lock" put in place and can then leave without fear that the IV solution will run dry or the needle will be knocked out during some other procedure. Utilizing this technique, patients do not have to have "keep-open" IVs. This greatly reduces the nursing care time for those patients not requiring a continuing IV.

"Heparin lock" needles are left in place for a total of up to 4 to 5 days, even in severely granulocytopenic patients, without significant problems. There have been no episides of thromobophlebitis or sepsis associated with this technique after use in over 1000 patient trials.

SUMMARY

Supportive care of children with malignancy requires eternal vigilance. A major key to success in the treatment of children with malignancy is to prevent them from developing the significant secondary problems of infection or problems resulting from defects in blood components. Continued improvement in the diagnosis and treatment of infection and also the techniques for replacement of blood components should provide improved results in the therapy. Frequent examination and testing to promptly detect or prevent complications, followed by the immediate administration of proper supportive care, are vital factors in determining the ultimate successful treatment of the patient.

REFERENCES

1. Abell, C., and Holland, P.: Acute toxoplasmosis complicating leukemia, Am. J. Dis. Child. **118**:782-787, 1969.
2. Armstrong, D., Young, L. S., Meyer, R. D., and Blevins, A. H.: Infectious complications of neoplastic disease, Med. Clin. North Am. **55**:729-745, 1971.
3. Aur, R. J. A.: Treatment of parasitic infestation in children with malignant neoplasms, J. Pediatr. **78**:129-131, 1971.
4. Bodey, G. P.: Fungal infections complicating acute leukemia, J. Chronic Dis. **19**:667-687, 1966.
5. Bodey, G. P., Buckley, M., Sathe, Y. S., and Freireich, E. J.: Quantitative relationships between circulating leukocytes and infection in patients with acute leukemia, Ann. Intern. Med. **64**:328-340, 1966.
6. Bodey, G. P., Freireich, E. J., and Frei, E., III: Studies of patients in a laminar air flow unit, Cancer **24**:972-980, 1969.
7. Bodey, G. P., Gehan, E. A., Freireich, E. J., and Frei, E., III: Protected environment—prophylactic antibiotic program in the chemotherapy of acute leukemia, Am. J. Med. Sci. **262**:138-151, 1971.
8. Bodey, G. P., and Hersh, E. M.: The problem of infection in children with malignant disease. In Neoplasia in Childhood. A collection of papers presented at the Twelfth Annual Clinical Conference on Cancer, 1967, at The University of Texas M. D. Anderson Hospital and Tumor Institute at Houston, Chicago, 1969, Year Book Medical Publishers, Inc., pp. 135-154.
9. Bradshaw, M., Myerowitz, R. L., Schneerson, R., Whisnant, J. K., and Robbins, J. B.: *Pneumocystis carinii* pneumonitis, Ann. Intern. Med. **73**:775-777, 1970.
10. Brainerd, H. D., Hanna, L., and Jawetz, E.: Methisazone in progressive vaccinia, N. Engl. J. Med. **276**:620-622, 1967.
11. Brunell, P., Miller, L. H., and Lovejoy, F.: Zoster in children, Am. J. Dis. Child. **115**:432-437, 1968.
12. Brunell, P. A., Ross, A., Miller, L. H., and Juo, B.: Prevention of varicella by zoster immune globulin, N. Engl. J. Med. **280**:1191-1194, 1969.
13. Cangir, A., and Sullivan, M. P.: The occurrence of cytomegalovirus infections in childhood leukemia, J.A.M.A. **195**:616-622, 1966.
14. Cangir, A., Sullivan, M. P., Sutow, W. W., and Taylor, G.: Cytomegalovirus syndrome in children with acute leukemia, J.A.M.A. **201**:612-615, 1967.
15. Christy, J. H.: Treatment of gram-negative shock, Am. J. Med. **50**:77-86, 1971.
16. Clarysse, A. M., Cathey, W. J., Cartwright, G. E., and Wintrobe, M. M.: Pulmonary disease complicating intermittent therapy with methotrexate, J.A.M.A. **209**:1861-1864, 1969.

17. Cohen, S. N.: Toxoplasmosis in patients receiving immunosuppressive therapy, J.A.M.A. 211:657-660, 1970.

18. Corrigan, J. J., Jr., and Jordan, C. M.: Heparin therapy in septicemia with disseminated intravascular coagulation, N. Engl. J. Med. 283:778-782, 1970.

19. Djerassi, I., Kim, J., and Suvansri, U.: Filtration-leukopheresis for separation of granulocytes from single normal donors (Abstract), Proc. Am. Assoc. Cancer Res. 112:28, March, 1971.

20. Dupuy, J. M., Kourilsky, F. M., Fradelizzi, D., Feingold, N., Jacquillat, Cl., Bernard, J., and Dausset, J.: Depression of immunologic reactivity of patients with acute leukemia, Cancer 27:323-331, 1971.

21. Einzig, S., Hong, R., and Sharp, H. L.: Successful treatment of Pneumocystis carinii in as immunologically deficient acute lymphatic leukemia patient, Cancer 23:658-662, 1969.

22. Fass, R. J., and Perkins, R. L.: 5-Fluorocystine in the treatment of cryptococcal and Candida mycoses, Ann. Intern. Med. 74:535-539, 1971.

23. Feigin, R. D., Guggenheim, M. A., and Johnsen, S. D.: Vaccine-related paralytic poliomyelitis in an immunodeficient child, J. Pediatr. 79:642-647, 1971.

24. Fernbach, D. J., Nora, A. H., and Simonsen, L. G.: Recognizing and treating neutropenic infection, Postgrad. Med. 45:167-173, Feb., 1969

25. Fortuny, I. E., Tempero, K. F., and Amsden, T. W.: Pneumocystis carinii pneumonia diagnosed from sputum and successfully treated with pentamidine isethionate, Cancer 26:911-913, 1970.

26. Freireich, E. J.: Continuous flow in vivo blood cell separator, Lab. Management 6:1-7, April, 1968.

27. Freireich, E. J., Judson, G., and Levin, R. H.: Separation and collection of leukocytes, Cancer Res. 25:1516-1520, 1965.

28. Freireich, E. J., Levin, R. H., Whang, J., Carbone, P. P., Bronson, W., and Morse, E. E.: The function and fate of transfused leukocytes from donors with chronic myelocytic leukemia in leukopenic recipients, Ann. N. Y. Acad. Sci. 113:1081-1089, 1964.

29. Freireich, E. J., Shively, J. A., and DeJongh, D. S.: Platelet replacement. In Neoplasia in childhood. A collection of papers presented at the Twelfth Annual Clinical Conference on Cancer, 1967, at The University of Texas M. D. Anderson Hospital and Tumor Institute at Houston, Chicago, 1969, Year Book Medical Publishers, Inc., pp. 125-133.

30. Gatmaitan, B. G., Carruthers, M. M., and Lerner, A. M.: Gentamicin in treatment of primary gram-negative pneumonias, Am. J. Med. Sci. 260:90-94, 1970.

31. Goodell, B., Jacobs, B., Powell, R. D., and DeVita, V.: Pneumocystis carinii: The spectrum of diffuse interstitial pneumonia in patients with neoplastic diseases, Ann. Intern. Med. 72:337-340, 1970.

32. Gravina-Sanvitale, G., Gravina, E., and Panizon, F.: Immunoglobulin in childhood acute leukemia, Acta Paediatr. Latina 23:137-146, May-June, 1970.

33. Gruhn, J. G., and Sanson, J.: Mycotic infections in leukemic patients at autopsy, Cancer 16:61-73, 1963.

34. Hersh, E. M., Bodey, G. P., Nies, B. A., and Freireich, E. J.: Causes of death in acute leukemia, J.A.M.A. 193:105-109, 1965.

35. Hryniuk, W., Foerster, J., Shojania, M., Bercovitch, L., and Chow, A.: Disseminated herpes zoster infections controlled with low doses of cytosine arabinoside (Abstract), Blood 38:788, 1971.

36. Jameson, B., Gamble, D. R., Lynch, J., and Kay, H. E. M.: Five-year analysis of protective isolation, Lancet 1:1034-1040, 1971.

37. Johnson, H. D., and Johnson, W. W.: Pneumocystis carinii—pneumonia in children with cancer, J.A.M.A. 214:1067-1073, 1970.

38. Karpatkin, M.: Diagnosis and management of disseminated intravascular coagulation, Pediatr. Clin. North Am. 18:23-38, 1971.

39. King, O. Y., and Wilbur, J. R.: New techniques in ambulatory intravenous infusions (abst.), Ambulatory Pediatric Association, Eleventh Annual Meeting, April, 1971, p. 44.

40. Klein, E., Farber, S., and Djerassi, I.: Control and prevention of hemorrhage: platelet separation, Cancer Res. 25:1504-1509, 1965.

41. Levitan, A. A., and Perry, S.: The use of an isolator system in cancer chemotherapy, Am. J. Med. **44**:234-242, 1968.
42. Markley, K.: Vaccine prophylaxis for pseudomonas infections, Ann. Intern. Med. **74**:140, 1971.
43. Masi, M., and Vivarelli, F.: Serum levels of immunoglobulins in childhood acute lymphoblastic leukemia, Clin. Pediatr. **52**:185-198, May, 1970.
44. McCredie, K. B., and Freireich, E. J.: Increased granulocyte collection from normal donors with increased granulocyte recovery following transfusion (Abstract), Proc. Am. Assoc. Cancer Res. **12**:58, March, 1971.
45. McCredie, K. B., Freireich, E. J., Hersh, E. M., Curtis, J. E., and Kaizer, H.: Early bone marrow recovery after chemotherapy following the transfusion of peripheral blood leukocytes in identical twins (Abstract), Proc. Am. Assoc. Cancer Res. **11**:54, March, 1970.
46. Middleman, E. A., Watanabe, A., Kaizer, H., and Bodey, G. P.: Antibiotic combinations for infections in neutropenic patients, Cancer **30**:573-579, 1972.
47. Miller, D. G.: Patterns of immunological deficiency in lymphomas and leukemias, Ann. Intern. Med. **57**:703-716, 1962.
48. Mitus, A., Holloway, A., Evans, A. E., and Enders, J. F.: Attenuated measles vaccine in children with acute leukemia, Am. J. Dis. Child. **103**:413-418, 1962.
49. Penland, W. Z., Jr., and Perry, S.: Portable laminar-air flow isolator, Lancet **1**:174-176, 1970.
50. Pinkel, D.: Chickenpox and leukemia, J. Pediatr. **58**:729-737, 1961.
51. Plotkin, S. A., and Stetler, H.: Treatment of congenital cytomegalic inclusion disease with antiviral agents, Antimicrob. Agents Chemother. **9**:372-379, 1969.
52. Prager, D., Bruder, M., and Sawitsky, A.: Disseminated varicella in a patient with acute myelogenous leukemia: Treatment with cytosine arabinoside, J. Pediatr. **78**:321-323, 1971.
53. Pratt, C. B., and Dugger, D. L.: Treatment of Pseudomonas infections in leukemic children with carbenicillin and colistin, Curr. Ther. Res. **13**:182-187, March, 1971.
54. Robbins, J. B.: *Pneumocystis carinii* pneumonitis, Pediatr. Res. **1**:131-158, March, 1967.
55. Rosner, F., Valmont, I., Kozinn, P., and Caroline, L.: Leukocyte function in patients with leukemia, Cancer **25**:835-842, 1970.
56. Saslaw, S.: Cephalosporins, Med. Clin. North Am. **54**:1217-1228, 1970.
57. Schimpff, S., Satterlee, W., Young, V. M., and Serpick, A.: Empiric therapy with carbenicillin and gentamicin for febrile patients with cancer and granulocytopenia, N. Engl. J. Med. **234**:1061-1065, 1971.
58. Schneider, M., Schwarzenberg, L., Amiel, J. L., Cattan, A., Schlumberger, J. R., Hayat, M., De Vassal, F., Jasmin, Cl., Rosenfeld, Cl., and Mathe, G.: Pathogen-free isolation unit —three years' experience, Br. Med. J. **1**:836-839, 1969.
59. Siegel, S. E., Lunde, M. N., Gelderman, A. H., Halterman, R. H., Brown, J. A., Levine, A. S., and Graw, R. G., Jr.: Transmission of toxoplasmosis by leukocyte transfusion, Blood **37**:388-394, 1971.
60. Strauss, R. R., Paul, B. B., Jacobs, A. A., Simmons, C., and Sbarra, A. J.: The metabolic and phagocytic activities of leukocytes from children with acute leukemia, Cancer Res. **30**:480-488, 1970.
61. Sutherland, R. M., Inch, W. R., and McCredie, J. A.: Phytohemagglutinin (PHA)-induced transformation of lymphocytes from patients with cancer, Cancer **27**:574-578, 1971.
62. Western, K. A., Perera, D. R., and Schultz, M. G.: Pentamidine isethionate in the treatment of *Pneumocystis carinii* pneumonia, Ann. Intern. Med. **73**:695-701, 1970.
63. Yankee, R. A., Grumet, F. C., and Rogentine, G. N.: Platelet transfusion therapy, N. Engl. J. Med. **281**:1208-1212, 1969.
64. Young, L. S., Louria, D. B., and Armstrong, D.: Gentamicin in the treatment of severe, hospital-acquired gram-negative infections, Trans. N. Y. Acad. Sci. (ser. II) **29**:579-588, 1967.

CHAPTER 8

Principles of total care— psychologic support[*]

DANIEL M. LANE

To cure sometimes, to relieve often, to comfort always.

No words better describe the work of the pediatric oncologist. Most of this book on childhood cancer addresses itself to the phrase "to cure sometimes." Here I will consider the aspects of care reflected in the phrases "to relieve often" (the control of pain) and "to comfort always" (psychologic support). In a sense, the other chapters concern the science of oncology. This chapter deals with the art of oncology. It has been divided into three sections: (1) the control of pain, with major emphasis on systemic drug therapy (most childhood cancer is widely disseminated when pain appears), (2) the psychologic care of the child and his family and the roles of medical and paramedical personnel, and (3) some socioeconomic factors affecting the health care of the child with cancer.

CONTROL OF PAIN

The management of pain in children is rarely considered to be a separate problem in pediatric practice, as evidenced by its absence even from the index of a currently available book on pediatric therapy.[5] Children, especially young children, do not communicate the nature or extent of their pain as clearly as adults, and this complicates its management. In addition, children may express feelings of anxiety and fear by reporting specific physical pain. Because of the complexity of the problem, the discussion is limited in this section to the management of children with cancer who complain of specific pain. Since these patients also tend to suffer from marked anxiety, pain of possible psychologic origin and its management will be briefly considered.

When pain is present in childhood cancer, it is most commonly due to widespread disease. Consequently, systemic analgesic drugs are usually most effective. Almost every physician has his own preference of drugs for controlling pain, usually based on his familiarity with them. No one regimen is necessarily better than another. However, certain categories of drugs are appropriate for certain kinds of pain, and these fall into three major groups. First, the sedatives and tranquilizers are useful for pain of psychogenic origin. Second, the mild

---

*This chapter was completed during the tenure of a National Institutes of Health Special Research Fellowship (5 FO3 HE43135-03) from the National Heart and Lung Institute. I gratefully acknowledge not only the editorial assistance but also the personal interest and understanding of Mrs. Barbara G. Cox, who contributed so much to the creation of this chapter.

analgesics are beneficial to relieve minor pain problems. Finally, the strong analgesics are indicated when pain is severe enough to disable the child.[1]

Sedatives and tranquilizers, neither of which have specific pain-relieving actions, play a special role in the control of pain. Many children with cancer become extremely anxious, either about the disease itself or about what will happen to them in the future. And often this fear finds expression in the form of somatic pain, especially at night. Thus these compounds are generally most effective in conditions in which pain symptoms interfere with sleep. However, since pain can also reflect progression of the child's disease, differentiation between organic pain and psychogenic pain may be of critical importance. The use of sedatives or tranquilizers can help solve this dilemma, as well as make the child more comfortable. However, doses sufficient to sedate the child are unlikely to produce adequate relief if a metastatic lesion is present. For this reason, the use of sedatives should be seriously considered whenever a new pain symptom appears in a patient who was previously free of pain. The choice of drugs makes little difference, but the barbiturates are probably best because of their low cost and well-defined effects.

Tranquilizers, besides reducing anxiety, can sometimes potentiate the activity of the analgesic drugs. The tranquilizers used for this purpose are too numerous to describe here, but the phenothiazines constitute the largest group. The antiemetic effect of the phenothiazines is an additional benefit in the care of the child with cancer, since nausea and vomiting are frequently associated with both the basic disorders and various forms of cancer therapy. My experience has been primarily with promethazine, but other phenothiazines function equally well. Standard dosage regimens are satisfactory in most cases, although doses may have to be increased if anxiety is severe and no apparent increase in side effects ensues.

The mild analgesics can be divided into two major groups: (1) the aspirin and aspirin-related compounds and (2) codeine and drugs of equivalent effectiveness. Compounds in the aspirin family are of little use in the treatment of cancer pain, since their potency is usually inadequate. This is equally true for phenacetin and acetaminophen. Aspirin and related compounds are primarily useful as antipyretic agents. Aspirin can produce a feeling of well-being by reducing fever, but it seldom brings about effective pain control. Moreover, the use of aspirin may be hazardous for patients with thrombocytopenia because of its recently noted effect on platelet aggregation in the primary hemostatic mechanism. Because of this problem, aspirin should be used strictly as an antipyretic and then only with caution when the platelet count is normal. In the presence of thrombocytopenia, dextropropoxyphene hydrochloride (Darvon) can be used alone as a mild analgesic and acetaminophen (Tempra, Tylenol) substituted as an antipyretic.

Codeine or drugs of equivalent potency (the second group of mild analgesics) are most helpful in malignant conditions in which pain is neither severe nor of long duration. For example, codeine can relieve the bone pain associated with proliferation of leukemic cells in the bone marrow before treatment has had time to control the disease. In properly selected patients, routine dosages are usually adequate. Increasing dosages of codeine tend only to increase its sedative effect without increasing the level of analgesia. Of the mild analgesics available for pain control, codeine is most recommended. Other drugs of equivalent potency probably elicit no more satisfactory a response, nor are they less expensive. Dextropropoxyphene hydrochloride is the most widely used codeine substitute and probably should be tried when codeine is poorly tolerated by the patient.

The strong analgesic drugs are the most commonly needed compounds to control pain in the child with cancer because in children pain is ordinarily a late manifestation of the disease—when it appears, it is severe. By this time, neoplasia has become rapidly progressive and widespread. Consequently, the problem of sedation created by the more potent analgesic drugs is offset by their marked capacity to alleviate pain. Although many potent analgesic drugs are available, I prefer two in particular: meperidine and morphine. Despite relatively poor absorption by mouth, meperidine is nevertheless better absorbed than other drugs in this category of analgesics. Moreover, it is most readily controlled. Children tolerate meperidine well, and it is convenient for outpatient use. Dosage recommendations should be followed closely, however, since the variable intestinal absorption and the capacity for respiratory depression can combine to produce severe complications. Morphine, on the other hand, is ideal when parenteral therapy is indicated. No drug has yet offered better pain relief, although some more recently developed strong analgesics such as dihydromorphinone (Dilaudid) are more potent on a milligram for milligram basis. Its duration of action and extremely effective control of pain make it an excellent drug for use in children. It should be saved until late in the disease, however, since little else is available after morphine has lost its effect. Initially, the dose should be as low as possible to obtain maximal benefit before progressive tolerance to the drug develops. The appropriate time to start morphine still depends on the judgment of the physician caring for the child and his confidence in the need for a drug this potent.

In addition to drug therapy, special procedures can be used to control pain due to tumor growth, including anesthetic procedures, neurosurgery, and radiation therapy.[4] Unfortunately, these techniques may be less effective in childhood cancer than in adult cancer because severe pain is characteristically associated with wide dissemination of the disease in children. Nevertheless, the possible benefits of these procedures should be weighed in every child suffering from pain. Even transient relief may be worth the effort invested.

Anesthetic procedures are generally of two kinds: (1) peripheral nerve blocks and (2) subarachnoid blocks. Pain due to regional involvement can often be effectively alleviated by peripheral nerve blocks. Also, temporary blocks with local agents can help determine whether permanent destruction of particular nerves will afford sensory relief. If a local block proves to be temporarily effective, permanently effective agents or neurosurgery can be resorted to for long-term relief of regional pain. If pain involves the viscera, pelvis, or more than one or two dermatomes, local anesthesia will be inadequate, and treatment must be directed to the spinal roots and canal. In these cases, subarachnoid blocks with alcohol, phenol, or supercooled saline slush may be effective, providing significant pain relief for periods of weeks to months. Both peripheral and subarachnoid blocks should be performed by an anesthesiologist or neurosurgeon skilled in the techniques necessary to obtain satisfactory results.

Neurosurgical procedures can also afford significant pain relief. Rhizotomy, the surgical interruption of the posterior spinal roots as they emerge from the spinal cord, can be performed on one or both sides to interrupt pain perception. Again, however, if the tumor involvement responsible for the pain is widespread, the procedure required would be too extensive and would not be feasible. For the relief of intractable pain, spinothalamic cordotomy is the most common of the neurosurgical procedures. This operation involves the surgical interruption of the fairly well-delineated spinothalamic tract located within the anterolateral quadrant of the spinal cord contralateral to the side of the pain. In addition, the anatomic source of the pain also determines the location of the fibers within the tract itself. By careful anatomic analysis, very precise pain relief can be obtained. Although this procedure is rarely performed for the relief of pain in children, it should perhaps be more often considered for patients whose prognosis is extremely poor. Finally, intracranial surgery can be done to relieve pain, including prefrontal lobotomy. Basically, prefrontal lobotomy prevents the patient from recognizing pain, without interfering with the source of the pain itself. Except in most unusual circumstances, however, it would be hard to consider a procedure of this magnitude for a child with malignant disease, since it involves a major surgical procedure on a patient with a very short survival time as opposed to the adult for whom survival may be much longer. If neurosurgical intervention is being considered for the control of pain, a neurosurgical colleague should closely cooperate in evaluating the child's problem and then undertake the surgery if it seems advisable.

Radiation therapy can be valuable in the control of pain, especially in radiosensitive tumors. Radiation is used most often to control pain from local lesions in widely disseminated disease when adequate control of the disease by other means has been lost. Two anatomic areas, the bones and the head and neck region, are especially responsive to radiation therapy. Obviously, single pain-producing lesions at any site are also amenable to the approach. Again, however, the physician should consult a radiotherapist before considering pain control by this method in any given patient.

No matter what means are used to control pain in the child with cancer, the physician should commit himself to an aggressive approach—the goal being to reduce the anxiety of his patient and to make him as comfortable as the tools of medicine will allow.

PSYCHOLOGIC CARE

No aspect of pediatric oncology depends more on personal opinion and less on scientific fact than the psychologic management of the child with cancer. Nor is the physician the only person responsible for this important area of medical care. All medical and paramedical personnel who come into contact with the family are (or should be) involved.

Despite the tremendous activity in cancer research, little study has been devoted to the psychologic needs of the cancer patient. Emphasis has rested almost entirely on treatment of the malignancy per se. What research on psychologic care has been done has been based primarily on personal observation, rather than documentation by carefully controlled studies designed to determine whether one approach is superior, inferior, or equivalent to another. Consequently, no proved guidelines can be offered in this section. I can only discuss general principles of management as validated by my own experience, present some of the controversy, and briefly consider the roles of some of the individuals surrounding the child and family.

The principles of management outlined here are modified from those developed by Green[6] and serve as an excellent guide to the major responsibilities of the pediatric oncologist. They include medical competence, availability, preparation for future events, participation of the child and his family, and hope.

Medical competence. The physician who treats children with malignant diseases must possess the medical skills required to cope with the serious clinical problems that arise in childhood cancer. But he must also be confident of his abilities so that the extreme pressures brought to bear on him, particularly by the family, will not divert him from a sound course of action. The parents of a seriously ill child have a natural desire to "shop" for the best help they can get. Knowing this, the physician should not regard it as a personal reflection on his abilities and let his confidence be shaken. Self-doubt swayed by the demands of parents and patients may cripple what was originally good judgment.

The physician's ability to give competent health care may be limited by deficiencies over which he has little or no control. He may lack adequate hospital support such as transfusion services or treatment facilities such as radiotherapeutic equipment. Whenever the pediatric oncologist finds himself in these straits, he should strive to correct whatever deficiencies block him from giving his patient optimum care. He may find it necessary to seek some services for the child outside the local community. If the physician himself lacks any of the many skills necessary to deal with childhood cancer, he should make whatever effort is needed to close gaps in his knowledge and gain the needed skill.

In other words, the pediatric oncologist must have confidence in his hospital, in his co-workers, in his clinics, in his techniques, and in himself. The parents will sense the high quality of service their physician is providing, feel that they are doing all that is possible for their child, and make the oncologist's job less difficult by offering their full cooperation. If the physician cannot meet these requirements, he should refer the child to a physician who can.

Availability. Perhaps no obligation is more difficult for the physician of a child with incurable cancer than that of making himself readily available to the child and family throughout the course of the disease. Yet to fail in this responsibility is a major omission in therapy. If for some reason the physician is temporarily unavailable, he should provide the family with an adequate substitute. The need of the child and family for their physician's support is especially pressing in the terminal stages of the disease. At this very time, however, the physician is most inclined to abandon the patient, both emotionally and physically. The evidence literally lies before him of his inability to cure a patient, and he is faced with the frustrating and demoralizing experience of clinical defeat, especially poignant when a child is involved. If the physician steadfastly continues to treat the child from a purely medical standpoint, he may find himself subtly depersonalizing his relationship with the child and family, shifting the burden of psychologic support to someone else.

At no time are the needs of the child and family for total care more urgent. And no area of oncology leads to more patient and family dissatisfaction than the physician's inability to meet these needs. If the physician can face his natural feelings of failure with honesty and see his role in a broader light, he can minimize the psychologic price of dealing with a dying child and anguished parents. He has a dual role: to control the pathologic disease process insofar as possible, but also "to comfort always." Thus the care he gives must be both continuous and personalized, so that the family is assured of his presence and support to the end. Having met this obligation, the physician will pay a psychologic price to be sure; but he will find that this is far outweighed by the personal satisfaction derived from giving his best to the child and family throughout the course of the disease.

Preparation for future events. As the child's disease progresses, certain medical events become fairly predictable. By preparing the family for these changes in their child's physical condition, the physician can help them avoid a great deal of anxiety. A new symptom or side effect of therapy will not frighten them as much if they expect it and are given some time in advance to adjust to it. Many highly emotional, even hysterical, scenes can be circumvented by diplomatic preparation of the patient and family. For example, when remission is successfully induced by steroid therapy in acute leukemia, the patient's general condition improves dramatically, but cessation of the drug is accompanied by loss of appetite. Unless the parents are told what to expect, they often become disturbed because they see their child improving and yet notice that he does not eat. They become confused and anxious. By forewarning them of such expected changes in the child's condition, the physician is more likely to ease the course of a long and difficult sequence of events.

Participation of the child and his family. The child and his family should be encouraged to play as active a role as possible in the management of the disease. They should not be allowed to be passive observers, at the mercy of a disease process that only the physician can comprehend and handle. All their questions should be answered openly. In fact, questions should be encouraged. If they want to know the name of a drug, how it works, and how effective it is, their physician should give them a full explanation in terms they can understand. The child can be given a sense of participation by taking oral drugs himself, rather than having a nurse or parent give them to him. In this way, he will feel that he is actually helping himself to improve. Furthermore, by being included as an active participant in medical efforts to alleviate his disease, he will accept other therapeutic procedures more readily. The parents can sometimes be instructed in the administration of parenteral drugs, giving them a sense of constructive contribution to the child's welfare. Or they can cooperate in other aspects of daily care that medical personnel would ordinarily undertake while the child is hospitalized. This is a strengthening experience for both the child and parents. The child sees his trusted parents caring for him and cooperating with the hospital staff, and the parents feel that they are actively promoting the welfare of the child, not standing by helplessly while others care for him.

Hope. No single individual can better keep the germ of hope alive in the child and family than the physician. Underneath, everyone may sense that death is inevitable, but the physician can divert their thoughts from the ultimate event to an acceptance of life on day-to-day terms. Although a general philosophy of openness and honesty is advocated for the physician, reassurance should be offered whenever it can honestly be given. He should emphasize the positive aspects of management, for example, the fact that a remission may be induced, during which the child may become symptom free for an appreciable length of time, even years in some children.

Occasionally, however, the physician may find himself caught in a situation in which the naked truth helps no one, and a white lie seems a small price to pay for the psychologic comfort it brings. At the bedside of a small dying child asking, "Doctor, am I going to die now?" I can see little virtue in telling the cold truth.

To sustain themselves throughout the course of incurable cancer, the child and his family must have the benefits of whatever hope the physician can offer them. They must know that the physician is doing all he can to prolong the life of the child, make him comfortable, and give him psychologic support. The physician, on the other hand, must try to turn their attention away from the specter of death and help them see the child as having an illness that must be dealt with day by day, not all at once.

Age of the child and the meaning of death. The management of the child with a life-threatening or fatal disorder is complicated by the fact that disease and death mean different things to children of different ages. Thus the child must be dealt with in a manner appropriate to his psychologic development.[2]

Children under 6 years old have no clear concept of death. They imagine it as some vague state of limbo that follows severe trauma, from which the victim can somehow return to normal. Perhaps from their experiences with television, these children think of death as immediate, painful, and violent, but transitory. No matter what happens to the hero, he always reappears on the next episode. The child himself feels immune from such a fate, knowing that his parents and the other adults responsible for his security will protect him from danger. Certainly he has no concept of slow deterioration of the body, culminating in death. So when he thinks about death, he views it not as a permanent change, but as a reversible process. In this age group, children show little fear of the possibility of personal death. Rather, they are frightened by the medical or surgical procedures that they may have to undergo because they fear physical pain. It is the parents of the young child who need psychologic support more than the child himself.

From 6 years of age to adolescence, the concept of death becomes more real. A child in this age group, faced with the prospect of death, rapidly establishes the normal denial defenses characteristic of the adult in the same plight. He also develops the capacity to understand that death means the loss of loved ones. Unlike the adolescent and young adult, however, this youngster imagines an ill-defined continuation of physical existence after death, a bewildering sort of going-on-alone. The management of children in this age group should be directed toward separation fears superimposed on the normal denial response. The child must be reassured repeatedly that he will not be left alone. Parents, other relatives, and friends should be encouraged to offer maximum support throughout the disease. If relatives or friends temporarily rally around the child and then disengage, this is worse than if they had never offered their support at all. The child's worst fears then appear to be justified. On the other hand, if his separation fears can be relieved, the child will deal more effectively with his progressive disease, and his denial mechanism will support him.

Death is most difficult to approach in the adolescent age group. The teenager fully understands the "end-of-self" implicit in death and its permanent nature. Unfortunately, he has also developed a keen sense of personal destiny by this age. He feels the drive to pursue life with all his energies. In this age group the physician for the first time encounters the spoken or mute question, "Why did this have to happen to me?" The adolescent's anguish is deepened by his tendency to interpret imminent death as a punishment for some great sin or for what he views as a generally guilty past. The problem is further aggravated by the conflicts that children in this age group experience over dependency versus self-sufficiency. They are beginning, at this point in life, to assert their independence from parents and other authority figures—a necessary step in healthy psychologic growth. Being sick means that they must regress back into childlike dependence and let others care for them. The denial of the possibility of ultimate death does offer some support, but not as effectively as in earlier life. As a result, the adolescent faced with death has a typical psychologic course characterized by widely swinging emotions and a frequently overwhelming rage that his destiny—life—is being snatched from him at the moment he was about to embark on it.

To tell or not to tell. An understanding of the psychologic reactions to death in the major age groups can give the pediatric oncologist some insight into whether he should tell the child of his diagnosis—or how much he should tell. There are currently two major schools of thought on this subject, which might be called "The School of Tell" and "The School of Don't Tell." Karon and Vernick,[7] proponents of the former, believe that the physician should be as open and direct as possible about informing the child of his prognosis. Conversely, Evans[3] is opposed to telling the child anything that would arouse fears of death. Perhaps the conflict stems partly from the different patient populations with which these workers have dealt. In my opinion, the psychologic management of a child with cancer should be grounded on the responses to death that are characteristic of his age group, as well as the child's individual personality.

For the child under 6 years of age, who has little grasp of the concept of death or its permanence, little can be gained by informing him of his prognosis. In many cases, it arms him with something with which to extract added solicitude from his parents. Children sense when they have the ammunition to get what they want. In the case of the child with cancer, the anxiety of the parents is greatly increased by this kind of attention-getting behavior, and the child benefits very little. In fact, extremely anxious parents will eventually make their child more anxious. Therefore I recommend that nothing about prognosis be discussed with the child under 6 years of age.

The school-age child presents a somewhat more difficult problem. In this age group the concept of death is developing, and the defense mechanism of denial can only partially support the sick child. The physician has little hope of making the child fully understand his medical problem. Because of this, his efforts are best directed at simply explaining to the child the immediate reasons for him to cooperate. The child should be told no more than he is willing to ask. And information should be presented in terms just adequate to satisfy his curiosity. As discussed earlier, psychologic support should be focused primarily on relieving the child's anxieties about separation from loved ones.

For the adolescent the approach to management must be altered considerably. The physician who is caring for an adolescent with cancer and thinks the patient is ignorant of his diagnosis and probable prognosis is only fooling himself. Because the child senses the truth, he should be told as much about his disease and its prognosis as he wants to know. If an adolescent is left in confusion about his condition and his physician or parents are unwilling to communicate openly and honestly with him, he will be frustrated, fearful, and lonely. Certainly he will find his fate much harder to endure. Frequently, an adolescent in this situation will become so disturbed that his psychologic difficulties erupt in intractable behavior. He may refuse to come to the hospital for treatment, for example. Obviously, this precludes optimum medical management of the child's disease. The adolescent should be treated much as though he were an adult, with the right to know everything he wants to and the privilege of dealing with his future accordingly. The adolescent is starting to branch out independently. His life is no longer centered around his family. Until sound psychologic data prove otherwise, I recommend an open and honest approach to the adolescent with cancer. The initial emotional price will be high for both the patient and his physician, but in the long run the patient will better adapt to his disease and cooperate with medical personnel.

Dealing with the family. Unless the child's pediatrician or the family physician discovers that the child has cancer, the first contact that the physician has with the family occurs at the time of diagnosis. The child may be brought to the physician for any one of many reasons, either directly or by referral. The circumstances under which the physician and family first meet can be critical to their relationship thereafter. Within the guidelines already discussed, each physician must adopt an approach that is most comfortable for him and is compatible with his personality.

Some specific recommendations can be made about dealing with the family in this important initial stage of the physician-family relationship:

1. The diagnosis should be determined as rapidly and thoroughly as possible. When a question exists about the diagnosis, all possible alternatives should be investigated exhaustively before a conference is arranged with the parents. The parents should not be left with the impression that diagnostic measures are being delayed or that they are being kept waiting unnecessarily.

2. When the diagnosis has been established, a private meeting should be arranged between the parents, physician, and possibly those medical personnel who have been or will be involved in the child's care. The child, of course, should be absent, although he may be present at subsequent meetings.

3. The diagnosis should be presented to the family and explained in clear, unambiguous terms. Information discussed with the family should include not only what is known about the malignancy but also what is not known. Being told that the causes of most childhood cancers and the time of their onset have not been determined can relieve the parents of a great deal of anxiety about their own role in the child's disease. The physician should make certain that the parents have understood his explanation. Although gentleness and empathy are important, anything less than complete honesty at this point can result in

misunderstandings that become a source of pain or resentment later in the disease. The unpleasant task that the physician faces should not tempt him to circumvent the necessity to be frank.

4. The physician should offer brief comments about the expected course of the disease and problems that are likely to arise. However, no predictions should be made about the expected survival time. Parents inevitably ask how long their child will live, but a specific answer should be avoided. A general discussion of survival statistics is appropriate and may even be demanded by the patient's family.

5. The family should be encouraged to deal with the child's disease as though it were a medical disorder that was not fatal. They should be advised to try to take each day as it comes and avoid the idea of death until the terminal stages of the disease. They should try to put death out of their minds altogether when the child is clinically free of disease.

This piece of advice is extremely important to the well-being of the family during long symptom-free periods of remission, particularly in acute leukemia. Also, it gives the family time to unconsciously prepare themselves for episodes likely to lead to the child's death.

6. At the initial conference, the physician should strongly urge the parents to ask questions as often as they desire. A useful suggestion is to have them write down questions as they come to mind, rather than trying to remember them during office visits. This technique is especially helpful during the period immediately after the first visit (when the parents learn the diagnosis), since they usually remember very little of what was said to them—except the fact that their child has cancer.

7. If the patient has siblings, the parents should be warned not to wrap themselves up in their sick child and ignore the problems of the other children, who will continue to have the usual troubles of everyday life. The siblings should be expected to sacrifice some attention for their sick sister or brother, but complete absorption in that child by the parents is pathologic and can create problems that persist long after the affected child has died.

Even when parents have suspected the diagnosis previously, they respond to confrontation with the established fact with shock and disbelief. Soon afterward, they begin experiencing overwhelming feelings of guilt. They ask themselves repeatedly what they might have done that caused their child to develop cancer. Occasionally, this is accompanied by feelings of anger and hostility directed outward at the world for this cruel blow to the family. The physician may find this reaction particularly difficult to cope with when it happens to be directed at him or other medical personnel. Fortunately, this phase ends shortly. In its wake comes a period of depression and an urge to comfort and help their child. It is at this point that the physician and family can join hands, working together to provide the best possible care for the child. The physician should neither overlook nor turn aside this opportunity.

With the passing of time, the physician should keep the family closely informed about the medical problems currently being handled and the relative seriousness of each. The parents should be encouraged to ask questions, no matter how foolish they may seem. If they read something in the newspapers or get information from friends about their child's disease that raises questions in their minds, they should feel free to consult the physician. Otherwise, if a new chemotherapeutic agent is described in the newspapers for the treatment of leukemia, for example, they may wonder why their child is not receiving it. They may fear that their physician is not staying abreast of current developments and that their child is being deprived of the benefits of this new drug. By keeping the lines of communication fully open, the physician can reassure the parents about the quality of care their child is getting and ensure continued physician-family cooperation.

The greatest stress for both the physician and family arises in the terminal stages of the child's disease. For the family, this means that they must begin to accept the fact that their child is going to die and that neither their efforts nor those of the physician can save him. Usually the parents undergo some anticipatory grief—a period of bereavement before death actually occurs. This helps them accept the real event afterward. At the same time they may begin resuming interests outside their child and make plans for life after their child has died. How effectively the parents can accept the death of their child depends primarily on their psychologic makeup.

For the physician, too, this is a traumatic time. Accepting the death of the child means not only an emotional loss but a personal defeat. It is not surprising that the physician experiences an urge to abandon his patient emotionally and physically at this time to relieve the pain of the imminent loss. The physician should fight this temptation with all his resources. The child and family need him most at this critical time and deserve his skills to the end. Moreover, the rewards of seeing the family through the entire course of the disease are worth the emotional price.

Ideally, the physician's responsibility to the family extends beyond the child's death. Certain responsibilities are self-evident: requesting autopsy permission, informing the family of the probable cause of death, and signing the death certificate. Less well appreciated are the responsibilities to the family for days, weeks, or even months after the child's death. If at all possible, the physician should see the family and discuss the autopsy findings as soon as they are available. In addition, he should encourage the parents to communicate their needs and feelings with him during the period of bereavement. He may be able to offer support that will ease them through this stressful time. He can also be alert for the serious psychiatric problems that sometimes result from the death of a child and arrange for counseling. The grief felt by everyone associated with a child who has died can be temporarily overwhelming. But the nature and duration of the responses have limits beyond which they can be considered abnormal. The pediatric oncologist would do well to review the study of Parkes,[8] who has classified normal versus pathologic grief reactions.

The role of other medical personnel. Much of what has been said about the physician's role in caring for the dying child, especially the comments about the tendency to desert the child and his parents in the final hours when their needs are greatest, also applies to other individuals directly involved in the child's care: nurses, nurses' aids, technicians, dieticians, hospital volunteers, psychiatrists, office personnel, interns, and residents. In the typical hospital environment, each person tends to perform his or her role independently of other workers, helping the child by providing a particular service, but failing to communicate with other personnel who also care for the child. There is little communication across professional lines. In addition, each hospital worker tends to repress his or her painful emotions about dealing with dying children. As a group, medical personnel tend to be success oriented—"success" being defined as "cure." They derive their major satisfactions from making sick people well. They are not geared to helping sick people die. To compound the problem, they are usually ill informed about the process of death and have their own unresolved conflicts about the meaning of death itself. When the child does die, they usually respond as isolated individuals, with age-appropriate responses. This conventional approach is entirely unsatisfactory in the management of the dying child.

A team approach is far more effective.[9] Medical and paramedical personnel working together in mutual understanding not only give the child and family far greater psychologic support but also reinforce one another. The team should include all the individuals directly involved in the child's care, with equal status for each. If a hierarchy of "importance" exists, true cooperation within the team is difficult, and the contributions, such as those of the nurses' aide, may be minimized. Every member should communicate openly with the others and verbalize his feelings at the appropriate times. Each must accept the fact that his role as a professional worker involves the ability to relieve and comfort, as well as specific therapeutic skills. In addition, all team members must understand and accept the emotional cost that is inescapable if they are to provide this very difficult type of medical care.

The secretary who arranges appointments, the receptionist who admits the child to the hospital, the nurses' aide who helps him bathe in the morning, the laboratory technician who comes in to draw blood—all are important figures to the child and the family. It is they who make arrangements run smoothly, add to the comfort of the child in their individual ways, and give the family confidence that everyone is working together to provide optimum care. In such a setting, both the child and family are led to feel that they are surrounded by competent and understanding professional workers functioning as a team in the child's best interests.

SOCIOECONOMIC FACTORS

Cost. The total care of the child with cancer is expensive. It requires frequent prolonged hospitalization, extensive treatment facilities, special support capabilities, repeated outpatient visits, and the administration of expensive drugs. Weeks of radiation therapy may be required as a part of treatment. Recent efforts have been made to lower the expense such as domiciliary care, but the irreducible minimum still remains high. Those who care for the child must undertake the obligation to make every effort to reduce these costs without compromising the quality of care. Childhood cancer probably exacts a greater toll in terms of time, money, and emotional energy than any other single group of disorders.

The community. The community from which the child comes can be an important source of support during the course of the child's illness, especially in rural areas. Their eagerness to help can be of particular assistance when blood donors are needed for platelet support programs or routine blood donations.

However, the community can also have detrimental effects on the child and family. Many times it becomes very emotional about the child with cancer—printing maudlin newspaper articles and otherwise overwhelming the family at a time when they need to collect themselves and adjust quietly to the grim facts of their child's disease. In addition, community support is usually episodic and inconsistent, which keeps the family off-balance. Perhaps the most damaging type of community involvement—one from which the family must be protected—is the oversolicitous advances of friends, neighbors, and relatives. Instead of being warmly supportive, these individuals often approach the parents in a hand-wringing fashion, offering tearful sympathy and consolation that weakens, not strengthens. Sometimes the child and parents almost have to go into seclusion to maintain their sanity. The physician should be sensitive to this aspect of the family's problem and assist them in whatever way he can. There is no way to completely prevent individuals in the parents' community of friends and relatives from knowing about their child's diagnosis, but every effort should be made to limit the number of persons who are informed about it. This difficulty gradually improves as the parents adjust to their child's problem and the community loses interest in the tragic aspects of the disease.

Religion. In my experience with children dying of cancer, religion has tended to offer little support to the child and his family unless they are very devout. The family's religion has its most significant influence in how it colors their view of death. The physician who appreciates the religious background of the family is better equipped to help them cope with their grief reaction as it is modified by their concept of death. Although effective support from a clergyman or rabbi is uncommon, some unusually gifted individuals do help families through this crisis. Their demeanor or words may bring the family closer to the realization and calm acceptance of impending death. The prudent physician who cares for dying children will seek out capable clergymen to assist him when families can benefit from their help.

REFERENCES

1. AMA drug evaluations, ed. 1, Chicago, 1971, American Medical Association.
2. Easson, W. M.: Care of the young patient who is dying, J.A.M.A. **205**:203-207, 1968.
3. Evans, A. E.: If a child must die. . . . N. Engl. J. Med. **278**:138-142, 1968.
4. Finneson, B. E.: Diagnosis and management of pain syndromes, Philadelphia, 1969, W. B. Saunders Co.
5. Gellis, S. S., and Kagan, B. M.: Current pediatric therapy, vol. 4, Philadelphia, 1970, W. B. Saunders Co.
6. Green, M.: Care of the dying child, Pediatrics **40**:492-497, 1967.
7. Karon, M., and Vernick, J.: An approach to the emotional support of fatally ill children, Clin. Pediatr. **7**:274-280, 1968.
8. Parkes, C. M.: Bereavement and mental illness. Part 2. A classification of bereavement reactions, Br. J. Med. Psychol. **38**:13-26, 1965.
9. Sheldon, A., Ryser, C. P., and Kraut, M. J.: An integrated family orientated cancer care program: the report of a pilot project in the socio-emotional management of chronic disease, J. Chronic Dis. **22**:743-745, 1970.

ADDITIONAL REFERENCES OF RELATED INTEREST

1. Easson, W. M.: The dying child, Springfield, Ill., 1970, Charles C Thomas, Publisher.
2. Kennell, J. H., Slyter, H., and Klaus, M. H.: The mourning response of parents to the death of a newborn infant, N. Engl. J. Med. **283**:344-349, 1970.

3. Klagsbrun, S. C.: Cancer, emotions, and nurses, Am. J. Psychiatry 126:1237-1244, 1970.
4. Koenig, R. R.: Anticipating death from cancer—physician and patient attitudes, Mich. Med. 68:899-905, 1969.
5. Moore, D. C., Holton, C. P., and Marten, G. W.: Psychologic problems in the management of adolescents with malignancy, Clin. Pediatr. 8:464-473, 1969.
6. Schowalter, J. E.: Death and the pediatric house office, J. Pediatr. 76:706-710, 1970.
7. Wiener, J. M.: Attitudes of pediatricians toward the care of fatally ill children, J. Pediatr. 76:700-705, 1970.

CHAPTER 9

Natural history of acute leukemia*

DONALD J. FERNBACH

The emergence of leukemia as one of the most publicized targets of modern medical research is a tribute to the impressive progress made in controlling the common infectious diseases once ranked as the prevailing cause of death among children. Leukemia is the most common malignant disease of prepubertal children and has stimulated increasingly productive medical investigation. The connotation of doom has been dispelled and replaced with a positive attitude based on a demonstrated prolongation of survival and the reasonable expectation that more effective therapy is forthcoming.

DEFINITION

Leukemia is a protean group of diseases of unknown cause that have in common a high fatality rate due to complications of bone marrow failure or infiltration of tissues because of a generalized proliferation of immature or abnormal leukocytes or both.

The bone marrow is presumed to be the site of origin of leukemia, whereas the lymphomas appear to arise in extramedullary sites with involvement of the bone marrow as a secondary or metastatic event. Some of the myelogenous, monocytic, or monomyelogenous leukemias may present with prominent extramedullary tissue infiltration but with an inconclusive bone marrow pattern. This group is responsible for many of the diagnostic problems that confound the clinician. Fortunately for the pediatric diagnostician, atypical cases are uncommon, and the diagnosis of primary acute leukemia can be made easily by aspiration of bone marrow from almost any accessible site.

HISTORICAL ASPECTS

Dameshek and Gunz[34] have credited the first accurate description of leukemia to Velpeau,[139] who examined the body of a 63-year-old florist who died in 1827 after a 2-year illness. The patient had symptoms of abdominal swelling and at autopsy was found to have an enlarged liver and spleen and blood that resembled "laudable pus, mixed with blackish coloring matter, rather than blood."

There is ample reason to believe that leukemia existed as a disease long before the nineteenth century, but an incredible reluctance to use the microscope in clinical medicine probably accounts for its relatively recent discovery. In 1839 Barth sent a specimen of blood obtained at autopsy to Donné, who re-

*The research for this chapter was supported in part by USPH research grants CA-07357 and CA-03161 and the Research Hematology Fund, Texas Children's Hospital.

ported that most of the cells present were "mucous globules."[37, 38] It is probable that Donné later became the first person to examine the blood of a leukemic individual during life; he felt that these "mucous globules" probably represented pus.

In 1845 leukemia was firmly established as a distinct clinical entity by Bennett[7] and by Virchow[141] in independent papers published a month apart. Bennett adhered to the principle that the peculiar changes in the blood represented a "suppuration of the blood," whereas Virchow held the contrary opinion that this phenomenon was not "pyemic." He referred to this as "weisses Blut." Additional case studies were quickly accumulated[28, 55] and by August, 1846, Virchow[142] was convinced that the disease was not the result of a purulent reaction but was due instead to an excess production of the "colorless globules" normally present in the blood. The following year he introduced the term *leukemia,* and in 1856 he presented a summary of the pathology of this disease that, except for his emphasis on a splenic origin, is essentially unchanged to this day.[143-145]

From the available descriptions, most of the early cases appear to have been chronic myelogenous leukemia. The first case report of acute leukemia has been credited to Friedreich[54] in 1857. Again, after this observation other reports quickly appeared, and within 30 years of Velpeau's crude description, the major clinical types and the pathology of leukemia had been described. In 1863 Damon[35] presented a monograph that included what was probably the first published photograph of a child with leukemia.

Neumann's observation,[99, 100] reported in 1870, that the bone marrow was responsible for the formation of leukocytes and that the red blood corpuscles and the white blood corpuscles probably originated from different precursor cells within the marrow was undoubtedly another milestone event. However, Erlich's discovery[41] of cell staining techniques in 1891 made possible a long series of studies of cellular details that are still being evaluated. In spite of the tremendous value of Erlich's work, Dameshek and Gunz[34] commented, "Erlich's stains probably added to rather than relieved the difficulties of classifying the leukemias." Regrettably, as will be seen, this statement is still applicable.

EPIDEMIOLOGY

Incidence. The mortality rate of acute leukemia in children has been scrutinized for a long time and perhaps more so since the beginning of the nuclear age. However, there are innumerable variables in statistical surveys that may contribute to erroneous conclusions, some of which are difficult to reconcile.

Cooke[26] reviewed the mortality rates from 1930 to 1949, based on figures from the vital statistics of the United States Bureau of the Census, and his results suggested a progressive increase in the leukemic mortality rate; however, he noted that the rise was less from 1940 to 1949 than from 1930 to 1940. Because the diagnosis was not dependent on bone marrow examination during this latter period, patients without leukocytosis could have been excluded and patients who presented with unusual complaints might have been misdiagnosed. He concluded that the increase was primarily due to improved diagnostic methods rather than an absolute increase in incidence.

In those countries where the leukemia mortality has been tabulated by the World Health Organization, the apparent trend continued upward from 1940 to 1960.[63] Considerable variation was noted among countries, as well as in geographic areas of the same countries. In 1966 Segi and Kurihara[120] tabulated data accumulated from 24 countries. Among males, Denmark had the highest rate (approximately 8.0/100,000), the United States (whites) was second of 24 countries, and Chile had the lowest rate. Among females, Israel had the highest mortality rate (approximately 6.3/100,000), the United States (whites) was sixth, and Japan had the lowest rate. Obviously, validity of reporting is an important factor in assessing this type of statistic.

In the United States the increased mortality rate among whites of all ages began to level off in 1940 (1955 for nonwhites).[60] In Harris County, Texas, the annual incidence* of leukemia in children 0 to 14 years of age from 1958 to 1970 was 3.86/100,000 children.[103] This figure approximates the United States average. Comparison of age, sex, and race-specific rates show that the leukemia mortality is higher in the northern United States and lower in the southern United States.[147] Comparison by geographic area showed an excessive mortality in the West North Central, Middle Atlantic, and Pacific regions, which is a pattern reflecting three states—Minnesota, New York, and California.[147] These differences appear to correlate with the density of physicians and also with increasing age at death, which suggests that variations in certain aspects of medical practice and care may account for the geographic variations observed. Martin[90] found no difference in the overall death rates relative to the degree of urbanization by studying communities of five different sizes. Observed variations were attributed to the large non-white population in several of the areas involved.[90] However, the discrepancy between white and nonwhite leukemia mortality rates may be largely related to social and economic rather than racial factors.[88] Hewitt[73] similarly reported higher mortalities in the upper as compared with the lower social groups in England.

Age patterns. In a compilation of material obtained from 33 pediatric services, Cooke[25] (1942) described the specific age pattern of childhood leukemia, which is essentially the same as that seen on most leukemia services today. Approximately 40% of 1500 cases occurred in children between 3 and 5 years of age (Fig. 9-1).[25] In their monograph on "Perspectives in the Epidemiology of Leukemia," Kessler and Lilienfeld[79] give reference to Court Brown and Doll[27] for the first recorded peak in the childhood mortality at ages 2 to 4 years in England and Wales during the 1920's. In a detailed examination of mortality data for children under 5 years of age in the United States, Walter and Gilliam[147] (1956) stated that a comparable peak in the mortality was not as obvious among white males until 1931-1941 and not among white females until the later 1940's. Burnet,[21] in reviewing these data, indicated that the first definite age peak in the United States appeared in children born in 1943 and 1944. The disparity between these data and those of Cooke in 1942 probably reflects the statistical methodology applied. This would be academic now except for the possibility that a change in the biologic pattern of the disease might incriminate

---

*In most epidemiology studies statistics are derived from *mortality* rates. The *incidence* data in Harris County are derived from *diagnosis* rather than from death certificates and are therefore presumably more accurate.

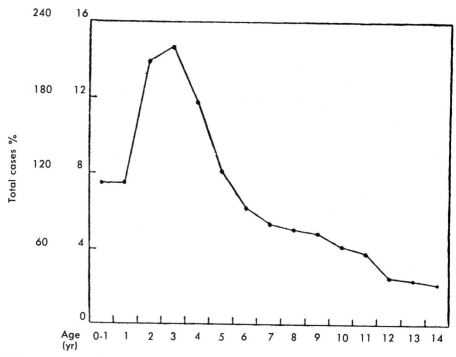

Fig. 9-1. Age incidence of acute leukemia. (From Cooke, J. V.: J.A.M.A. **119**:549, 1942.)

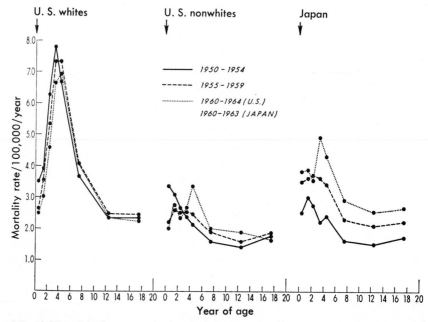

Fig. 9-2. Childhood leukemia mortality rate by age and calendar period in the United States and Japan. (From Fraumeni, J. F., Jr., and Miller, R. W.: J. Natl. Cancer Inst. **38**:597, 1967.)

an environmental leukemogenic agent. Overall childhood leukemia mortality rates by age show a consistent pattern among United States whites over three time periods (Fig. 9-2).[53] During the same time periods there was an interesting change in United States nonwhites and Japanese, both of whom began to develop similar age peaks (between 2 and 6 years of age) during the 1960-1963 period.[53]

The parallel relationship between the peak age of childhood leukemia and that of common childhood infectious diseases stimulated much consideration of the possibility that leukemia might be caused by an infectious agent. This contention has not been supported by analysis of the data.[108] Antecedent infection is commonly associated with the disease, although in most cases the infection may be secondary to the disease, which has not yet been diagnosed. There has been speculation that certain infections may adversely affect the hematopoietic mechanism at an opportune moment. The infrequent occurrence of leukemia and its lack of demonstrated communicability place doubt as to any sole specific infectious origin.[93]

Sex factor. Cooke's series[25] revealed a predominance of boys over girls in all except the first year of life. A definite rise in the proportion of males was noted between 6 and 7 years of age (68.8%) and was maintained with minor fluctuations thereafter through 15 years of age. The predominance of boys over girls after the first year of age has been observed in virtually every series reported.

Ethnic factors. Several reports between 1947 and 1955 indicated that the recorded death rate from leukemia was less frequent among American Negroes than among whites.[59, 110, 117, 121] In a careful study of the ethnic differences in the frequency of leukemia in Brooklyn, New York, and from data collected in an earlier investigation, MacMahon and Koller[88] concluded that the incidence of leukemia among whites and nonwhites was similar. When analyzed, the age-standardized leukemia mortality rate of 1.3:1, white to nonwhite, appeared to relate more to socioeconomic status than to racial factors. They also concluded that the frequency of leukemia death was almost twice as high among the Jewish population as among the non-Jewish population. The difference was constant for acute and chronic myelogenous leukemia and for chronic lymphocytic leukemia, but apparently the data were inadequate to evaluate acute lymphatic leukemia. The factors that may influence such statistics are many. For example, it was noted that the Jewish population was more likely to seek medical care than members of the non-Jewish population. The increased exposure to leukemogenic factors such as x-irradiation, drugs, and possibly other unknown contributory etiologic factors must therefore be considered. No evidence was found to link variations in the occupation, nutrition, or other environmental factors with leukemogenesis.

Leukemia clusters. One of the more popularized leukemia clusters occurred in Niles, Illinois, between the years 1957 and 1960.[69, 118] The observed incidence of acute leukemia in children was five times the expected rate for the population density. Extensive studies, including serologic tests for leukemia antigens, have thus far failed to reveal any common denominator. In most instances clusters have been discovered retrospectively, when detailed statistical evaluation is almost impossible. For this reason, a number of prospective studies have been organized through the United States Public Health Service.[23]* From the results accumulated to date, it is not possible to attribute any significance to reported clusters, which appear to reflect chance phenomenon. However, neither the presence nor absence of clusters eliminates the possibility of a virus relationship with acute leukemia, particularly if there is a long latent incubation period.

The relationship between the incidence of disease and dates of birth has been thoroughly analyzed.[79] The failure of these studies to reveal any periodicity suggests that if a virus is involved in the cause of leukemia in children, it is independent of season or year of birth.[51, 130]

Mortality versus incidence. Because of the effect of modern chemotherapy, there is a growing gap between reported *mortality* data and the actual *incidence* data. This is presently more obvious for some of the solid tumors than for leukemia. Most current studies agree that the 2- to 6-year age group has a better prognosis in terms of the duration of survival and that the *mortality* data (primarily from death certificates) and *incidence* data therefore cannot be viewed as they were prior to the age of chemotherapy. The difference between the actual incidence and the mortality data is shown in Table 9-1.[103] The difference between the true incidence figures in the left column and the mortality figures in the right column reflects the survival rate in a given time period. This is most dramatic with retinoblastoma but is also illustrated by Wilms' tumor and rhabdomyosarcoma. The importance of prospective studies and reliable incidence data is obvious for many reasons, and support for the continuous accumulation of this information is strongly recommended.

---

*The Leukemia Section, Epidemiology Branch, Center for Disease Control, United States Public Health Service. The leukemia surveillance program involves a total population of 10,662,656 in four states (Colorado, Connecticut, Rhode Island, Utah) and four metropolitan areas (Kansas City, Atlanta, Harris County, Texas, Nassau County, New York).

Table 9-1. Malignancy in children: Harris County incidence (1958-1970)* compared with United States mortality (1960-1966)†

| | Cases per 100,000 per year | |
Diagnosis	Harris County	United States
Leukemia	3.72	3.45
Central nervous system tumors	1.85	1.14
Lymphoma	1.25	.54
Neuroblastoma	0.90	.51
Wilms' tumor	0.85	.38
Bone tumor	0.48	.29
Rhabdomyosarcoma	0.27	.16
Retinoblastoma	0.24	.06
Other	1.01	.62
Total‡	10.57	7.15

*Data from O'Connor, D.: Center for Disease Control, 1972.
†Data from Miller, R. W.: Fifty-two forms of childhood cancer: United States mortality experience, 1960-1966, J. Pediatr. **75:**686, 1969.
‡Excludes malignant reticuloendothelioses.

HEREDITY AND FAMILIAL FACTORS

In 1947 Videbaek[140] called attention to the possibility of genetic factors in a study that demonstrated a disproportionate number of leukemic familial aggregates. Although studies on groups of children by Amiotti[5] in 1953 and Steinberg in 1957[131] and 1960[132] failed to support Videbaek's observation, several other studies (not restricted to children) by Stewart[133] in 1961 and by Rigby and associates[113] in 1966 have supported Videbaek's findings. Kessler and Lilienfeld[79] estimate that there have been 100 case reports of familial aggregates of leukemia in the literature. Some involve multiple sibships, and others extend over several generations.

Holton and Johnson[74] reported the first unusual occurrence of chronic myelogenous leukemia in two sets of siblings. Both sets resembled the infantile (Philadelphia chromosome-negative) type of chronic myelogenous leukemia. The occurrence of such a rare entity in two families would tend to support the role of heredity in some instances. The continuing accumulation of case histories of this type accompanied by detailed cytogenetic evaluation and by verification of familial aggregates as they occur may resolve many of the existing doubts.

In an attempt to improve on earlier studies that lacked adequate control groups, Nora[102] surveyed 60 families of children with leukemia and used a control group of well children matched for sex, age range, ethnic group, and socioeconomic background. The results as shown in Table 9-2 reveal a statistically significant difference between the control group and the patient group when the heterogeneous entity of "cancer" is dealt with separately. Acute and chronic myelogenous and acute and chronic lymphatic leukemia were admixed within families. The lack of contact among family members with leukemia is evidence against the direct spread of an infectious agent.[93] Miller[95] has suggested that there is a fourfold risk to the siblings of leukemic children over the population risk. The apparent risk to relatives in Nora's study is approximately the same.

Chromosome defects and leukemia. In 1956 Krivit and Good[81] reported a relationship between Down's syndrome and acute leukemia. In a detailed review Ingalls[76] presented data associating Down's syndrome with older mothers. Subsequent identification of the trisomy 21 defect in Down's syndrome has also been correlated with advanced age of the mother.[135] The report by Stark and Mantel[129] that leukemia mortality increases with maternal age was consistent with these findings except that their data revealed a paradoxical decline in leukemia mortality by increasing birth order. In a more recent evaluation of 802 leukemia deaths in children between 1 and 9 years of age, Fasal[46] concluded

Table 9-2. Number of family members with leukemia or cancer: Texas Children's Hospital Study

	Leukemia group 60 families	Control group 60 families	P
Leukemia	16	4	< 0.05
Other cancer	117	106	> 0.90
Total family members	3273	2909	

that neither birth order nor maternal age had a statistically significant effect on the risk of death from leukemia.

Regardless of these statistical variations, all of which were derived from complicated retrospective analyses, the marked increase of acute leukemia in Down's and in other clinical syndromes associated with chromosomal abnormalities indicates the importance of genetic factors in determining predisposition to acute leukemia[95, 154] (Chapter 2).

Maternal leukemia and pregnancy. In 1953 Harris[67] reviewed 119 cases of leukemia complicating pregnancy; no cases of leukemia occurred in the offspring of these women. The most common type of maternal disease observed in Harris' series of 119 cases was chronic myelogenous leukemia (70), followed by acute myelogenous (30), acute lymphatic (13), chronic lymphocytic (3), and lastly, acute monocytic leukemia (3). Lingeman's review[87] in 1968 included additional cases; however, by then 2 cases of leukemia occurring in infants of leukemic mothers had been reported—the first by Cramblett[29] in 1958 and the second by Bernard in 1964.[9] Cramblett's patient developed acute lymphoblastic leukemia at 9 months of age; the mother had symptoms at about the seventh month of gestation that were suspected in retrospect to represent the onset of lymphatic leukemia, but the diagnosis was not confirmed until 8 days postpartum.[29] Bernard's patient developed acute leukemia at 5 months of age; the mother's diagnosis was made at the time of delivery.[9] If a leukemogenic agent was transmitted vertically, a higher incidence of leukemia would be expected among the offspring of mothers with leukemia, but this has not been observed. In one of the groups reviewed by Lingeman, 34 of 48 babies of leukemic mothers survived the neonatal period, and some were observed for as long as 18 years. None developed leukemia, and no evidence of leukemia was found in 12 autopsied babies of the 14 who died. The time of onset of leukemia varied considerably during these pregnancies; all morphologic types of leukemia were observed; and the nonspecific mortality rate of the infants of these mothers was high.[87]

Neonatal leukemia. Although relatively rare, neonatal leukemia is of particular importance in the study of leukemogenesis. If an infectious agent is involved in the cause of leukemia, the occurrence of the disease would limit the possible incubation time to 9 months. The prospect of coning down on the causative factors places emphasis on quick recognition and diagnosis of the illness in the newborn. This must be approached cautiously because the hematopoietic system of the newborn is extremely labile, and leukemoid responses are relatively common.

In a review of the literature in 1950, Taylor and Geppert[134] found only 16 cases of "verified congenital leukemia." All except 1 were myelogenous. In 1957 Pierce[108] brought this number up to 22 and also identified the emerging pattern of association of neonatal leukemia with Down's syndrome and other congenital defects. Since it is now known that rubella and other virus infections of the mother can infect the fetus with resultant congenital malformations, including hematologic abnormalities, this observation supports the possibility that a viral factor could be involved in leukemogenesis. In a 1967 report of a child with congenital leukemia who had chromosome abnormalities, Zussman and associates[155] increased the number of reported neonatal leukemia cases to at least 50, all of which had acute leukemia. In evaluating the neonatal leukemias, it is difficult to omit speculation on the role of viruses and the relationship with chromosomal defects, acquired or inherited.

Twinning. The occurrence of disease in an identical twin is an established means of evaluating the importance of heredity and environment. From Mac-Mahon and Levy's study,[89] the *risk* of the identical twin of a leukemic proband developing leukemia is 25%. Seventy-seven cases of leukemia were found in 72 twin sets. Of the 5 pairs in which both twins had the disease, all were of like sex and presumed to be monozygous. All had acute leukemia—2 pairs had acute lymphatic, 1 pair had acute myeloid, and 2 pairs were unclassified. In 2 pairs the onset was simultaneous; in the others the intervals between diagnoses were 3, 12, and 21 months. Because this was a retrospective study, the determination of zygosity was mostly circumstantial. A collaborative prospective study in which the zygosity of the twins and the diagnosis of leukemia are precisely established would be a significant contribution.[106] The use of mixed lymphocyte cultures appears to have value in this respect, since cells from normal identical twins do not interact. Thus far, this technique has been applied unsuccessfully in 4 sets of twins in a search for tumor-specific antigen when one of the twins in each set had leukemia.[115] With equivalent environmental influences, differences between monozygotic or between dizygotic twins might help define the role of genetics, and careful studies of these patients may eventually aid in the identification of a leukemogenic agent.

Leukemia susceptibles. It is now apparent that there are individuals in the general population who are at greater risk than others for developing leukemia. These "leukemia susceptibles" are listed in Table 9-3.[95] It is not possible to dismiss the role of heredity because some genetic aberrations have been associated with a higher incidence of leukemia. Other genetic factors appear to be of acquired rather than of inherited origin. By avoiding classic Mendelian patterns and by not restricting the search to a single causative factor, the possible interaction of genetic and environmental factors can be viewed with greater flexibility. The interaction of multiple factors is reinforced by the report of Gibson and

Table 9-3. Groups at exceptionally high risk of leukemia*

Group	Approximate risk	Time interval
Identical twins of children with leukemia	1 in 5†	Weeks or months
Radiation-treated polycythemia vera	1 in 6	10-15 years
Bloom's syndrome	1 in 8‡	< 30 years of age
Hiroshima survivors who were within 1000 meters of the hypocenter	1 in 60	12 years
Down's syndrome	1 in 95	< 10 years of age
Radiation-treated patients with ankylosing spondylitis	1 in 270	15 years
Sibs of leukemic children	1 in 720	10 years
U. S. Caucasian children < 15 years of age	1 in 2880	10 years

*From Miller, R. W.: Persons with exceptionally high risk of leukemia, Cancer Res. 27:2420, 1967.

†Of 22 identical twins with leukemia, the co-twin was affected in five instances.

‡Three leukemics among 23 persons with Bloom's syndrome.

associates,[58] who studied the risk of developing acute leukemia in children 1 to 4 years of age. Four factors were evaluated: (1) mother's irradiation before conception, (2) in utero irradiation of the child, (3) previous history of reproductive wastage, and (4) early childhood viral diseases. The children exposed to all four factors had the highest risk, which was 4.64 times that of the nonexposed group. The risk for leukemia was significantly greater only when there was concordance of the two types of events—irradiation and some pathologic insult. Henceforth, it would be more productive to consider a multifactorial inheritance scheme in which leukemia is the result of an interaction between hereditary or genetic predisposition and environmental influences.[102]

The report of Fialkow and associates,[50] who infused HL-A–matched bone marrow cells of a brother into his 16-year-old sister who had acute leukemia, is of great importance. Leukemic cells reappeared 62 days after the transplant, but cytogenetic studies showed that the leukemic cells were the *male donor* cells. Among the possibilities to explain this result, the activation of a leukemogenic agent (i.e., virus) in susceptible donor cells or the transfer of an agent from host to donor cells must be considered. The implication of this study relative to the pathogenesis of acute leukemia is obvious.

As stated in Chapter 2, the cause of leukemia is unknown and although patterns of susceptibility are being identified, the role of viruses in human leukemia is still unproved. A detailed discussion on the academic question as to whether leukemia is a true neoplastic disorder is given by Dameshek and Gunz in their book, *Leukemia*.[34] At this time the majority of pathologists, hematologists, and oncologists appear content to consider this disease to be neoplastic.

CLASSIFICATION

In the period after the introduction of tissue staining techniques by Erlich,[41] a number of names were proposed to describe the different clinical syndromes of leukemia. Acute leukemia has been traditionally divided into three classic groups: lymphatic, myelocytic, and monocytic. Each title, regardless of the synonym used, implies a specific cell of origin. In children with acute leukemia, 50% to 100% of the initial bone marrow cells may be primitive and poorly differentiated. Subdivision into specific cellular types has resulted in considerable controversy, and there is no universally accepted nomenclature. Since it is apparent that the morphologic diagnosis is of some value in prognosis, the need for a consistent and common classification has become increasingly important. For these reasons, no attempt will be made to offer another method of classification here. The reader is simply advised to consider leukemia in children as a nosologic entity and to view the commonly used nomenclature as a subjective conclusion derived from the experience and judgment of the observer. Even the time-honored differentiation between *acute* ("blastic") and *chronic* ("differentiated") leukemia, although not difficult to make, reflects obsolete terminology. Many of the typical "chronic leukemias" have undergone blastic transformation, and the patients have died within weeks of diagnosis, whereas many of the "acute" leukemia patients have survived in excess of 5 years. Chronic myelogenous leukemia is discussed in Chapter 12.

Although several cases of chronic lymphocytic leukemia have been listed by Shimkin[122] and Dale,[33] this disease is virtually nonexistent in children.

Table 9-4 shows a comparison of the distribution of cases during the first decade of chemotherapy.[33, 108, 137] Table 9-5 shows a more current review of greater numbers of patients from groups participating in large chemotherapy programs.[52, 109] In the majority of current clinical studies the distinction is essentially made between "acute lymphoid leukemia" and "acute nonlymphoid leukemia." The terms *lymphatic, lymphocytic, lymphoblastic, lymphoid,* and *lymphoblastoid* are generally used synonomously, and acute stem cell or acute unclassified (undifferentiated) leukemia has also been accepted by many hematologists as the same disease type. Similarly, the terms *granulocytic, myelocytic, myelogenous,* and *myeloblastic* have been used synonomously, except that in many cases myelomonocytic, erythrocytic, and monocytic leukemias have been lumped together as one group. The rarities referred to as *eosinophilic, basophilic,* or *megakaryocytic* leukemia have been excluded from mention here.

The persistent inconsistency in Tables 9-4 and 9-5 is obvious and is not a reflection on the integrity of the investigators, who are aware of the problem, but an illustration of the depth and the effect of the problem. Several of the groups have omitted use of the term *stem cell* in the lymphoid category and the term *monomyelogenous* in the nonlymphoid category. However, these are minor variations when the differences in the percentages of acute myelogenous leukemia are compared. None of these methods of classification permits a direct comparison of the results of treatment programs between research units. Engaging the problem, Fraumeni[52] reported the results of a review of 1200 cases from the Children's Cancer Research Foundation based on a classification schema included in the article, which revealed fewer stem cell or unclassified leukemias and more myelogenous forms than either of the other two groups. When the cases were classified and correlated with survival patterns, the unclassified group had a survival pattern midway between the relatively favorable lymphatic leu-

Table 9-4. Acute leukemia in children: comparison of morphologic classification by major groups in prechemotherapy and early chemotherapy eras

Classification	Dale—1949[33] (72 cases)		Tivey—1954[137] (445 cases)		Pierce—1957[108] (232 cases)	
Lymphoid*	64%		80%		84%	
Lymphatic	—			70%	—	
Stem cell		64%	—			84%
Unclassified	—			10%	—	
Nonlymphoid*	32%		20%		16%	
Myelogenous (granulocytic)		31%	15%			6%
Monomyelogenous	—		—		—	
Monocytic		1%	5%			5%
Erythroleukemia	—		—		—	
Leukosarcoma	—		—			4%
Reticuloendothelial	—		—			1%
Chronic	4%		—		—	
Myeloid		3%	—		—	
Lymphocytic		1%	—		—	

*Arbitrary groups that conform to most current chemotherapy group divisions.

Table 9-5. Acute leukemia in children: recent comparison of morphologic classification by cooperative chemotherapy study groups

Classification	CCSG-A—1969[109] (1770 cases)		SWCCSG— 1970 (745 cases*)		Children's Cancer Research Foundation— 1971 (1200 cases†)
Lymphoid	78%		86%		68%
Acute lymphocytic		44%		54%	44%
Acute stem cell		—		16%	—
Acute unclassified		34%		16%	24%
Nonlymphoid	19%		13%		32%
Acute myelogenous (granulocytic)		8%		9%	24%
Acute monomyelogenous		—		2%	—
Acute monocytic		8%		2%	8%
Acute erythroleukemia		1%		—	—
Acute leukosarcoma		2%		—	—
Acute reticuloendothelial		—		—	—
Chronic myelogenous	1%	1%	—	—	— —
Classification not stated	2%	2%	1%	1%	— —

*Chronic myelogenous leukemia and patients with primary diagnosis of lymphosarcoma excluded. Also excluded were 271 patients of one institution that did not make specific cytologic diagnoses.
†Acute leukemia types only; 133 with the initial diagnosis of lymphosarcoma were excluded.

Table 9-6. Median survival times of children with acute leukemia in England and Wales (1963-1967)*

Region†	All cases		Lymphocytic		Myelocytic		Not specified	
	Number of cases	Median‡	Number of cases	Median	Number of cases	Median	Number of cases	Median
A	29	25	20	41	8	1	1	68
B	41	23	21	23	16	21	4	7
C	174	25	106	27	59	20	9	2
D	51	23	40	26	10	15	1	26
E	71	22	47	27	9	7	15	16
F	243	26	174	28	51	24	18	10
G	70	29	47	33	21	16	2	21
H	85	25	68	26	15	8	2	1
I	48	25	37	32	8	17	3	6
J	167	28	103	32	55	23	9	11
K	46	22	28	33	16	20	2	22
Total	1025	26	691	29	268	18	66	11
Study group	220	64	188	71	31	17	1	16

*From Committee on Leukaemia and the Working Party on Leukaemia in Childhood: Duration of survival of children with acute leukaemia, Br. Med. J. 4:7-9, 1971.
†Excluding study group.
‡Median = median survival time in weeks.

kemia and the relatively unfavorable myelogenous leukemia, a fact that they were unable to reconcile. With conventional terminology, the acute lymphocytic group also showed a taller age peak when compared to either of the other groups mentioned. Table 9-6 shows the variations in the reporting from 11 different registries in England and Wales.[2] The influence these variations would have on statistical evaluation of the survival time requires no discussion.

In separate studies to determine the comparable accuracy of participating hematologists, Lee from Acute Leukemia Cooperative Group B and Thurman from the Pediatric Division of the Southwest Cancer Chemotherapy Study Group (SWCCSG) circulated slides for diagnosis by different investigators.[84, 136] The results of the two studies were similar. The cytologic characterization of acute leukemia in Group B had a reproduciblity of about 70%. This improved to 90% by applying a set of cytologic characteristics to separate acute leukemia into only two groups, which fit the consensus diagnosis of either acute lymphatic or acute myeloid leukemia.

In 1963, Gunz and Burry[66] noted that the authors of the seventh revision of the *International Causes of Death* accepted the diagnostic problems associated with these diseases and merely provided one category for all forms of acute leukemia, excluding acute monocytic leukemia and erythroleukemia (erythraemia, Di Guglielmo's disease). These authors agreed with others, however, in demonstrating that there was a difference in the survival according to cell type. Those classified as having myelogenous leukemia lived for shorter periods than did the others.

Mathé,[91] who heads the World Health Organization Reference Center for Leukemia, has proposed a totally new subdivision of acute leukemia based on the initial diagnostic bone marrow material prepared with Giemsa staining. Although the data are not adequate for statistical analysis, he has proposed subdivision within each cell line based on the degree of differentiation. This includes a myeloblastic-lymphoblastic variety of granulocytic leukemia that reportedly has a survival curve falling between the more differentiated prolymphocytic and granulocytic leukemias. Another aspect of Mathé's work is that the classification of each case derives not from the gross pattern of the smears but from the percentage of the different types of blasts present. In support of this concept he presents data to show the apparent disappearance of one cell line and the emergence of another in the same patient at a later time. In our own patients there have been numerous instances in which the cells of the marrow in relapse were different than the original cells.

Acute monocytic leukemia is a rare entity in children. Mathé omitted discussion of this in his article because few cases had been studied. The monoblast and the myeloblast are difficult to differentiate, and the clinical compromise is to use the term *myelomonocytic* or *monomyelocytic* leukemia, which suggests that the leukemia process involves two completely separate cell lines. This concept caused Osgood[104] to remark that, "while this is theoretically possible, the picture is far too frequent for this explanation to be plausible." It was his opinion that most of these cases actually represented acute monocytic leukemia. To aid in the differential diagnosis, he suggested the use of the peroxidase stain, phase microscopic examination for promonocytic motility, tissue culture of the blood, and tissue biopsy other than bone marrow, if possible.[16] The urine muramidase (lysozyme) level may have some value, but it is not consistently elevated in either mono-cytic or monomyelocytic leukemia.[105, 109, 151]

The use of cytochemical techniques—PAS, Sudan black, peroxidase, aryl sulfatase, and various naphthol esterase compounds—has failed to show spec-ificity.[68, 80] Abbrederis and associates[1] reported a high correlation of acute lymphocytic leukemia with a positive PAS reaction, a correlation of acute mye-logenous leukemia with Sudan black positivity, and a correlation of acute mono-cytic leukemia with various naphthol esterase reactions, but none of the reactions are absolute. Boysen[15] failed to confirm the work of Lawrinson and Gross[82] and Ekert and Denett[40] with aryl sulfatase.

After reviewing a consecutive series of 170 children and adolescents with acute leukemia from Leukemia Group B, Lee now believes that a continuous quantitative relationship exists between certain characteristics (amount of cyto-plasm, azurophilic granules, nucleoli, and chromatin) and that these interrelation-ships may provide a better model for prognosis than the traditional lympho-blast-myeloblast differentiation.[83] From the trend in the current literature, this view is gaining support.[8, 52, 66, 98, 122]

It is difficult to account for long-term remissions and survival in some chil-dren with myelogenous or monocytic leukemia, regardless of the therapy. It is no less difficult to account for short-term responses in children with acute lymphocytic leukemia. Unknown individual variables obviously play an im-portant role in each case. Generalizations regarding prognosis may still be made on the basis of morphologic diagnosis, but this is less than adequate in the direct confrontation between the clinician and a given child with leukemia.

CLINICAL CONSIDERATIONS, DIAGNOSIS, AND DIFFERENTIAL DIAGNOSIS

At the risk of oversimplification, the clinical features of typical primary acute leukemia may be summarized as follows: (1) bone marrow failure due to dis-placement of the normal hematopoietic elements by leukemic cells and (2) infiltration of other tissues by leukemic cells that have been released from, or proliferate outside of the bone marrow. The consequences of bone marrow failure depend on the severity of involvement but are the same, regardless of the cause: (1) *anemia* due to inadequate erythrocyte production, (2) *infection* due to inadequate neutrophil production, and (3) *bleeding* due to inadequate platelet production. Excursion of leukemic cells from the marrow or proliferation of these cells outside the marrow may result in elevated peripheral leukocyte counts or selective infiltration of almost any tissue of the body or both. Most commonly, the organs of the reticuloendothelial system are involved with re-sultant hepatomegaly, splenomegaly, and lymphadenopathy. Because of the po-tential ability to infiltrate all types of tissues, acute leukemia has to be considered as another of the classic "great imitators," in which the diagnosis depends on the astuteness of the clinician who makes few assumptions and maintains a high index of suspicion.

Perhaps the most significant factor in the modern approach to diagnosis is that clinicians more frequently request an early examination of bone marrow. Hence an awareness of the behavioral patterns of acute leukemia has resulted in the prompt diagnosis of many cases in which the diagnosis might have been significantly delayed 30 years ago. Dating the actual onset of the disease in a given case is not possible and probably will not be until the etiologic factor(s) are identified. Furthermore, the actual time of onset has become less important to therapists because the duration of the illness prior to starting therapy seems to have relatively little influence on the response to treatment. The incidence of the usual presenting symptoms is given in Table 9-7.

Presenting patterns of disease. The symptomatology of acute leukemia varies little with the cell type. The most common complaints that bring the child to the physician are *fever, pallor, purpura,* and/or *pain.* The onset may be insiduous or abrupt, and children may present with any or all of these complaints in varying degrees of severity. In many cases the symptoms date back only a few days, but in others they may have been present weeks or months before medical attention was sought. In the extreme case the onset may be fulminant, with high temperature, marked prostration, anemia, vague or localized aches and pains, and numerous petechiae or ecchymoses. The rapidity with which these symptoms progress varies greatly. In our experience the child is usually first seen with relatively few symptoms or physical findings, but this will depend on the type of referral and the type of institution.

Children seem to tolerate chronic anemia with fewer symptoms than do adults, but in acute blood loss the characteristic symptoms of tachycardia, air hunger, apprehension, restlessness, and thirst may be the same. In impending shock the pulse rate is one of the most important vital signs to monitor because it will rise long before any change occurs in the blood pressure. Restlessness is often overlooked in small children whose behavior after admission may be attributed mistakenly to the psychologic effects of the changed environment. Epistaxis is not uncommon when the child is severely thrombocytopenic, and many children will swallow varying amounts of blood while lying in bed. Swallowed blood is nauseating, and vomiting may follow. The psychologic effect of hematemesis on the child and parents can be profound. Intestinal bleeding may result in melena, grossly bloody, foul-smelling stools, and diarrhea, depending on the rate of blood loss. Digested blood may cause considerable flatus and gaseous distention.

Agranulocytic infection may develop rapidly in the presence of extreme neutropenia. Because of the availability of platelet transfusions the number of

Table 9-7. Frequency of the more common presenting complaints

Finding	Percent
Fever	61
Pallor	55
Hemorrhage	52
Anorexia	33
Fatigue	30
Bone pain	23
Abdominal pain	19
Joint pain	15
Lymphadenopathy	15
Weight loss	13

early deaths due to hemorrhage has been reduced. Most of the deaths that occur during the first few days of hospitalization now are probably due to agranulo-cytic septicemia. In the absence of neutrophils the normal surface bacterial flora of the entire gastrointestinal tract, the upper respiratory passages, and the skin may become aggressive pathogens. In a defenseless host the absence of neutro-phils may result in unrecognized infection that would have been quickly identi-fied in the presence of a normal purulent response. The gingivae may lose their normal sheen and appear swollen, dull gray, or erythematous. Bacterial invasion of the membranes lining the upper airway often results in an irritation that causes the young child to pick at lips or nose with resultant abrasions that may bleed because of the accompanying thrombocytopenia. Epistaxis is not uncom-mon if the area of irritation involves the nasal mucocutaneous junction. A bron-chial cough and rhonchi may develop, both of which may be aggravated if there are enlarged hilar lymph nodes. Many children complain of vague abdominal pain, presumably due to areas of inflammation or nodal involvement within the intestinal tract. Some children may complain of pain during attempted defeca-tion as the result of proctitis. These latter lesions are not easy to visualize unless the perianal area is examined carefully by everting the anorectal area in order to visualize the mucocutaneous junction. Any break in the skin is a potential opening for bacterial invasion; it is therefore not unusual to see paronychia, infected insect bites, or agranulocytic cellulitis secondary to minor abrasions. Deep infection may be seen in the sites of intramuscular injections where medi-cations were administered prior to diagnosis. At this stage the peripheral blood counts and physical findings are almost universally abnormal, although there are marked variations from child to child.

A computer analysis of the presenting characteristics of children seen by participating members of the SWCCSG is shown in Table 9-8.[56] Note that in

Table 9-8. Presenting characteristics of 1024 patients with acute leukemia (1958-1971) in the Southwest Cancer Chemotherapy Study Group

Characteristic	Percent	Characteristic	Percent
Age (yr)		Blasts (%)	
< 2	14	< 65	25
2-5	47	65-84	22
6-10	24	85-94	28
≥ 11	15	95 or more	25
WBC (/mm³)		Platelets (/mm³)	
< 10	34	< 20	29
10-24	25	20-49	23
25-49	22	50-99	20
≥ 50	19	100 or more	29
Hemoglobin (grams/100 ml)		Liver enlarged	79
< 7	44	Spleen enlarged	69
7-11	43	Nodes (cervical) enlarged	62
> 11	14	Nodes (inguinal) enlarged	54
Sex (males)	57	Nodes (axillary) enlarged	47
Race (white)	85		
Hemorrhage (yes)	48		

59% of the cases the leukocyte count was below 25,000/mm³ and that 34% of the patients had white cell counts below 10,000/mm³. Leukopenia is a characteristic feature of leukemia in children and does not reflect a different disease (commonly referred to in the past as *aleukemic leukemia*). In our own series of 398 patients, 205 (51%) had leukocyte counts below 10,000/mm³; the hemoglobin level was normal in 15%; and the platelet count was normal (over 100,000/mm³) in 29%. On occasion, children presenting with a complaint such as pain may have normal peripheral blood counts and normal leukocyte differentials when first seen.

It can be seen that hepatosplenomegaly is a more consistent clinical feature than lymphadenopathy. The significance of this has never been clear, particularly for lymphocytic leukemia, although it is now possible to speculate that the involved cell is of bone marrow origin, a concept that has been given credibility by the work of Wilson and Nossal[150] regarding the "t" and "b" lymphocytes. As with the peripheral blood findings, it is worth emphasizing that children may present without any abnormal physical findings.[56]

Of the 398 patients seen on our service, 25 presented with fever of unknown origin in the absence of any other clinical features of leukemia. The diagnosis was established by examination of the bone marrow. Six children admitted with confirmed septicemia were found to have leukemia only after they failed to respond to appropriate antibiotic therapy. Five children were seen with central nervous system complaints and were found to have leukemia after examination of the cerebrospinal fluid revealed a predominance of mononuclear cells. One child who had meningococcal meningitis and died within 24 hours of admission was found to have acute leukemia at necropsy. Three children admitted for evaluation of severe recurrent epistaxis in the presence of normal platelet counts were found to have leukemia after becoming neutropenic.

Eighteen other children were evaluated for bone pain associated with specific radiologically visible bone lesions. One was thought to have had osteomyelitis because of swelling and induration over the area of involved bone; the others had a presumptive diagnosis of rheumatoid arthritis. None of these children had other obvious evidence of leukemia, and the diagnosis was made only after examination of the bone marrow. Because of the high frequency with which these children present with arthralgia (up to 10%), rheumatoid arthritis is a common differential diagnosis.

Diagnosis. The diagnosis of acute leukemia is not usually difficult to establish. The bone marrow is often hypercellular with 60% to 100% blast cells. Scattered normal myeloid or erythroid precursors may be seen, most likely residua of the previously normal marrow. Megakaryocytes are usually absent but occasionally will be the only residual normal appearing cells amid a sea of blast forms. Based on criteria stated later, a minimum of 25% blast cell forms is considered adequate to establish the diagnosis, but this is commonly an all-or-none diagnosis, and the pattern is obvious. Abnormal cells are usually found in the peripheral blood, but this is an area fraught with errors in judgment, since bizarre mononuclear cells are not infrequently seen in the peripheral blood of children with viral illnesses. If blasts or unidentified cells are encountered in the peripheral blood, the diagnosis should be confirmed or documented by bone marrow examination, regardless of other findings. It is a fallacy that a blood transfusion will alter the bone marrow pattern. However, it is preferable to withhold therapy whenever possible until a positive diagnosis is established. Most importantly, chemotherapy should not be started until the diagnosis has been proved.

In rare instances the diagnosis of myelogenous, monocytic, or other atypical leukemia may be difficult if the bone marrow is not clearly blastic or if the marrow is too densely packed to aspirate with a needle. When a needle aspiration of the marrow is unsuccessful and all factors point to leukemia, it may be worthwhile to obtain an open surgical bone biopsy or to biopsy the tissue that appears to be involved. Discussion of leukemia variants is continued in Chapter 12.

Most hematologists have records on patients who have some type of "preleukemic" disorder. Depending on the situation and the parents, it is advisable to at least alert them of the ultimate possibility of leukemia. This is particularly important in any case in which the bone marrow is hypoplastic or aplastic and possibly also in those cases with unexplained megaloblastic changes. These cases are rare, and in our experience the time interval between suspected disease and confirmed disease has been as long as 2 years. Leukopenia with chronic neutropenia may also terminate in classic leukemia, and the same precautions about warning the family should be given considertion. "Improvement" that might result from the use of corticosteroid therapy sometimes creates a false sense of success until the "remission" terminates with leukemia. Thus the apparently favorable response in such a situation may actually presage a bad prognosis.

On occasion a child may present with hematologic abnormalities that defy diagnosis by all techniques. In such cases it is often wise to withhold specific therapy and to observe the child at regular intervals until some change in the clinical condition forces action. Fortunately, such cases are most uncommon.

COMPLICATIONS

The complications that stem from bone marrow failure require little comment beyond mentioning that productivity of the three major hematopoietic tissues involved may vary in the extreme from case to case. As in other conditions such as aplastic anemia, the level of thrombocytopenia may or may not correlate with the degree of capillary fragility or observed bleeding. Some children with platelet counts below $10,000/mm^3$ may have no capillary fragility, whereas others may be severely purpuric at higher levels. Coexisting infection is an influencing factor, and bleeding is usually more profound in the presence of systemic infection. On occasion, particularly in more advanced disease, disseminated intravascular coagulation may contribute to the hemorrhagic diathesis; therefore it is wise to evaluate the prothrombin time, partial thromboplastin time, fibrinogen level, and the level of fibrinogen-split products whenever this possibility is suspected. Hypoprothrombinemia may follow prolonged antibiotic therapy, any cause for malabsorption, and hepatic parenchymal damage from chemotherapy and may result in bleeding in the absence of thrombocytopenia. A therapeutic dose of vitamin K (also diagnostic) will usually result in a prompt response in these cases.

Fever occurring in a child with acute leukemia should be considered the result of infection, regardless of the presence or absence of clinical findings and particularly when associated with neutropenia.[48, 123] Infection is the most common and most serious complication of leukemia. The administration of *bacteriostatic* antimicrobial agents such as the tetracyclines may enhance the overgrowth of fungal organisms, which often results in severe esophagitis with dysphagia and substernal pain.[39] Mediastinitis invariably follows perforation of the esophagus. As has been mentioned in Chapter 7, *bactericidal* therapy should be used whenever possible.[48]

Viral infections occurring during active disease or aggressive antileukemic therapy, which is also immunosuppressive, may be overwhelming, particularly with varicella, vaccinia, rubeola, herpes simplex, cytomegalovirus, and herpes zoster.* As mentioned in Chapter 7, all live virus vaccinations are contraindicated in these patients. Varicella, rubeola, and other virus infections are not invariably fatal, but the illness may be markedly prolonged. In the two former conditions, severe pneumonia or encephalitis may occur as terminal events. Complications may occur weeks or months after the primary infection.

The immunoglobulin levels, as measured during the course of acute leukemia, have shown an immediate drop in IgG, IgM, and IgA during the induction phase, with gradual return to normal or slightly subnormal levels thereafter.[62, 112] Gooch[62] has shown that children with leukemia are capable of response to infection even during relapse.

It seems reasonable to assume that the interaction of many factors accounts for the decreased resistance of leukemic patients to severe infection in advanced disease.[72] Relative malnutrition or debilitation, quantitative reduction of the bone marrow reserve, and the immunosuppressive effects of chemotherapy undoubtedly contribute to reduced host resistance, but prolonged depression of the absolute neutrophil count below 500 cells/mm³ is probably the single most important factor.

It is not possible to exclude the simultaneous development of leukemia in the marrow and in extramedullary organs of children with leukemia. However, the general behavioral pattern suggests that involvement of tissues other than bone marrow most likely reflects infiltration in the metastatic sense.[101] Infiltration of many organs may occur during periods when the bone marrow is in complete remission. Problems of managing extramedullary leukemic involvement of organs such as the central nervous system, peripheral nervous system, testes, ovaries, kidneys, skin, and gastrointestinal tract are discussed separately in Chapter 11. Involvement of the breasts is uncommon and usually occurs only in adolescent or pubescent girls.

The occurrence of extramedullary disease has been investigated during life and at autopsy. It appears to be occurring with greater frequency as the life-span of the leukemic child is extended. A postmortem study by Nies and associates[101] revealed that 10 of 15 patients without evidence of bone marrow involvement had evidence of leukemia elsewhere. The kidney and liver were the most commonly involved organs; all but two patients had involvement in more than one site. In an in vivo study by Mathé,[92] multiple biopsies of the bone marrow, liver, kidneys, and testicles were obtained, and examinations of the cerebrospinal

---

*References 22, 57, 78, 97, 124, 138.

fluid and skeleton were made. Of the 31 patients evaluated during a period of clinical "complete remission," 12 (38%) had loci of leukemic cells in one or more sites outside the marrow. In our experience gonadal or renal involvement is common, although symptoms are rare; occasionally the involvement is sufficient to cause loss of function or discomfort, and radiotherapy is required for relief. We have biopsy documentation in one case in which a bizarre infiltration of the liver occurred during bone marrow remission and was similarly treated by irradiation. The liver enlarged so quickly that it was thought at first that the child had a hepatic vein thrombosis. Pericardial tamponade and myocardial infiltration have been reported as presenting complaints in rare cases.[77, 114] A 7-week-old infant who presented with priapism had myelogenous leukemia.[64]

In our series several children presented with unilateral or bilateral proptosis similar to neuroblastoma; other children with leukemic involvement of the conjunctiva have been seen, as well as others with retinal hemorrhage and presumed retinal infiltrates. Infiltration involving almost all areas of the eye has been reported, and it is possible that many lesions have been missed because of the difficulty in examining the eyes in small children. Allen and Straatsma[3] report ocular involvement of various types in 38 (50%) of 76 patients who died of leukemia or related disorders. Retinal hemorrhage is probably the most frequent ocular complication.

Manifestations related to the bones and joints are frequent in children. Migratory joint pains combined with leukemic involvement of the heart or with cardiac symptoms secondary to anemia or lymphadenopathy may be mistaken for rheumatic fever.[127] Commonly, the bone and joint pains are migratory, vague, and without associated areas of swelling or inflammation. Many of these cases fail to show roentgenographic changes. Conversely, changes are frequently seen in the absence of bone or joint pain during the evaluation of children known to have leukemia. The vague bone pain described by some children has been assumed to be the result of encroachment of the bone marrow space by leukemic cells. This type of pain may disappear dramatically after starting therapy. The characteristic intramedullary pain that occurs during the sudden aspiration of bone marrow in normal children is frequently absent in children with leukemia, although it usually returns during remission. This pain typically radiates down the sciatic nerve distribution if the posterior iliac spine is used as the site of aspiration.

The radiologic features of leukemia are variable, but several features are characteristic: osteolytic lesions involving the medullary cavity and cortex, subperiosteal new bone formation along the ribs and long bones, transverse bands of rarefication at the metaphyses of the long bones, and, rarely, osteosclerotic lesions with or without osteolytic lesions. Bone lesions, although not diagnostic, are found in over half the children with leukemia at the time of diagnosis. Curtis,[31] using panoramic radiographs, has shown abnormalities of the jaw in 62.9% of 214 children examined.

Involvement of almost every portion of the intestinal tract has been reported. Al-Rashid and Harned[4] recently wrote about a 12-year-old boy with presumed esophageal infiltration that caused dysphagia but resolved promptly after radiotherapy. Others have described infiltration lesions of the small intestine, appendix, and colon[44, 111] and selective infection of the cecum.[146] One of our patients died of infection as the result of marked debilitation attributed to malabsorption, which was explained at postmortem examination by multiple infiltrates in the small intestine in spite of complete bone marrow and peripheral blood remission.

Leukemic involvement of the lungs is rarely of significance. Bodey found microscopic infiltrates in 66% of 50 cases, which included 20 children less than 10 years of age.[14] The peribronchiolar and peribronchial areas were the most commonly involved. In 2 cases (age not stated) the lesion, which was big enough to be visible to the naked eye, appeared to consist of a mass of leukemic cells occluding the lumen of a vessel. Perivascular infiltrates were seen with greater frequency in patients with acute myelogenous leukemia.

Because of interest in the role of the thymus, Gilmartin[61] reviewed the radiographs of children with acute leukemia and found an "abnormal thymic shadow" in 15%. The diagnosis was not confirmed other than by radiographs, but 5 of 12 patients with apparent thymic enlargement reportedly had an abnormal thymic shadow before the peripheral blood changes occurred.

The increasing incidence of central nervous system involvement (CNS) in children is one of the apparent changes in the natural history of the disease that seem to relate directly to the increased duration of remission and increased survival time. In a study of leukemic children treated from 1944-1948, Evans reported a 10% incidence of CNS complications.[42] In 1945 Leidler and Russell[86] found microscopic or gross evidence of leukemic involvement of the CNS in 83% of the patients autopsied, but only 35% had shown symptoms of involvement during life. In 1970 the overall incidence of symptomatic CNS involvement was 51% of 209 children in Children's Cancer Study Group A.[43] According to Evans the incidence was 56% in patients with acute lymphocytic leukemia and 25% for those with other forms of leukemia. Further details on the diagnosis and treatment of what has became one of the most common complications of childhood leukemia are discussed in Chapter 11.

Pleocytosis occurring during the course of acute leukemia is presumed to be due to leukemic infiltration of the leptomeninges. CNS complications were observed in 795 of 5788 leukemia and lymphoma patients of all ages reviewed by Williams, Diamond, and Craver.[149] Of these, only 23 represented infectious meningitis. The possibility of infection has to be considered in each case, despite the low frequency with which it is observed. A case of mumps meningoencephalitis was reported by Rupprecht and Naiman,[116] a case of group D streptococcal meningitis has been reported,[126] and one of our patients had meningococcal meningitis. If the patient is only capable of mounting a "blastic" cellular response, an infectious meningitis might be unrecognized because of the absence of polys. In many instances of "tumor" meningitis the cerebrospinal fluid glucose will be low, and the protein will be elevated. To evaluate the differential diagnosis, a study was conducted on our service during 1969.[49] Seventy-seven specimens of cerebrospinal fluid were obtained from 32 children with acute leukemia at the time of diagnosis, at intervals during remission, and during relapse. During the year, seventeen episodes of CNS leukemia involvement occurred in 12 children. Specimens were inoculated in routine bacterial culture media, examined for fungi, and tested for viral content in tissue culture cells of human aorta, human embryonic kidney, human diploid fibroblasts (WI-38), HEP-2, and rhesus or African green monkey kidney. No bacterial agents or viral agents were isolated. This study confirmed the fact that pleocytosis occurring in children with acute leukemia is most likely due to the disease, but it certainly does not rule out an occasional infectious meningitis.

Of 23 patients who were observed serially to necropsy, 19 (80%) reportedly had abnormal tracings sometime during the disease regardless of the presence or absence of pleocytosis or of symptoms of CNS disease. The 4 children who had normal tracings throughout had distinctive CNS involvement at autopsy. Three of the 19 patients with abnormal tracings had no evidence of CNS infiltration at autopsy; the remaining 16 patients all had leukemic involvement of the CNS.[47]

Metabolic abnormalities are usually secondary to therapy that causes interference with renal or hepatic function, but unusual complications may follow leukemic infiltration. Hyperuricemia with subsequent uric acid nephropathy is an uncommon complication that is usually associated with a rapid drop in the initial leukemia cell count after therapy[125] (Chapter 16). Factitious hypoglycemia has been observed in patients with extreme leukocytosis unless the blood cells are removed from the specimen immediately after drawing blood from the patient.[94] The blood glucose is presumably consumed rapidly by the leukemic cells. Diabetes insipidus has also been reported.[96]

CHANGING PATTERNS OF DISEASE

After the introduction of folic acid antagonists by Farber and associates,[45] an increasing number of antileukemic drugs have resulted in significant prolongation of the duration of remission and survival times. Improved methods of utilizing blood components, particularly platelets, and an impressive accumulation of potent antimicrobial agents have provided formidable treatment with which to control many of the complications already described.

In an analysis of 414 patients of all ages, Hersh[71] reviewed the changes in the cause of death for two time periods: 1954-1959 and 1960-1963. The incidence of death due to hemorrhage alone dropped from 22% to 14%, whereas the incidence of death due to infection alone rose from 25% to 44%. Since death is rarely due to a single distinctly identifiable cause in patients with leukemia, combinations of factors were also considered. The overall incidence of hemorrhage as a complicating cause of death decreased from 67% to 37%, a fact that was attributed to the increasingly more liberal use of platelet transfusions. The overall incidence of infection as a complicating cause of death has remained essentially unchanged at approximately 70%. Infection is still the predominant primary cause of death in childhood leukemia in spite of the fact that many of the children who would have been lost early during their illnesses undoubtedly survived to achieve remission because of the use of effective antibacterial therapy, as well as transfusion therapy. However, a difference in the types of microorganisms involved was noted. Fatal staphylococcal infection declined from 23.5% to 3.1%, whereas the occurrence of fungal infection rose from 8.3% to 23.2%. The elimination of staphylococcal infection was attributed to the introduction of the more potent semisynthetic penicillin compounds. *Candida* species caused the greatest majority of the fungal infections reported.

The type and the incidence of the microbial flora responsible for serious infection vary among services from that reported by Hersh, but not greatly. A list of the organisms identified at death in 238 autopsied children at Texas Children's Hospital indicates the prevalence of *Pseudomonas* organisms but a lower incidence of significant fungal infection. Isolated disseminated moniliasis was uncommon (less than 5%), but secondary infection of the esophagus, mouth, and scattered areas of the gastrointestinal tract was seen frequently (Table 9-9). The rigid avoidance of bacteriostatic agents and the strict adherence to bactericidal antibiotic therapy may have influenced these figures. This series was obtained from 398 children seen on our service between the years 1954 and 1970. There were 122 deaths attributed to infection, 74 deaths attributed to hemorrhage, and the remainder due to combinations of other causes. In most cases a combination of hemorrhage and infection was noted, but for our purposes the individual reason most likely to have caused the death is stated. Hughes,[75] reporting on a series of 199 deaths in children with leukemia between 1962 and 1969, gives an incidence of microbial infections almost identical to ours. The persistence of *Pseudomonas aeruginosa* as a leading infectious agent is relatively unchanged in spite of the availability of several potent antimicrobial agents—colistin, carbenicillin, and gentamicin. The increase in fungal infection and more recently in protozoal *(Pneumocystis carinii)* and viral (cytomegalovirus)

Table 9-9. Microorganisms found at death in autopsies of 238 children with acute leukemia (1954-1970)[*]

Type	Number of patients	
Bacterial	141 (69%)	
Pseudomonas aeruginosa		64
Escherichia coli		22
Staphylococcus aureus		16
Staphylococcus epidermidis		1
Aerobacter aerogenes		3
Clostridium species		3
Klebsiella pneumoniae		7
Gamma streptococci		9
Alpha streptococci		5
Beta streptococci		3
Diplococcus pneumoniae		2
Neisseria meningitidis		1
Proteus morganii		1
Proteus vulgaris		1
Proteus mirabilis		1
Paracolobactrum aerogenoides		1
Mycobacterium tuberculosis		1
Fungal	44 (22%)	
Candida species		38
Cryptococcus neoformans		2
Mucor species		4
Viral	10 (5%)	
Varicella		3
Rubeola		4
Cytomegalovirus		3
Protozoal	9 (4%)	
Pneumocystis carinii		9

[*]Most information obtained from autopsy reports of the Department of Pathology, Texas Children's Hospital.

infections may reflect the immunosuppressive effects of some of the newer combinations of antileukemic agents and probably progressive subtle debilitation of the host after repeated remission and relapse.[65, 70, 119] The effect of newer antibacterial agents in predisposing to opportunistic fungal infection remains to be evaluated.

Postmortem findings. The generalized nature of acute leukemia is distinctly demonstrated by reviewing the organ involvement in 238 autopsied patients seen on our service. The microscopic findings are listed in order of occurrence (Table 9-10).

Selected tissues not listed in our experience have been reported elsewhere, and organs such as the eye, which is not examined as a routine part of the postmortem procedure in our pathology department, have been discussed under clinical features.

In almost every group of autopsy studies of children with acute leukemia, there are cases in which no evidence of the disease can be found. Some of these represent children who have died of other causes during complete remission or whose disease pattern has in some way been altered. Myelofibrosis has been

Table 9-10. Tissue involvement found at death in autopsies of 238 children with acute leukemia (1954-1970)*

Reticuloendothelial system		Respiratory system	
Spleen	150	Lung	32
Bone marrow	139†	Pleura	6
Lymph nodes	120	Trachea	3
Thymus	11	Larynx	1
Gastrointestinal system		Bones	6
Liver	137	Cardiovascular system	
Gut	42	Heart (not specified)	18
Pancreas	41	Epicardium	18
Gallbladder	11	Myocardium	15
Peritoneum	4	Pericardium	3
Esophagus	3	Endocardium	2
Appendix	2	Endocrine glands	
Stomach	1	Pituitary	4
Genitourinary system		Thyroid	3
Kidney	136	Parathyroid	3
Testes	42	Adrenal medulla	3
Ovary	27	Skin and appendages	9
Uterus	15	Miscellaneous	
Vagina	11	Muscle	7
Bladder	6	Orbit	2
Cervix	3	Buccal mucosa	1
Ureter	2	Gingivae	1
Epididymis	2	Tongue	1
Central nervous system		Middle ear	1
Meninges	89	Fat	1
Brain-related structures	14	Diaphragm	1

*Most information obtained from autopsy reports of the Department of Pathology, Texas Children's Hospital.
†Because of the aggressive use of chemotherapy, bone marrow involvement is becoming a less frequent finding at autopsy.

observed in several patients at the time of initial diagnosis and confirmed by open surgical bone biopsy; postmortem examination revealed the classic features of acute leukemia without myelofibrosis. Conversely, two children with classic acute leukemia at diagnosis had no findings other than myelofibrosis at autopsy. Seven children had diffuse marrow hypoplasia in the absence of infiltrative disease; other unusual findings included toxic hepatitis, hepatic fibrosis, pancreatitis, toxic epidermal necrolysis, and uric acid infarction of the kidneys. These findings most likely reflect direct or secondary toxic manifestations of cytotoxic chemotherapy. Disseminated tuberculosis was found unexpectedly in one child who died in 1970. The origin of the primary infection was never found.

As the duration of remission and the life-span of children with acute leukemia have been prolonged, subtle changes in the clinical patterns have also developed. The increased incidence of CNS infiltration has been directly attributed to the longer survival (Chapter 11).[43] The appearance of extramedullary infiltrates in other areas of the body has also become more obvious. Local infiltration resembling lymphosarcoma in behavior has been observed in some children who have remained in hematologic remission for years.

Until recently, it has been customary to minimize extramedullary disease with regard to the definition of relapse. Because the behavioral patterns are changing, the criteria for evaluating response may require revision (Chapter 11).

PROGNOSIS

Lehndorff[85] was perhaps overexuberant when he stated, "The most important achievement of modern hematology is the proof that leukemia is a reversible affliction." But there is no argument that children with acute leukemia are responsive to therapy.

Prechemotherapy era. In an early review (1929) of 141 cases, Warren found that 18.5% of patients were dead within 2 weeks of onset of symptoms and 84% were dead by 8 weeks.[148] Warren reported "no essential difference in the clinical picture of acute leukemia, whether the case had been diagnosed as acute myelogenous or lymphogenous leukemia." In 1933 Cooke[24] reported that 88% were dead within 6 months and 100% by 9 months. Tivey[137] found reports of spontaneous remissions dating back to 1878 but noted that the criteria for determining remission varied considerably. He concluded from the available data that the difference in the survival time between children and adults with acute leukemia was negligible. For a group of 218 children, the median survival from the onset of symptoms to death was 3.3 months. Table 9-11 shows the survival data by cell type at diagnosis. In another detailed review, Southam and associates[128] devised criteria for determining remission and evaluated 38 patients between 1924 and 1949 who supposedly had achieved remission before or without antifolate therapy. There were 20 adults and 18 children in this group who were treated with "supportive measures," arsenic, marrow extracts, urine extracts, feces extracts, pentonucleotides, exsanguinating transfusions, and simple blood transfusions. Each form of therapy was tried, most of them with the hope that a maturation factor might be involved. In spite of some remissions, only 6 patients survived more than a year after the onset of symptoms. In their own series of 150 patients who were treated prior to the advent of folic acid antagonists, only thirteen remissions (8.7%) were noted, of which only 4% were complete. Only two reports of second responses were found. The longest survivor was a 50-year-old man with acute monocytic leukemia who lived in excess of 220 weeks. The mean survival time was 20.3 weeks; 90% were dead by 36 weeks. There was no apparent difference between the mean survival time in children and in adults. Burchenal[20] summarized 825 patients in 1965; only 9 survived as long as 12 months, and none of these was alive after 24 months. Skimkin[122] reported that all 286 patients seen at the University of California Hospital between 1913 and 1947 were dead by 19 months.

After the first reports of the apparent effectiveness of folate antagonists, ACTH, and hydrocortisone, Bierman[10] attempted to obtain background data on the response rate to irradiation, transfusion therapy, and antibiotic therapy in a controlled study. The average survival time was 5.6 months if no treatment was given, 5.8 months after irradiation therapy, 6.0 months after transfusion therapy, and 8.9 months after transfusion and antibiotics were used in combination. It was concluded that the improvement in the latter group was statistically significant. In the following year Diamond and Luhby[36] reviewed 300 children, 90% of whom had "blast cell" leukemia, who had been seen over a 25-year period. An occurrence of 9.6% "spontaneous" remissions was noted. Complete remissions (4.5%) averaged 10 weeks, and partial remissions (5.2%) averaged 8 weeks in duration. Survival time averaged 29.7 weeks for those achieving complete remission and 23.6 weeks for partial remission. Three-fourths of the complete remissions occurred during 1945-1947 when antibiotics became available. They concluded that the use of antibiotics may have prevented severe infections from becoming fatal. Of the 300 children, only 2 survived for 14 months, and all were dead by 24 months.

Bassen and Kohn,[6] in presenting an unusual case, stress the fact that in most instances remissions were preceded by a marked leukopenia and hypoplasia of the bone marrow. Their patient had four spontaneous remissions, each of which was preceded by agranulocytosis and hypoplasia or aplasia of the marrow. They raised the issue—which is of obvious importance—that the ability to control or to arrest the leukemic process is inherent in some leukemic patients. Bierman[11] supported this concept further with a report of 11 children with acute leukemia who went into clinical and hematologic remission after infection with *Staphylococcus aureus*, varicella, or feline agranulocytosis virus during the course of the disease. The remissions were of short duration, and there

Table 9-11. Acute leukemia in children: median survival time (prechemotherapy data)

	Onset of symptoms to death		Diagnosis to death		Onset of symptoms to diagnosis	
	Number of patients	Months	Number of patients	Months	Number of patients	Months
Acute lymphatic	171	3.6	18	3.5	40	1.2
Acute myelocytic	41	4.2	12	1.2	30	1.2
Acute monocytic	20	2.6	3	—	5	—
All types	572	2.7	37	2.4	142	1.2

is no indication that the survival time was prolonged. The same group had investigated the responses of children with leukemia to corticosteroid therapy and found objective evidence of remission in 7 of 15 children treated.[12] The average survival time of 6.8 months was the same in 59 patients either untreated or treated with irradiation or transfusions. In light of present knowledge, the response rate of more than half the patients to steroid therapy probably reflects the action of these drugs for *induction* but not for *maintenance* of remission.

Remission. In almost all the previously mentioned reports the development of moderate to severe peripheral leukopenia and bone marrow hypoplasia is cited as preceding remission. This is the same sequence that is observed on virtually all modern induction treatment regimens. The leukemic cells first disappear (presumably eradicated), and at first the bone marrow appears hypocellular (vacated), but regeneration and repopulation by erythroid precursors follow rapidly. This is followed closely by myeloid repopulation and by the reappearance of megakaryocytes. Generally these changes are accompanied by a rapid return of the peripheral blood counts to normal levels. Within a relatively short time, usually several weeks, the blood and bone marrow show no demonstrable traces of the leukemic process (complete remission). Platelet counts often rise before significant megakaryocytic repopulation is observed.

The peculiar variation in the reported incidence of observed spontaneous remissions, which in Tivey's review[137] ranged from 0% to 10%, most likely reflects the infrequent use of bone marrow examination in the earlier cases as well as the lack of common criteria for the evaluation of responses. In his evaluation of the spontaneous remissions in 54 children, the majority were preceded by some type of "insult"—46% followed infection, 24% followed exsanguinating transfusion or blood transfusion, and 3.4% followed surgery (thymectomy, splenectomy). Some remissions were observed in which no antecedent cause could be implicated. Since the trauma to the body from infection or surgery could result in an adrenal stress response, it is presumed that this might be an explanation for such cases. The degree of similarity between the duration of remission from corticotropic hormones and "spontaneous remission" supports this suggestion.

Relapse. The reason for the reappearance (relapse) of the disease after widely varying intervals is still poorly understood, but it is the subject of much attention in studies of the mechanism of drug action, drug resistance, and cellular kinetics.

For many years it was the practice of most hematologists to observe the course of children with acute leukemia by periodic physical examination and by peripheral blood counts only. Prior to the advent of effective therapy it hardly seemed necessary to do more. However, it is apparent that changes in the peripheral blood are likely to become obvious only after the bone marrow has been largely replaced by leukemic cells. The rapidity with which bone marrow changes can occur is variable, but a normal appearing marrow can be almost completely replaced by blasts within 28 days. In other cases the percentage of blasts in the marrow may increase slowly over several months before deterioration in the peripheral blood counts can be detected. This area needs further study in relation to cellular kinetics and for determination of the optimal interval at which to obtain marrow specimens. At present, serial examination of the bone marrow is useful to the clinician to anticipate relapse and to consider changes in therapy. By observing changes in the marrow, it is usually possible to reinduce remission before serious symptoms develop, thereby avoiding many unnecessary hospitalizations. Our practice has been to obtain posterior iliac crest marrow specimens every 4 weeks. This is an arbitrary interval, and as further information becomes available, it may not be necessary to obtain specimens this often. However, it is a relatively simple procedure that can be done easily with the patient under local anesthesia. The preparation of the patient and the technique are illustrated in Fig. 9-3. Other sites may serve equally as well, but aspiration of the sternal bone marrow is a hazardous procedure that should be avoided in children.

Occasionally, by doing serial marrow examinations as described, patients have been encountered who remained in bone marrow relapse for as long as a year while maintaining normal peripheral blood counts. Aspiration of marrow from multiple sites only confirms relapse. Not all of the problems with these children can be explained easily.

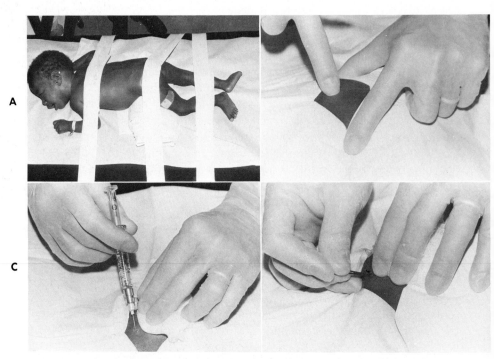

Fig. 9-3. A, Positioning of child for posterior iliac bone marrow puncture with three strips of 2-inch tape and a folded sheet to elevate pelvis. **B,** Posterior iliac spine. **C,** Local anesthesia with 2% procaine hydrochloride (intradermally and intraperiosteally). **D,** Puncture with No. 11 blade. **E,** Fixation of No. 15 Türkel trochar into posterior iliac spine. **F,** Left hand immobilizes trochar as biopsy needle is inserted. **G,** Biopsy obtained by rotary motion of needle. The dark tip of the cartilage plug represents red marrow. **H,** Hard aspiration of marrow content. **I,** Aliquot of marrow from which smears will be made and stained. (Photographs by Manfred Gygli, Medical Photography, Texas Children's Hospital.)

Chemotherapy era. Although a few long-term survivors were reported before effective chemotherapy was made available, the diagnosis of acute leukemia was inadequately documented in all but a small number of the early case reports. In several institutional reviews, reference is made to the longer survival time of those patients who achieved complete or partial remission on drug therapy. This significant concept is now the elemental basis of modern therapy (Chapter 10). Achieving a complete remission status is prerequisite to long-term survival.

To avoid controversy that may relate to the results of specific studies, Fig. 9-4 shows the trends in overall survival rates for 2702 children less than 10 years of age taken from the End Results Section, Biometry Branch, National Cancer Institute report dated May, 1970.[32] The report was controlled against the possibility that the improvement in survival may have resulted from changes in

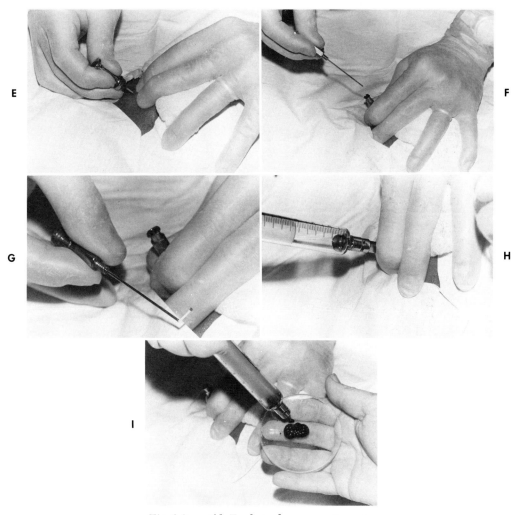

Fig. 9-3, cont'd. For legend see opposite page.

diagnostic criteria. No great difference was noted if the graph was plotted to include all types of acute leukemia or was limited to acute lymphatic leukemia. As the known incidence rates leveled off in the mid-1950's, the survival trend continued upward. This supports the conclusion that the improved survival time is due to changes in therapeutic management.

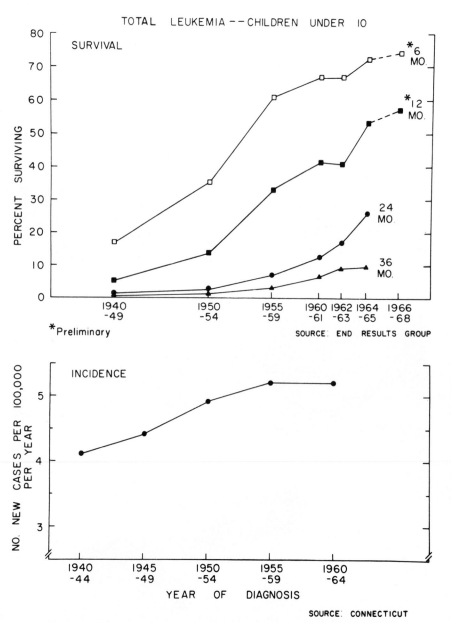

Fig. 9-4. Comparison of the trends in survival and incidence rates in acute leukemia. (From Cutler, S. J., and Axtell, L. M.: End Results Section, Biometry Branch, National Cancer Institute, May, 1970.)

In 1969 Pierce[109] reported the results of a study of epidemiologic factors in 1770 children with acute leukemia who had been treated by members of Children's Study Group A between 1946 and 1957. A characteristic peak age of incidence extending from 2 to 5 years was found in acute lymphoid leukemia, whereas the peak was absent in other morphologic groups. An almost identical age peak was found for white and Negro children, confirming earlier mention in this chapter that socioeconomic factors were probably more contributory to earlier differences in ethnic groups, but further comment on the role of ethnic or racial origin in survival was omitted for lack of adequate data. In the Group A study the most favorable prognosis was found in children with acute lymphoid leukemia who were diagnosed between 2 and 6 years of age and had leukocyte counts below 4000/mm³ at the onset.[109] The median survival time for all children with acute lymphoid leukemia was extended between 1957 and 1964 but not for other types of leukemia. However, the 10% survival figure improved for all types of leukemia during this period. Zippin[152] reviewed 873 cases of acute leukemia and reported a sex differential that was not considered in either of the reports just discussed; the best survival for any age-sex group was in girls 4 to 10 years of age. In Israel, Modan[98] closely examined age, sex, and

Table 9-12. Factors possibly related to survival in 1024* children with acute leukemia (1958-1971), Southwest Cancer Chemotherapy Study Group

Factor	Patients	Dead	Percentiles (wk)			Surviving (%)		
			75	50	25	1 yr	2 yr	5 yr
Age								
< 2	83	74	10	28	59	26	13	1
2-5	338	263	32	68	130	61	32	6
6-10	168	148	20	42	88	44	21	4
11 or over	82	72	10	38	72	41	11	4
WBC (/mm³)								
< 10	204	168	37	73	133	65	34	6
10-24	169	136	22	41	94	43	21	5
25-49	152	126	20	42	89	48	23	6
⩾ 50	138	117	22	41	84	44	19	2
Type								
ALL† + stem cell	343	276	30	60	112	54	26	5
AML‡	96	83	9	24	57	29	9	2
Unclassified	240	204	27	56	110	54	26	2
Hemorrhage								
Yes	217	177	22	46	76	46	17	3
No	213	190	27	52	97	50	22	4
Sex								
Male	386	320	24	52	98	50	24	6
Female	297	247	24	52	104	50	26	2
Race								
White	576	482	25	54	108	52	27	5
Nonwhite	107	85	22	49	97	46	23	3

*Total number of patients within each group varies according to availability of information collected retrospectively.
†ALL = Acute lymphocytic leukemia.
‡AML = Acute myelogenous leukemia.

tumor type relationships and found the survival of girls to be superior to boys in brain tumors and lymphomas but failed to find that sex influenced survival in children with acute leukemia.

Data from the Southwest Cancer Chemotherapy Study Group obtained from 1024 patients were also reviewed to evaluate prognostic and survival variables[56] (Table 9-12). The usual male prominence was noted, but there was no difference in the overall survival between the sexes. In order, the most favorable prognostic characteristics obtained from the Southwest Group data are (1) cell type (lymphoid), (2) age at diagnosis (between 2 and 6 years), and (3) leukocyte count (less than 10,000/mm³). The poor prognosis related to higher leukocyte counts in other reports was less apparent when all cell types were combined to evaluate this variable. Utilizing the investigator's diagnosis, the Group also examined acute "lymphocytic" and acute "unclassified" leukemia separately but found no difference in the survival pattern. Because of the obvious and inexplicable differences in the various studies, both Fraumeni[52] and Modan[98] specifically emphasize that the imprecise morphologic classification of acute leukemia is a gross handicap to studies on this scale.

In 1956 the National Cancer Institute addressed itself to the problem of developing common criteria for evaluating response, particularly because of the rapidly proliferating clinical studies of the various study groups.[13] The original criteria have subsequently been modified, and the most recent criteria in use by the Southwest Group are as follows[30]:

1   Criteria for rating categories
    Qualitative or quantitative changes that appear to be the operation of normal homeostatic mechanisms or physiologic responses of the patients to nonleukemic stimuli rather than a part of the disease should not be considered abnormalities, for example, secondary to medication or the normoblastic hyperplasia seen in early phases of remission.
1.1   Bone marrow (category M)
1.1.1   Ratings for subcategories (all ages)

Category M rating	Blast cells[*] (%)	Lymphocytic lymphocytes + blast cells[†] (%)	Granulocytic + other types leukemic + blast cells[*] (%)
1	0-5	0-40	0-5
2	6-25	41-69	6-39
3	> 25	> 69	> 39

1.1.2   Ratings for category M
    Rating of category M will be determined by the most abnormal subcategory found. Bone marrows qualifying for M_1 ratings must contain qualitative and quantitative normal erythropoiesis, granulopoiesis, and megakaryopoiesis.
1.2   Hemogram (category H)
1.2.1   Ratings for parameters

Category H rating	Hemoglobin, grams/100 ml				Neutrophilic granulocytes (all ages)	Percent blast cells[*] (all ages)	Platelet count, cells/mm³ (all ages)
	Child		Adult				
	< 2	> 2	M	F			
1	10	11	12	10	1500	0	100,000 normal

[*]This term includes blast cells as well as all cells that cannot be classified as either blast cells or more mature normal elements and "leukemic cells," "pathologic lymphocytes," and stem cells.
[†]Include childhood undifferentiated leukemia with the lymphocytic group. Percentage values given for subcategory rating represent percentage of all marrow elements.

2		500	< 5	100,000
				decreased
3	< 7	500	≥ 5	25,000
				25% of
				normal

1.2.2. Ratings for category H

The rating for category H is determined by the sum of the ratings for all parameters (hemoglobin, neutrophilic granulocytes, blast cells, and platelets). Ratings indicating improvement in this category must not be ascribable to transfusion of any blood elements. Mononuclear cells must not exceed 7000/mm³ (10,000/mm³ for 2 years) for an H_1 rating. The appearance of 1% to 2% blast cells on an isolated count will not preclude an H_1 rating.

Category H rating	Sum of parameter rating
1	4
2	5-8
3	8

1.3 Physical findings (category P)

1.3.1 Ratings for subcategories

Each physical finding constitutes a subcategory. The degree of abnormality for each subcategory will be rated as follows:

    a. Liver
        1 = within normal limits for age
        2 = definite enlargement (to umbilicus)
        3 = enlargement below umbilicus
    b. Spleen
        1 = within normal limits for age
        2 = definite enlargement (to umbilicus)
        3 = enlargement below umbilicus
    c. Lymph nodes
        1 = within normal limits
        2 = definite enlargement
        3 = massive enlargement (grossly visible)
    d. Other leukemic organ involvement (if present, note and score separately: skin, central nervous system, kidney, lungs, etc.)
        1 = none
        2 = definite
        3 = marked

1.3.2 Ratings for category P

The final rating for category P is based on the sum of the numerical values given to each subcategory.

Category P rating	Sum of subcategory rating
1	4
2	5-8
3	> 8

1.4 Symptoms (category S)

Ratings for category S are determined by the activity status of the patient as follows:
1 = Asymptomatic and normal activity
2 = Symptomatic and normal activity
3 = Symptomatic and unable to work or attend school

4 = Symptomatic: < 50% of normal waking hours in bed
5 = Symptomatic: > 50% of normal waking hours in bed

2   Criteria for rating disease status

A. No evident disease = a rating of 1 in all categories (i.e., $M_1H_1P_1S_1$)

B. Moderate disease = a rating of 2 in one or more categories, but no rating of 3 in any category

C. Extensive disease = a rating of 3 in one or two categories

D. Extreme disease = a rating of 3 in more than two categories

3   Terms describing the response to therapy

Complete remission (CR) = improvement to disease status A

Partial remission (PR) = improvement to disease status B

Minimal remission (MR) = improvement to disease status C

No remission (NR) = no change in any status

Progressive disease (PD) = deterioration from initial disease status or, if initially in status D, documented deterioration in any category

Long-term survivors. By 1963, although it was already apparent that the overall survival of children with leukemia had been increased to a median survival time of approximately 12 months, there was a special group of patients who had survived longer than 5 years.[20, 153] In the interest of gaining information on the long-term survivors that might help in understanding the mechanism of therapy or differences in the disease, the Acute Leukemia Task Force began a worldwide survey to collect information on all patients surviving for more than 5 years from diagnosis. By 1967 records on 159 patients had been accumulated.[17] Because data were not available on the size of the leukemic population groups from which these patients had been culled, it was estimated that these cases represented something under 1% of all cases of acute leukemia. In 1964, when the preliminary data were presented by Burchenal,[20] the possibility was raised that these cases merely represented the tail of the survival curve and that they would eventually all die of leukemia. In 1970 Burchenal[19] presented another report on these same 159 patients. The 1967 group had included 31 adults; 17 were alive, and 14 had died after passing the 5-year mark. There were 128 children in the original group; 80 were living, and 48 were dead after the 5-year mark. These results among the adult patients were unchanged 2 years later. Among the children, there had been six deaths, one attributed to varicella in a child still on maintenance therapy. One childhood death occurred 12 years after diagnosis. Based on the loss rate proportionate to the population risk, Burchenal predicted that approximately 50% of patients who survived 5 years could be expected to survive 15 years. Between 5 and 6 years, 16% of the patients at risk died; between 6 and 7 years, 11% died; and between 7 and 8 years, 11% died. For the next 3 years the percentage dropped to 2% to 4% and then to zero for the remaining 5 years. It should be noted that the registry defined long-term survivors as "those patients who are surviving, usually without evidence of disease, for more than 5 years from the diagnosis." A review of the presenting diagnostic bone marrow specimens has failed to distinguish this group from any other with acute leukemia. So far, no specific factors have emerged nor have any common denominators been discovered that would aid in the recognition of a potential long-term survivor at the time of diagnosis. Table 9-13 shows the therapy in 108 living survivors.[18] The fact that a number of these patients had minimal therapy by present standards is strong evidence of the presence of some inherent factor in the individual patient that, aided perhaps by chemotherapy, has enabled the host to overcome the disease.

Of a total of 267 children with acute leukemia of all types seen at Texas Children's Hospital, thus far 9 (3%) have survived more than 5 years. Six children have been in continuous remission, and three have had repeated relapses and remissions. The longest survivor is a 16-year-old boy who has been off drugs for 10 years after 3 years of therapy and has been free of disease except for unexplained recurrent splenomegaly at wide intervals.

The first relapse is unquestionably a poor prognostic sign with regard to long-term survival, but the increasing number of patients who have survived in excess of 5 years with recurrent active disease is evidence of the effectiveness of the antileukemic agents now available. The existence of these patients, however, tends to shadow the prognostic value of "5-year survival." This definition, among others mentioned, may require revision.

The patient who dies soon after entry into the treatment series is not necessarily a therapeutic failure, and the patient who lives an extended period of time is equally not a therapeutic triumph. Both are expected manifestations of the disease and should be included in all series.*

SUMMARY

It is obvious that the introduction of effective antileukemic therapy has had a profound effect on the duration of survival. Not only have long-term com-

---

*From Tivey, H.: The natural history of untreated acute leukemia, Ann. N. Y. Acad. Sci. 60:322, 1954.

Table 9-13. Therapy in 108 patients living of 159 patients who survived in excess of 5 years*

Therapy	Number of patients
ST	6
ST + CTX	1
ST + Fowlers	1
MTX	1
MP	4
ST + MTX	14
ST + MP	40
MTX + MP	5
ST + MTX + MP	21
ST + MTX + MP + VCR	1
ST + MTX + MP (cyclic)	8
ST + MTX + MP (cyclic) + CTX	2
ST + MTX + MP (cyclic) + VCR	2
Miscellaneous	2

*From Burchenal, J. H.: Long-term survivors in acute leukemia. In Zarafonetis, C., editor: Proceedings of the International Conference on Leukemia-Lymphoma, Philadelphia, 1968, Lea & Febiger, pp. 469-474.
Key: ST = steroids; CTX = cyclophosphamide; MTX = methotrexate; MP = 6-mercaptopurine; VCR = vincristine.

plete remissions been observed with increasing frequency, but the duration of survival has been prolonged. Patients surviving in excess of 5 years or more are no longer rarities.

It is also obvious that there are painfully large gaps in understanding the cause and pathogenesis of this strange malady. Continuous objective appraisal is essential if the results of treatment are to be evaluated properly. Much subjectivity has already been eliminated by the ease with which bone marrow material can be obtained, and the whole treatment approach has become increasingly more deliberate.

Since it is now possible to reverse and to control this disease for varying periods of time and since the child with acute leukemia can be restored to normal function for long periods, there is good reason to hope for eventual long-term control or cure. Childhood leukemia can no longer be considered a hopelessly fatal disease.

REFERENCES

1. Abbrederis, F. S., Schmalzl, F., and Braunsteiner, H.: Zur Differential diagnose akuter Leukämien mittels zytochemischer Methoden, Schweiz. Med. Wochenschr. 99:1425, 1969.
2. Alexander, P., and the Committee on Leukaemia and the Working Party on Leukaemia in Childhood: Duration of survival of children with acute leukaemia, Br. Med. J. 4:7, 1971.
3. Allen, R. A., and Straatsma, B. R.: Ocular involvement in leukemia and allied disorders, Arch. Ophthalmol. 66:68, 1961.
4. Al-Rashid, R. A., and Harned, R. K.: Dysphagia due to leukemic involvement of the esophagus, Am. J. Dis. Child. 121:75, 1971.
5. Amiotti, P. L.: Sulla incidenza dei tumori nei familiari di bambini leucemici, Minerva Pediatr. 5:449, 1953.
6. Bassen, F. A., and Kohn, J. L.: Multiple spontaneous remissions in a child with acute leukemia, Blood 7:37, 1952.
7. Bennett, J. H.: Case of hypertrophy of the spleen and liver in which death took place from suppuration of the blood, Edinburgh Med. S. J. 64:413, 1845.
8. Bennett, J. M.: Myelomonocytic leukemias: A historical review and perspectives, Cancer 27:1218, 1971.
9. Bernard, J., Jacquillat, C., Chavelet, F., Boiron, M., Stoitchkov, Y., and Tanzer, J.: Leucémie aiguë d'une enfant de 5 mois née d'une mère atteinte de leucémie aiguë au moment de l'accouchement, Nouv. Rev. Fr. Hematol. 4:140, 1964.
10. Bierman, H. R., Cohen, P., McClelland, J. N., and Shimkin, M. B.: The effect of transfusions and antibiotics upon the duration of life in children with lymphogenous leukemia, J. Pediatr. 37:455, 1950.
11. Bierman, H. R., Crile, D. M., Dod, K. S., Kelly, K. H., Petrakis, N. L., White, L. P., and Shimkin, M. B.: Remissions in leukemia of childhood following acute infectious disease, Cancer 6:591, 1953.
12. Bierman, H. R., Kelly, K. H., Petrakis, N. L., and Shimkin, M. B.: Leukemia. Duration of life in children treated with corticotropin and cortisone, Calif. Med. 77:238, 1952.
13. Bisel, H. F.: Criteria for the evaluation of response to treatment in acute leukemia, Blood 11:676, 1956.
14. Bodey, G. P., Powell, R. D., Jr., Hersh, E. M., Yeterian, A., and Freireich, E. J.: Pulmonary complications of acute leukemia, Cancer 19:781, 1966.
15. Boysen, G.: An evaluation of aryl sulphatase activity in leukaemic cells, Scand. J. Haematol. 6:246, 1969.
16. Brooke, J. H., McNeese, J., and Osgood, E. E.: The gradient tissue culture method as an aid in classification of acute leukemias. In Jones, A. R., editor: Proceedings of the Sixth International Congress of the International Society of Hematology, Boston, 1956, Grune & Stratton, Inc.

17. Burchenal, J. H.: Formal discussion: Long-term survival in Burkitt's tumor and in acute leukemia, Cancer Res. **27**:2616, 1967.
18. Burchenal, J. H.: Long-term survivors in acute leukemia, In Zarafonetis, C., editor: Proceedings of the International Conference on Leukemia-Lymphoma, Philadelphia, 1968, Lea & Febiger, pp. 469-474.
19. Burchenal, J. H.: Features suggesting curability in leukemia and lymphoma. In Leukemia-lymphoma, Chicago, 1970, Year Book Medical Publishers, Inc., pp. 93-104.
20. Burchenal, J. H., and Murphy, M. L.: Long-term survivors in acute leukemia, Cancer Res. **25**:1491, 1965.
21. Burnet, M.: Leukemia as a problem in preventive medicine, N. Engl. J. Med. **259**:423, 1958.
22. Cangir, A., Sullivan, M. P., Sutow, W. W., and Taylor, G.: Cytomegalovirus syndrome in children with acute leukemia. Treatment with floxuridine, J.A.M.A. **201**:612, 1967.
23. Center for Disease Control Leukemia Surveillance Report No. 3, Washington, D. C., July, 1971, U. S. Department of Health, Education, and Welfare.
24. Cooke, J. V.: Acute leukemia in children, J.A.M.A. **101**:432, 1933.
25. Cooke, J. V.: Incidence of acute leukemia in children, J.A.M.A. **119**:547, 1942.
26. Cooke, J. V.: The occurrence of leukemia, Blood **9**:340, 1954.
27. Court Brown, W. M., and Doll, R.: Leukemia in childhood and young adult life: Trends in mortality in relation to aetiology, Br. Med. J. **1**:981, 1961.
28. Craigie, J.: Case of disease of the spleen in which death took place from the presence of purulent matter in the blood, Edinburgh Med. S. J. **64**:400, 1845.
29. Cramblett, H. G., Friedman, J. L., and Najjar, S.: Leukemia in an infant born of a mother with acute leukemia, N. Engl. J. Med. **259**:727, 1958.
30. Criteria for evaluating chemotherapy in acute leukemia (appendix), Cancer Chemother. Rep. **42**:27, 1964.
31. Curtis, A. B.: Childhood leukemias: Osseous changes in jaws on panoramic dental radiographs, J.A.D.A. **83**:844, 1971.
32. Cutler, S. J., and Axtell, L. M.: Trends in survival of leukemia patients: 1940-1968, Washington, D. C., May, 1970, End Results Section, Biometry Branch, National Cancer Institute, National Institutes of Health.
33. Dale, J. H., Jr.: Leucemia in childhood. A clinical and roentgenographic study of 72 cases, J. Pediatr. **34**:421, 1949.
34. Dameshek, W., and Gunz, F.: Leukemia, New York, 1958, Grune & Stratton, Inc.
35. Damon, H. F.: Leucocythemia (an assay that was awarded the Boylston Medical Prize of Harvard University for 1863), Boston, 1864, de Vries. Quoted in Dargeon, H. W.: Tumors of childhood; A clinical treatise, New York, 1960, Hoeber, Inc., p. 368.
36. Diamond, L. K., and Luhby, A. L.: Pattern of "spontaneous" remissions in leukemia of childhood observed in 26 of 300 cases, Am. J. Med. **10**:238, 1951.
37. Donné, A.: Cours de microscopie complementaire des etudes medicales, anatomie microscopique et physiologie des fluides de l'economie, Paris, 1844, J. B. Bailiere, p. 132.
38. Dreyfus, C.: Some milestones in the history of hematology, New York, 1957, Grune & Stratton, Inc., pp. 54-63.
39. Dukes, C. D., and Tettenbaum, I. S.: Studies on the potentiation of monilial and staphylococcal infections by tetracycline. In Antibiotics annual 1954-1955, New York, 1955, Medical Encyclopedia, Inc., p. 674.
40. Ekert, H., and Denett, X.: An evaluation of nuclear aryl sulphatase activity as an aid to the cytological diagnosis of acute leukaemia, Australas. Ann. Med. **15**:152, 1966.
41. Erlich, P.: Farbenanalytische Untersuchungen zur Histologie und Klinik des Blutes, Berlin, 1891, A. Hirschwald.
42. Evans, A. E.: CNS involvement in children with acute leukemia, Cancer **17**:256, 1964.
43. Evans, A. E., Gilbert, E. S., and Zandstra, R.: The increasing incidence of central nervous system leukemia in children, Cancer **26**:404, 1970.
44. Everett, C. R., Haggard, M. E., and Levin, W. C.: Extensive leukemic infiltration of the gastrointestinal tract during apparent remission in acute leukemia, Blood **22**:92, 1963.
45. Farber, S., Diamond, L. K., Mercer, R. D., Sylvester, R. F., Jr., and Wolff, J. A.: Temporary remission in acute leukemia in children produced by folic acid antagonist, 4-aminopteroyl-glutamic acid (aminopterin), N. Engl. J. Med. **238**:787, 1948.

46. Fasal, E., Jackson, E. W., and Klauber, M. R.: Birth characteristics and leukemia in childhood, J. Natl. Cancer Inst. **47**:501, 1971.

47. Fernbach, D. J., Kellaway, P., and Nichols, S.: The significance of abnormalities of the electrical activity of the brain in children with acute leukemia (in press).

48. Fernbach, D. J., Nora, A. H., and Simonsen, L. G.: Recognizing and treating neutropenic infection, Postgrad. Med. **45**:167-173, 1969.

49. Fernbach, D. J., and Phillips, C. A.: Virus screening studies of the cerebrospinal fluid of children with acute leukemia, Proc. Soc. Pediatr. Res. 77, 1965.

50. Fialkow, P. J., Thomas, E. D., Bryant, J. I., and Neiman, P. E.: Leukaemic transformation of engrafted human marrow cells in vivo, Lancet **1**:251, 1971.

51. Fraumeni, J. F., Jr., Ederer, F., and Handy, V. H.: Temporal-spatial distribution of childhood leukemia in New York State, Cancer **19**:996, 1966.

52. Fraumeni, J. F., Jr., Manning, M. D., and Mitus, W. J.: Acute childhood leukemia: Epidemiologic study by cell type of 1263 cases at the Children's Cancer Research Foundation in Boston, 1947-1965, J. Natl. Cancer Inst. **46**:461, 1971.

53. Fraumeni, J. F., Jr., and Miller, R. W.: Epidemiology of human leukemia—recent observations, J. Natl. Cancer Inst. **38**:593, 1967.

54. Friedreich, N.: Ein neuer Fall von Leukämie, Arch. path. Anat. **12**:37, 1857.

55. Fuller, H. W.: Particulars of a case in which enormous enlargement of the spleen and liver, together with dilatation of all the blood vessels of the body were found coincident with a peculiarly altered condition of the blood, Lancet **2**:43, 1846.

56. George, S., Fernbach, D. J., Vietti, T. J., Sullivan, M. P., Lane, D. M., Haggard, M. E., Berry, D. H., Lonsdale, D., and Komp, D.: Factors related to the survival for 1024 children with acute leukemia from 1958-1971, Pediatric Division, Southwest Cancer Chemotherapy Study Group (in press).

57. Gerard-Marchand, R.: Leucémie aigue et varicelle, Sem. Hôp. Paris **10**:574, 1955.

58. Gibson, R. W., Bross, I. D. J., Graham, S., Lilienfeld, A. M., Schuman, L. M., Levin, M. L., and Dowd, J. E.: Leukemia in children exposed to multiple risk factors, N. Engl. J. Med. **279**:906, 1968.

59. Gilliam, A. G.: Age, sex and race selection at death from leukemia and the lymphomas, Blood **8**:693, 1953.

60. Gilliam, A. G., and Walter, W. A.: Trends of mortality from leukemia in the United States, 1921-1955, Public Health Rep. **73**:773, 1958.

61. Gilmartin, D.: Leukemic involvement of the thymus in children, Br. J. Radiol. **36**:211, 1963.

62. Gooch, W. M., III, and Fernbach, D. J.: Immunoglobulins during the course of acute leukemia in children. Effects of various clinical factors, Cancer **28**:984, 1971.

63. Grais, M.: Mortality and morbidity from leukaemia and aleukaemia in specific countries, Bull. W.H.O. **26**:683, 1962.

64. Graivier, L., Gran, G., Rhoades, R. B., Reynolds, R. C., and Windmiller, J.: Priapism in a 7-week-old infant with chronic granulocytic leukemia, J. Urol. **105**:137, 1971.

65. Gruhn, J. C., and Sanson, J.: Mycotic infections in leukemic patients at autopsy, Cancer **16**:61, 1963.

66. Gunz, F. W., and Burry, A. F.: Cellular types in acute leukemia: Diagnosis and significance, J. Clin. Pathol. **16**:325, 1963.

67. Harris, L. J.: Leukaemia and pregnancy, Can. Med. Assoc. J. **68**:234, 1953.

68. Hayhoe, F. G. J., Quaglino, D., and Doll, R.: The cytology and cytochemistry of acute leukaemias. A study of 140 cases, Medical Research Council Special Report Series No. 304, London, 1964, H. M. Stationery Office.

69. Heath, C. W., Jr., and Hasterlik, R. J.: Leukemia among children in a suburban community, Am. J. Med. **34**:796, 1963.

70. Hendry, W. S., and Patrick, R. L.: Observations on thirteen cases of *Pneumocystis carinii* pneumonia, Am. J. Clin. Pathol. **38**:401, 1962.

71. Hersh, E. M., Bodey, G. P., Nies, B. A., and Freireich, E. J.: Causes of death in acute leukemia: A ten-year study of 414 patients from 1954-1963, J.A.M.A. **193**:105, 1965.

72. Hersh, E. M., Carbone, P. P., Wong, V. G., and Freireich, E. J.: Inhibition of the primary immune response in man by anti-metabolites, Cancer Res. **25**:997, 1965.

73. Hewitt, D.: Some features of leukaemia mortality, Br. J. Prev. Soc. Med. **9**:81, 1955.

74. Holton, C. P., and Johnson, W. W.: Chronic myelocytic leukemia in infant siblings, J. Pediatr. **72**:377, 1968.

75. Hughes, W. T.: Fatal infections in childhood leukemia, Am. J. Dis. Child. **122**:283, 1971.

76. Ingalls, T. H.: Etiology of mongolism, Am. J. Dis. Child **74**:147, 1947.

77. Jaffe, N., Traggis, D. G., and Tefft, M.: Acute leukemia presenting with pericardial tamponade, Pediatrics **45**:461, 1970.

78. Keidan, S., and Mainwaring, D.: Herpes zoster associated with leukemia and lymphoma in children, Clin. Pediatr. **4**:13, 1965.

79. Kessler, I. I., and Lilienfeld, A. M.: Perspectives in the epidemiology of leukemia. In Advances in cancer research, vol. 12, New York, 1969, Academic Press, Inc.

80. Krepler, V. P.: Zur Praxis der Klassifikation von Leukamien, Osterreichische Zschr. Krebsforsch., 1970.

81. Krivit, W., and Good, R. A.: Simultaneous occurrence of leukemia and mongolism, Am. J. Dis. Child. **91**:218, 1956.

82. Lawrinson, W., and Gross, S.: Nuclear arylsulfatase activity in primitive hemic cells, Lab. Invest. **13**:1612, 1964.

83. Lee, S. L.: Personal communication, October 18, 1971.

84. Lee, S. L., Livings, D., James, G. W., Schroeder, L., Selawry, O., and Stickney, J. M.: Morphological classification of acute leukemias, Cancer Chemother. Rep. **16**:151, 1962.

85. Lehndorff, H.: Leukemia one hundred years ago, Arch. Pediatr. **72**:26, 1955.

86. Leidler, F., and Russell, W. O.: The brain in leukemia, Arch. Pathol. **40**:14, 1945.

87. Lingeman, C. H.: Epidemiologic pathology of leukemias and lymphomas of man, Natl. Cancer Inst. Monogr. No. 32, 1968.

88. MacMahon, B., and Koller, E. K.: Ethnic differences in the incidence of leukemia, Blood **12**:1, 1957.

89. MacMahon, B., and Levy, M. A.: Prenatal origin of childhood leukemia. Evidence from twins, N. Engl. J. Med. **270**:1082, 1964.

90. Martin, D. C., Chin, T. D. Y., Larsen, W. E., Roth, A. E., and Werder, A. A.: Leukemia and lymphoma. An epidemiologic study in three midwestern states, 1950-1959, J. Kans. Med. Soc. **67**:361, 1966.

91. Mathé, G., Pouillart, P., Sterescu, M., Amiel, J. L., Schwarzenberg, L., Schneider, M., Hayat, M., De Vassal, F., Jasmin, C., and Lafleur, M.: Subdivision of classical varieties of acute leukemia. Correlation with prognosis and cure expectancy, Eur. J. Clin. Biol. Res. **16**:554, 1971.

92. Mathé, G., Schwarzenberg, L., Mery, A. M., Cattan, A., Schneider, M., Amiel, J. L., Schlumberger, J. R., Poisson, J., and Wajcner, G.: Extensive histological and cytological survey of patients with acute leukemia in "complete remission", Br. Med. J. **1**:640, 1966.

93. Milham, S., Jr.: Leukemia in husbands and wives, Science **148**:98, 1965.

94. Miller, A. P., Stool, J. A., and Brown, W. G.: Pseudohypoglycemia in a child with chronic myelogenous leukemia, Med. Rec. Ann. **59**:402, 1966.

95. Miller, R. W.: Persons with exceptionally high risk of leukemia, Cancer Res. **27**:2420, 1967.

96. Miller, V. I., and Campbell, W. G., Jr.: Diabetes insipidus as a complication of leukemia, Cancer **28**:666, 1971.

97. Mitus, A., Holloway, A., Evans, A. E., and Enders, J. F.: Attenuated measles vaccine in children with acute leukemia, Am. J. Dis. Child. **103**:243, 1962.

98. Modan, B., Virag, I., and Modan, M.: Survival in childhood malignancies: Assessment of the influence of age, sex, and tumor type, with emphasis on "long-term survivors," J. Natl. Cancer Inst. **43**:349, 1969.

99. Neumann, E.: Ein Fall von Leukämie mit Erkrankung des Knochenmarkes, Arch. Heilk. **11**:1, 1870.

100. Neumann, E.: Ueber myelogene Leukämie, Berl. Klin. Wochenschr. **15**:69, 87, 115, 131, 1878.

101. Nies, B. A., Bodey, G. P., Thomas, L. B., Brecher, G., and Freireich, E. J.: The persistence of extramedullary leukemia infiltrates during bone marrow remission of acute leukemia, Blood **26**:133, 1964.

102. Nora, A. H., Nora, J. J., and Fernbach, D. J.: Hereditary predisposition to leukemia. In Proceedings of the International Congress of the Twelfth International Society of Hematology, New York, 1968, p. 23.

103. O'Connor, D.: Incidence of childhood cancer in Harris County, Texas, 1958-1970, Atlanta, 1972, Center for Disease Control.

104. Osgood, E. E.: Acute monocytic leukemia as an explanation for "hiatus leukemicus" and "myelo-monocytic leukemia," Blood 33:268, 1969.

105. Osserman, E. F., and Lawlor, D. P.: Serum and urinary lysozyme (muramidase) in monocytic and monomyelocytic leukemia, J. Exp. Med. 124:921-955, 1966.

106. Pearson, H. A.: Leukemia in identical twins, N. Engl. J. Med. 268:1151, 1963.

107. Perillie, P. E., Kaplan, S. S., Lefkowitz, E., Rogaway, W., and Finch, S. C.: Studies of muramidase (lysozyme) in leukemia, J.A.M.A. 203:317, 1968.

108. Pierce, M. I.: The acute leukemias of childhood. In Zuelzer, W. W., editor: Symposium on Pediatric Hematology, Pediatr. Clin. North Am. 497-530, 1957.

109. Pierce, M. I., Borges, W. H., Heyn, R., Wolff, J. A., and Gilbert, E. S.: Epidemiological factors and survival experience in 1770 children with acute leukemia. Treated by members of Children's Study Group A between 1957 and 1964, Cancer 23:1296, 1969.

110. Pizzolato, P.: Leukemia in the Negro, J. Natl. Med. Assoc. 41:214, 1949.

111. Prolla, J. C., and Kirsner, J. B.: The gastrointestinal lesions and complications of the leukemias, Ann. Intern. Med. 61:1084, 1964.

112. Ragab, A. H., Lindquist, K. J., Vietti, T. J., Choi, S. C., and Osterland, C. K.: Immunoglobulin pattern in childhood leukemia, Cancer 26:890, 1970.

113. Rigby, P. G., Rosenlof, R. C., Pratt, P. T., and Lemon, H. M.: Leukemia and lymphoma, J.A.M.A. 197:95, 1966.

114. Roberts, W. C., Bodey, G. P., and Wertlake, P. T.: The heart in leukemia, Am. J. Cardiol. 21:388, 1968.

115. Rudolph, R. H., Mickelson, E., and Thomas, E. D.: Mixed leukocyte reactivity and leukemia: Study of identical siblings, J. Clin. Invest. 49:2271, 1970.

116. Rupprecht, L. M. T., and Naiman, J. L.: Meningitis due to mumps virus in a child with acute leukemia, Pediatrics 46:942, 1970.

117. Sack, M. S., and Seeman, I.: A statistical study of mortality from leukemia, Blood 2:1, 1947.

118. Schwartz, S. O., Greenspan, I., and Brown, E. R.: Leukemia cluster in Niles, Ill. Immunologic data on families of leukemic patients and others, J.A.M.A. 186:106, 1963.

119. Sedaghatian, M. R., and Singer, D. B.: *Pneumocystis carinii* in children with malignant disease, Cancer 3:772, 1972.

120. Segi, M., and Kurihara, M.: Cancer mortality for selected sites in 24 countries (1962-1963), No. 4, Sendai, Japan, 1966, Department of Public Health, Tohoku University School of Medicine.

121. Shimkin, M. B.: Hodgkin's disease. Mortality in the United States, 1921-1951; race, sex and age distribution; comparison with leukemia, Blood 10:1214, 1955.

122. Shimkin, M. B., Lucia, E. L., Oppermann, K. C., and Mettier, S. R.: Lymphocytic leukemia: An analysis of frequency, distribution and mortality at the University of California Hospital 1913-1947, Ann. Intern. Med. 39:1254, 1953.

123. Silver, R. T.: Infections, fever and host resistance in neoplastic diseases, J. Chronic Dis. 16:677, 1963.

124. Simpson, C. L., and Pinkel, D.: Pathology in leukemia complicated by fatal measles, Pediatrics 21:436, 1958.

125. Sinks, L. F., Newton, W. A., Jr., Nagi, N. A., and Stevenson, T. D.: A syndrome associated with extreme hyperuricemia in leukemia, J. Pediatr. 68:578, 1966.

126. Skeel, R. T., Wright, L. J., Levanthal, C. M., and Henderson, E. S.: Group D streptococcal meningitis masked by meningeal leukemia, Am. J. Dis. Child. 117:334, 1969.

127. Smith, C. H.: Leucemia in childhood with onset simulating rheumatic disease, J. Pediatr. 7:390, 1935.

128. Southam, C. M., Craver, L. F., Dargeon, H. W., and Burchenal, J. H.: A study of the natural history of acute leukemia with special reference to duration of disease and recurrence of remissions, Cancer 4:39, 1951.

129. Stark, C. R., and Mantel, N.: Effects of maternal age and birth order on the risk of mongolism and leukemia, J. Natl. Cancer Inst. **37**:687, 1966.
130. Stark, C. R., and Mantel, N.: Temporal-spatial distribution of birth dates for Michigan children with leukemia, Cancer Res. **27**:1749, 1967.
131. Steinberg, A. G.: A genetic and statistical study of acute leukemia in children. In Proceedings of the Third National Cancer Conference, Philadelphia, 1957, J. B. Lippincott Co., pp. 353-379.
132. Steinberg, A. G.: Genetics of acute leukemia in children, Cancer **13**:985, 1960.
133. Stewart, A.: Aetiology of childhood malignancies. Congenitally determined leukaemias, Br. Med. J. **1**:452, 1961.
134. Taylor, F. M., and Geppert, L. J.: Congenital myelogenous leukemia, Am. J. Dis. Child. **80**:417, 1950.
135. Thompson, J. S., and Thompson, M. W.: Genetics in medicine, Philadelphia, 1966, W. B. Saunders Co.
136. Thurman, W. G., Haggard, M. E., Fernbach, D. J., and Sullivan, M. P.: Letter to the editor: Bone marrow morphology study, Cancer Chemother. Rep. **30**:109, 1963.
137. Tivey, H.: The natural history of untreated acute leukemia, Ann. N. Y. Acad. Sci. **60**:322, 1954.
138. Toch, R.: The interaction of varicella and acute leukemia, Proc. Am. Assoc. Cancer Res. **2**:255, 1957.
139. Velpeau, A.: Rev. Med. **2**:218, 1827, quoted by Virchow, R.: Med. Ztg. **16**:9, 15, 1847.
140. Videbaek, A.: Heredity in human leukemia and its relation to cancer; a genetic and clinical study of 209 probands (thesis), Copenhagen, 1947, Eijnar Munksgaard.
141. Virchow, R.: Weisses Blut, N. Notiz. Geb. Nat. Heilk. **36**:151, 1845.
142. Virchow, R.: Weisses Blut und Milztumoren, Med. Ztg. **15**:157, 163, 1846.
143. Virchow, R.: Weisses Blut und Milztumoren, Med. Ztg. **16**:9, 15, 1847.
144. Virchow, R.: III. Die Leukämie. In Gesammelte Abhandlungen zur wissenchaftlichen Medizin, Frankfurt, 1856a, Meidinger Sohn & Co., p. 190.
145. Virchow, R.: IV. Die farblosen Blutkorperchen. In Gesammelte Abhandlungen zur wissenschaftlichen Medizin, Frankfurt, 1856b, Meidinger Sohn & Co., p. 212.
146. Wagner, M. L., Rosenberg, H. S., Fernbach, D. J., and Singleton, E. B.: Typhlitis: a complication of leukemia in childhood, Am. J. Roentgenol. Radium Ther. Nucl. Med. **109**:341, 1970.
147. Walter, W. A., and Gilliam, A. G.: Leukemia mortality. Geographic distribution in the United States for 1949-1951, J. Natl. Cancer Inst. **17**:475, 1956.
148. Warren, S. L.: Acute leukemia: A review of the literature and of twenty-eight new cases, Am. J. Med. Sci. **178**:490, 1929.
149. Williams, H. M., Diamond, H. D., and Craver, L. F.: The pathogenesis and management of neurological complications in patients with malignant lymphomas and leukemia, Cancer **11**:76, 1958.
150. Wilson, J. D., and Nossal, G. J. V.: Identification of human T and B lymphocytes in normal peripheral blood and in chronic lymphocytic leukaemia, Lancet **2**:788, 1971.
151. Youman, J. D., III, Saarni, M. I., and Linman, J. W.: Diagnostic value of muramidase (lysozyme) in acute leukemia and preleukemia, Mayo Clin. Proc. **45**:219-228, 1970.
152. Zippin, C., Cutler, S. J., Reeves, W. J., Jr., and Lum, D.: Variation in survival among patients with acute lymphocytic leukemia, Blood **37**:59, 1971.
153. Zuelzer, W. W.: Formal discussion: Long-term survivors, Cancer Res. **24**:1495, 1965.
154. Zuelzer, W. W., Thompson, R. I., and Mastrangelo, R.: Evidence for a genetic factor related to leukemogenesis and congenital anomalies: Chromosomal aberrations in pedigree of an infant with partial D trisomy and leukemia, J. Pediatr. **72**:367, 1968.
155. Zussman, W. V., Khan, A., and Shayesteh, P.: Congenital leukemia. Report of a case with chromosome abnormalities, Cancer **20**:1227, 1967.

CHAPTER 10

Management of acute leukemia*

TERESA J. VIETTI
ABDELSALAM H. RAGAB
VITA J. LAND

The management of acute leukemia has undergone profound changes in the last two decades, and there is every indication that even more drastic changes in the therapeutic regimen will take place in the next 10 years. Before 1948 no drugs were known to be significantly effective in treating this disease, and all children died within a few months of their diagnosis. At this time Farber and associates[23] described the therapeutic efficacy of aminopterin, a folic acid antagonist. Eventually aminopterin was replaced by another antifolate, methotrexate, which was less toxic and easier to regulate.[18, 87] The effectiveness of 6-mercaptopurine was subsequently described by Burchenal[12] in 1953. Pearson[85] noted in 1950 that cortisone and ACTH had antileukemic activity, but it was not until 1954 that Fessas[28] established the clinical efficacy of corticosteroids. It is now known that corticosteroids are effective agents to induce remission but do not significantly prolong the survival time when used as the sole agent.[87]

In addition to the discovery and development of effective chemotherapeutic compounds, there have been significant changes in the concept of what constitutes an optimal therapeutic regimen.† Thus initially a complete remission was induced with a single agent, therapy was stopped, and the patient was then observed until he had recurrent symptoms of his disease. It was then noted that if the antileukemic agent was continued after remission induction, the duration of remission was longer. Along with this observation, other studies indicated that some drugs were very effective remission *induction* agents but were of little value and were associated with considerable increase in toxicity when used to *sustain* remission. Conversely, some agents when used alone were relatively poor remission induction agents and were associated with enhanced toxicity but were effective for remission *maintenance*. Concomitantly with these observations, it was noted that a *combination* of agents was much more effective to induce remission. It was not until the past decade that effective therapeutic regimens utilizing a combination of agents have been described for remission maintenance.

As the duration of hematologic remission has lengthened, the incidence of

---

*This investigation was supported by the following grants: U.S.P.H. RR-00036, U.S.P.H. 5 R10 CA05587, U.S.P.H. 5 R10 CA11817, U.S.P.H. 5 PO2 CA10435, The Fern Waldman Memorial Fund, and the Leukemia Guild of Missouri and Illinois.
†References 7a, 16, 36, 46, 47, 53, 89, 102.

extramedullary relapse, especially central nervous system disease, has markedly increased. This has resulted primarily because there are anatomic areas of the body where drug diffusion is inadequate, and leukemic cells that have gained access to these areas are not exposed to cytocidal drug concentrations. These anatomic areas are called *pharmacologic sanctuaries,* and the therapy devised to attempt to eradicate disease in these areas is called *sanctuary therapy.* In the past, therapy was directed at treating overt disease after it had developed. During the past decade an attempt has been made to devise therapy that will prevent disease from developing in these areas; this has been termed *prophylactic sanctuary therapy.*

Many of the changes in therapy that have occurred in the past decade have been the result of a clearer understanding of tumor cell kinetics and the study of the effects of chemotherapeutic agents on experimental model systems in animals. This has been discussed in Chapter 5. Principal among the many unsolved problems is the development of drug resistance in both experimental animals and in man. Experimental immunotherapy and bone marrow transplants are effective in the treatment of animal malignancies; this form of therapy is just now being extensively evaluated in man and will be discussed briefly at the end of this chapter.

The advances that have been made in antileukemic therapy would not have been possible if similar advances had not been made in supportive care (see Chapter 7 for a more extensive review). The most significant advance, of course, was the discovery of antibiotics, which first became available for general use about 3 years before aminopterin was evaluated as an antileukemic agent. During the past decade another advance has been the development of methods to obtain platelet concentrates. Currently the problems of granulocyte isolation and concentration are under intensive investigation.

Most of the research centers in the United States follow the criteria for response that were formulated by a national committee (Chapter 9), but we still do not have any universally accepted criteria to determine the morphologic type of leukemia. To obviate this latter problem the Southwest Cancer Chemotherapy Study Group registers all the acute leukemias, regardless of morphologic type, for their protocols and reports their results on the basis of pooled data from this heterogeneous group of patients. Many of the other research centers attempt to separate out their patients into two broad classifications, one of which is designated acute lymphatic leukemia and the other acute myelogenous leukemia. Children with acute lymphatic, acute stem cell, and acute undifferentiated leukemia are placed in the acute lymphatic leukemia classification, whereas acute promyelocytic, acute myelogenous, acute monomyelogenous, acute erythroblastic, and acute monocytic leukemia are designated as acute myelogenous leukemia. Since it is well known that most patients who are classified as having acute lymphatic leukemia have a more favorable response to therapy than those who are classified as having acute myeloblastic leukemia, this seems a reasonable subdivision. The following review of the various therapeutic regimens will use these two classifications to discuss response to therapy. Eventually these two classifications will undoubtedly be further subdivided when our knowledge of morphology, cell biology, biochemistry, and effective therapy becomes more sophisticated.

REMISSION INDUCTION
Supportive therapy

The child whose bone marrow is replaced with 50% to 90% leukemic cells is almost invariably in a perilous condition because of severe granulocytopenia, thrombocytopenia, anemia, or all three. There is a great vulnerability to infection and life-threatening hemorrhage. The first objectives of the therapist must be to control the complications of the disease and at the same time induce remission by reduction of the blast cell population to permit regeneration of normal marrow elements and eventual return of the peripheral blood cells to adequate levels.

Many of these children are febrile on admission, and although fever may possibly be a direct symptom of the disease, it is usually due to infection. If fever is present, appropriate diagnostic studies such as blood, urine, nose, and throat cultures and chest roentgenogram should be obtained within a short period after admission and intensive bactericidal therapy instituted for both gram-negative and gram-positive sepsis. This therapy should be continued for at least 3 or 4 days after the child becomes afebrile, even if a causative agent is not identified.

In all children with severe granulocytopenia, some attempt at reverse isolation is advisable. The child should be confined to a private room, and visitors should be rigidly restricted. Strict isolation is not employed in our hospital, but all personnel wash their hands before handling the children and use antiseptic precautions such as povidone-iodine complex (Betadine) before puncturing the skin. Most children return to their home environment before their white blood counts become normal. Parents are advised to maintain social isolation within the limits of practicality until the granulocyte count is above 1000/mm³. Social isolation implies restriction to the immediate family environment and avoiding crowds such as might be encountered in school or stores and also isolation from friends or relatives with infections.

There are several schools of thought about managing thrombocytopenia. In our institution we do not treat thrombocytopenia unless there is clinical evidence of moderate to severe hemorrhagic diathesis, the platelet count is below 10,000/mm³, or there is evidence of severe infection. In these instances the platelet count can be usually increased to above 75,000/mm³ by the administration of platelet concentrates and fresh platelet-rich plasma. Four platelet concentrates per square meter of body surface area should increase the platelet count by 60,000/mm³, but if severe infection or bleeding is present, more may be required because of the increased consumption of platelets. Adequate control of bleeding can normally be attained by the administration of concentrates every other day or twice a week, but if severe complications are present, daily administration may be indicated. The value of platelet concentrates on a prophylactic basis remains to be established. If the platelet count is very low, especially if there is evidence of severe hemorrhagic diathesis, it is probably advisable that small children be fairly heavily sedated for traumatic procedures such as a venipuncture, bone marrow aspiration, or lumbar puncture. This may be especially true if the white blood cell count is over 50,000/mm³, since children and adults with this marked leukocytosis seem to be especially susceptible to intracranial hemorrhage.[86] Sometimes the platelet count cannot be increased because of the presence of platelet antibodies. Usually this problem is observed late in the course of the disease after repeated transfusions.

Anemia is one of the easiest complications to manage. Unless the child is actively bleeding, 10 ml/kg of packed red blood cells should be given at 8- to 24-hour intervals until the hemoglobin is above 10 to 12 gm/100 ml. If the child is in shock due to hemorrhage, saline solution should be given until blood is available, and then 20 ml/kg of whole blood (preferably fresh) should be given by rapid intravenous infusion. The patient's status should be reassessed at frequent intervals and more blood given when indicated.

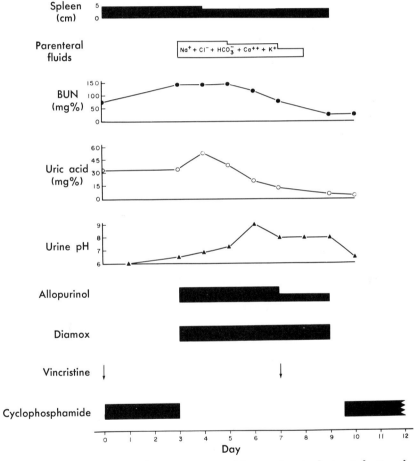

Fig. 10-1. Acute lymphoblastic leukemia: uremia and hyperuricemia during induction therapy. This illustration depicts the complication that occurred in a 15-year-old white boy whose remission was reinduced with daily oral cyclophosphamide and weekly vincristine therapy. The results of the BUN (75 mg/100 ml) and serum uric acid (34 mg/100 ml) drawn on admission were not obtained until the third hospital day. Repeat BUN, uric acid, and electrolytes were drawn, and allopurinol, acetazolamide (Diamox), and intensive fluid therapy with added sodium bicarbonate were initiated. Despite his rather impressive laboratory evidence of renal failure, his urinary output remained excellent. His subsequent course was uneventful, and he achieved remission in 4 weeks and remained in remission for 20 months.

Uric acid nephropathy, very rarely seen before chemotherapy is started and a fairly rare complication of therapy, presents such grave problems to the therapist that all efforts should be taken to avoid this complication. The stormy course that developed in a 15-year-old boy in relapse 2 days after vincristine and cyclophosphamide therapy was initiated to induce a remission is outlined in Fig. 10-1. Because we have observed a number of similar complications, four with fatal outcomes, we recommend the following preventive measures. At the time of the initial diagnosis or during subsequent relapse, blood urea nitrogen and uric acid levels should be drawn, and a regimen of 200 mg/M² of allopurinol in two or three divided doses should be begun. (Allopurinol is a xanthine oxidase inhibitor that prevents the metabolic breakdown of xanthine to uric acid.) If the serum uric acid is greater than 10 mg/100 ml or the child has a white count in excess of 75,000/mm³ or massive organomegaly or both, he

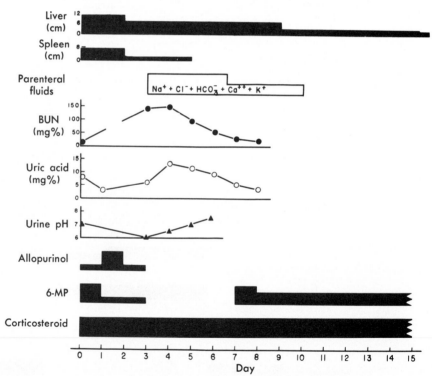

Fig. 10-2. Acute stem cell leukemia: uremia and possible xanthine nephropathy during induction therapy. This graph depicts the clinical course during the first 10 days of remission induction therapy in a 4-year-old white child with Down's syndrome. Because of massive hepatosplenomegaly and a serum uric acid level of 8.5 mg/100 ml, she was started on a regimen of 200 mg/M²/day of allopurinol. A high fluid intake (3000 ml/M²) was prescribed, but nausea and vomiting started on the second day. On the third day hypocalcemic tetany occurred, and she was noted to be mildly dehydrated. Blood electrolytes were checked, and she was noted to have a CO_2 of 10 mEq/L, Cl^- of 96 mEq/L, Na^+ of 128 mEq/L, a K^+ of 7.3 mEq/L, a Ca^{++} of 4.2 mg/100 ml, and a P of 21.3 mg/100 ml. Parenteral fluid therapy with added calcium gluconate and sodium bicarbonate was administered. The urine output remained adequate throughout, and uric acid crystals in the urine were never documented. A bone marrow aspirate on the fifteenth day revealed less than 5% blast cells.

should be hospitalized. Complete electrolytes should be obtained, and fluid therapy (3000 ml/M²/day) and alkalinization of the urine by administration of sodium bicarbonate (90 mEq/M²/day) should be started immediately before specific antileukemic therapy is begun. Each urine sample is checked for pH, and if it does not become alkaline within 6 hours, a carbonic acid anhydrase inhibitor (200 mg/M²/day of acetazolamide [Diamox]) should be administered. Once the serum uric acid level falls below 6 or 8 mg/100 ml, the sodium bicarbonate and the carbonic acid anhydrase inhibitor can be discontinued, but fluid therapy must be continued to prevent a xanthine nephropathy. Xanthine is soluble in acid urine, but the massive tissue breakdown that sometimes occurs during therapy can lead to excessive accumulation of this compound in the kidney if adequate diuresis is not maintained. This complication was thought probable in a 4-year-old child with Down's syndrome and acute lymphatic leukemia who had a serum uric acid level of 8.5 mg/100 ml on admission. The patient received allopurinol, which resulted in a prompt drop of uric acid levels to normal limits, but she developed uremia 5 days after admission. Her clinical course and treatment are outlined in Fig. 10-2.

Remission induction—single agent

Although it has been established that combinations of agents are more effective, a review of the action of single agents is essential to understand the effect

Table 10-1. Summary of remission induction with single agents

Agents	Suggested dosage schedule*	Route	Expected response rates† ALL (%)	AML (%)	Selected references
Prednisone	60 mg/M²/day, 4 divided doses	PO	60-75	10	7, 35, 68, 109,‡ 114
Vincristine	1.5-2 mg/M²/wk	IV	40-60	20	21, 43, 48, 58, 64
L-Asparaginase	200 IU/kg/day × 5 days q 2 wk or 300 IU/kg 3 ×/wk	IM or IV	40-60	10	6, 14, 17, 22, 73 81, 82, 101, 103
Daunorubicin	50 mg/M²/day × 5 days§	IV	40-50	30	6, 8, 55, 61, 63, 70
6-Mercaptopurine	2.5 mg/kg/day	PO	30-40	10-30	9, 26,‡ 31, 35, 49, 100
Methotrexate	3 mg/M²/day	PO	20-40	6‖	31, 52, 92, 98
Cyclophosphamide	5 mg/kg/day§	PO	40	—	27, 51,‡ 88
Cytosine arabinoside	25 mg/kg 2 ×/wk 100 mg/M²/4 hr infusion/day	IV IV	40 —	— 40	107 46

*See selected references. Induction therapy is given for 4 to 6 weeks.
†Complete marrow remission.
‡Data combined for acute lymphatic leukemia (ALL) and acute myelogenous leukemia (AML).
§Severe myelotoxicity may be observed.
‖Adults.

of therapy. Optimal dosages and schedules and the expected response to single agents are given in Table 10-1.

The *corticosteroids* are among the most effective single agents used to induce remission in children with acute lymphatic leukemia and have the advantage that there is little associated myelosuppression, Numerous studies have been done on various types of glucocorticoids, but no single agent has been proved demonstrably superior to another. The schedule of administration seems to be critical, and the drug is usually given frequently enough to maintain high plasma levels of the steroid. For prednisone we use a dosage schedule of 60 mg/M²/day given in four divided doses (minimum dose, 20 mg, and maximum dose, 60 mg). Corticosteroids given every other day or every fourth day were not as effective as when given daily in divided doses.[68] Similarly, moderate to massive daily doses (4 mg/kg/day up to 500 mg total dose per day) do not seem superior to 1 or 2 mg/kg/day.[68, 93] Response to corticosteroids is frequently dramatic, and marked reduction of massive organomegaly with decrease in blast cell count in the peripheral blood from 100,000/mm³ to 3,000/mm³ or less in 4 or 5 days is not unusual. If the blast count remains unchanged or continues to rise in the peripheral blood for 5 or 6 days and there is no reduction in organomegaly, the patient is unlikely to respond to prednisone. Toward the end of remission induction with corticosteroids, moderate hepatomegaly may be observed. This has been attributed to massive deposition of fat in the liver.[95] Hypertension and activation of latent diabetes can complicate steroid therapy; therefore blood pressure and urine should be checked regularly.

Despite the fact that prednisone is thought not to be myelosuppressive, the patient's platelets or normal granulocytes or both may decrease in the peripheral blood for the first week or two after therapy has been initiated. A case presentation of such response is depicted in Fig. 10-3. The reason for this effect is not certain, but it is wise to keep this in mind when treating with agents that are known to be myelosuppressive.

Corticosteroids induce remission in about 60% to 75% of patients with acute lymphatic leukemia.[7, 35, 68, 109, 114] If prednisone is stopped at the time the patient attains a complete remission, he has a 40% to 50% chance to respond to a second remission induction with prednisone alone.[109] If the patient is maintained on prednisone until relapse, he will not respond to a second reinduction with prednisone. Results in the treatment of monocytic leukemia or granulocytic leukemia with corticosteroids alone are much less favorable. Only about one patient in ten will achieve a remission.[7, 68, 114]

Vincristine is the second most effective remission induction agent in acute lymphatic leukemia and although it may cause myelosuppression, it is less myelosuppressive than other agents. Remission induction rates in most series vary between 40% and 50%.[21, 43, 48, 58, 64] Complete remission is usually achieved within 4 to 6 weeks of therapy. The recommended therapeutic regimen is 1.5 to 2 mg/M² by rapid intravenous infusion once a week. Many chemotherapists do not give more than a maximum single dose of 2 mg/wk to older children and adults because of marked increase in the side effects when the dose exceeds this amount. The response in acute myelogenous leukemia is less satisfactory, and only 10% to 20% of children will attain remission with this agent.[21, 64]

Many noxious side effects are associated with vincristine therapy. Severe jaw pain requiring narcotics may occur after the first or second dose of vincristine but usually does not recur after the third or fourth dose. One of the most serious side effects is severe obstipation, which occurs relatively frequently. Ideally, normal bowel movements should be reestablished before the next dose of vincristine is given. It is our opinion that stool softeners may help, but irritant laxatives are of no value. Severe neuropathy may occur early in the course of treatment in adults and in an occasional child. One child suffered generalized muscle weakness, loss of deep tendon reflexes, wristdrop, and foot drop after only two weekly doses of 2 mg/M² of vincristine.[24] Hyporeflexia *per se* is not an indication to stop therapy. We have continued therapy and stopped only if the child has trouble walking up stairs or picking up small objects, but this is rare with short-term therapy.

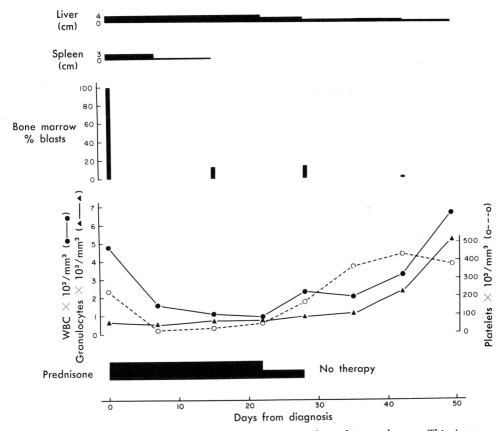

Fig. 10-3. Leukopenia and thrombocytopenia occurring with prednisone therapy. This 4-year-old girl in relapse was started on a regimen of 2.2 mg/kg/day of prednisone. The initial peripheral white blood cell count was 4800/mm³, and the platelet count was 234,000/mm³. The platelet and white blood count dropped to low levels within 1 week, and evidence of recovery did not ensue until after the third week of therapy. Note that although splenomegaly rapidly subsided, hepatomegaly did not disappear until after prednisone therapy was stopped. A bone marrow aspirate at 28 days revealed 14% blast cells, but a repeat aspirate at 42 days with no further therapy revealed 2% blast cells.

L-*Asparaginase* is currently undergoing extensive investigation. This agent will induce remission in 40% to 60% of the children with far advanced disease,* but because of the unpredictability of severe toxic side effects that are presumably secondary to impurities (anaphylactoid reactions, liver damage, pancreatitis, CNS toxicity), it has not yet been released for general use.† The types of observed toxic side effects vary considerably, depending on the pharmaceutical preparation.[22] 6-Mercaptopurine was found to suppress some of the hypersensitivity reactions observed with L-asparaginase obtained from Bayer,[81] but the administration of prednisone and vincristine along with L-asparaginase obtained from Squibb did not alter these side reactions.[67] The optimal therapeutic regimen remains to be established. Preliminary studies suggest that doses as small as 10 IU/kg/day for 28 days will induce a remission, but the duration of unmaintained remission is not as long as a remission induced with 1000 IU/kg/day.[103] Only about 1 in 10 patients with acute myelogenous leukemia will attain a remission.[14, 22, 82]

Daunorubicin and its hydroxymethyl analog *adriamycin* are both effective induction agents,‡ but both are associated with severe myelotoxicity, and their relative value in remission induction in acute lymphatic leukemia remains to be established. High dosage levels of 50 to 60 mg/M²/day of daunorubicin for 2 to 7 days will induce remission in over 40% of patients, but myelotoxicity is severe.[8] Not enough studies utilizing various therapeutic regimens are available to evaluate adriamycin, but studies in mouse leukemia indicate that it is superior to daunorubicin.[90] The rate of remission induction in acute myelogenous leukemia with daunorubicin is superior to most other agents,[8, 70] and this agent may prove to be of significant importance in this form of leukemia. Both drugs can cause severe myocardiopathy, but the occurrence of this toxicity in children is usually seen only if the total dose exceeds 500 mg/M².[72, 105]

6-Mercaptopurine given orally at a dosage of 2.5 mg/kg/day (75 mg/M²/day) will induce remission in approximately 30% to 40% of children with acute lymphatic leukemia[9, 12, 31, 49, 100] but only in 9% of children with acute myelogenous leukemia.[31] The initial responses are slower than those observed with prednisone or vincristine, and the duration of therapy required to obtain remission may be as long as 6 weeks. The principal toxic side effect of 6-mercaptopurine is severe myelosuppression, but this is rarely observed during the remission induction period. Oral ulceration is rarely observed. Some patients occasionally have abdominal pain, which disappears when they have a bowel movement. Usually, this pain is not significant, but occasionally it is necessary to reduce the drug dosage. If allopurinol is administered with 6-mercaptopurine, it is necessary to reduce the dosage of 6-mercaptopurine to one-fourth the estimated dosage, since this compound interferes with the metabolism of 6-mercaptopurine and its subsequent detoxification.

The value of *methotrexate* in inducing remission is inferior to the drugs already discussed.[31, 52, 92, 98] A regimen of daily oral methotrexate (3 mg/M²) is probably as effective as one in which the drug is given two times per week

*References 6, 14, 22, 73, 81, 82, 101, 103.
†References 17, 22, 67, 73, 82, 103.
‡References 6, 8, 55, 61, 63, 70, 98, 111a.

(30 mg/M²) to induce remission in acute lymphatic leukemia. In one study, 60% of the patients treated with daily oral methotrexate attained a remission after relapse on 6-mercaptopurine,[98] but other investigators have observed remission rates of only 20% to 30%.[31, 52, 92, 98] In acute myelogenous leukemia the remission induction rate is very poor, especially with daily oral therapy.[31] Better results were obtained when the drug was given every 6 hours for 5 days; the complete remission rate in this series was 16% in adult patients.[111] Methotrexate may cause myelosuppression during remission induction. Its principal side effect is mucosal ulceration and diarrhea, and therapy must stop immediately if these complications develop. The parents should be instructed to check the child's

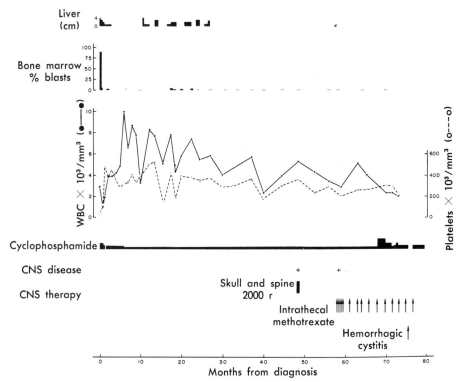

Fig. 10-4. Cyclophosphamide: an effective agent for induction and maintenance therapy in acute childhood leukemia. This 11-year-old white boy presented with moderate hepatomegaly, thrombocytopenia, and granulocytopenia. After bone marrow aspirate revealed almost total replacement by lymphoblasts, he was started on a regimen of 5 mg/kg/day of oral cyclophosphamide. One month later a marrow aspirate revealed he was in complete remission. Cyclophosphamide was continued, and he has remained in complete marrow remission for the past 4½ years but developed evidence of central nervous system disease 3½ years after the initial diagnosis. He received 2000 rads to the craniospinal axis but had evidence of recurrent central nervous system disease within 8½ months. Central nervous system remission was reinduced with six doses of 12.5 mg/M² of intrathecal methotrexate, and central nervous system remission is now maintained with intrathecal methotrexate given every 8 weeks. He has had only one bout of hemorrhagic cystitis, which occurred after 76 months of cyclophosphamide therapy. (Case history courtesy Drs. G. B. Humphrey and D. M. Lane at the University of Oklahoma Medical Center.)

mouth daily for evidence of oral ulceration and report this complication to the physician. If renal function is impaired, a lower dose must be used, since methotrexate is excreted primarily by the kidney.

Cyclophosphamide is superior to other alkylating agents in its effectiveness in the treatment of acute childhood leukemia.[27, 51, 88, 104] Unfortunately, some investigators have questioned its value, but the Southwest Cancer Chemotherapy Study Group observed a complete remission rate of 40% on a therapeutic regimen of 5.0 mg/kg/day orally.[51] This exceeds the remission induction rates of either 6-mercaptopurine or methotrexate and approaches that of prednisone or vincristine. Different dosages or different therapeutic regimens have not been found to be as effective.[57, 88] From the evidence it appears that pessimism concerning the efficacy of this drug in treatment of acute lymphatic leukemia is unwarranted. Fig. 10-4 presents the course of a 7-year-old boy whose remission was induced and then maintained with cyclophosphamide alone. He has remained in complete hematologic remission for the last 4 years but has had several CNS relapses. Cyclophosphamide alone has not been found to be an effective agent to induce remission in acute myelogenous leukemia.[57]

The principal toxic effect of cyclophosphamide is leukopenia, but this is rapidly reversible on cessation of therapy. The complication that causes the most severe problems is hemorrhagic cystitis. The cystitis is due to a high concentration of the active metabolite in the bladder, which has a direct toxic effect on the mucosal cells. To prevent the cystitis, cyclophosphamide should be given in the morning and fluids forced throughout the day, especially in the summer months. It may help to have the child take a large glass of water before going to bed and the parents awaken him during the night to void. If hematuria develops, the drug must be stopped at once and not resumed until the urine is free of red cells. If the cystitis recurs, an intravenous pyelogram with voiding cystograms should be obtained and if there is evidence of mucosal hypertrophy and contracted bladder, therapy should be discontinued.

The results with cytosine arabinoside in induction of remission in acute lymphatic leukemia[59, 107, 112] have been somewhat disappointing, particularly since it seems to be such an effective agent in mouse leukemia[91]; but it is still one of the most effective single agents used to induce remission in acute myelogenous leukemia.[20, 46] Many therapeutic regimens have been evaluated, and all seem to be associated with moderate to severe myelotoxicity.

There are many other agents that have been evaluated in remission induction of acute leukemia, but to date the results have not been satisfactory. 5-Fluorouracil and 5-fluoro-2-deoxyuridine given on a daily intravenous schedule induced a remission in one out of six children with acute lymphatic leukemia who had an adequate trial of therapy,[44] but toxicity was severe, and other studies have been abandoned. Thioguanine given daily was no more effective than 6-mercaptopurine and because absorption was erratic and cross-resistance to 6-mercaptopurine was demonstrable,[13] further attempts to evaluate this drug were abandoned until recently. With the demonstration that its mechanism of action is different from 6-mercaptopurine and that there may be a synergistic action when given with cytosine arabinoside,[37] interest has been renewed. Although methylglyoxal bis(guanylhydrazone) dihydrochloride (methyl GAG) is an effective agent in acute myelocytic leukemia,[71] the toxicity is so severe that no further clinical investigation has been undertaken with this agent.

Remission induction—multiple agents

As we have mentioned, combination therapy is always preferable to single-agent therapy. Goldin and Mantel[41] reviewed the theoretical justification for use of combination therapy. Briefly, these are therapeutic synergism between

Table 10-2. Summary of remission induction with multiple agents

Agents	Suggested dosage schedule*	Route	Expected response rates† ALL (%)	AML (%)	Selected references
Prednisone	60 mg/M²/day 4 ÷ doses	PO	85		39, 92, 99‡
Vincristine	2 mg/M²/wk	IV			
Prednisone	60 mg/M²/day 4 ÷ doses	PO	80	—	26,‡ 32, 65
6-Mercaptopurine	2.5 mg/kg/day	PO			
Prednisone	60 mg/M²/day 4 ÷ doses	PO	80	—	65
Methotrexate	3 mg/M²/day	PO			
Prednisone	60 mg/M²/day 4 ÷ doses	PO	76	—	26‡
Cyclophosphamide	5 mg/kg/day	PO			
Prednisone	60 mg/M²/day 4 ÷ doses	PO	65§	—	56
Daunomycin	25 mg/M²/day × 3/wk	IV			
Prednisone	60 mg/M²/day 4 ÷ doses	PO	95	—	61, 75, 108
Vincristine	1.5 mg/M²/wk	IV			
Daunomycin	50 mg/M²/wk	IV			
6-Mercaptopurine	3 mg/kg/day	PO	43	13	31
Methotrexate	3 mg/M²/day	PO			
Vincristine	2 mg/M² × 1	IV	90	—	36
Amethopterin	20 mg/M²/days 1 and 4	IV			
6-Mercaptopurine	60 mg/M²/day × 8	PO			
Prednisone	40 mg/M²/day × 8	PO			
Prednisolone	1 Gm/M²/day × 5	PO	95	45	45, 46
Oncovin	2 mg/M²/day × 1	IV			
Methotrexate	7.5 mg/M²/day × 5	IV			
Purinethol	500 mg/M²/day × 5	IV			
Prednisone	60 mg/M²/day 4 ÷ doses	PO	80-90	—	101
Vincristine	2 mg/M²/wk	IV			
Asparaginase	200 IU/kg/day × 5 days	IV			
Vincristine	1.5 mg/M² × 1	IV	—	45	97
Cyclophosphamide	25 mg/M² q 8 hr × 12	IV			
Cytosine arabinoside	25 mg/M² q 8 hr × 12	IV			
Vincristine	1.5 mg/M²/wk	IV	52§	—	25‡
Cyclophosphamide	5 mg/kg/day	PO			

*See selected references. Induction therapy is given for 4 to 6 weeks.
†Complete marrow remission.
‡Data combined for acute lymphatic leukemia (ALL) and acute myelogenous leukemia (AML).
§Previously treated patients.

two agents, prevention or delay of development of drug resistance, allowance of drug therapy below single tolerated dose levels, or achievement of simultaneous cytocidal effect from two different compounds. (See Chapter 6.)

The following description of the results of combination therapy is summarized in Table 10-2.

The combination of *prednisone + vincristine* has been shown to be the most effective therapeutic schedule[39, 92, 99] to induce remission in acute lymphatic leukemia of childhood. Not only is a complete remission attained in over 85% of the children, but also the toxicity associated with this remission induction therapy causes little myelosuppression. About 20% of children with acute myelocytic leukemia will attain a remission with this combination of agents.

Prednisone in combination with *6-mercaptopurine,*[*] *methotrexate,*[65] *daunorubicin,*[56] or *cyclophosphamide*[26] are all equally effective in inducing remission in children with acute lymphatic leukemia, with remission rates ranging from 80% to 90% of patients. Other combinations of therapy such as *VAMP* (vincristine + amethopterin + 6-mercaptopurine + prednisone)[36] and *POMP* (the same agents except in a different dosage schedule—Purinethol + Oncovin + methotrexate + prednisolone[45] are probably not much more effective than the prednisone + vincristine, and there is an enhanced toxicity. *Prednisone + vincristine + daunorubicin,* when used in the initial remission induction regimens, is said to induce remissions in as many as 100% of patients[61, 75]; but other studies comparing the triple regimen with vincristine + prednisone alone to reinduce remission did not find it to be superior to prednisone + vincristine.[108] The myelosuppression associated with the triple therapy was much more severe. Only a very few results are available to evaluate the effectiveness of asparaginase when used in combination therapy with vincristine and prednisone,[101] but these are promising. Vincristine + cyclophosphamide is an efficient remission induction combination, but there is considerable myelotoxicity.[25]

The results with combination therapy in the remission induction of acute myelocytic leukemia have until recently been almost as discouraging as attempted remission inductions with single agents. *Prednisone + 6-mercaptopurine* induced remissions in only 3% of 77 adult patients with acute myelogenous leukemia,[106] and it was thought that prednisone probably had an adverse effect. The results with *6-mercaptopurine + methotrexate,*[31] *6-mercaptopurine + 6-methylmercaptopurine riboside,*[33] and *6-mercaptopurine + methyl GAG*[10] were somewhat better, and *POMP* was reported to induce remission in 70% of 51 children with acute myelogenous leukemia.[46]

When *cytosine arabinoside* was combined with other agents, however, definite improvement was noted. Recent studies indicate that combinations of *vincristine + arabinosyl cytosine + cyclophosphamide* (VAC),[97] *cytosine arabinoside + thioguanine,*[37] or *cyclophosphamide + vincristine + cytosine arabinoside + prednisone* (COAP)[34] are very effective in inducing remission in acute myelogenous leukemia. Except for VAC, the available reports relate to clinical trials in adults with acute myelogenous leukemia.

---

[*]References 26, 32, 65, 98, 116, 117.

Management of extramedullary leukemia

Occasionally a child presents at the time of initial diagnosis with leukemic infiltration of the meninges and massive infiltration of the kidneys, testes, ovaries, or other areas. The complications are discussed in Chapter 9, and therapeutic management is fully discussed in Chapter 11.

REMISSION MAINTENANCE

After a complete remission status has been attained, it has been difficult for some parents to understand that further therapy is necessary. It has now been established that if therapy is stopped at this point, most patients will relapse within 3 to 4 months. Only a few patients will remain in remission for longer than 6 months, and only rarely will a child live longer than 5 years without further treatment. That apparent cures do occur is illustrated by Fig. 10-5, which

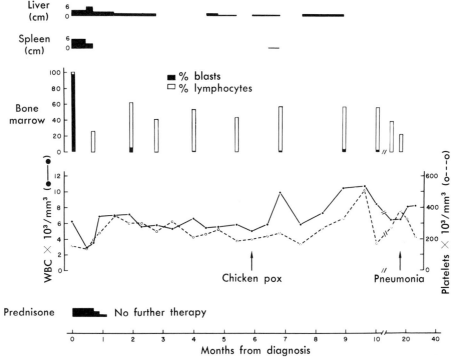

Fig. 10-5. Prolonged remission after 4 weeks of prednisone therapy. This 2½-year-old white boy presented with a 1-month history of increasing lethargy and pallor. He was extremely pale and had moderate hepatosplenomegaly. The hemoglobin was 2.8 gm/100 ml; the platelet count was 159,000/mm³, and the differential revealed 33% blasts. His bone marrow was almost completely replaced by primitive undifferentiated stem cells that had a scant amount of cytoplasm and a bilobed, "kidney-shaped" nucleus with a granular chromatin pattern. Prednisone, 2.2 mg/kg/day in four divided doses was administered. Within 3 weeks his spleen could not be palpated, his blood counts were normal, a marrow aspirate revealed less than 5% blasts, and he was thought to be in complete remission. He has had no evidence of recurrence of his disease for the past 9 years and has received no additional antileukemic therapy. It is interesting that he has had intermittent bone marrow lymphocytosis up to 60%. (Case history courtesy Drs. D. M. Lane and G. B. Humphrey, Department of Pediatrics, The University of Oklahoma Medical Center, Oklahoma City.)

gives a graphic illustration of a boy who has been completely free of his disease for 8 years after an initial remission induction of only 3 weeks of prednisone therapy.

The magnitude of the problem still facing the physician after remission has been induced can easily be visualized in biologic terms of the logs of reduction of leukemic cell population.[30, 96] If we assume that the child had approximately 10^{12} leukemic cells at the onset of remission induction,[15] the leukemic cell population has to be reduced to only 10^{10} cells to obtain a complete remission. It has been theorized that in order to cure the child, the leukemic cell population must be reduced to below 10^0, that is, the last leukemic cell must be destroyed. This was discussed further in Chapter 1. It has also been postulated that once the leukemic population is reduced below 10^5, if the child has some degree of immunologic resistance to his disease, the endogenous immune defense mechanism may eliminate the remaining malignant cells. Conversely, even though every last leukemic cell has been eradicated, the leukemogenic agent may still be present, and leukemia may recur. The recurrence of leukemia after 2 years or more without therapy may be the result of such an event.

While the child is in remission, he should be seen periodically so that his condition can be monitored for evidence of early relapse or drug toxicity. During the first several months of remission maintenance, the child is seen at weekly intervals for history, physical examination, and a complete blood count. After several months, he is seen every 2 weeks if there is no evidence of complication; after a year, the child is seen once a month but continues to have a complete blood count every 2 weeks as long as he remains in complete remission. Marrow morphology is examined at monthly intervals for the first 6 to 12 months and then every 2 to 3 months thereafter unless there is evidence of marrow relapse or leukemic infiltration of other organs. If a change of therapy is contemplated, regardless of the reason, a bone marrow aspirate should be examined.

Remission maintenance—single agent

Initially, the effectiveness of single agents will be presented, but, again, combination therapy is proving to be much more effective. (A summary of the effective remission agents is given in Table 10-3.) *Prednisone,*[60] *vincristine,*[64] L-*asparaginase,*[82] and probably *daunorubicin* are of little value as maintenance drugs. Not only is the remission of short duration but also the toxic side effects are intolerable. If the agent is used for continuous maintenance therapy until the patient relapses, permanent resistance to the drug develops, and it cannot be used again for remission induction. We have observed a number of children treated with continuous prednisone therapy after their initial remission induction. These children develop Cushingoid features, severe osteoporosis, and compression fractures of the vertebrae. These complications may be augmented by the child's disease and perhaps by additional chemotherapy, but we have never observed this problem in children who have not received long-term prednisone therapy. The roentgenograms of the vertebral column in a child with this complication are shown in Fig. 10-6. There is no indication for continuous prednisone administration during maintenance therapy of acute leukemia in children.

Table 10-3. Acute lymphatic leukemia remission maintenance: single agents

Agents	Optimal dosage schedule	Route	Expected MDR* (days)	Selected references
Methotrexate	3 mg/M²/day	PO	100	31, 92
	30 mg/M² 2 × wk†	IM, PO	300	92, 1
	3-5 mg/kg every 2 wk	IV	348	79
	15 mg/M²/day for 5 days every 2 wk for 8 mo†	IV	315	54
6-Mercaptopurine	2.5 mg/kg/day	PO	150	26,‡ 31, 35
Cyclophosphamide	5.0 mg/kg/day†	PO	120	26‡
Cytosine arabinoside	12 mg/kg 2 × wk	IV	130§	59, 107

*MDR = the median duration of remission.
†Severe toxicity may be observed and the dose revised downward.
‡Results for acute lymphatic leukemia and acute myelogenous leukemia combined.
§This is for acute myelogenous leukemia; the remaining are for acute lymphatic leukemia.

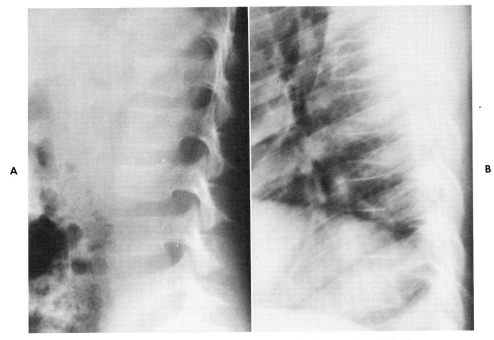

A   B

Fig. 10-6. Roentgenograms of thoracic vertebrae (**A**) and lumbar vertebrae (**B**). These roentgenograms reveal the severe osteoporosis that occurred in an 8-year-old white boy who had been on continuous prednisone therapy since his initial diagnosis 1½ years previously. He had severe radicular pain and was unable to walk. In addition to the prednisone, he had initially received intermittent short-term sequential therapy with 6-mercaptopurine, methotrexate, vincristine, and cyclophosphamide; at the time these x-ray films were taken, he was in marrow relapse. Prednisone was discontinued, and remission was induced with methotrexate. There was some improvement in his back pain, but this was a recurrent complication during the rest of his life.

Methotrexate is thought by many to be the most effective single agent to maintain remission.[31, 92] For many years methotrexate was given daily by mouth at a dosage level of about 3 mg/M². After Goldin observed that a twice-weekly schedule was much more effective in prolonging the survival of mice with early experimental mouse leukemia (L1210),[42] a clinical trial in acute lymphatic leukemia of childhood was undertaken after remission was induced with prednisone + vincristine, comparing methotrexate given twice weekly (30 mg/M² intramuscularly) with a daily schedule of 3 mg/M²/day by mouth. The median duration of remission was 11 months when given two times per week as compared with 2 months when given daily.[92]

A study comparing oral versus intramuscular methotrexate given two times per week indicated that there was no difference in the median duration of remission,[1] and methotrexate is now most frequently given orally two times per week. Good results have been obtained with methotrexate given intravenously at 2-week intervals at a dosage level of 3 to 5 mg/kg.[79] Furthermore, the hepatic fibrosis, bone complications (osteoporosis, fracture), and pneumonitis that are sometimes observed when methotrexate is given on a twice-weekly schedule are much less frequent when it is given once every 2 weeks.[77] Recently, Holland and Glidewell[54] have reported that 20% of children receiving intensive methotrexate therapy (15 to 18 mg/M²/day for 5 days every 2 weeks for 8 months) will remain in remission in excess of 2 years. Djerassi and co-workers have reported prolonged remissions in children receiving intensive methotrexate therapy for 2 days every 28 days.[19] These observations have not yet been confirmed.

Remissions in childhood acute leukemia maintained with daily oral *6-mercaptopurine** are probably equal in length to those obtained by methotrexate, and the toxic side effects other than myelosuppression are much fewer. The optimum dosage schedule is 2.5 mg/kg/day by mouth until relapse. Three courses of 1000 mg/M²/day of 6-mercaptopurine intravenously for 5 days during the first 50 days of remission and then stopped has been reported to be almost as effective.[53] Results from a current ongoing study by the Southwest Cancer Chemotherapy Study Group indicate that the median duration of remission is shorter in children receiving oral daily 6-mercaptopurine for a 2-month or a 6-month period as compared with children on continuous 6-mercaptopurine therapy to relapse.[98] To date, 6-mercaptopurine remains the most effective single agent to sustain remission of acute myelogenous leukemia.[46]

Cyclophosphamide given on a daily oral schedule of 5 mg/kg/day has been reported as effective as 6-mercaptopurine to sustain remission,[26] but because of its toxic side effects (hemorrhagic cystitis, alopecia), it is the third drug of choice. Fig. 10-7 illustrates the effectiveness of cyclophosphamide therapy in a 14-year-old boy with acute leukemia. Fig. 10-8 is the urogram of a 9-year-old boy in whom cyclophosphamide therapy was discontinued because of a contracted spastic bladder. To attain an optimal therapeutic benefit, it is necessary to administer the drug at a maximally tolerated dosage level that will keep the white blood cell count between 1500 and 4000/mm³. Unlike 6-mercaptopurine and methotrexate, if severe leukopenia (below 1000/mm³)

---

*References 9, 12, 26, 31, 35, 49, 100.

develops, rapid recovery within 4 to 7 days of cessation of therapy almost invariably ensues.

Most studies evaluating cytosine arabinoside[59, 112] as a maintenance agent have been disappointing. An exception was the study by Traggis and colleagues.[107] After remission had been induced with cytosine arabinoside, the children were placed on a regimen of 15 mg/kg twice weekly. The median duration of remission for this group was 130 days.

Remission consolidation and maintenance—multiple agents

Since no single drug has been found that will sustain prolonged remission in the majority of patients, many different combinations of agents have been investigated in an attempt to either completely eradicate all the malignant cells or, if this is not possible, to suppress recurrence of the disease. Some of the earlier reported studies were designed to prevent the development of resistance to chemotherapeutic agents by simultaneous administration of several agents

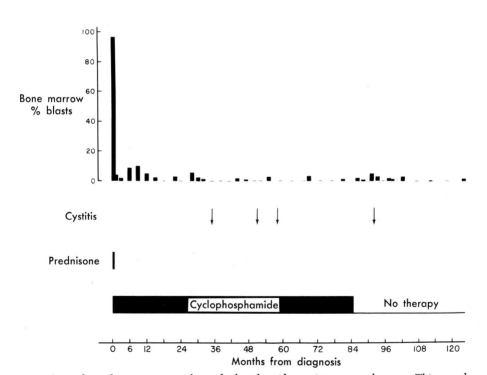

Fig. 10-7. Prolonged remission with cyclophosphamide maintenance therapy. This graph depicts the clinical course of a white boy in whom the diagnosis of acute lymphoblastic leukemia was made in 1961 at 3⅔ years of age. Remission was induced with 2.2 mg/kg/day of prednisone and 5 mg/kg/day of cyclophosphamide, and the boy was then maintained on a regimen of cyclophosphamide. Cyclophosphamide therapy was temporarily discontinued on three occasions because of hematuria. Intravenous pyelograms and voiding cystograms showed no evidence of bladder contraction or other urinary tract pathology, and the medication was resumed within 2 weeks after each bout of hematuria. Chemotherapy was stopped after 85 months, and he has remained in continuous bone marrow remission up to the present time (February, 1973—almost 12 years since the initial diagnosis).

(Table 10-4) or cycling (Table 10-5) the agents at periodic intervals. Subsequent studies comparing cyclic with sequential use of the same agents did demonstrate that the median duration of remission was longer in the cyclic therapy group but the median duration of survival and the number of long-term survivors was the same for both groups.[5, 32, 65, 98] Children's Cancer Study Group A evaluated the addition of dactinomycin and nitrogen mustard to the

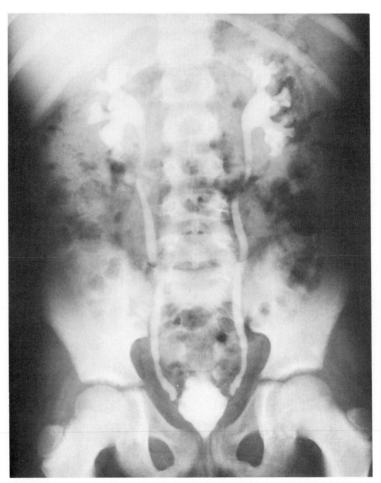

Fig. 10-8. Contracted bladder and ureterectasis secondary to cyclophosphamide therapy. This urogram reveals the contracted bladder and ureterectasis that occurred in a 9-year-old white boy receiving cyclophosphamide therapy. After a diagnosis of acute lymphatic leukemia was made, he was started on a regimen of 2.2 mg/kg/day of prednisone and 5 mg/kg/day of cyclophosphamide. After 1 month of therapy he was in complete remission; prednisone was stopped, and he was maintained on cyclophosphamide. Hematuria developed 4 weeks later, but cyclophosphamide therapy was continued for another 18 days. This urogram was obtained, and cyclophosphamide therapy was stopped, then restarted 10 days later after the hematuria ceased. He had no recurrence of his hematuria. Cyclophosphamide therapy was permanently discontinued 1 month later because of bone marrow relapse. (From Gellman, E., Kissane, J., Frech, R., Vietti, T., and McAlister, W.: J. Can. Assoc. Radiol. **20**:99-101, 1969.)

cyclic regimen of alternating 6-mercaptopurine with methotrexate at 8-week intervals. These studies suggest that there was an increase in the median duration of remission in those patients receiving dactinomycin + nitrogen mustard as compared with a control group.[69]

The VAMP (vincristine + amethopterin + 6-mercaptopurine + prednisone) protocol was originally designed to eradicate all leukemic cells, incorporating the tolerated doses of drugs into combination therapy. Remission was induced with this combination and intermittent courses given for 4 months, after which therapy was stopped. By using data from another study that suggested that the average doubling time of the leukemic cell population was around 4 days, Frei[30]

Table 10-4. Remission maintenance: multiple agents in combination

Agents		Dosage schedule	Route	Duration therapy	MDR* (days)	Selected references
6-Mercaptopurine		3 mg/kg/day	PO	Until	112	31
Methotrexate		3 mg/M²/day	PO	relapse		
Vincristine	V	2 mg/M²/on day 1 only	IV			
Amethopterin	A	20 mg/M²/days 1 and 4	IV, IM	5 mo	245	36
6-Mercaptopurine	M	60 mg/M²/day	PO			
Prednisone	P	40 mg/M²/day × 8	PO			
Purinethol	P	500 mg/M²/day × 5	IV			
Oncovin	O	2 mg/M²/on day 1 only	IV	14 mo	405	45
Methotrexate	M	7.5 mg/M²/day × 5	IV			
Prednisolone	P	1 Gm/M²/day × 5	IV			
Cytosine arabinoside		120 mg/M²/wk	IM	Until	233†	97
Cyclophosphamide		75 mg/M²/day	PO	relapse		

*MDR = the median duration of remission.
†This MDR is for children with acute myelogenous leukemia. The others are for children with acute lymphatic leukemia.

Table 10-5. Remission maintenance: cyclic therapy

Agents	Dosage schedule	Route	Time interval for complete cycle	MDR or MDS*	References
6-Mercaptopurine	2.5 mg/kg/day	PO (12 wk)	24 wk	MDR (11 mo†)	116
Methotrexate	3 mg/M²/day	PO (12 wk)			
Methotrexate	3.3 mg/M²/day	PO (6 wk)			
Vincristine	2.0 mg/M²/wk	IV (6 wk)			
Prednisone	60 mg/M²/day	PO (6 wk)	30 wk	MDS (17.8 mo)	65
Cyclophosphamide	50 mg/M²/day	PO (6 wk)			
6-Mercaptopurine	70 mg/M²/day	PO (6 wk)			
Vincristine	2-3 mg/M²/wk	IV (6 wk)			
6-Mercaptopurine	65 mg/M²/day	PO (12 wk)	30 wk	MDS (22 mo†)	5
Cyclophosphamide	75 mg/M²/day	PO (6 wk)			
Methotrexate	3.2 mg/M²/day	PO (6 wk)			

*MDR = the median duration of remission; MDS = the median duration of survival.
†Extrapolated data.

theorized that the VAMP regimen reduced the leukemic population to less than ten cells. Subsequently, using a different therapeutic regimen of the same agents, POMP was given to induce remission and was continued for a total of 14 months. The median duration of remission for this group of patients was 13.5 months.[45] We have used both VAMP and POMP regimens for remission induction and maintenance therapy in patients who have previously relapsed on both 6-mercaptopurine and methotrexate. Although most patients either failed to achieve remission or the remissions were of short duration, about 20% have had complete remissions for 6 months or more.

After remission induction with prednisone and vincristine and 1 week of consolidation therapy with high-dose 6-mercaptopurine, methotrexate, and cyclophosphamide, Pinkel and colleagues placed the patients on a regimen of continuous oral 6-mercaptopurine, and methotrexate and cyclophosphamide were given once weekly.[39, 89] They obtained median remission durations similar to those observed with the POMP regimen. In one of their protocols they reduced drug therapy by half to determine whether it was necessary to utilize maximal therapeutic doses during therapy. These children did significantly less well than children who received the maximal dosage schedule.[4]

Some of the most effective regimens that are now being evaluated currently utilize "intermittent reinduction" or "reinforcement therapy" with prednisone and vincristine in combination with continuous maintenance therapy.[54, 98] Bernard and Boiron,[6] using a maintenance regimen similar to that of Pinkel and colleagues, except that prednisone and vincristine were given every 6 months and cyclophosphamide was omitted, reported a median duration of remission in excess of 3 years. The Southwest Cancer Chemotherapy Study Group has just completed a study in which 6-mercaptopurine alone was used for maintenance and prednisone and vincristine were given for 1 month every 3 months. Our results appear to parallel the more intensive chemotherapeutic regimens, and preliminary evaluation indicates that the median duration of hematologic remission was 80 weeks.[98] Good results were also obtained by Acute Leukemia Group B.[54] This cooperative group used methotrexate for continuous maintenance, and prednisone and vincristine were administered at 6-week intervals for 8 months. Therapy was then stopped and the patients followed up until relapse; 30% have been in unmaintained remission for more than 2½ years since starting treatment. (See Table 10-6.)

"Sanctuary" therapy

Attention has recently been directed to "sanctuary" therapy. Relapse in many of the long-term survivors has been heralded by the development of meningeal leukemia.[3, 32, 78] Single or multiple injections of intrathecal methotrexate[78] did not prolong the total duration of survival, but there was a decrease or delay or both in the occurrence of central nervous system disease. Management of extramedullary disease is completely discussed in Chapter 11. Prophylactic sanctuary therapy is currently under intensive investigation. In a very small study by Nesbit, 2400 rads were given to the craniospinal axis, liver, spleen, and gonads of patients; 3 of the 10 children so treated have been in complete remission for longer than 6½ years.[80, 94] In a recent study reported by Pinkel and co-workers, in addition to an intensive systemic maintenance regimen, 2400 rads were given to the skull and 12 mg/M² of intrathecal methotrexate was given twice weekly for five doses.[4] Over 63% of the children who were entered on this study have survived for 31 months or longer from the date of diagnosis. Recently this group has reported on a comparative study of radiation therapy to the entire craniospinal axis as compared with no radiation therapy. Those patients receiving radiation therapy have remained in complete remission longer than the control patients.[3]

MANAGEMENT OF RELAPSE

Patients who have responded to previous prednisone-vincristine induction therapy and have not been on maintenance therapy with these two drugs have better than a 70% to 80% chance of responding to a second remission induction, 60% to 70% chance for a third remission, and 50% to 60% chance for a fourth remission.[99] Fig. 10-9 gives the clinical course of a 3½-year-old boy who had repeated remission inductions with prednisone and vincristine.

If the child fails to respond to prednisone and vincristine, L-asparaginase either alone or in combination with other agents would be the next therapy of choice. Cytosine arabinoside given at a dosage level of 25 mg/kg twice weekly intramuscularly has been reported to be an effective remission induction regimen

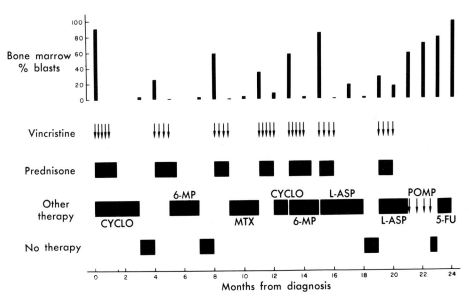

Fig. 10-9. Repeated remission inductions with vincristine and prednisone. This illustration depicts the clinical course of a 3½-year-old Negro boy with acute lymphocytic leukemia. He expired within 24 months, during which time he had six complete remissions and one partial remission, all of which were induced with weekly intravenous vincristine and daily oral prednisone over a month's duration. 6-Mercaptopurine and L-asparaginase were also administered during the fifth and sixth inductions, respectively, and L-asparaginase was administered during the induction of the last partial remission. His final relapse occurred 21 months after diagnosis and did not respond to the eighth trial of vincristine and prednisone as part of a POMP protocol. Attempts to induce remission with 5-fluorouracil and high-dose intravenous cyclophosphamide were unsuccessful. This patient's remissions—maintained or unmaintained—were never longer than 3 months.

in patients resistant to other remission induction regimens.[107] Daunorubicin is effective but is associated with severe toxicity.[8, 63, 70] Initial trials with adriamycin are promising,[98, 111a] although considerable myelotoxicity has been observed.

After the remission has been reinduced, any of the other agents previously mentioned under maintenance can be used if the child's disease is not known to be resistant to these drugs. In general, the second and third remissions are generally not as long as the initial remission, but numerous exceptions have been observed.

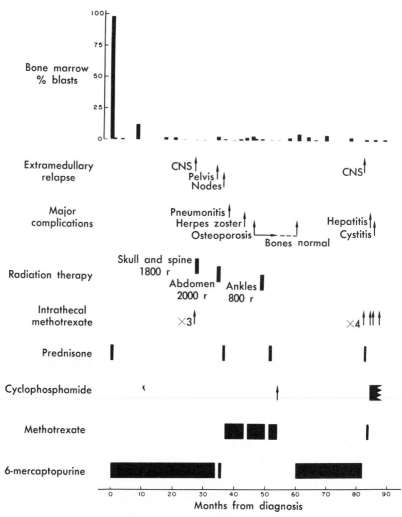

Fig. 10-10. Complications observed during long-term therapy for acute lymphoblastic leukemia. This graph depicts the clinical course of a white girl who was diagnosed at 7 years of age and has remained in continuous bone marrow remission since her initial remission induction with prednisone and 6-mercaptopurine. She has had four documented extramedullary relapses; two episodes of meningeal leukemia; massive infiltration of the uterus, ovaries, and adnexal tissue; and leukemic involvement of the cervical lymph nodes.

As the duration of hematologic remissions increases, the occurrence of extra-medullary relapses has become an increasing problem. Fig. 10-10 is a graph of a 14-year-old girl who has had two episodes of meningeal infiltration, invasion of the uterus and ovaries, and infiltration of her lymph nodes, but no evidence of marrow relapse since her initial remission induction.

DURATION OF THERAPY

A decade ago, the median duration of survival was only 10 to 12 months. Now the problem is arising with increasing frequency as to how long therapy should be continued with children who have been in continual complete re-mission for 2 or more years since their initial diagnosis. This question is com-pletely unanswered at the present time. A small group of patients from Chil-dren's Cancer Study Group A who had been in continuous remission for 3 or more years were randomized to continuous therapy versus no further therapy.[66] The results to date do not suggest any difference between the two groups. This is being expanded into a much larger study, but obviously a long time will be required before we are able to answer this question.

IMMUNOTHERAPY

Immunotherapy is one of the most fascinating new approaches to the treat-ment of acute leukemia. A number of investigators have shown that growth of a tumor in the experimental animal can be retarded by pretreatment of the host before grafting the tumor. This may be performed either by inoculation of irradi-ated tumor cells[40] or by adjuncts such as BCG,[2, 83, 84] *Corynebacterium par-vum,*[115] and *Bordetella pertussis* vaccine.[113] It is noted that when grafting was accomplished with a small number of leukemic cells (10^5), active immunotherapy (BCG, irradiated leukemia cells, or both) was effective in curing some animals even when started *after* the cells were inoculated.[76] It was therefore postulated that if the number of leukemic cells in the body were sufficiently reduced, active immunotherapy might play a significant role in reducing this number even further and hopefully curing the patient.

There has been some controversy as to whether leukemic cells carry specific antigens on their surface membrane. Viza and colleagues[110] have reported that cells taken from patients in relapse and stored in liquid nitrogen were able, when inactivated, to stimulate autologous lymphocytes in the mixed lymphocyte culture obtained when the patient was in remission. This occurred in 4 of 5 acute leukemia patients. Hirschhorn and Fudenberg[50] found that inactivated leukemic cells from one monozygotic twin produced significant stimulation of lymphocytes from the other (healthy) twin.

Mathé[74] reported on 30 patients included in a trial of immunotherapy. All had acute lymphoblastic leukemia. After remission was induced, numerous diagnostic aspirations were performed (including multiple bone marrow bi-opsies; biopsies of the kidneys, liver, and testicles; and examination of CSF and EEG) to verify that the patients were in "complete" remission. This was followed by multiple chemotherapeutic agents, sequential intrathecal metho-trexate, and irradiation of the CNS (1000 rads). At this time all chemotherapy was stopped, and the patients were randomized into four treatment groups: (1) patients receiving no further treatment (controls), (2) patients receiving

Table 10-6. Remission maintenance: reinforcement therapy

Agent(s) used for continuous therapy	Dosage schedule	Route	Reinforcement	Dosage schedule	Route	Frequency	Response*	References
6-Mercaptopurine	75 mg/M²/day	PO	Vincristine / Prednisone	2 mg/M²/wk x 4 wk / 60 mg/M²/day × 4 wk	IV / PO	Every 3 mo	MDR (80 wk)	98
6-Mercaptopurine / Methotrexate†	90 mg/M²/day / 15 mg/M²/wk	PO / IM	Vincristine / Prednisone	1-2 mg/M²/wk × 3 / 120 mg/M²/day × 15 days	IV / PO	Every 6 mo	MDS (37 mo)	6
6-Mercaptopurine‡ / Methotrexate / Cyclophosphamide	50 mg/M²/day / 30 mg/M²/wk / 200 mg/M²/wk	PO / IV / IV	Vincristine / Prednisone	1.5 mg/M²/wk × 3 / 40 mg/M²/day × 15 days	IV / PO	Every 10 wk	75% in CR over 1 yr	4
Methotrexate	15 mg/M²/day × 5 every 2 wk		Vincristine / Prednisone	2 mg/M²/wk × 3 / 40 mg/M²/day × 15 days	IV / PO	Every 3 wk	40% in CR unmaintained over 1 yr	54

*MDS = the median duration of survival; MDR = the median duration of remission; CR = the complete remission.
†Three of the doses of methotrexate were given intrathecally.
‡Patients given "consolidation therapy" followed by 2400 rads to skull and 5 doses of intrathecal methotrexate.

BCG vaccination, (3) patients receiving irradiated leukemic cells, and (4) patients receiving a combination of BCG and leukemic cells. By 125 days, all 10 untreated patients had relapsed. Of the group receiving immunotherapy, 7 of the 20 were still in remission more than a year after stopping therapy. There was no difference between patients receiving BCG (five relapses in 8 patients), leukemic cell inoculations (three relapses in 5 patients), and both treatments (five relapses in 7 patients). Since then, newer protocols have been devised adding *Corynebacterium parvum* to the immunotherapy, together with the drugs vincristine and amantadine. Although these preliminary reports are encouraging, immunotherapy cannot be accepted as a mode of treatment until other centers are able to confirm these results.

BONE MARROW TRANSPLANTATION

The successful use of allogeneic bone marrow grafts in the treatment of accidentally irradiated persons led many investigators to try this form of therapy in the treatment of acute leukemia.[62] The prime goal of such treatment was to permit the use of very high doses of radiation therapy or chemotherapy in an effort to destroy all leukemic cells. It was hoped that the infused donor cells would repopulate the patient's marrow. An ancillary beneficial effect would be the destruction of any remaining leukemic cells by specific graft versus host reaction of the donor's lymphocytes against the host's leukemic cells.

One of the main stumbling blocks in this approach is the problem of tissue rejection. If this procedure is carried out between identical twins, there will be no rejection phenomena because the donor and recipient have similar histocompatibility (HL-A) antigens. If, however, the donor and recipient differ in their HL-A antigens, the patient's lymphocytes will react against the infused donor cells (host versus graft reaction). Similarly, the infused immunocompetent lymphocytes will react against the recipient's tissue cells (graft versus host disease). Since the patient is generally severely immunosuppressed at the time of the bone marrow transplant, either by total body radiation or chemotherapy, it is the latter complication that becomes a serious problem. Graft versus host reactions in the recipient are generally characterized by an ill-defined syndrome of scaly erythematous skin reaction, alopecia, diarrhea, jaundice with disturbed liver function, weight loss, severe infection, bone marrow failure, and finally death. There have been many attempts to eliminate or at least diminish these reactions, including the use of cyclophosphamide or antilymphocyte globulin. Another approach is to separate immunocompetent cells from the marrow graft, by either velocity sedimentation or density gradient centrifugation, and exclude them from the transplant graft.

Closely matched family siblings offer the best chances of a successful graft. The sibling has a reasonable chance (1 in 4) of being HL-A identical to the patient. Extensive tissue typing by antisera and mixed lymphocyte cultures must be performed to ensure that the donor and recipient are closely matched. Then, with the donor under general anesthesia, multiple bone marrow aspirations are performed. At least 10^9 cells must be collected, and these marrow cells are then infused intravenously (with special precautions taken to prevent marrow embolism) into the immunosuppressed patient.

The results so far have not been very encouraging. Out of 834 patients treated in this manner, only 14 were still alive when last reported.[11] Survival in these 14 patients varied from 16 days to 660 days. Five patients were alive more than 200 days after the transplant. Recently, a case was reported of a 16-year-old girl with acute lymphoblastic leukemia that was resistant to all chemotherapy who was given 1000 rads whole-body radiation.[29] This was followed by infusion of marrow from an HL-A matched brother. Blood counts showed successful graft, and male only (XY) donor cells could be identified. Recurrent leukemia was evidenced 62 days after transplant. Cytogenetics revealed that the leukemia recurred in the XY normal donor cells. This case suggests the possibility of a leukemogenic factor (possibly a virus), which induced the leukemic transformation of her brother's cells. If this observation is reproduced, the concept of curing leukemia by the "total cell kill" approaches will have to be completely reevaluated.

Although the results to date of bone marrow transplantation are not very encouraging, principally because of graft versus host disease, some information has been gathered from this procedure. If immunologic rejection can be modified, this method of therapy may be of great value in the treatment of acute leukemia.

SUMMARY OF THERAPY

Great strides have been made in the management of acute lymphatic leukemia. Almost 90% of the children falling under this classification will achieve remission with a relatively simple regimen of vincristine and prednisone, and current analysis of the data from some maintenance regimens indicates that the median duration of survival will be in excess of 3 to 4 years. There is an increasing number of 5-year survivors who have had no evidence of recurrence of their disease.

Advances in the treatment and management of the child with acute myelogenous leukemia have been much more disheartening. The number of children in this classification who achieve remission is increasing, but adequate maintenance regimens remain to be described.

A definitive therapeutic regimen for the management of acute leukemia was not outlined in this chapter because it may well be that by the time this book is in print our concepts of optimal treatment will have changed considerably. A review of the effect of single agents on the disease and on the patient was presented, not because this would be considered reasonable therapy, but because the clinician taking care of a child receiving multiple agents should know the therapeutic potential and toxicity of each drug. Because the concepts of optimal therapy are changing so rapidly, it is wise for the physician who rarely sees a child with acute leukemia to consult one of his colleagues at a medical center so that his patient can have the best that recent medical advances have to offer.

Most of the treatment schedules in use today involve a regimen of chemotherapeutic drugs either intermittently or continuously for at least 2 years. Hopefully, in the near future other therapeutic modalities will be proposed by the tumor biologists that will achieve even more favorable results, but without the toxicity that is associated with long-term cytocidal therapy.

REFERENCES

1. Acute Leukemia Group B: Acute lymphocytic leukemia in children: maintenance therapy with methotrexate administered intermittently, J.A.M.A. **207**:923-928, 1969.
2. Amiel, J. L.: Immunotherapie active non-specifique par le B. C. G. de la leucémie virale E G₂ chez des receveurs isogeniques, Rev. Fr. Etud. Clin. Biol. **12**:912-914, 1967.
3. Aur, R. J. A., Simone, J. V., Hustu, H. O., and Verzosa, M. S.: A comparative study of central nervous system irradiation and intensive chemotherapy early in remission of childhood acute lymphocytic leukemia, Cancer **29**:381-391, 1972.
4. Aur, R. J. A., Simone, J., Hustu, H. O., Walters, T., Borella, L., Pratt, C., and Pinkel, D.: Central nervous system therapy and combination chemotherapy of childhood lymphocytic leukemia, Blood **37**:272-281, 1971.
5. Australian Cancer Society's Childhood Leukemia Study Group: Cyclic drug regimen for acute childhood leukemia, Lancet **1**:313-318, 1968.
6. Bernard, J., and Boiron, M.: Current status: treatment of acute leukemia, Semin. Hematol. **7**:427-440, 1970.
7. Bernard, J., Boiron, M., Weil, M., Levy, J. P., Seligman, M., and Najean, J.: Etude de la remission complete des leucémies aiguës, Nouv. Rev. Fr. Hematol. **2**:195, 1962.
7a. Bernard, J., Jacquillat, C., and Weil, M.: Treatment of the leukemias, Semin. Hematol. **9**:181-192, 1972.
8. Bernard, J., Jacquillat, C., Weil, M., Boiron, M., and Tanzer, J.: Present results on daunorubicine (rubidomycin, daunomycin). In Mathé, G., editor: Recent results in cancer research: advances in the treatment of acute (blastic) leukemias, New York, 1970, Springer-Verlag New York, Inc.
9. Boggs, D., Wintrobe, M. W., and Cartwright, G. E.: The acute leukemias, Medicine **41**:163-225, 1962.
10. Boiron, J., Jacquillat, C., and Weil, M.: Combination of methylgloxal-bis-(guanylhydrazone) (NSC-32946) and 6-mercaptopurine in acute granulocytic leukemia, Cancer Chemother. Rep. **45**:69, 1965.
11. Bortin, M. D.: A compendum of reported human bone marrow transplants, Transplantation **9**:571-587, 1970.
12. Burchenal, J. H., Murphy, M. L., Ellison, R. R., Sykes, M. P., Tan, C. C., Leone, L. A., Karnofsky, D. A., Craver, L. F., Dargeon, H. W., and Rhoads, C. P.: Clinical evaluation of a new antimetabolite, 6-mercaptopurine, in the treatment of leukemia and allied diseases, Blood **8**:965-999, 1953.
13. Cancer Chemotherapy National Service Center: Thioguanine and thioguanosine, Cancer Chemother. Rep. **11**:202-213, 1961.
14. Carbone, P. P., Haskell, C. M., Canellos, G. P., Leventhal, B. G., Block, J., Serpick, A. A., and Selawry, O. S.: Asparaginase: early clinical and toxicology studies. In Mathé, G., editor: Recent results in cancer research: advances in the treatment of acute (blastic) leukemias, New York, 1970, Springer-Verlag New York, Inc.
15. Clarkson, B. D.: Clinical techniques for evaluating antileukemic efficacy. In Siegler, P. E., and Moyer, J. H., III, editors: Animal and clinical pharmacologic techniques in drug evaluation, Chicago, 1967, Year Book Medical Publishers, Inc.
16. Clarkson, B. D., and Fried, J.: Changing concepts of treatment in acute leukemia, Med. Clin. North Am. **55**:561-600, 1971.
17. Crowther, D., Bateman, C. J. T., Vartan, C. P., Whitehouse, J. M. A., Malpas, J. S., Fairly, H. G., and Bodley-Scott, R.: Combination chemotherapy using L-asparaginase, a daunorubicin, and cytosine arabinoside in the treatment of adults with acute myelogenous leukemia, Nature (Lond.) **229**:168-171, 1971.
18. Delmonte, L., and Jukes, T. H.: Folic acid antagonists in cancer chemotherapy, Pharmacol. Rev. **14**:91-135, 1962.
19. Djerassi, I., Farber, S., Esshagh, A., and Neikirk, W.: Continuous infusion of methotrexate in children with acute leukemia, Cancer **20**:233-242, 1967.
20. Ellison, R. R., Holland, J. F., Weil, M., Jacquillat, C., Boiron, M., Bernard, J., Sawitsky, A., Rosner, F., Gussoff, B., Silver, R. T., Karanas, A., Cuttner, J., Spurr, C. L., Hayes, D. M., Blom, J., Leone, L. A., Haurani, F., Kyle, R., Hutchinson, J. L., Forcier, R. J.,

and Moon, J. H.: Arabinosyl cytosine: a useful agent in the treatment of acute leukemia in adults, Blood **32**:507-523, 1968.

21. Evans, A. E., Farber, S., Brunet, S., and Mariano, P. J.: Vincristine in the treatment of acute leukemia in children, Cancer **16**:1302-1306, 1963.

22. Fairley, G. H.: Clinical experience with L-asparaginase and side effects. In Mathé, G., editor: Recent results in cancer research: advances in the treatment of acute (blastic) leukemias, New York, 1970, Springer-Verlag New York, Inc.

23. Farber, S., Diamond, L. K., Mercer, R. D., Sylvester, R. F., Jr., and Wolff, J. A.: Temporary remissions in acute leukemia in children produced by folic acid antagonist, 4-aminopteryl-glutamic acid (aminopterin), N. Engl. J. Med. **238**:787-793, 1948.

24. Fernbach, D. J.: Personal communication.

25. Fernbach, D. J., Donaldson, M., Lane, D., Lonsdale, D., and Vietti, T. J.: The treatment of advanced acute leukemia in children with concomitant vincristine sulfate and cyclophosphamide. In Jaffe, E. R., editor: Proceedings of the Twelfth International Society of Hematology, New York, 1968, p. 8.

26. Fernbach, D. J., Griffith, K. M., Haggard, M. E., Holcomb, T. M., Sutow, W. W., and Vietti, T. J.: Chemotherapy of acute leukemia in childhood: comparison of cyclophosphamide and mercaptourine, N. Engl. J. Med. **275**:451-456, 1966.

27. Fernbach, D. J., Sutow, W. W., Thurman, W. G., and Vietti, T. J.: Clinical evaluation of cyclophosphamide, a new agent for the treatment of children with acute leukemia, J.A.M.A. **182**:30-37, 1962.

28. Fessas, P., Wintrobe, M. M., Thompson, R. B., and Cartwright, G. D.: Treatment of acute leukemia with cortisone and corticotropin, Arch. Intern. Med. **94**:384-401, 1954.

29. Fialkow, P. J., Thomas, E. D., Bryant, J. I., and Neiman, P. E.: Leukaemic transformation of engrafted human marrow cells in vivo, Lancet **1**:251-255, 1971.

30. Frei, E., III, and Freireich, E. J.: Progress and perspectives in chemotherapy of acute leukemia. In Goldin, A., Hawking, F., and Schnitzer, R. J., editors: Advances in chemotherapy, New York, 1965, Academic Press, Inc.

31. Frei, E., III, Freireich, E. J., Gehan, E., Pinkel, D., Holland, J. F., Selawry, O., Haurani, F., Spurr, C. L., Hayes, D. M., James, G. W., Rothberg, H., Sodee, D. G., Rundles, R. W., Schroeder, L. R., Hoogstraten, B., Wolman, I. J., Traggis, D. G., Cooper, T., Gendel, B. R., Ebaugh, F., and Taylor, R. (Acute Leukemia Cooperative Group B): Studies of sequential and combination antimetabolite therapy in acute leukemia: 6-mercaptopurine and methotrexate, from the Acute Leukemia Group B, Blood **18**:431-454, 1961.

32. Frei, E., III, Karon, M., Levin, R. H., Freireich, E. J., Taylor, R. J., Hananian, J., Selawry, O., Holland, J. F., Hoogstraten, B., Wolman, I. J., Abir, E., Sawitsky, A., Lee, S., Mills, S. D., Burget, E. O., Jr., Spurr, C. L., Patterson, R. B., Ebaugh, F. G., James, G. W., III., and Moon, J. H.: The effectiveness of combinations of antileukemia agents in inducing and maintaining remission in children with acute leukemia, Blood **26**:642-656, 1965.

33. Freireich, E. J., Bodey, G. P., Harris, J. E., and Hart, J. S.: Therapy for acute granulocytic leukemia, Cancer Res. **27**:2573, 1967.

34. Freireich, E. J., Bodey, G. P., Hart, J. S., Whitecar, J. P., Jr., and McCredie, K. B.: Current status of therapy for acute leukemia. In Ultmann, J. E., Griem, M. L., Kirsten, W. H., and Wissler, R. W., editors: Recent results in cancer research: current concepts in the management of leukemia and lymphoma, New York, 1971, Springer-Verlag New York, Inc.

35. Freireich, E. J., Gehan, E., Frei, E., III, Schroeder, L. R., Wolman, I. J., Anbari, R., Burgert, E. O., Mills, S. D., Pinkel, D., Selawry, O. S., Moon, J. H., Gendel, B. R., Spurr, C. L., Storrs, R., Haurani, F., Hoogstraten, B., and Lee, W.: The effect of 6-mercaptourine on the duration of steroid-induced remission in acute leukemia: a model for evaluation of other potentially useful therapy, Blood **21**:699-716, 1963.

36. Freireich, E. J., Henderson, E. S., Karon, M. R., and Frei, E., III: The treatment of acute leukemia considered with respect to cell population kinetics. In University of Texas M. D. Anderson Hospital and Tumor Institute: Proliferation and spread of neoplastic cells, Baltimore, 1968, Williams & Wilkins Co.

37. Gee, T. S., Yu, K. P., and Clarkson, B. D.: Treatment of adult acute leukemia with arabinosyl cytosine and thioguanine, Cancer 23:1019-1032, 1969.

38. Gellman, E., Kissane, J., Frech, R., Vietti, T., and McAlister, W.: Cyclophosphamide cystitis, J. Can. Assoc. Radiol. 20:99-101, 1969.

39. George, P., Hernandez, K., Hustu, O., Borella, L., Holton, C., and Pinkel, D.: A study of "total therapy" of acute lymphocytic leukemia in children, J. Pediatr. 72:399-408, 1968.

40. Glynn, J. P., Humphreys, S. R., Trivers, G., Bianco, A. R., and Goldin, A.: Studies on immunity to leukemia L1210 in mice, Cancer Res. 23:1008-1015, 1963.

41. Goldin, A., and Mantel, N.: The employment of combinations of drugs in the chemotherapy of neoplasia: a review, Cancer Res. 17:635-654, 1967.

42. Goldin, A., Venditti, J. M., Humphreys, S. R., and Mantel, N.: Modification of treatment schedules in the management of advanced mouse leukemia with amethopterin, J. Natl. Cancer Inst. 17:203-212, 1956.

43. Haggard, M. E., Fernbach, D. J., Holcomb, T. M., Sutow, W. W., Vietti, T. J., and Windmiller, J. A.: Vincristine in acute leukemia of childhood, Cancer 22:438-444, 1968.

44. Hartmann, J. R., Origenes, M. L., Jr., Murphy, M. L., Sitarz, A., and Erlandson, M.: Effects of 2'deoxy-5-fluorouridine and 5-fluorouracil on childhood leukemia, Cancer Chemother. Rep. 34:51-54, 1964.

45. Henderson, E. S.: Combination chemotherapy of acute lymphocytic leukemia of childhood, Cancer Res. 27:2570-2572, 1967.

46. Henderson, E. S.: Treatment of Leukemia, Semin. Hematol. 6:271-319, 1969.

47. Henderson, E. S., and Samaha, R. J.: Evidence that drugs in multiple combinations have materially advanced the treatment of human malignancies, Cancer Res. 29:2272-2280, 1969.

48. Heyn, R. M., Beatty, E. C., Jr., Hammond, D., Louis, J., Pierce, M., Murphy, M. L., and Severo, N.: Vincristine in the treatment of acute leukemia, Pediatrics 38:82-91, 1966.

49. Heyn, R. M., Brubaker, C. A., Burchenal, J. H., Cramblett, H. G., and Wolff, J. A.: The comparison of 6-mercaptopurine with the combination of 6-mercaptopurine and azaserine in the treatment of acute leukemia in children: results of a cooperative study, Blood 15:350-359, 1960.

50. Hirschhorn, K., and Fudenberg, H. H.: Cited by Viza, D. C. et al.: Leukemia antigens, Lancet 2:493-494, 1969.

51. Holcomb, T. M.: Cyclophosphamide (NSC-26271) in the treatment of acute leukemia in children, Cancer Chemother. Rep. 51:389-392, 1967.

52. Holland, J. F.: Symposium on the experimental pharmacology and clinical use of antimetabolites. VIII. Folic acid antagonists, Clin. Pharmacol. Ther. 2:374-409, 1961.

53. Holland, J. F.: Progress in treatment. In Dameshek, W., and Dutcher, R. M., editor: Perspectives in leukemia, New York, 1968, Grune & Stratton, Inc.

54. Holland, J. F., and Glidewell, O.: Complementary chemotherapy in acute leukemia. In Mathé, G., editor: Recent results in cancer research: advances in the treatment of acute (blastic) leukemias, New York, 1970, Springer-Verlag New York, Inc.

55. Holton, C. P., Lonsdale, D., Nora, A. H., Thurman, W. G., and Vietti, T. J.: Clinical study of daunomycin (NSC-82151) in children with acute leukemia, Cancer 22:1014-1017, 1968.

56. Holton, C. P., Vietti, T. J., Nora, A. H., Donaldson, M. H., Stuckey, W. J., Jr., Watkins, W. L., and Lane, D. M.: Daunomycin and prednisone for induction of remission in advanced leukemia, N. Engl. J. Med. 280:171-174, 1969.

57. Hoogstraten, B.: Cyclophosphamide (Cytoxan) in acute leukemia, Cancer Chemother. Rep. 16:167-171, 1962.

58. Howard, J. P.: Response of acute leukemia in children to repeated courses of vincristine (NSC-67574), Cancer Chemother. Rep. 51:465-469, 1967.

59. Howard, J. P., Albo, V., and Newton, W. A., Jr.: Cytosine arabinoside: results of a cooperative study in acute childhood leukemia, Cancer 21:341-345, 1968.

60. Hyman, C. B., Borda, E., Brubaker, C., Hammond, D., and Sturgeon, P.: Prednisone in childhood leukemia. Comparison of interrupted and continuous therapy, Pediatrics 24:1005-1008, 1959.

61. Jacquillat, C., Weil, M., Boiron, M., and Bernard, J.: Traitment des leucémies aiguës par la rubidomycin, Union Med. Can. **97**:8-12, 1968.

62. Jammet, H., Pendic, B., Schwarzenberg, L., Duplan, J. F., Maupin, B., Latarjet, R., Larrieu, M. K., Kalic, D., and Djuric, Z.: Transfusions et greffes de moelle osseuse homologue chez des humains irradiés à forte dose accidentellement. Rev. Fr. Etude Clin. Biol. **4**:226, 1959.

63. Jones, B., Holland, J. F., Morrison, A. R., Lee, S. L., Sinks, L. F., Cuttner, J., Rausen, A., Kung, F., Pluss, H. J., Haurani, F. I., Patterson, R. B., Blom, J., Burgert, E. O., Jr., Moon, J. H., Chevalier, L., Sawitsky, A., Albala, R., Forcier, J., Falkson, G., and Glidewell, O.: Daunomycin in the treatment of resistant acute lymphoblastic leukemia, Cancer Res. **31**:84-90, 1971.

64. Karon, M., Freireich, E. R., Frei, E., III, Taylor, R., Wolman, I. J., Djerassi, I., Lee, S. L., Sawitsky, A., Hananian, J., Selawry, O., James, D., Jr., George, P., Patterson, R. B., Burgert, O., Haurani, F. I., Oberfield, R. A., Macy, C. T., Hoogstraten, B., and Blom, J.: The role of vincristine in the treatment of childhood acute leukemia, Clin. Pharmacol. Ther. **7**:332, 1966.

65. Krivit, W., Brubaker, C., Thatcher, L. G., Pierce, M., Perrin, E., and Hartmann, J. R.: Maintenance therapy in acute leukemia of childhood: comparison of cyclic vs. sequential methods, Cancer **21**:352-356, 1968.

66. Krivit, W., Gilchrist, G., and Beatty, E. C.: The need for chemotherapy after prolonged complete remission in acute leukemia of childhood, J. Pediatr. **76**:138-141, 1970.

67. Land, V., Sutow, W. W., Fernbach, D. J., Lane, D. M., and Williams, T. E.: Toxicity of L-asparaginase in children with advanced leukemia, Cancer **30**:339-347, 1972.

68. Leikin, S. L., Brubaker, C., and Hartmann, J. R.: Varying prednisone dosage in remission induction of previously untreated childhood leukemia, Cancer **21**:346-351, 1968.

69. Leikin, S., Brubaker, C., Hartmann, J., Murphy, M. L., and Wolff, J.: The use of combination therapy in leukemia remission, Cancer **24**:427-432, 1969.

70. Leukemia and Hematosarcoma Cooperative Group of the European Organisation for Research on the Treatment of Cancer: Rubidomycin (or daunomycin): a clinical evaluation. In Mathé, G., editor: Recent results in cancer research: advances in the treatment of acute (blastic) leukemias, New York, 1970, Springer-Verlag New York, Inc.

71. Levin, R. H., Henderson, E., Karon, M., and Freireich, E. J.: Treatment of acute leukemia with methylglyoxal-bis-guanylhydrazone (methyl-GAG), Clin. Pharmacol. Ther. **6**:31, 1965.

72. Macrez, C., Marneffe-Lebrequier, H., Ripault, J., Clauvel, J. P., Jacquillat, C., and Weil, M.: Accidents cardiaques observés au cours des traitements par la rubidomycine, Pathol. Biol. (Paris) **15**:949-953, 1967.

73. Mathé, G., Amiel, J. L., Clarysse, A., Hayat, M., and Schwarzenberg, L.: The place of the L-asparaginase in the treatment of acute leukemias. In Mathé, G., editor: Recent results in cancer research: advances in the treatment of acute (blastic) leukemias, New York, 1970, Springer-Verlag New York, Inc.

74. Mathé G., Amiel, J. L., Schwarzenberg, L., Schneider, M., Cattan, A., Schlumberger, J. R., Hayat, M., and deVassal, F.: Chemotherapy of acute lymphoblastic leukemia. In Proceedings of the Sixth International Congress of Chemotherapy: Progress in antimicrobial and anticancer chemotherapy, Baltimore, 1970, University Park Press.

75. Mathé, G., Hayat, M., Schwarzenberg, L., Amiel, J. L., Schneider, M., Cattan, A., Schlumberger, J. R., and Jasmin, C. L.: Haute frequence et qualite des remissions de la leucémie aiguë lymphoblastique chez l'enfant, Arch Fr. Pediatr. **25**:181-188, 1968.

76. Mathé, G., Pouillart, P., and Lapeyraque, F.: Active immunotherapy of L1210 leukemia applied after the graft of tumor cells, Br. J. Cancer **23**:814-824, 1969.

77. Mauer, A. M.: Personal communication, 1971.

78. Melhorn, D. K., Gross, S., Fisher, J., and Newman, A. J.: Studies on the use of "prophylactic" intrathecal amethopterin in childhood leukemia, Blood **36**:55-60, 1970.

79. Nagao, T., Lampkin, B. C., and Mauer, A. M.: Maintenance therapy in acute childhood leukemia, J. Pediatr. **76**:134-137, 1970.

80. Nesbit, M. E.: Personal communication.

81. Nesbit, M. E., Chard, R., Ertel, I., Lahey, E., Karon, M., and Hammond, G. D. for

Children's Cancer Study Group A.: Reduction of sensitivity reactions produced by L-asparaginase by combination with 6-mercaptopurine, Proc. Am. Assoc. Cancer Res. **12**:39, 1971.

82. Oettgen, H. F., Stephenson, P. A., Schwartz, M. K., Leeper, R. D., Tallal, L., Tan, C. C., Clarkson, B. D., Golbey, R. B., Krakoff, I. H., Karnofsky, D. A., Murphy, M. L., and Burchenal, J. H.: Toxicity of E. coli L-asparaginase in man, Cancer **25**:253-278, 1970.

83. Old, L. J., Benacerraf, B., Clarke, D. A., Carswell, E. A., and Stockert, E.: The role of the reticuloendothelial system in the host reaction to neoplasia, Cancer Res. **21**:1281-1300, 1961.

84. Old, L. J., and Clarke, D. A.: Effect of bacillus Calmette-Guérin infection on transplanted tumours in mice, Nature (Lond) **184**:291-292, 1959.

85. Pearson, O. H., and Eliel, L. P.: Use of pituitary adrenocorticotropic hormone (ACTH) and cortisone in lymphomas and leukemias, J.A.M.A. **144**:1349, 1950.

86. Phair, J. P., Anderson, R. E., and Namiki, H.: The central nervous system in leukemia, Ann. Intern. Med. **61**:863-875, 1964.

87. Pierce, M. I.: The acute leukemias of childhood. In Kaplan, S., editor: Pediatr. Clin. North Am. **4**:497-530, 1957.

88. Pierce, M. I., Shore, N., Sitarz, A., Murphy, M. L., Louis, J., and Severo, N.: Cyclophosphamide therapy in acute leukemia of childhood, Cancer **19**:1551-1560, 1966.

89. Pinkel, D.: Five-year follow up of "total therapy" of childhood lymphocytic leukemia, J.A.M.A. **216**:648-652, 1971.

90. Sandberg, J. S., Howsden, F. L., DiMarco, A., and Goldin, A.: Comparison of the antileukemic effect in mice of adriamycin (NSC-123127) with daunomycin (NSC-82151), Cancer Chemother. Rep. **54**:1-7, 1970.

91. Schabel, F. M., Jr.: In vivo leukemic cell kill kinetics and "curability" in experimental systems. In The University of Texas M.D. Anderson Hospital and Tumor Institute at Houston, The proliferation and spread of neoplastic cells, Baltimore, 1968, The Williams & Wilkins Co.

92. Selawry, O. S.: New treatment schedule with improved survival in childhood leukemia: intermittent parenteral vs. daily oral administration of methotrexate for maintenance of induced remission, J.A.M.A. **194**:75-81, 1965.

93. Shanbrom, E., and Miller, S.: Critical evaluation of massive steroid therapy in acute leukemia, N. Engl. J. Med. **266**:1354-1358, 1962.

94. Sharp, H. L., Nesbit, M. E., D'Angio, J., and Krivit, W.: Addition of local radiation after bone marrow remission in acute leukemia in children, Cancer **20**:1403-1404, 1967.

95. Sharp, H. L., Nesbit, M. E., White, J. G., and Krivit, W.: Renal and hepatic pathology following initial remission of acute leukemia induced by prednisone, Cancer **20**:1395-1402, 1967.

96. Skipper, H. E., Schabel, F. M., Jr., and Wilcox, W. S.: Experimental evaluation of potential anticancer agents. XIII. On the criteria and kinetics associated with "curability" of experimental leukemia, Cancer Chemother. Rep. **35**:1-111, 1964.

97. Sonley, M. J., Nesbit, M., Thatcher, L. G., Karon, M., and Hammond, G. D. for Children's Cancer Study Group A.: Cytosine arabinoside, cyclophosphamide and vincristine in children with acute myelogenous leukemia, Am. Assoc. Cancer Res. **12**:87, 1971.

98. Southwest Cancer Chemotherapy Study Group: Unpublished data.

99. Starling, K., Lane, D. M., Sutow, W. W., Monto, R. W., and Thurman, W. G.: Third and fourth remission induction with prednisone and vincristine in children with acute leukemia (letter to editor), Cancer Chemother. Rep. **54**:293-300, 1970.

100. Sullivan, M. P., Beatty, E. C., Jr., Hyman, C. B., Murphy, M. L., Pierce, M. I., and Severo, N. C.: A comparison of the effectiveness of standard dose 6-mercaptopurine, combination 6-mercaptopurine and DON, and high-loading 6-mercaptopurine therapies in treatment of the acute leukemias of childhood: results of a cooperative study, Cancer Chemother. Rep. **18**:83-95, 1962.

101. Sutow, W. W., Gracia, F., Starling, K. A., Williams, T. E., Lane, D. M., and Gehan, E. A.: L-Asparaginase therapy in children with advanced leukemia, Cancer **28**:819-824, 1971.

102. Sutow, W. W., Sullivan, M. P., and Taylor, G.: Status of present treatment for acute leukemia in children, Cancer Res. **25:**1481-1490, 1965.
103. Tallal, L., Tan, C., Oettgen, H., Wollner, N., McCarthy, M., Helson, L., Burchenal, J., Karnofsky, D., and Murphy, M. L.: E. Coli L-asparaginase in the treatment of leukemia and solid tumors in 131 children, Cancer **25:**306-320, 1970.
104. Tan, C. C., Phoa, J., Lyman, M., Murphy, M. L., Dargeon, H. W., and Burchenal, J. H.: Hematological remissions in acute leukemia with cyclophosphamide, Blood **18:**808, 1961.
105. Tan, C., Tasaka, H., Yu, K. P., Murphy, M. L., and Karnofsky, D.: Daunomycin, an antitumor antibiotic, in the treatment of neoplastic disease, Cancer **20:**333-353, 1967.
106. Thompson, I., Hall, T. C., Maloney, W. C.: Combination therapy of adult acute myelogenous leukemia: experience with the simultaneous use of vincristine, amethopterin, 6-mercaptopurine and prednisone, N. Engl. J. Med. **273:**1302-1307, 1965.
107. Traggis, D. G., Dohlwitz, A., Das, L., Jaffe, N., Moloney, W. C., and Hall, T. C.: Cytosine arabinoside in acute leukemia of childhood, Cancer **28:**815-818, 1971.
108. Vietti, T. J., Starling, K., Wilbur, K., Lonsdale, D., and Lane, D. M.: Vincristine, prednisone and daunomycin in acute leukemia of childhood, Cancer **27:**602-607, 1971.
109. Vietti, T. J., Sullivan, M. P., Berry, D. H., Haddy, T. B., Haggard, M. D., and Blattner, R. J.: The response of acute childhood leukemia to an initial and a second course of prednisone, J. Pediatr. **66:**18-26, 1965.
110. Viza, D. C., Bernard-Degani, O., Bernard, C., and Harris, R.: Leukemia antigens, Lancet **2:**493-494, 1969.
111. Vogler, W. R., Huguley, C. M., Jr., and Rundler, R. W.: Comparison of methotrexate and 6-mercaptopurine-prednisone in treatment of acute leukemia in adults, Cancer **20:**1221, 1967.
111a. Wang, J. J., Cortes, E., Sinks, L. F., and Holland, J. F.: Therapeutic effect of toxicity of adriamycin in patients with neoplastic disease, Cancer **28:**837-843, 1971.
112. Wang, J. J., Selawry, O. S., Bodey, G. P., and Vietti, T. J.: Prolonged infusion of arabinosyl cytosine in childhood leukemia, Cancer **25:**1-6, 1970.
113. Wissler, R. W., Craft, K., Kesden, D., Polisky, B., and Dzoga, K.: Inhibition of the growth of the Morris Hepatoma (5123) in Buffalo rats using a mixture of pertussis vaccine and irradiated tumors. In Dausset, J., Hamburger, J., and Mathé, G.: Advances in transplantation, Proceedings of the First International Congress of Transplantation Society, Baltimore, 1968, The Williams & Wilkins Co.
114. Wolff, J. A., Brubaker, C. A., Murphy, M. L., Pierce, M. I., and Severo, N.: Prednisone therapy of acute childhood leukemia: prognosis and duration of response in 330 treated patients, J. Pediatr. **70:**626-631, 1967.
115. Woodruff, M. F. A., and Boak, J. L.: Inhibitory effect of injection of *Corynebacterium parvum* on the growth of tumor transplants in isogenic hosts, Br. J. Cancer **20:**345-355, 1966.
116. Zuelzer, W. W.: Implications of long-term survival in acute leukemia of childhood treated with composite cyclic therapy, Blood **24:**477-494, 1964.
117. Zuelzer, W. W.: Therapy of acute leukemia in childhood. In Zarafonetis, C. J. D., editor: Proceedings of the International Conference on Leukemia-Lymphoma, Philadelphia, 1968, Lea & Febiger.

CHAPTER 11

Extramedullary leukemia

MARGARET P. SULLIVAN
MARTIN HRGOVCIC

OCCULT LEUKEMIA DURING MARROW REMISSION

The ability to achieve long-term bone marrow control in a substantial number of children with acute leukemia has focused attention on extramedullary aspects of the disease as (1) impediments or obstacles to cure of the disease and (2) major causes of morbidity during marrow remission.

Incidence and implications. After induction of apparent complete marrow remission in 31 patients, Mathé[41] sampled multiple suspected sites of occult disease and also obtained electroencephalograms and radiographs of the skeletons. Evidence of residual leukemic disease was found in 12 of 31 patients surveyed; 6 patients had involvement of two or more sites. The bone marrow and liver (4 patients) showed residual activity most frequently. Electroencephalograms were interpreted as indicating central nervous system (CNS) involvement in 3 patients, and a cerebrospinal fluid (CSF) cytology study was positive in one other instance, raising the incidence of residual CNS disease activity to that shown by bone marrow and liver.

An investigation of a similar nature conducted by Sharp and co-workers[64-66] provided for sampling of the CSF, liver, and kidneys after remission had been induced with prednisone alone. Two of the ten patients studied were found to have hepatic involvement, and two additional patients had renal involvement.

Evidence of residual leukemia during marrow remission has been presented by Nies and associates[49] from a different group of patients, that is, patients expiring during remission and undergoing postmortem examination. Among the 15 patients studied, 10 had evidence of extramedullary leukemia. Most frequent involvement occurred in the kidneys (6 patients) and liver (5 patients). Testicular involvement was present in 3 of the 4 males included in the study group. This site was not studied by Sharp and associates and was found to be positive in only 1 of the 13 cases of the Mathé series.

The meninges have been a frequent site for termination of remission in patients receiving cyclic and "total therapy." One M. D. Anderson Hospital (MDAH) patient who has continued in her initial marrow remission for over 8½ years developed meningeal leukemia 7 years and 8 months from time of initial diagnosis while on maintenance treatment with a cyclic 6MP and methotrexate program. Ovarian or testicular infiltration was the first symptom of relapse in 8 of 139 long-term survivors entered in the Registry of Long-Term Survivors.[12]

TREATMENT OF EXTRAMEDULLARY RESIDUAL DISEASE AND PROPHYLACTIC EXTRAMEDULLARY THERAPY

In the French study an attempt was made to eradicate residual disease by doubling drug dosages for 1 month and superimposing intrathecal methotrexate therapy if the central nervous system was involved.[41] Despite intensified therapy, disease reactivation was significantly earlier in patients having a positive survey for residual disease. Patients with three or more positive occult sites with residual bone marrow disease had particularly rapid recurrences.

All patients of Sharp and co-workers were given radiation, 1200 rads to the brain, spinal cord, liver, spleen, and both kidneys, while prednisone therapy was continued at half dosage; thereafter methotrexate and 6-mercaptopurine were administered in a cyclic fashion.[65] Exacerbation of leukemic disease was noted in 7 of the 10 radiated patients within 5 to 16 months (median of 11 months). The shortest remissions occurred in the two children with the heaviest involvement of a single organ. Length of continuing remission for the three remaining children ranged from 14 to 22 months. Meningeal leukemia developed in 3 of the 10 irradiated patients; it should be noted that all 10 patients had normal CSF examinations before and after irradiation of the brain and spinal cord. The data were interpreted as showing little alteration of ultimate outcome by the radiation given.

In view of these studies, serious attempts to cure leukemic disease must provide for the eradication of residual disease in extramedullary sites by (1) intensification of systemic chemotherapy, which may place the patient at considerable risk unless a protective environment is provided; (2) employment of local radiation in dosages exceeding the 1200 rads administered by Sharp and colleagues; (3) use of combination radiation and chemotherapy for the one site where such treatment is feasible, namely, the central nervous system; or (4) reliance on the patient's own immunologic responses, unimpaired by immunosuppressive drugs or stimulated by such agents as BCG or *Corynebacterium parvum*.

Because of prominent symptoms and increasing incidence (now above the 50% level),[7, 19] the central nervous system has received greatest clinical attention. A single dose (0.9 mg/kg) of prophylactic intrathecal methotrexate (IT MTX) incorporated into initial therapy for acute leukemia has not significantly altered the incidence of subsequent meningeal leukemia as compared with control groups (54% vs. 68%); however, the onset of meningeal leukemia appears to have been delayed in the prophylactic therapy group, which showed an average time to onset of meningeal leukemia of 11.9 months, as compared with 7.6 months for the control group.[42] Among 30 children completing "total therapy," which included irradiation to the cranium (2400 rads plus 12 mg/M^2 IT MTX × 5), 6 (20%) have developed CNS leukemia.[7] In three instances CNS disease terminated remissions of 23 to 30 months; in the other three children, CNS leukemia followed marrow relapse by 2, 5, and 7 months. "Total therapy" supplemented by radiation to the cerebrospinal axis (2400 rads) reduced the incidence of remission termination by CNS leukemia to 6.6% (3 of 45 children), as compared with 51% (25 of 49 children) in the nonirradiated group.[7] At the time of this report the median duration of this study was "about 1 year." Five of the nonradiated and one of the radiated children have subsequently shown marrow relapse.

In 1971 the Pediatric Division of the Southwest Cancer Chemotherapy Study Group began evaluating the effectiveness of "triple IT therapy" (methotrexate plus hydrocortisone and cytosine arabinoside × 4) with triple IT maintenance therapy every 8 weeks for 1 year in comparison with triple IT therapy as just mentioned supplemented with cranial radiation (2400 rads).[2] CNS prophylactic programs are also being devised by other study groups and centers, and the results of these studies will be most useful in devising comprehensive care for the leukemic patient.

OVERT EXTRAMEDULLARY LEUKEMIA

Clinical manifestations of leukemia involving structures other than bone marrow are being recognized with increasing frequency both in remission and relapse. In an effort to determine the incidence of infiltration in sites other than bone marrow currently thought to be of clinical significance and to compare the therapeutic effectiveness of various treatment modalities, the records of 172 children who expired at the M. D. Anderson Hospital and Tumor Institute in the 15-year period from 1954 to 1968 have been examined. In rare instances children had prominent manifestations of extramedullary leukemia, but autopsy was not performed. Data from these children have been included to obtain a more comprehensive picture of the magnitude of the clinical problem. The autopsy study group contained 94 boys and 78 girls (Table 11-1). The relative increase in numbers of children with acute granulocytic leukemia and with leukemia arising from lymphosarcoma is probably a reflection of the type of referrals made to a categoric institution, particularly when there has been a manifest interest in certain clinical diagnoses. The findings in this study group will be considered with reference to the site(s) of extramedullary involvement. Those sites that appear to have greatest clinical and theoretical significance have been selected for review.

Table 11-1. Age and histologic type of acute leukemia in the MDAH study group

Age	Number and percent of patients
Age under 2 years	21 (12%)
2 to 8 years	91 (53%)
8 to 12 years	25 (14%)
Over 12 years	35 (20%)
Total	172

Histologic type	Number and percent of patients
Lymphocytic (ALL)	84 (49%)
Unclassified (AUL)	14 (8%)
Monocytic or myelomonocytic (AML/AMML)	18 (10%)
Granulocytic (AGL)	38 (22%)
Leukemia from lymphosarcoma	18 (10%)
Total	172

Nervous system infiltrates

Incidence. Infiltration of the central nervous system is now being detected clinically in about half the children with acute lymphocytic leukemia.[7, 19] Disease within the nervous system is thought to develop because of a failure of systemically administered antileukemic agents to cross the blood-brain barrier in therapeutic amounts. In our group, 44% of the patients demonstrated CNS involvement at autopsy or had a clinical history of meningeal leukemia. CNS infiltrates were not related to sex in this group of patients, and the predisposition for males previously reported was not confirmed.[45] Age showed no influence on the occurrence of the syndrome in our patients. When type of acute leukemia was considered, the percentages of patients with meningeal leukemia were as follows: acute lymphocytic—46%, acute unclassified—35%, acute monocytic and acute myelomonocytic—22%, acute granulocytic—48%, and acute leukemia arising from lymphosarcoma—58%. Approximately 50% of our patients were in bone marrow remission when CNS leukemia became apparent. The occurrence of cerebrospinal pleocytosis at the time of initial diagnosis has been documented in two studies in 4 of 47 children (8%) and in 9 of 123 children (7%).[22a, 42] In the latter series, 49 children had cerebrospinal fluid white blood cell counts of 10 or less/mm³ (range, 1 to 10/mm³; median, 2/mm³), and 9 had mononuclear cell counts exceeding 10/mm³ (range, 25 to 4014/mm³; median, 109/mm³).[22a] Children with peripheral white blood cell counts of 10,000/mm³ or more at the time of diagnosis are reported to have an increased incidence of meningeal leukemia when compared with children with lower initial white blood cell counts.[42]

Signs and symptoms. Children affected with meningeal leukemia show signs and symptoms of meningeal irritation and of increased intracranial pressure suggestive of brain tumor but lacking in localizing signs. The frequency of various signs and symptoms among 656 children pooled from five series has been summarized by Kanner and co-workers.[36] The most frequent symptoms are headache, vomiting, and pain and stiffness in the back and neck. Polyphagia and excessive weight gain are dramatic but infrequent symptoms that may occur

Table 11-2. Clinical patterns produced by nervous system infiltrations in children with leukemia

Pattern		Number and percent of patients
Meningeal		39 (42.4%)
Meningeal variants		30 (32.6%)
Hypothalamic	(6)	
Cranial nerve	(12)	
Cerebellar	(4)	
Cranial and spinal nerve	(2)	
Spinal nerve	(5)	
Peripheral nerve	(1)	
Dural		2 (2.2%)
Silent		21 (22.8%)
Total		92 (100.0%)

in the absence of obvious signs of increased intracranial pressure. The importance of weight gain in the early detection of meningeal leukemia has been stressed.[31] Papilledema occurs in approximately half the patients. Other less frequent presenting signs include suture separation, sixth and seventh cranial nerve palsies, and tremor. In approximately one third of the patients from MDAH there were findings indicating involvement of structures other than the leptomeninges. These additional sites included the dura, hypothalamus, cerebellum, cranial or spinal nerves or both, nerve roots, and peripheral nerves (Table 11-2). Of the cranial nerves, the seventh was most often affected. In several children both seventh nerves were involved sequentially. Paresis of the sixth cranial nerve, a reflection of increased intracranial pressure, was of lesser frequency. Involvement of the second, third, fourth, and eighth cranial nerves was uncommon. Of the spinal nerves, involvement of the lumbar sacral plexus nerves was recognized most often by symptoms of pain radiating from the back down the legs to the feet, weakness in the legs, and difficulty in voiding.

Twenty-one patients were found who had no clinical evidence of CNS involvement during life but were found to have leukemic infiltrates within the nervous system at autopsy. In many instances the infiltrate was described as minimal or focal. However, marked infiltration was also found.

Diagnosis. The diagnosis of meningeal leukemia is dependent on the demonstration of increased numbers of mononuclear cells (more than $10/mm^3$) or the presence of blast cells in the CSF. CSF WBC counts exceeding $1000/mm^3$ were not unusual in our study material; the highest CSF WBC count found in our group was $12,900/mm^3$. Smears prepared using the Shandon-Elliott Cytocentrifuge* have shown the presence of blast cells when the CSF WBC count was within normal limits and even when zero. Use of this technique would appear to be a significant advance in the diagnosis of occult meningeal leukemia.

Spinal fluid pressure is usually elevated, often markedly so. Since no blocks occur in the ventriculosubarachnoid system, pressure is uniform throughout, and cautious lumbar punctures can be performed without risk. The protein level may be elevated at the time meningeal leukemia is diagnosed; an increase in protein level during a course of intrathecal therapy is relatively common. At diagnosis, glucose levels may be normal or decreased. In the past, decrease in CSF glucose levels has been attributed to glucose utilization by leukemic cells, but rarely did there appear to be a correlation between the height of the CSF WBC count and the glucose level. Recently, increased glucose utilization by the brain resulting from increased glycolysis and a defective glucose transport system has been shown to be the primary causative factor in low spinal fluid sugar levels in bacterial meningitis.[43] Low CSF glucose levels may occur through similar mechanisms in meningeal leukemia.

Pathology. The pathologic features of the nervous system involvement in meningeal leukemia have been described in great detail.[15, 45, 71, 76] The changes of early involvement are minimal. The dura usually shows only slight thickening and grayish discoloration. Occasionally nodules may be identified, and, very rarely, a large transdural plaque may be found compressing the underlying brain. The leptomeninges may appear thickened and somewhat milky in ap-

---

*Shandon Scientific Co., Inc., Sewickley, Pa.

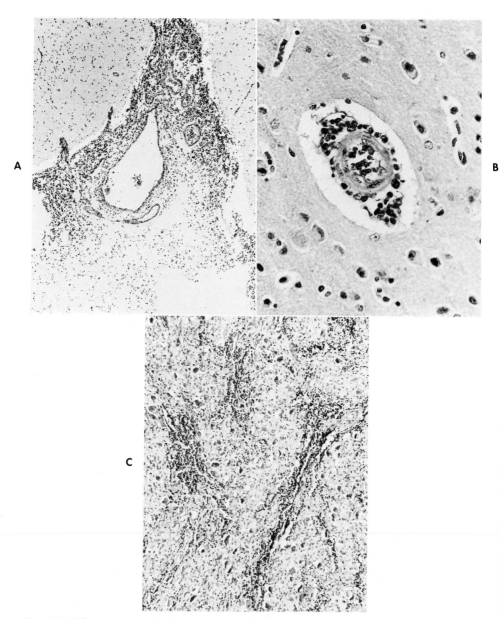

Fig. 11-1. Photomicrographs showing leukemic infiltrates within the nervous system. **A,** Spinal cord showing moderately severe infiltration of the leptomeninges and subarachnoid space. The pia shows artifactual separation from the cord; extensions of the subarachnoid into the substance of the cord, however, are clearly discernible (×31). **B,** Leukemic cells within the Virchow-Robin space (×850). **C,** Leukemic infiltrate in ganglion (×50). **D,** Spinal cord and cauda equina. Residual or recurrent leukemic infiltrate of leptomeninges with fibrosis following low-dose radiation therapy. Leukemic cells are clearly visible in perineurium (×31). (Courtesy Medical Communications, the University of Texas at Houston, M. D. Anderson Hospital and Tumor Institute.)

pearance, with leveling of the succal depressions. Hydrocephalus, now considered to result from neglect or long-standing refractory meningeal leukemia, is seldom seen, although it occurred with fair frequency when this syndrome was first recognized.

Microscopic infiltrations of the dura, leptomeninges, and perivascular spaces vary in intensity from scant to dense. Infiltrations within the brain are rare, excepting the area postrema and the tuber cinereum. The pineal gland, pituitary gland, and choroid plexus are sometimes affected as well. A marked association has been observed between the degree of infiltration in the arachnoid and in these areas in humans.[76] It has been speculated that nonneural structures have some influence on the rate of CSF production and that leukemic infiltrates in these areas may affect the rate of CSF production by the choroid plexus.[76] An alternate hypothesis postulates increased CSF production and hydrocephalus on the basis of choroid plexus irritation by abnormal cellular constituents of the CSF. This mechanism is thought to be operative in subarachnoid hemorrhage.

Although dural involvement has been noted in 70% of patients with acute lymphocytic leukemia studied postmortem, the degree of infiltration was most often slight to moderate.[45] Arachnoid infiltrations occurred in only half as many children but were of greater intensity. With involvement of the meninges, either cerebral or spinal, there is infiltration of the arachnoid membrane with leukemic cells, and the subarachnoid space is more or less filled with leukemic cells. The pia is closely adherent to the brain and spinal cord, extending into the depths

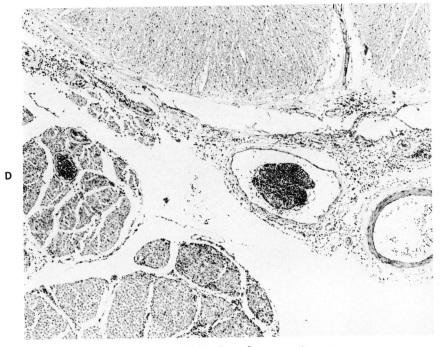

D

Fig. 11-1, cont'd. For legend see opposite page.

of fissures and sulci. Perivascular (Virchow-Robin) spaces surround the vessels as they enter the brain substance. The inner walls of these spaces are formed by extensions of the arachnoid. The outer walls are continuous with the pia, with the intervening channel open to the subarachnoid space. Through these spaces tissue fluids are brought to the surface and enter the subarachnoid space. As shown in the photomicrographs (Fig. 11-1), leukemic cells may be found within the brain in these extensions of the subarachnoid space. Infiltrates within the Virchow-Robin spaces have not been found without accompanying infiltrates in the subarachnoid space. However, there may be fairly intensive involvement of the arachnoid with little or no infiltrate within Virchow-Robin spaces.

Autopsy data on the frequency of leukemic infiltrates within the spinal meninges is scanty, but there is increasing evidence that spinal involvement is fairly frequent. Clinical symptoms have in several cases directed attention to the dorsal root ganglia, spinal nerves, and peripheral nerves as possible sites of leukemic involvement. Postmortem examination of these structures has demonstrated the presence of leukemic cells, either residual or recurrent, after radiation therapy as illustrated in Fig. 11-1, D.

Pathogenesis. The lack of correlation between disease activity in the bone marrow and central nervous system suggests that disease progression in the central nervous system is autonomous. The pathogenesis of disease in this pharmacologically isolated compartment is not certain. Small islands of totipotent mesenchymal elements occurring in the normal meninges have been described as possible sites for the in situ development of leukemic meningitis in lymphocytic disease.[5] Meningeal leukemia of the granulocytic type could therefore be of metastatic origin.[5]

A second area of speculation is afforded by Kappers' demonstration of hematopoiesis in the cerebral leptomeningeal mesenchyme of the 18 mm, 6½-week human embryo. Hematopoiesis in this site is transient and is not observed in the 8-week embryo.[37] The potential for hematopoietic activity may persist, however, within the choroid plexus and the meninges and might be subject to recall by the leukemic stimulus. Recall of fetal function through activation of unused genes that are normally expressed at an early stage of development has been documented in both experimental and human tumor systems.[1, 11, 17, 27, 28]

In L1210-bearing mice inoculated subcutaneously, leukemic cells enter the arachnoid by direct migration and grow through the perivascular and perineural tissues that bridge the subdural space.[76] By analogy, a similar route of spread has been postulated for humans.

Treatment. Lumbar puncture with limited spinal fluid drainage often results in dramatic relief of symptoms and subsequent improvement in spinal fluid findings.[15, 19] Palliation is assumed to occur through the same poorly understood mechanism when subarachnoid hemorrhage is treated with lumbar punctures. Although such treatment may relieve the urgency of the clinical situation, the benefits are of short duration. Lumbar punctures with removal of fluid, once advocated as a form of therapy for meningeal leukemia, are no longer recommended except for the introduction of intrathecal medications and for interval palliation of intracranial hypertension if required.

Adrenocorticosteroids, administered orally, will favorably affect CNS leukemia if systemic resistance to this class of agents has not been established.[67, 70]

No blood-brain barrier exists for these compounds.[52, 62] Infiltrates in deeper nervous system structures and in nerves and nerve roots are also favorably affected. Therapeutic response is prompt. In critical situations of impending blindness or paralysis, adjuvant steroid therapy may effect a more rapid response than either radiation or intrathecal MTX alone. Dexamethasone, 0.2 mg/kg/day in divided doses for 2 days, has been recommended for relief of the acute symptoms of meningeal leukemia.[44] Marked palliation is afforded by this regimen, which does not alter papilledema or eliminate blast cells from the CSF.

Radiation therapy has been of great value in controlling symptoms of meningeal leukemia and is especially useful when deep structures of the brain are involved.[15, 19, 31, 54, 70] Reported radiation dosages to the cranium have ranged from 400 to 2000 r given over periods of 5 to 10 days. The duration of symptomatic control after such therapy has ranged from 3 to 4 months. In a systematic study conducted by the Pediatric Division of the Southwest Cancer Chemotherapy Study Group, irradiation of the skull, 500 and 1000 rads tumor dose, was found to be ineffective therapy for meningeal leukemia when spinal fluid findings were used as an objective measure of response. Radiation therapy to the entire cerebrospinal axis, tumor dose 1000 rads, and combination therapy employing irradiation to the cerebrospinal axis, 1000 rads, plus two priming and one consolidating dose of IT MTX, resulted in spinal fluid remission rates of 92% and 100%, respectively. Neither of these regimens, however, was superior to conventional IT MTX in duration of CNS remission, duration of existing bone marrow remission, survival, or number of subsequent CNS relapses.[73]

Experience at the Los Angeles Children's Hospital suggests that improvement in results may be obtained by treating the entire cerebrospinal axis with radiation doses ranging from 2000 to 2500 rads.[32] Among 7 children so treated, the median duration of CNS remission was 9.6 months. At the M. D. Anderson Hospital, 14 children have been given cerebrospinal irradiation in this dosage range. During the posttreatment period the CSF was monitored by periodic lumbar punctures, and the duration of the radiation-induced remissions was shown to range from 48+ days to 286 days (median 112 days).[13] Treatment was well tolerated by those children in bone marrow remission. Children in bone marrow relapse required supportive care with whole blood components or antibiotics or both.

Radiation therapy has been of particular benefit in treating leukemic infiltrates of the facial nerve and of spinal nerves and nerve roots. In most instances, radiation doses of approximately 1000 rads delivered to the seventh nerve through portals that included the peripheral course of the nerve have resulted in complete restoration of function. Inverted "T" fields have been used to treat infiltrates of spinal nerves when the lumbar plexus appears involved. Pain is usually greatly reduced after the first treatment, followed gradually by full restoration of function.[71] Low-dose therapy previously reported has been abandoned in favor of modest doses in the 1500- to 2000-rads range.

The feasibility of intrathecal methotrexate therapy for meningeal leukemia was demonstrated by studies in dogs.[80, 81] A commonly employed dosage schedule for children calls for injection of 0.5 mg/kg MTX into the subarachnoid space every 4 to 5 days until the CSF WBC count falls to normal levels.[46] Simultaneously administered citrovorum factor (Leucovorin) can be used for protection from systemic toxicity. A good symptomatic response to therapy may be expected in two thirds or more of the children treated. Mean durations of such responses have been reported as 2½ and 5 months.[19, 33, 46, 54] Remissions as judged by a normal CSF WBC count tend to be at least 1 month shorter than the symptomatic responses.[73]

Characteristics of the IT MTX response in 50 patients were analyzed by the Southwest Cancer Chemotherapy Study Group. In this group, 40 (78%) achieved complete CNS remission. Treatment failures, which occurred in 22% of patients, were attributable to toxicity that limited therapy, involvement of deeper brain structures, or involvement of the seventh cranial nerve. The duration of IT MTX remissions ranged from 6 to 414 days (median, 87 days).[73] Evidence of MTX toxicity was seen in 24 of the children. The most common toxic side effects were fever, ulceration of the oral mucosa, nausea or vomiting or both, headache, and increasing stiffness of the back and neck. In no case was toxicity life threatening.

Paresis of one leg has been reported in one patient,[9] paraplegia has occurred in 6 patients,[8, 53, 60, 75] and paresis of all four extremities was reported in another child.[10] Two additional cases of paraplegia, one of which terminated fatally, have occurred at this hospital. Paresis of one leg and paraplegia have now been observed in patients given IT cytosine arabinoside.[9, 60] It has been postulated that the preservative common to both preparations may be responsible for the demyelination that has been observed.[60]

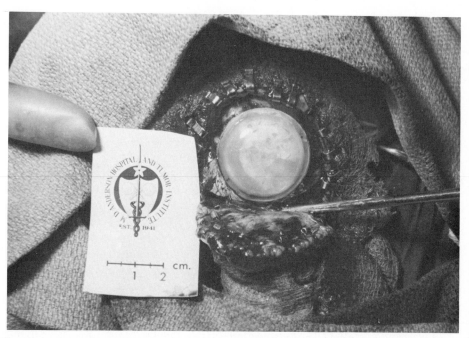

Fig. 11-2. Ommaya reservoir in place on periosteum with catheter extending into lateral ventricle. Note CSF level in reservoir. Scalp flap ready for replacement. (Courtesy University of Texas, M. D. Anderson Hospital and Tumor Institute, Houston, Texas.)

The greater activity of aminopterin when compared with MTX stimulated interest at one time in the intrathecal use of this preparation.[49, 57] Response rates exceeding 90% with median durations of remission of 9 weeks[49] and 5.4 months[31] have been reported. Remissions were established with fewer intrathecal treatments than with MTX, but the need for citrovorum protection was more urgent.

In an effort to obtain more effective drug distribution within the CSF, the Ommaya reservoir was used for direct delivery of chemotherapeutic agents into the ventricular fluid.[51, 59] Reservoirs were inserted into 4 leukemic children at the M. D. Anderson Hospital (Fig. 11-2). Use of the reservoir for monitoring the CSF and for instillation of medication was far more acceptable to the patients than lumbar puncture. The number of injections required to establish remission and the durations of the resultant CNS remissions, however, were similar to those for MTX injected into the lumbar sac.

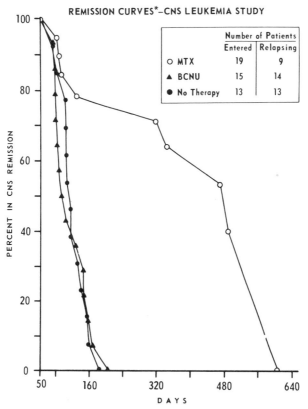

Fig. 11-3. Curves showing duration of CNS remissions for children receiving IT MTX maintenance, BCNU maintenance, and no maintenance therapy. Remissions were measured from the last day of remission induction therapy to relapse. The curves include only those patients in CNS remission at the time of randomization to maintenance therapy (about 50 days after remission induction). Approximately 25% of patients relapsed prior to randomization. (From Sullivan, M. P., Vietti, T. J., Haggard, M. E., Donaldson, M. H., Krall, J. M., and Gehan, E. A.: Blood **38:**683, 1971.)

Intensive efforts have been directed toward the development of compounds that will pass the blood-brain barrier and permit treatment of meningeal leukemia with systemically administered compounds. Essential physical characteristics of such agents include (1) nonionization in aqueous solutions at pH 7 and (2) lipid solubility.[58] The compound 1,3-bis(2-chloroethyl)-1-nitrosourea (BCNU) possesses these attributes and has been effective in controlling L1210 leukemia implanted intraperitoneally or intracerebrally.[61, 68] Clinical trials with BCNU in patients with meningeal leukemia have shown the compound to be effective in treating autonomous leukemic disease in the CNS.[56] In one study dosages of 150 mg/M^2 BCNU intravenously for 3 days resulted in marked thrombocytopenia, even though systemic antileukemic therapy has been discontinued.[34] Dosages of 100 mg/M^2 given intravenously at intervals of 8 weeks were not associated with delayed toxicity and did not interfere with other chemotherapy.[16]

The Pediatric Division of the Southwest Cancer Chemotherapy Study Group compared the effectiveness of 100 mg/M^2 BCNU intravenously every 8 weeks and 12 mg/M^2 IT MTX every 8 weeks as "maintainers" following conventional CNS remission induction.[74] A control "no-therapy" maintenance group was also included. The median durations of remission among the maintenance groups were as follows: MTX, 488 days; BCNU, 94 days; and "no therapy," 116 days (Fig. 11-3). Differences in medians between MTX and each of the other regimens were highly significant in favor of MTX ($< .01$). Headaches, fever, vomiting, or all three were experienced by approximately one third of the children after one or more of their maintenance treatments. In general, symptoms tended to increase in severity as maintenance continued. Similar symptoms have been encountered by others giving IT MTX.[10, 47] Despite such toxicity, which may necessitate discontinuation of therapy, IT MTX maintenance can be recommended for consideration for all children with CNS leukemia.

Pyrimethamine (Daraprim), a substituted pyrimidine that is a folic acid antagonist, has been reported to pass the blood-brain barrier when given orally. CSF levels are 10% to 25% of plasma levels.[25a] There is a case report of pyrimethamine-induced CNS remissions of 6 and 7 months in a patient with "subleukemic" acute myeloblastic leukemia.

In recent years the application of the principles of combination chemotherapy to systemic therapy of acute lymphocytic and acute granulocytic leukemia has resulted in marked improvement in survival. The potential of combination intrathecal chemotherapy in treating meningeal leukemia is now being explored.[72] Hydrocortisone (HDC) is being used intrathecally in an effort to reduce the toxic side effects of IT MTX; some augmentation of antileukemic effect may also occur. Cytosine arabinoside (CA) has been added to the regimen for antileukemic effect. Intrathecal CA, 30 mg/M^2, 15 mg/M^2 MTX, and 15 mg/M^2 HDC given in combination appear to be as well tolerated as IT MTX alone. Preliminary studies suggest a more rapid response to triple IT therapy as shown in the comparison of two successive CNS episodes in an infant with acute lymphocytic leukemia in Fig. 11-4.

Genitourinary tract infiltrates

Renal masses. The incidence of renal infiltration in leukemia has been reported to be as high as 66% in autopsy studies.[69] Among the 172 children in

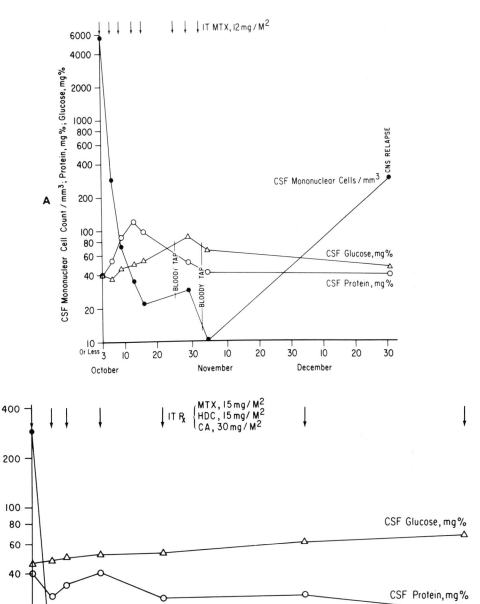

Fig. 11-4. A, Response to intensive IT MTX therapy; duration of CNS remission from normalization of CSF WBC count less than 2 months. **B,** Response to triple IT CNS remission induction therapy followed by triple maintenance therapy; remission duration of 4 months documented on May 4, 1971, when all therapy was discontinued. (Courtesy University of Texas, M. D. Anderson Hospital and Tumor Institute, Houston, Texas.)

our series, infiltrates at the microscopic level were reported in 63 of 94 (67%) boys and 48 of 78 (61%) girls. Children 8 to 12 years of age showed slightly less renal involvement (42%) than did children of all other age groups (66% to 70%). Of those whose leukemia evolved from lymphosarcoma, 83% developed renal masses; the percentage with kidney involvement varied from 57% to 66% among the other histologic types of leukemia.

Postmortem examinations that included renal weights in 158 of our cases showed these values to be more than one and a half times normal for 60% of the children. Slight enlargement (one and one-half to two and one-half times normal weight) was found in 38% of children; moderate enlargement (two and one-half to five times normal weight) was seen in 13%; and massive enlargement (five to more than fifteen times normal weight) was found in 7% of the patients. Patients with renal infiltrates are apparently symptom free, since they offer no complaint. Elevation of the blood urea nitrogen level occurs as a late effect. Electrolyte disturbances with high potassium levels may develop when infiltrated kidneys are presented with a high uric acid load. Renal size in our patients was not monitored during life by periodic pyelographic studies, and the clinical diagnosis of renal infiltrates rested on palpation of enlarged kidneys or on findings from a pyelograph fortuitously obtained. Often palpation of the kidneys is made somewhat difficult by anterior and caudal displacement of liver and spleen by the enlarging renal masses; the lower poles of the kidneys are usually first palpated as flank masses. Infiltrations of the kidneys usually occur late in the course of leukemic disease, but marked enlargement of the kidneys has been noted at the time of diagnosis.[82] Involvement in our patients has usually been symmetrical as it has been in most of the reported cases.

Microscopically, the leukemic infiltrate is diffusely distributed throughout the renal cortex with less intense or minimal involvement of the medulla. Nodular infiltrates occur infrequently. Individual nephrons are often widely separated, and the tubules may be compressed and show some degeneration (Fig. 11-5). Glomeruli may be well preserved or may show degeneration. During marrow relapse, abnormal white blood cells may be observed in glomerular tufts.

Associated alterations in renal function are rare in children, but minimal depression of the glomerular filtration rate, renal plasma flow, and tubular maximum para-aminohippurate secretion have been noted.[24] Studies at this hospital showed normal renal function test values for 6 of 8 children with renal masses; the two remaining children showed reduced renal function (Table 11-3). In patient M. M., only Tm_{PAHA} was affected; in J. C., all three parameters were greatly reduced, and acute renal failure was precipitated by the function tests. Episodes of azotemia have been reported by several investigators.[24, 82]

The development of palpable renal masses has been considered an unfavorable prognostic sign, since uremia will ultimately develop.[54] Chemotherapy employing agents excreted by the kidneys poses serious clinical problems. For example, methotrexate in standard doses may produce marked systemic toxicity in children with renal infiltrates.

Urograms in cases of moderate to severe leukemic infiltration of the kidneys will show enlargement of the renal shadows and an increase in the thickness of the renal cortex; calyces may show compression, elongation, and distortion (Fig. 11-6). The changes demonstrable by urography resemble those found in

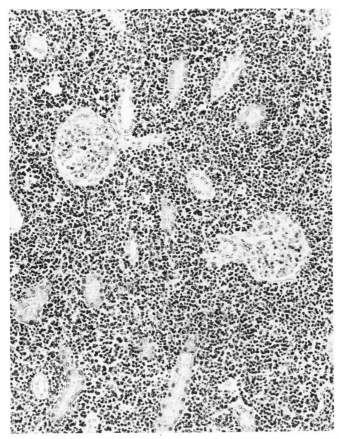

Fig. 11-5. Photomicrograph of section of renal parenchyma. Glomeruli and tubules are widely separated by intense leukemic infiltrate (×85). (Courtesy Medical Communications, the University of Texas at Houston, M. D. Anderson Hospital and Tumor Institute.)

Table 11-3. Renal function studies in leukemic children with renal masses*

Patient	GFR (ml/min/M²)	ERPF (ml/min/M²)	Tm$_{PAHA}$ (ml/min/M²)
E. H.			
(12-29-59)	61	308	47
(1-22-60)	42	121	37
(3-10-60)	97	381	70
E. G.			
(3-22-60)	80	429	73
(5-6-60)	101	464	73
A. K.	64	332	51
R. L.	63	308	58
T. K.	88	329	84
J. C.	14	40	8
M. M.	75	288	21
D. R.	99	443	74
Normal children	55-75	300-400	45

*Courtesy C. W. Daeschner, M.D., Pediatric Metabolic Laboratory, Galveston, Texas.

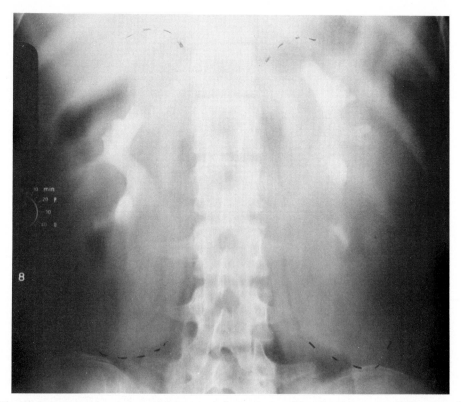

Fig. 11-6. Intravenous urogram (planogram) from 16-year-old girl with acute undifferentiated leukemia of 1½ years' duration. Kidneys are markedly enlarged by leukemic infiltrates, but the calyceal system is relatively normal, and the appearance does not yet suggest polycystic kidneys. (Courtesy Medical Communications, the University of Texas at Houston, M. D. Anderson Hospital and Tumor Institute.)

polycystic disease of the kidneys,[18, 29, 77] Base line and serial intravenous urograms have been advocated to detect early renal enlargement.[63] Periodic surveillance of the kidneys would seem indicated.

Decrease in renal size by palpation or urography with associated improvement in renal function has been reported after effective systemic chemotherapy and local irradiation.[63, 77, 82] Radiation dosages and dosimetry for treatment of this extramedullary site have not yet been standardized. At the M. D. Anderson Hospital, 9 leukemic children with renal enlargement have been given radiation therapy to the kidneys after a rising blood urea nitrogen level had been documented (Table 11-4). Improvement in renal function or measurable decrease in kidney size or both occurred in 5 patients. The degree and duration of improvement were of clinical significance only in J. C. and L. J. Earlier, more aggressive treatment would seem indicated, particularly in those children in marrow remission in whom the renal involvement is autonomous. Treatment of only one kidney serves no clinical purpose and is to be discouraged.

Renal enlargement with urographic findings similar to those resulting from infiltration has also been attributed to interstitial edema and to extensive pa-

Table 11-4. Radiation therapy for leukemic infiltration of the kidneys

Patient	Fields treated	Duration radiation therapy	Radiation dose	Outcome of radiation therapy
P. R.	Both kidneys	14 days	205 r, given dose	BUN 92 mg-39 mg
M. R.	Right kidney	10 days	370 r, tumor dose	Decrease in renal size
G. R.	Right kidney	2 days	275 r, given dose	No improvement
J. C.	Both kidneys	12 days	450 r, given dose	Relief of acute renal failure
T. N.	Both kidneys	7 days	600 r, given dose	Reversal rising BUN
L. M.	Both kidneys	26 days	1618 rads, tumor dose	Sustained reversal uremia
L. G.	Both kidneys	16 days	720 rads, tumor dose	No improvement
R. G.	Both kidneys	12 days	1000 rads, tumor dose	Slight decrease in renal size
A. B.	Both kidneys	20 days	1525 rads, tumor dose	Slight decrease in renal size

renchymal hemorrhage.[40] The etiology of the edema was not determined, and no specific therapy was recommended.

Enlargement of the kidneys without evidence of leukemic infiltration was reported in 15% of 108 cases of leukemia in a postmortem study in 1955.[69] A morphologic explanation for the enlargement was not apparent, but renal hypertrophy as a result of pterin (sic) therapy was postulated. Renal and hepatic enlargement not due to leukemic infiltrates has subsequently been reported in one third of 57 leukemic patients in an autopsy series.[25] Increase in mass was attributed to hyperplasia or hypertrophy of parenchymal cells or both. Documentation of the changes found in the size and number of the renal components is awaited. It has been postulated that one or more of the following mechanisms may stimulate renal and hepatic hypertrophy: (1) increased metabolic load resulting in compensatory hypertrophy; (2) secretion by neoplastic cells of a product that induces hypertrophy, for example, the tumor extract toxohormone, derived from tumors of some experimental systems; or (3) homologous or secondary disease following multiple fresh whole blood transfusion.[24] Evidence of renal dysfunction associated with noninfiltrative enlargement of the kidneys has not been forthcoming, and specific therapy for this phenomenon does not seem indicated. In our autopsy material this type of renal enlargement has been most rare, having been recognized in only 1 of the 172 children in the postmortem study.

Testicular infiltrates. The reported incidence of microscopic infiltration of the testicles ranges from 48% to 92%.[23, 26, 30] In the study conducted at this institution a much lower incidence of 27.7% was noted. Twenty-one of 26 (80%) of these boys also showed renal involvement. Frequent involvement of other extramedullary sites has been noted by others.[26, 30] Among the various histologic types of leukemia, testicular infiltrates in the Anderson material were most frequent in boys with acute monocytic and myelomonocytic leukemia, occurring in 45% of these children. No testicular infiltrates were noted in boys with leukemia arising from lymphosarcoma. Involvement varied from 12% to 30% in the remaining histologic types of leukemia. Boys from 8 to 12 years of age had the lowest percentage of testicular infiltrates (i.e., 15%), whereas involvement varied from 26% in boys 2 to 8 years of age to 40% in boys over 12 years of age.

Infiltrated testicles apparently escape clinical notice until organ size is several times normal. Only 6 of our 26 boys with autopsy evidence of testicular leukemia were noted to have clinical involvement of the testes during life. Since the infiltrative process is painless, patients may be aware of increasing size and firmness of the testicles but fail to mention these changes to the parents or to the physician. Only when involvement is massive will patients complain of heaviness or "a dragging feeling." Clinically, involvement is usually asymmetrical; however, the testicle that appears normal in size will also show leukemic infiltrates microscopically.[23] The diffuse nature of the infiltrate that does not significantly involve the tunica albuginea is illustrated in a photomicrograph (Fig. 11-7).

Testicular leukemia appears to have some autonomy, since the masses are frequently noted during bone marrow remission,[23, 26] and lymphosarcoma of the testicle has been a terminating event for several long-term survivors.[12] A

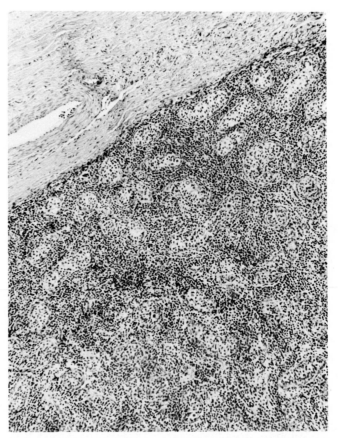

Fig. 11-7. Photomicrograph of section of immature testis. An intense, diffuse leukemic infiltrate surrounds the seminiferous tubules. The tunica albuginea is not significantly involved (×50). (Courtesy Medical Communications, the University of Texas at Houston, M. D. Anderson Hospital and Tumor Institute.)

"blood-gonad" barrier similar to that known for colchicine has been postulated for chemotherapeutic agents.[23] This barrier, however, must be only partial, since we have observed a decrease in testicular size in several patients after large single doses (1000 mg/M[2]) of cyclophosphamide and after 28 days of "reinforcement therapy" with vincristine sulfate (2 mg/M[2]/week × 4) plus prednisone (60 mg/M[2]/day × 28). Regressions have been only partial, and eventually further increase in size becomes evident.

Orchidectomy has been employed for diagnostic purposes and for treatment of massively enlarged organs. More limited biopsy techniques should be encouraged, and radiation should be employed in the maximum dose tolerated by the organ when the objective of treatment is cure of the disease. Prior to radiation, testicular size should be reduced insofar as possible with chemotherapy. Radiation in the dose of 1200 rads has been reported as controlling testicular size with no interference with sexual maturation.[23] Doses of 1200 to 1500 rads usually result in permanent sterility. Since the interstitial cells of Leydig are more resistant to radiation, testosterone production is not affected, and no alterations in sexual maturation occur. Sterility must be accepted as a side effect of therapy, and it is unrealistic to expect local testicular cure with doses of 1200 rads when doses of 2000 to 2500 rads fail to cure meningeal leukemia once it becomes overt. Postmortem studies after radiation of the testicles have shown extensive fibrosis.[26]

Prostatic infiltrates. Leukemic infiltrations of the prostate in children, having attracted no attention in the medical literature, are assumed to be most rare. Involvement of this organ was found at autopsy in only 2 of our 94 boys. Neither had associated symptoms during life. A recent patient who complained of frequency, dysuria, and dribbling was found to have prostatic and pelvic node enlargement, as well as testicular enlargement. Local radiation therapy produced prompt alleviation of symptoms and regression of all masses.

Ovarian infiltrates. Ovarian infiltrates occur with low frequency in autopsy series; 9 of 78 (11.5%) of our girls showed involvement of the gonads. One child also had infiltrates of the uterus. In addition, a child with uninvolved ovaries was reported as having uterine involvement.

Among 80 girls with acute leukemia studied postmortem at another institution, 41% were found to have leukemic infiltrates in the genital organs. The number of girls showing involvement of a specific organ was as follows: ovary, 29; uterus, 13; both uterus and ovaries, 9; fallopian tubes, 1; and vagina, 3.[67a]

The termination of remission with lymphosarcoma of the ovary in long-term survivors draws particular attention to gonadal involvement.[12] Among our living patients, there is a girl now 8 years of age who received remission induction therapy with vincristine and prednisone for acute unclassified leukemia beginning July 14, 1967. Daily oral cyclophosphamide maintenance therapy was given from August 11, 1967, to October 6, 1967. The girl was then observed without therapy and remained in complete marrow remission. A pelvic mass was palpated March 3, 1969. Exploratory laparotomy 10 days later showed leukemic infiltrates of the ovaries, tubes, uterus, broad ligaments, and pelvic nodes. Hysterectomy and bilateral salpingo-oophorectomy were performed. Purinethol maintenance with periodic vincristine-prednisone reinforcement was instituted, and the girl continues in her original marrow remission.

Gastrointestinal tract infiltrates

Gross leukemic infiltrates of the gastrointestinal tract have been reported in 25% of an autopsy series containing patients with all types of leukemia and in 18% of an acute leukemia series containing patients of all ages.[14, 55] At the microscopic level the incidence of gastrointestinal involvement has been reported as high as 63%.[48] In the M. D. Anderson Hospital autopsy study, 27% of the children showed leukemic infiltrates of the gastrointestinal tract, gross or microscopic. Involvement was slightly greater in boys than in girls, 33% vs. 21%. Forty-three percent of children less than 2 years of age had gastrointestinal infiltrates, which were found in only 20% to 29% of older children, the percentage of involvement decreasing with advancing age. The increased incidence in early childhood may be associated with the increased lymphoid mass in the younger age group. In the M. D. Anderson series, gastrointestinal involvement occurred in similar percentages of children with acute lymphocytic and acute granulocytic leukemia, 28% vs. 27%. Involvement was noted in only 17% of those children whose leukemia arose from lymphosarcoma. Leukemic infiltration of the bowel has been reported during bone marrow remission.[21] Usually involvement of sites other than the cecum cannot be established with certainty prior to autopsy.

Leukemic infiltration of the esophagus is apparently infrequent but has been noted in 12% of patients with acute leukemia.[55] Esophageal involvement occurred in 8% of the children in the M. D. Anderson Hospital group.

The stomach has been considered a common site of involvement, and infiltrates in this organ are usually confined to the mucosa and submucosa. Commonly, plaquelike thickenings and nodular elevations are seen. Diffuse infiltration of the stomach may produce cordlike rugae that give the stomach the general appearance of brain tissue. In the Anderson series, gastric infiltrates accounted for 33% of the involvement of the gastrointestinal tract.

Among our patients the small bowel was a frequent site for infiltrates, with 58% of the children with gastrointestinal leukemia having infiltrates in this segment. An increasing incidence of involvement occurred with increasing distance from the pylorus. Often the infiltrate was restricted to normally occurring lymphoid follicles and Peyer's patches. Plaques, nodules, and polypoid masses were sometimes noted.

An impressive number of M. D. Anderson Hospital children, 34 of 48, showed infiltrates of either the colon (17), cecum (15), or appendix (2). The clinical and radiologic features of necrotizing colitis involving the cecum, referred to as "typhlitis," have been described in 19, or 10%, of leukemic children in an autopsy series.[79] Clinically this syndrome seems to progress from vague right lower quadrant fullness and discomfort to the development of a partially obstructive mass with hemorrhage into the tissues as well as the bowel lumen. The ulcerated surface of the mass serves as a portal of entry for bacteria and fungi, and septicemia is a common event. Perforation of the bowel also occurs. Usually the appendix is uninvolved. Leukemic infiltrate limited to the appendix occurs and has been associated with acute appendicitis.[35] Two cases of appendicitis with perforation and 12 cases of typhlitis occured in the M. D. Anderson series. Curiously, leukemic infiltrates were not described in 4 cases of typhlitis. Fatal septicemia developed in 8 of the 12 children with typhlitis. The causative organism was a *Pseudomonas* species in 4 cases and *Escherichia coli* in 3 cases. In the remaining case, the organism was not identified. Monilial invasion of the cecal lesions was not uncommon, but the organism did not become disseminated in this group of children. The pathogenesis of this form of necrotizing colitis is not understood; it has been suggested that it is related to chemotherapy-induced regression of leukemic masses, which leaves the mucosa eroded and subject to infection.[3]

Since infection of endogenous origin is now a leading cause of death in acute leukemia, further study of leukemia of the bowel seems imperative to eliminate this important portal of entry for infectious organisms.

Pulmonary parenchymal infiltrates

Leukemic lung infiltrates have been reported as occurring in 14% to 30% of patients with all types of leukemia.[22, 78] In a more recent study pulmonary infiltrates were found in 32% of patients with acute lymphocytic leukemia, 27% of those with acute granulocytic leukemia, and 46% of those with acute

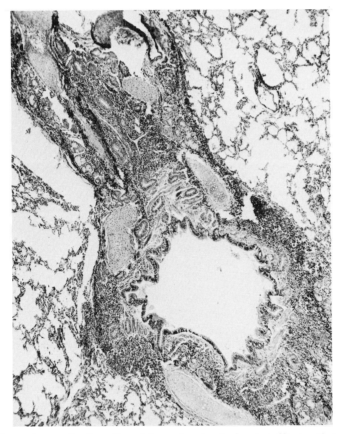

Fig. 11-8. Photomicrograph of section of lung showing leukemic infiltrates that are primarily peribronchial in location (×20). (Courtesy Medical Communications, the University of Texas at Houston, M. D. Anderson Hospital and Tumor Institute.)

monocytic leukemia.[38] Among the 52 children in the Anderson study who were noted to have lung infiltrates, leukemia arising from lymphosarcoma was most often associated with pulmonary involvement. Fifty-two percent of children with this type of leukemia had pulmonary infiltrates at autopsy; 40% of children with acute monocytic or acute myelomonocytic leukemia showed these changes (Fig. 11-8). Forty-three percent of infants showed lung involvement, as did 33% of children 2 to 8 years of age. Thereafter, age was not related to the occurrance of leukemic infiltrates in the lung.

Klatte[38] has described the following patterns of pulmonary infiltrates: (1) involvement of the interalveolar septa separating the capillaries from the alveolar walls, (2) perivascular and peribronchial infiltrates, and (3) dilatation and packing of venules, capillaries, and arterioles with leukemic cells. If infarcts were present, they were usually infiltrated about the periphery. Infiltrates are usually of microscopic proportions; gross lesions as occurred in one of our children have been extremely rare.[4]

Radiographic findings consisted of increased markings in 7 of the 33 cases in the Klatte series.[38] In our material no meaningful correlation could be made between the final radiograph of the chest and the autopsy findings because of the time interval between the two events or the quality of the final film, often a portable.

The pulmonary tissues have received no attention as a possible site of autonomous extramedullary disease, even though this site was found to be positive for leukemic cells in 2 of the 10 children dying in complete remission.[50] Since undiagnosed pulmonary disease is becoming a major problem in the care of leukemic children, needle biopsy in problem cases would seem indicated to rule out leukemic infiltrates as well as exotic infection.

REFERENCES

1. Abelev, G. I., Assecritova, I. V., Kraevsky, N. A., Perova, S. D., and Perevodchikova, N. I.: Embryonal serum alpha-globulin in cancer patients: diagnostic value, Int. J. Cancer 2:551, 1967.
2. Acute Leukemia in Childhood Protocol No. 9, Southwest Cancer Chemotherapy Study Group, Headquarters, Houston, Texas.
3. Amromin, G. D.: Digestive tract. In Pathology of leukemia, New York, 1968, Harper & Row, Publishers, pp. 291-308.
4. Amromin, G. D.: Heart, lungs and urinary tract. In Pathology of leukemia, New York, 1968, Harper & Row Publishers, pp. 239-262.
5. Amromin, G. D.: Nervous system, including orbital contents, middle and inner ear, semicircular canals. In Pathology of leukemia, New York, 1968, Harper & Row, Publishers, pp. 263-290.
6. Amromin, G. D., and Solomon, R. D.: Necrotizing enteropathy, J.A.M.A. 182:23-29, 1962.
7. Aur, R. J. A., Simone, J., Hustu, H. O., Walters, T., Borella, L., Pratt, C., and Pinkel, D.: Central nervous system therapy and combination chemotherapy of childhood lymphocytic leukemia, Blood 37:272-281, March, 1971.
8. Back, E. H.: Death after intrathecal methotrexate, Lancet 2:1005, 1969.
9. Bagshawe, K. K., Magrath, I. T., and Golding, P. R.: Intrathecal methotrexate, Lancet 2:1258, 1969.
10. Baum, E. S., Koch, H. F., Corby, D. G., and Plunket, D. C.: Intrathecal methotrexate, Lancet 1:649, 1971.
11. Boyse, E. A., and Old, L. J.: Some aspects of normal and abnormal cell surface genetics, Annu. Rev. Genet. 3:269, 1969.

12. Burchenal, J. H.: Geographic chemotherapy—Burkitt's tumor as a stalking horse for leukemia: Presidential address, Cancer Res. 26:2393-2401, 1966.

13. Castro, J. R.: Personal communication.

14. Cornes, J. S., Jones, T. G., and Fisher, G. B.: Leukaemic lesions of the gastrointestinal tract, J. Clin. Pathol. 15:305-312, 1962.

15. D'Angio, G. J., Evans, A. E., and Mitus, A.: Roentgen therapy of certain complications of acute leukemia in childhood, Am. J. Roentgenol. Radium Ther. Nucl. Med. 82:541-553, 1959.

16. Djerassi, I., Abir, E., Royer, G. L., Jr., and Treat, C. L.: Long-term remissions in childhood acute leukemia: use of infrequent infusions of methotrexate; supportive roles of platelet transfusions and citrovorum factor, Clin. Pediatr. 5:502-509, 1966.

17. Edynak, E. M., Old, L. J., Vrana, M., and Lardis, M.: A fetal antigen in human tumors detected by antibody in the serum of cancer patients, Proc. Am. Assoc. Cancer Res. 11: 22, 1970.

18. Egan, R. L., and Dodd, G. D.: Roentgen characteristics of the malignant lymphomas and leukemias in childhood, Tex. State J. Med. 53:775, 1957.

19. Evans, A. E., D'Angio, G. J., and Mitus, A.: Central nervous system complications of children with acute leukemia, J. Pediatr. 64:94-96, 1964.

20. Evans, A. E., Gilbert, E. S., and Zandstra, R.: The increasing incidence of central nervous system leukemia in children, Cancer 26:404-409, 1970.

21. Everett, C. R., Haggard, M. E., and Levin, W. C.: Extensive leukemic infiltration of the gastrointestinal tract during apparent remission in acute leukemia, Blood 22:92-99, July, 1963.

22. Falconer, H., and Leonard, M. E.: Pulmonary involvement in lymphosarcoma and lymphatic leukemia, Am. J. Med. Sci. 195:294-301, 1938.

22a. Fernbach, D. J.: Personal communication.

23. Finklestein, J. Z., Dyment, P. G., and Hammond, G. D.: Leukemic infiltration of the testes during bone marrow remission, Pediatrics 43:1042-1045, 1969.

24. Frei, E., III, Bentzel, C. J., Rieselbach, R., and Block, J. B.: Renal complications of neoplastic disease, J. Chronic Dis. 16:757, 1963.

25. Frei, E., III, Fritz, R. D., Price, E., Moore, S. W., and Thomas, L. B.: Renal and hepatic enlargement in acute leukemia, Cancer 16:1089-1092, 1963.

25a. Geils, G. F., Scott, C. W., Jr., Baugh, C. M., and Butterworth, C. E., Jr.: Treatment of meningeal leukemia with pyrimethamine, Blood 38:131-137, Aug., 1971.

26. Givler, R. L.: Testicular involvement in leukemia and lymphoma, Cancer 23:1290-1295, 1969.

27. Gold, P.: Circulating antibodies against carcinoembryonic antigen of the human digestive system, Cancer 20:1663, 1967.

28. Gold, P., and Freedman, S. O.: Specific carcinoembryonic antigens of the human digestive system, J. Exp. Med. 121:467, 1965.

29. Gowdey, J. F., and Neuhauser, E. B. D.: Roentgen diagnosis of diffuse leukemic infiltration of kidneys in children, Am. J. Roentgenol. Radium Ther. 60:13, 1948.

30. Haggar, R. A., MacMillan, A. B., and Thompson, D. C.: Leukemic infiltration of testis, Can. J. Surg. 12:197-201, 1969.

31. Haghbin, M., and Zuelzer, W. W.: A long-term study of cerebrospinal leukemia, J. Pediatr. 67:23-28, 1965.

31a. Hardisty, R. M., and Norman, P. M.: Meningeal leukemia, Arch. Dis. Child. 42:441-447, 1967.

32. Hittle, R.: Personal communication.

33. Hyman, C. B., Bogle, J. M., Brubaker, C. A., Williams, K., and Hammond, D.: Central nervous system involvement by leukemia in children. II. Therapy with intrathecal methotrexate, Blood 25:13-22, Jan., 1965.

34. Iriarte, J. V., Hananian, J., and Cortner, J. A.: Central nervous system leukemia and solid tumors of childhood. Treatment with 1,3-bis (2-chloroethyl-)-1-nitrosourea (BCNU), Cancer 19:1187-1194, 1966.

35. Johnson, W., and Borella, L.: Acute appendicitis in childhood leukemia, J. Pediatr. 67: 595-599, 1965.

36. Kanner, S. P., Wiernik, P. H., Serpick, A. A., and Walker, M. D.: CNS leukemia mimicking multifocal leukoencephalopathy, Am. J. Dis. Child. 119:264-266, 1970.
37. Kappers, J. A.: Structural and functional changes in the telencephalic choroid plexus during human ontogenesis. In The cerebrospinal fluid, Ciba Foundation Symposium, Boston, 1958, Little, Brown & Co.
38. Klatte, E. C., Yardley, J., Smith, E. B., Rohn, R., and Campbell, J. A.: The pulmonary manifestations and complications of leukemia, Am. J. Roentgenol. Radium Ther. Nucl. Med. 89:598-609, 1963.
39. Leef, F., Kende, G., and Ramot, B.: Testicular leukemia, Pediatrics 45:338, 1970.
40. Lusted, L. B., Besse, B. E., Jr., and Fritz, R.: The intravenous urogram in acute leukemia, Am. J. Roentgenol. 80:608, 1958.
41. Mathé, G., Schwarzenberg, L., Mery, A. M., Cattan, A., Schneider, M., Amiel, J. L., Schlumberger, J. R., Poisson, J., and Wajcner, G.: Extensive histological and cytological survey of patients with acute leukemia in "complete remission," Br. Med. J. 1:640-642, 1966.
42. Melhorn, D. K., Gross, S., Fisher, B. J., and Newman, A. J.: Studies on the use of "prophylactic" intrathecal amethopterin in childhood leukemia, Blood 36:55-60, July, 1970.
43. Menkes, J. H.: The causes for low spinal fluid sugar in bacterial meningitis: another look, Pediatrics 44:1-3, 1969.
44. Mitus, A.: Dexamethasone: its effectiveness in the treatment of the acute symptoms of meningeal leukemia, Am. J. Dis. Child. 117:307-312, 1969.
45. Moore, E. W., Thomas, L. B., Shaw, R. K., and Freireich, E. J.: The central nervous system in acute leukemia; a post mortem study of 117 consecutive cases, with particular reference to hemorrhages, leukemic infiltrates and meningeal leukemia, Arch. Intern. Med. 105:451, 1960.
46. Murphy, M.: Leukemia and lymphoma in children, Pediatr. Clin. North Am. 6:611-638, 1959.
47. Naiman, J. L., Rupprecht, L. M., Tanyeri, G., and Philippidis, P.: Intrathecal methotrexate, Lancet 1:571, 1970.
48. Naruki, N.: Studies on the pathologic anatomy of the digestive tract in leukemia (abstract), Nagoya Med. J. 76:129-143, 1958.
49. Nies, B. A., Bodey, G. P., Thomas, L. B., Brecher, G., and Freireich, E. J.: The persistence of extramedullary leukemic infiltrates during bone marrow remission of acute leukemia, Blood 26:133-141, Aug. 1965.
50. Nies, B. A., Thomas, L. B., and Freireich, E. J.: Meningeal leukemia. A follow-up study, Cancer 18:546-553, 1965.
51. Ommaya, A. K.: Subcutaneous reservoir and pump for sterile access to ventricular cerebrospinal fluid, Lancet 2:983-984, 1963.
52. Oppenheimer, J. H., and Riester, W. H.: Influence of cortisone on leptomeningeal reaction induced by talc, Proc. Soc. Exp. Biol. Med. 83:844-847, 1953.
53. Pasquinucci, G., Pardini, R., and Fedi, F.: Intrathecal methotrexate, Lancet 1:309, 1970.
54. Pierce, M. I.:: Neurologic complications in acute leukemia in children, Pediatr. Clin. North Am. 9:425-442, 1962.
55. Prolla, J. C., and Kirsner, J. B.: The gastrointestinal lesions and complications of the leukemias, Ann. Intern. Med. 61:1084-1103, 1964.
56. Rall, D. P., Ben, M., and McCarthy, D. M.: 1,3-bis(-2-chloro-ethyl)-1-nitrosourea, Proc. Am. Assoc. Cancer Res. 4:55, 1963.
57. Rall, D. P., Rieselbach, R. E., Oliverio, V. T., and Morse, E.: Pharmacology of folic acid antagonists as related to brain and cerebrospinal fluid, Cancer Chemotherap. Rep. 16:187-190, 1962.
58. Rall, D. P., and Zubrod, C. G.: Mechanism of drug absorption and excretion. Passage of drugs in and out of the central nervous system, Annu. Rev. Pharmacol. 2:109-128, 1962.
59. Ratcheson, R. A., and Ommaya, A. K.: Experience with the subcutaneous cerebrospinal fluid reservoir: preliminary report of 60 cases, N. Engl. J. Med. 279:1025-1031, 1968.
60. Saiki, J. H., Thompson, S., Smith, F., and Atkinson, R.: Paraplegia following intrathecal chemotherapy, Cancer 29:370-374, 1972.

61. Schabel, F. M., Jr., Johnston, T. P., McCaleb, G. S., Montgomery, J. A., Laster, L. R., and Skipper, H. E.: Experimental evaluation of potential anticancer agents. VIII. Effects of certain nitrosoureas on intracerebral L 1210 leukemia, Cancer Res. **23**:725-733, 1963.

62. Shane, S. J., Clowater, R. A., and Riley, C.: The treatment of tuberculous meningitis with cortisone and streptomycin, Can. Med. Assoc. J. **67**:13-15, 1952.

63. Shapiro, J. H., Ramsey, C. G., Jacobson, H. G., Botstein, C. C., and Allen, L. B.: Renal involvement in lymphomas and leukemias in adults, Am. J. Roentgenol. **88**:928-941, 1962.

64. Sharp, H. L., and Nesbit, M. E.: Renal and hepatic infiltration after initial remission of acute leukemia, Proc. Am. Assoc. Cancer Res. **7**:64, 1966.

65. Sharp, H. L., Nesbit, M. E., D'Angio, G. J., and Krivit, W.: Addition of local radiation after bone marrow remission in acute leukemia in children, Cancer **20**:1403-1404, 1967.

66. Sharp, H. L., Nesbit, M. E., White, J. G., and Krivit, W.: Renal and hepatic pathology following initial remission of acute leukemia induced by prednisone, Cancer **20**:1395-1402, 1967.

67. Shaw, R. K., Moore, E. W., Freireich, E. J., and Thomas, L. B.: Meningeal leukemia: a syndrome resulting from increased intracranial pressure in patients with acute leukemia, Neurology **10**:823-833, 1960.

67a. Simonsen, L., and Fernbach, D. J.: Personal communication, 1971.

68. Skipper, H. E., Schabel, F. M., Jr., Trader, M. W., and Thompson, R. J.: Experimental evaluation of potential anticancer agents. VI. Anatomical distribution of leukemic cells and failure of chemotherapy, Cancer Res. **21**:1154-1164, 1961.

69. Sternby, N. H.: Studies in enlargement of leukemic kidneys, Acta Haematol. **14**:354, 1955.

70. Sullivan, M. P.: Intracranial complications of leukemia in children, Pediatrics **20**:757-781, 1957.

71. Sullivan, M. P.: Leukemic infiltration of meninges and spinal nerve roots, Pediatrics **32**: 63-72, 1963.

72. Sullivan, M. P., Sutow, W. W., Taylor, H. G., and Wilbur, J. R.: Intrathecal (IT) combination chemotherapy for meningeal leukemia using methotrexate (MTX), cytosine arabinoside (CA), and hydrocortisone (HDC), Proc. Am. Assoc. Cancer Res. **12**:45, March, 1971.

73. Sullivan, M. P., Vietti, T. J., Fernbach, D. J., Griffith, K. M., Haddy, T. B., and Watkins, W. L.: Clinical investigations in the treatment of meningeal leukemia: radiation therapy regimens vs conventional intrathecal methotrexate, Blood **34**:301-319, Sept., 1969.

74. Sullivan, M. P., Vietti, T. J., Haggard, M. E., Donaldson, M. H., Krall, J. M., and Gehan, E. A.: Remission maintenance therapy for meningeal leukemia: intrathecal methotrexate vs intravenous bis-nitrosourea, Blood **38**:680-688, 1971.

75. Sullivan, M. P., and Windmiller, J.: Side effects of amethopterin (methotrexate) administered intrathecally in the treatment of meningeal leukemia, Med. Rec. Ann. **50**:92-101, March, 1966.

76. Thomas, L. B.: Pathology of leukemia in the brain and meninges: postmortem studies of patients with acute leukemia and of mice given inoculations of L 1210 leukemia, Cancer Res. **25**:1555-1571, 1965.

77. Tucker, A. S., Newman, A. J., and Persky, L.: The kidney in childhood leukemia, Radiology **78**:407, 1962.

78. Vieta, J. O., and Craver, L. F.: Intrathoracic manifestations of lymphomatoid diseases, Radiology **37**:138-159, 1941.

79. Wagner, M. L., Rosenberg, H. S., Fernbach, D. J., and Singleton, E. B.: Typhlitis: a complication of leukemia in childhood, Am. J. Roentgenol. Radium Ther. Nucl. Med. **109**:341-350, 1970.

80. Whiteside, J. A., Philips, F. S., Dargeon, H. W., and Burchenal, J. H.: Intrathecal amethopterin in neurological manifestations of leukemia, Arch. Intern. Med. **101**:279-285, 1958.

81. Wollner, N., Murphy, M. L., and Gordon, C. S.: A study of intrathecal methotrexate, Proc. Am. Assoc. Cancer Res. **3**:74, 1959.

82. Zuelzer, W. W., and Flatz, G.: Acute childhood leukemia: a ten-year study, Am. J. Dis. Child. **100**:886-907, 1960.

CHAPTER 12

Chronic myelogenous leukemia and other myeloproliferative disorders*

DANIEL M. LANE

Because the more common acute leukemias are considered elsewhere, chronic myelogenous leukemia and those conditions that either present like leukemia or ultimately lead to leukemia will be reviewed here. The major features that these disorders may share with the typical leukemias of childhood include depression of normal cellular elements, leukemic blasts in the peripheral blood, uncontrolled proliferation of one or more major cell lines, varying degrees of organomegaly, and, ultimately, conversion to a frankly blastic leukemia. Table 12-1 lists the major clinical entities closely resembling acute leukemia along with their typical findings in the bone marrow. As a group, they constitute what are usually called the *myeloproliferative disorders*.

Whereas the acute childhood leukemias are characterized by an abnormal proliferation of immature cells incapable of developing into the mature form, the myeloproliferative disorders are characterized (at least early in the disease) by the capacity of the hematopoietic cells to mature. This ability to produce the mature form of a given cell line separates the chronic forms from the acute forms and may confuse the clinician caring for the affected child. The myeloproliferative disorders are rare in children when compared with their incidence in adults. This is important for the clinician to remember, since other disorders may produce signs and symptoms compatible with leukemia variants in children. The physician caring for a child whom he believes to have a myeloproliferative disorder should diligently investigate all other possibilities before assigning this diagnosis. Often the time spent in attempting to rule out a benign or non-hematologic cause will be rewarded with the discovery of one of these much less serious disorders.

Chronic myelogenous leukemia, erythroleukemia, and polycythemia vera will be covered in depth. Myeloid metaplasia, which is basically myelofibrosis with extramedullary hematopoiesis, may represent a late manifestation of either acute or chronic myelogenous leukemia and will not be considered further, since it is extremely rare in children. Hemorrhagic thrombocythemia, also called *megakaryocytic leukemia,* is difficult to separate from the thrombocythemia occurring as a part of the myeloproliferative syndromes and is so infrequent as to be of

---

*This chapter was completed during the tenure of a National Institutes of Health Special Research Fellowship (5 FO3 HE43135-03) from the National Heart and Lung Institute.

no concern in the pediatric patient. Finally, conditions that may present findings suggestive of either an acute leukemia or a myeloproliferative disorder will be reviewed briefly at the end of the chapter.

CHRONIC MYELOGENOUS LEUKEMIA

The management of chronic myelogenous leukemia (CML) is difficult to discuss because two separate disease entities must be considered together. One

Table 12-1. Myeloproliferative disorders and their differential features (bone marrow)

Disorders	Hemato-poietic cellularity	Erythroid series	Granulo-cytic series	Megakaryo-cytic series	Comments
Chronic myeloge-nous leukemia	Increased	Decreased	Markedly increased	Decreased	Frequently terminates as acute myeloge-nous leukemia
Erythroleukemia (Di Guglielmo's syndrome)	Increased	Increased early	Increased	Decreased	Leukemic blasts pres-ent at diagnosis; in-crease as disease progresses
Polycythemia vera	Increased	Markedly increased	Increased	Normal	All cellular elements usually increased, at least early
Myeloid meta-plasia (myelo-fibrosis)	Decreased	Decreased	Decreased	Decreased	Defect appears to be in hematopoietic cells, not in fibro-blastic cells
Hemorrhagic thrombo-cythemia	Increased	Normal or decreased	Normal or decreased	Increased	Frequently precip-itated by splenec-tomy (due to re-duced platelet destruction)

Table 12-2. Differences between adult and juvenile forms of chronic myelogenous leukemia*

Characteristic	Adult form	Juvenile form
Age of maximum incidence	10-12 yr	1-2 yr
Philadelphia chromosome	Always present	Absent
Fetal hemoglobin levels	Normal	15%-50%
Splenomegaly	Marked	Moderate to marked
Lymphadenopathy with suppuration	Occasional	Frequent
Skin rash	Absent	Frequent
White blood cell count at onset	Frequently > 100,000/mm³	Rarely > 100,000/mm³
Thrombocytopenia at onset	Uncommon	Common
Blast forms in peripheral blood	Uncommon	Occasional
Megakaryocytes in bone marrow	Often increased	Usually decreased
Response to therapy	Frequent	Rare

*Slightly modified from Bloom, G. E., Gerald, P. S., and Diamond, L. K.: Chronic myelog-enous leukemia in an infant: serial cytogenetic and fetal hemoglobin studies, Pediatrics **38:**295-299, 1966.

type of childhood CML produces a clinical picture inseparable from that seen in the adult form, including the presence of a Philadelphia chromosome in the patient's leukocytes. The other type, known as the juvenile form, probably represents a mixture of disorders characterized by the proliferation of myeloid elements without a demonstrable Philadelphia chromosome. The major features of the two forms are summarized in Table 12-2, especially when a feature is useful in separating one type from the other. Fortunately, the management of both disorders is much the same; hence both will be discussed as a single entity.

Chronic myelogenous leukemia accounts for about 5% of childhood leukemia.[5] The incidence is equal between the sexes, but the age distribution is uneven. The peak incidence of the adult form is found in preadolescence, whereas the juvenile form is most frequent around 2 years of age. The cause of CML remains to be determined, although the chromosomal abnormalities reported strongly implicate a genetic defect. Familial disorders have been reported in which the clinical findings were compatible with CML.[7] However, a report has also appeared of the disorder being found in only one of a set of identical twins, which is more compatible with an acquired disorder.[4] More information must be gathered about this disorder before its varieties can be satisfactorily classified and a specific cause attached to each.

Clinically, the disease begins insidiously, with generalized malaise and weakness usually appearing as the first symptoms. They may be associated with recurrent infections, intermittent febrile episodes, and skin rashes. The first sign of the disease most commonly is a protuberant abdomen, although lymphadenopathy and hepatosplenomegaly also constitute initial signs. The physician's suspicions are most likely to be aroused by the finding of splenomegaly, often to a marked degree, with few or no other physical findings.

Diagnosis may be a problem. Often the final diagnosis is established only after a long period of observation, especially if the child is relatively asymptomatic at the onset of his disease. Physical examination usually reveals a protuberant abdomen with an enlarged spleen (often massive) and varying degrees of hepatomegaly. Lymphadenopathy is common, but the severity varies. Skin rashes and skin infections may also be found. Late in the course, generalized debilitation can become an impressive feature. Bleeding occurs only when marked thrombocytopenia is present.

A tentative diagnosis of CML depends on finding a persistent, marked elevation of the peripheral white blood cell count with a predominance of myeloid cells, both mature and immature. Although blast forms are often seen in peripheral blood late in the disease, they are uncommon at the times of diagnosis. Bone marrow examination reveals a hypercellular marrow with a marked predominance of myeloid cells, usually neutrophilic, and an increase in the more immature myeloid cells. Megakaryocytes are present, although their number may be either increased or decreased. Early in the disease the erythroid series is usually little affected, but later a decrease is typical. Anemia is uncommon, but thrombocytopenia is fairly frequent. The thrombocytopenia is usually related to the degree of hypersplenism manifested by the patient until progression of the leukemic proliferation displaces the megakaryocytes from the bone marrow.

Determination of the level of the enzyme alkaline phosphatase in neutrophilic leukocytes has been useful in the diagnosis of CML. Measured either histochemically or chemically, levels are usually markedly reduced during periods of activity and normal during periods of remission in this disorder. CML can be differentiated from leukemoid reactions (as in Down's syndrome), acute lymphocytic leukemia, and glucocorticoid effects, in which levels are moderately elevated, as well as from polycythemia vera and idiopathic thrombocythemia, in which levels are markedly elevated. Difficulties with the use of the leukocyte alkaline phosphatase assay arise when evaluating disorders in which the level is below normal (as in infectious mononucleosis, aplastic anemia, idiopathic thrombocytopenic purpura, and androgenic hormone effects) or is absent (as in acute myelogenous leukemia). A better understanding of what is being measured will be necessary before more definitive use of this test is possible.

More definitive diagnosis depends on further laboratory investigation, the most specific study being an evaluation of the karyotype of the white blood cells. The best preparations are obtained from bone marrow samples, but peripheral blood samples are also satisfactory. Children with the adult form of CML have an abnormal chromosome in the number 21-22 group,[3] generally known as the Philadelphia chromosome (Ph^1). This abnormal chromosome is one of the small acrocentrics having a deletion of approximately half its long arm. Although cells of the granulocytic series are the most common carriers of the Philadelphia chromosome, the erythroid and megakaryocytic lines may also demonstrate this abnormal chromosome. The fact that cells from other tissues of the body do not carry the Ph^1 chromosome suggests that the etiologic agent in CML affects only those cells that are hematopoietic in origin.

A less specific but very helpful study in children consists of measuring the percent of fetal hemoglobin in the total circulating hemoglobin. In the juvenile form of CML, elevations in the range from 15% to 50% are common and probably are diagnostic.[2] How the elevated fetal hemoglobin relates to the etiology of the disease can only be speculated on at this time. Additional confirmation of the difference between chromosome-negative and chromosome-positive forms of CML is possible through studies on serum, leukocyte, and urinary levels of muramidase.[11] The presence of muramidase in the urine is apparently diagnostic of the chromosome-negative type.

Unfortunately, the results of these studies are sometimes negative in childhood CML. Although a poorer prognosis is generally associated with such cases, some children survive for years. The major problem arising when these tests are negative is the physician's inability to reach a diagnosis; he may have to exercise a great deal of patience before he can obtain confirmatory evidence of CML. The prime responsibility of the physician in such situations is to be sure that no other disease is producing the same clinical picture suggestive of CML.

Three major entities must be considered carefully in the differential diagnosis: chronic infection, autoimmune disorders, and a systemic disease whose course has been modified by drug administration. Chronic infection, especially with tuberculosis, should be specifically ruled out. As in CML, elevation of the peripheral white blood cell (WBC) count, bone marrow myeloid hyperplasia, and splenomegaly are common to many infectious disorders early in the disease process. A possible infectious cause should be carefully sought before one concludes that the child has CML. The autoimmune disorders, especially rheumatoid arthritis, also share the features of CML. Although the involvement of multiple systems in autoimmune disease usually separates it from CML, the initial findings may be similar. The third major group of disorders to be differentiated from CML are those in which the administration of drugs, especially glucocorticoids and antipyretics, has modified the course of a systemic disease. For example, in hypogammaglobulinemia steroids can alter the clinical picture, and yet organomegaly with chronic infection can continue to be present, Extensive studies are justified when the findings are atypical for CML and chronic drug administration has been a part of the previous medical management.

The clinical management is determined by three basic features of the disease. First, the leukocyte count is markedly elevated with tissue infiltration by the leukocytes. It is difficult to determine if the elevated count contributes to the course of the disease, but reduction of the count is usually associated with an improved clinical status. Second, marked splenomegaly occurs, producing varying degrees of hypersplenism and significantly hastening the course of the disease by depression of circulating cellular elements, especially the platelets. In addition, the large spleen can cause mechanical problems, most often by impinging on the stomach. Third, CML eventually converts to a more acute form of leukemia, the so-called "acute blastic transformation" of chronic myelogenous leukemia. The natural course of a child's disease may be benign, requiring almost no therapy, until the rather sudden onset of acute leukemia in a form essentially inseparable from acute myelogenous leukemia. However, from this point onward the course is rapidly progressive, and the disorder responds more poorly to therapy than does primary acute myelogenous leukemia. In caring for the child with CML, treatment should be based on the progression of these three major features.

The treatment of CML in children is difficult and complicated primarily because one often cannot be sure whether the patient actually needs therapy for his disease. Consequently, this discussion will be restricted to disease complications for which specific therapy is available, including hypersplenism (and its associated effects on the peripheral blood), marked elevations of the peripheral WBC count with tissue infiltration, and the so-called "blastic transformation" to a more acute form of leukemia.

The hypersplenic syndrome is the clinical condition characterized by leukopenia, thrombocytopenia, and anemia, which are not directly due to the leukemic process. Splenomegaly, however, is presumed to result from leukemic infiltration. This syndrome may be controlled in one of two ways: by radiation therapy or by splenectomy. Radiation therapy will lower the white cell count and reduce the size of the spleen, but unfortunately the responses are usually transient, and irradiation fails to effect long-term control of the problem. Splenectomy will relieve the hypersplenism and probably is the best approach. However, if the enlarged spleen is not the cause for peripheral blood changes, obviously no improvement will ensue, and the disease may progress more rapidly. In addition, splenectomy increases the risk of overwhelming septicemia. The younger the patient, the greater this risk. In my experience, splenectomy has been the definitive approach, although the course of the basic disease apparently continues undeterred.[8]

Marked elevations of the peripheral WBC count should initially be treated with busulfan. The dosage will vary according to the patient's response and his ability to tolerate the drug. Melphalan has recently been reported to be effective in a child with CML initially unresponsive to busulfan.[13] An initial dose of 2 mg/day elicited a response, but 4 mg daily was necessary to achieve complete remission. Failure to control the disease with one of these agents suggests that the disease may be changing in character, requiring more aggressive therapy.

Acute blastic transformation is responsible for at least 75% of the deaths in CML.[9] Its onset is characterized symptomatically by increasing fatigability, fever, and bone pain and physically by increasing organomegaly. Laboratory findings reveal anemia, thrombocytopenia, and increased immature myeloid cells, often blastic, in both the peripheral blood and bone marrow. Although data on the results of treatment of childhood varieties of CML during acute blastic transformation are limited, the clinical experience with adults has been discouraging. Therapy is less effective than in acute myelogenous leukemia (AML), which CML in the blastic phase resembles morphologically. Even when agents recently found to be effective in AML such as cytosine arabinoside are used, the responses are short lived and unimpressive. For specific dosage recommendations, the reader should refer to pp. 104 and 111 and Chapter 10.

The prognosis for CML in childhood is difficult to define because this entity occurs so infrequently and comprises a more heterogeneous group of disorders than does the adult form. Once acute blastic transformation has taken place, the child is unlikely to survive for more than 3 to 4 months. Before this change, however, survival may vary from a few months to years. Thus the child's physician must not only exercise caution in assessing the prognosis but must also aggressively treat intercurrent problems.

ERYTHROLEUKEMIA (DI GUGLIELMO'S DISEASE)

Erythroleukemia (EL) cannot be defined as a specific entity because no consistently characteristic clinical and hematologic features have been found in all cases. The findings that are considered most diagnostic are the combination of an erythroid hyperplasia and a leukemic process in the bone marrow. However, the extent of the erythroid hyperplasia and the type of leukemic process can vary greatly, obscuring the diagnosis. A possible explanation for this variation might be that both a malignant erythroid cell line and a malignant leukocytic cell line are present. Most evidence suggests that only a leukemic cell line is responsible, with the erythroid cells increased in response to a reduced number of circulating erythrocytes. If this is indeed the case, the leukemic process must not suppress the production of red cells as it ordinarily does in other forms of leukemia. The facts that blood transfusion sufficient to achieve normal hemoglobin levels can suppress erythroid hyperplasia and that the percentage of erythroid cells decreases due to replacement by leukemic cells as the disease progresses strongly support this concept.[1] Consequently, erythroleukemia and its management will be considered on the assumption that the disease is a leukemia variant in which erythroid hyperplasia early in the disease is a characteristic diagnostic feature.

The incidence of EL is impossible to determine in children because of its rarity and the difficulty in defining precisely what it is. In one series of 600 cases of acute leukemia (all ages) collected over a 9-year period, only 20 were diagnosed as erythroleukemia.[12] Four of the 20 patients were under 15 years old and had an acute form of leukemia associated with an increase in the erythroid series. Obviously, then, the overall incidence is very low, and the disease causes diagnostic difficulty by confusing physicians who are familiar with the more common types of leukemia.

EL begins much like the other forms of leukemia—with malaise, fatigue, weakness, and febrile episodes as the first symptoms. By the time the child is brought in for a physical examination, he is usually pale, chronically or acutely ill, and may have petechiae and ecchymoses. Almost invariably, the abdomen is enlarged. Less consistently, splenomegaly with hepatomegaly is found. Although lymphadenopathy is generally present, enlarged nodes are so common in children that their significance is often questionable.

Diagnosis is dependent on hematologic data from studies of both the peripheral blood and bone marrow. Anemia is less common than in erythroleukemic adults. Nucleated red blood cells in the peripheral blood are diagnostically significant, as well as anisocytosis and poikilocytosis. Thrombocytopenia is always evident late in the disease but may be absent in its early stages. An elevated white blood cell count with a marked left shift is most frequently seen, although the levels are sometimes normal or reduced. Blasts are observed in the peripheral blood with increasing regularity as the disease progresses but may be inapparent at the time of diagnosis.

The specific diagnosis of EL is based primarily on bone marrow cytological studies. Leukemic blasts are observed in the hypercellular marrow and usually are myelocytic, although myelomonocytic forms are seen. Proliferation of the erythroid series is increased, with bizarre and abnormal forms, including multinucleated and megaloblastoid erythroblasts.

The ratio of erythroid to myeloid (or blast) cells varies considerably at the time of diagnosis, but the general pattern is a decrease in erythroid cells with a concomitant increase in leukemic blasts, leading ultimately to a completely leukemic marrow. Megakaryocytes also progressively decrease as the marrow is replaced with leukemic cells. It is the presence of both erythroid hyperplasia and leukemic proliferation that is characteristic of this disorder. Unfortunately, no specific test to diagnose EL is available, although periodic acid–Schiff (PAS) staining has been reported to be helpful.[6]

Disorders to be considered in the differential diagnosis of childhood EL include acute lymphocytic leukemia (ALL) with erythroid hyperplasia, hemolytic anemias, and bacterial infections with associated hemolytic anemia. Since erythroid hyperplasia commonly occurs in ALL after responses to therapy, partially treated patients may present a clinical picture that misleads the physician into considering EL as a possible diagnosis. The marked erythroid hyperplasia (with abnormal peripheral blood erythrocytes), especially early in the disease when few blasts are present, can strongly suggest a hemolytic anemia. Fortunately or unfortunately, the progressive increase in leukemic blasts will solve this diagnostic dilemma. Occasionally, the marked migration of mature granulocytes from the bone marrow in a bacterial infection may be associated with a hemolytic anemia. This can result in the appearance of very early granulocytic precursors and erythroid hyperplasia in the bone marrow, suggestive of EL. With infections the acute nature of the patient's illness and the subsequent course should eliminate EL as a diagnosis.

The management of EL is the same as that for acute myelogenous leukemia, since the leukemic blasts are of either the myelocytic or myelomonocytic type. Supportive measures should be diligently applied, since a few patients survive for long periods (possibly because their leukemia is actually a chronic form).

For most patients, however, the prognosis is very poor; 6 months of survival is generally considered the upper limit. The small percentage of patients who live for unusually long periods probably owe their extended survival more to the nature of their disease process than to the therapy. The response to therapy is usually poor, even with the newer agents such as cytosine arabinoside, which has been effective in acute myelogenous leukemia. Development of increasingly effective chemotherapeutic agents may improve the prognosis.

POLYCYTHEMIA VERA

Childhood polycythemia vera (PV) is exceedingly rare, having been documented in only 3 or 4 children under 15 years old.[10] However, because so many different disorders are associated with an elevated hemoglobin, one should be able to differentiate between true PV and other disorders.

Normal erythrocyte production is controlled by variation in the secretion of erythropoietin (ESF), a circulating glycoprotein that stimulates the proliferation of erythroid precursors. Polycythemia vera is a disease state in which erythroid hyperplasia occurs in the absence of an increase in ESF secretion. Consequently, PV will be defined here as an absolute increase in the red blood cell (RBC) mass without an appropriate increase in the secretion of erythropoietin. Disorders associated with an increased ESF are considered secondary polycythemias, as are elevated hemoglobin levels due to hypoxic disorders, even though an elevated plasma ESF may not be demonstrable in the latter.

The cause of polycythemia vera is unknown, but apparently it is related to other myeloproliferative syndromes, since the platelet and leukocyte levels are elevated in most cases of PV. The release of increased amounts of ESF plays no etiologic role, as shown by repeated assays of plasma and urine. Probably the cause of PV will be uncovered when the causes of other proliferative disorders involving the hematopoietic system are elucidated, whether they be viruses, radiation, chromosomal damage, or currently unknown agents.

Easy fatigability is the most common clinical symptom, but dizziness, blurring of vision, and headache also occur frequently. Physical signs include hepatosplenomegaly, bleeding, redness of the mucous membranes, and facial blush. No other major symptoms and signs are consistently apparent, although other findings such as shortness of breath have been reported. This symptom complex is so uncommon in children that when it occurs the diagnosis of polycythemia should be considered early.

In the presence of these signs and symptoms, the diagnostic process usually starts with a complete blood count, including determination of hemoglobin, hematocrit, white blood count with differential, and platelet count. All these values are elevated in polycythemia vera, including the leukocytes and platelet counts. The hemoglobin level is 16 gm/100 ml or higher. Bone marrow examination reveals a marked erythroid hyperplasia with a normoblastic maturation pattern. There should be no shift in granulopoiesis toward immature forms in the bone marrow. Definitive diagnosis of polycythemia, or erythrocytosis, depends on the demonstration of an expanded red blood cell mass above the level appropriate for the body surface of the child. The plasma volume is also usually above normal limits, but the red cell mass is the major determinant for the presence of a true erythrocytosis.

The physician attempting to pinpoint the cause of an elevated hemoglobin and hematocrit level in a child should search for problems that might be treatable as early as possible with a minimum exposure to potentially dangerous diagnostic procedures. Since defective oxygenation due to either cardiac or pulmonary disease frequently produces an elevated hematocrit in children, arterial oxygen saturation studies should be performed before the red cell volume is measured. If oxygen saturation is found to be low, polycythemia vera need not be investigated further. If the oxygen saturation is normal, the red cell mass and plasma volume should be determined to verify the existence of a true increase in the red cell mass. A normal red cell mass in a child with an elevated hematocrit is necessarily associated with a reduced plasma volume, and further studies should shift toward explaining the contracted plasma volume.

An elevated red cell mass with normal oxygen saturation is due either to increased secretion of erythropoietin or to polycythemia vera. The latter can usually be diagnosed only by the process of elimination, that is, by excluding all possible causes of abnormal ESF secretion. The major causes of such defective secretion are renal disorders (including tumors) and a wide variety of other malignant tumors. Consequently, careful evaluation of the kidney is critical, including an intravenous pyelogram (IVP) and additional studies as indicated. If the IVP reveals any abnormality, it should be followed up by further investigation for renal cysts, hydronephrosis, or a tumor. In addition, a careful search should be made for the presence of intracranial, hepatic, and adrenal tumors that have been reported to be associated with erythrocytosis. If these efforts prove fruitless, no further tests are necessary, and watchful waiting is the best remaining course. However, plasma and urinary erythropoietin levels can be measured if laboratory facilities are readily available. These studies help eliminate polycythemia from the differential diagnosis only if the levels are elevated, since the values usually remain within normal limits in PV. The finding of elevated levels should stimulate a more aggressive search for other possible causes of the increased secretion.

A few specific disorders to be considered in the differential diagnosis are worth special mention. Benign familial erythrocytosis, a rare disorder affecting children, is associated with a true elevation of the red cell mass but differs from polycythemia vera by producing fewer symptoms, no splenomegaly, and normal platelet and leukocyte counts. The hypoxic disorders, already mentioned, include such entities as cyanotic congenital heart disease, a major disease category itself. Pulmonary disorders due either to inadequate diffusion or to shunts can produce polycythemia. Special consideration must be given to the possibility of hemoglobinopathies and enzymatic deficiencies, either congenital or acquired. Finally, the need for a careful search for malignant tumors cannot be overemphasized when a child has an elevated red cell mass coexisting with a normal arterial oxygen saturation.

The treatment of PV depends primarily on which cell types are increased, especially when the increase has resulted in clinical manifestations. If erythrocytosis is present and is producing the only symptoms, then phlebotomy to

Table 12-3. Disorders to be considered in the differential diagnosis of childhood leukemia*

				Hematology				
	Hepatic and/or splenic enlargement	Generalized lymphadenopathy	Purpura or hemorrhage	Anemia	Thrombocytopenia	Leukocytosis	Immature leukocytes in peripheral blood	Blasts in bone marrow
I. Infections								
Pyogenic bacterial infection	+	+	−	Occasional	−	+ (N)	+	−
Tuberculosis	+	+	−	−	−	+ (N)	+	−
Syphilis	+	+	−	+	−	+ (N)	+	−
Toxoplasmosis	+	+	−	−	−	+ (N)	+	−
Brucellosis	+	+	−	−	−	+ (N)	+	−
Histoplasmosis	+	+	−	−	−	+ (N)	+	−
Leptospirosis	+	+	−	Occasional	−	+ (L)	+	−
Infectious mononucleosis	+	+	−	Occasional	−	+ (L)	+	−
Infectious lymphocytosis	Rare	Rare	−	−	−	+ (L)	−	−
Cytomegalic inclusion disease	+	+	−	−	−		−	−
Visceral larval migrans (or parasitic tissue invasion)	+	−	−	+	−	+ (E)	+	−
Malaria	+	+	−	+	−	−	+	−
II. Miscellaneous								
Autoimmune disorders (e.g., rheumatoid arthritis, lupus erythematosus)	+	+	−	+	−	+ (N)	+	−
Malignancies (lymphomas, neuroblastoma, rhabdomyosarcoma)	+	+	+	+	+	+	+	+
Lipid storage disorders (especially Gaucher's disease)	+	+	Late in disease	+	Late in disease	+	+	−
Histiocytosis	+	+	+	+	−	+	+	−
Hemolytic anemias	+	+	−	+	−	+	+	−
Iron-deficiency anemia	+	+	−	+	−	+	+	−
Megaloblastic anemias	+	−	−	+	−	+	+	−
Aplastic anemia (either acquired or congenital)	Occasional	+	+	+	+	−	+	−
Idiopathic thrombocytopenic purpura	Occasional	Occasional	+	Occasional	+	+	−	−
Chronic granulomatous disease	+	+	−	+	−	+	+	−

*The signs and symptoms appearing in the column headings are consistently present in childhood leukemia.
Key: + = present; − = absent; N = neutrophilic; L = lymphocytic; E = eosinophilic.

maintain the hematocrit below 50 is adequate therapy. Increases in the granulocytic and megakaryocytic series result in a more complicated problem. Thrombocythemia with an associated hypercoagulability in particular requires more aggressive treatment. In the child or adolescent, alkylating agents are the preferred modality. Because of its shorter duration of effect and its ability to affect all three major cell lines, melphalan (L-phenylalanine mustard) is probably the agent of choice over busulfan, chlorambucil, or cyclophosphamide. Radioactive phosphorus should probably not be used in children, since it offers no advantage over the alkylating agents other than ease of administration and control. Its major disadvantage is the long-term effect that radioactivity may have on the child's growing tissues. Although not a primary manifestation, hyperuricemia and gout may occur, for which allopurinol is adequate therapy.

Because of its extreme rarity in children, polycythemia vera cannot be assigned a prognosis. The greatest danger in managing suspected polycythemia is that the physician may not proceed with differential diagnostic studies assiduously enough and thereby overlook a different, potentially curable lesion until it is too late.

DISORDERS PRESENTING AS POSSIBLE LEUKEMIA

In addition to the previous disorders, which are actually the less common varieties of hematopoietic proliferative disorders, a large group of diseases share basic features with acute and chronic leukemia. Table 12-3 lists many of the diseases that may present the signs and symptoms of leukemia. Infections are particularly important because they can be confused with chronic myelocytic leukemia, acute lymphocytic leukemia, or even the very rare eosinophilic leukemia, depending on the etiology. Autoimmune disorders, especially when the disorder presents in a very active stage, can cause considerable confusion. Other malignancies may be so similar that differentiation is almost impossible before extensive tissue studies are completed. This is especially true for lymphosarcoma, disseminated neuroblastoma, and disseminated rhabdomyosarcoma. The last several disorders listed are included primarily because they share major findings with leukemia, although differentiation is basically fairly easy after initial studies are completed.

Special attention should be brought to bear on the "dangerous duo" so common in acute leukemia, anemia and thrombocytopenia. Only two entities in Table 12-3 frequently share these two findings with acute leukemia. Both groups, the malignancies and aplastic anemias, also share a very poor prognosis with leukemia. In addition, disseminated intravascular coagulation (DIC), a complex disorder associated with thrombocytopenia and a hemolytic anemia, can develop during the course of most of the diseases listed in Table 12-3. DIC must be diagnosed and treated early in its course if a successful outcome is to be obtained. Finding both anemia and a low platelet count in a child who is ill should be a cause for extreme concern, since the diagnosis is most likely to be a very serious disorder.

Leukemia, both acute and chronic, can masquerade as many different diseases just as the latter may appear to be leukemia. Since the various disorders are so numerous and the opportunities for making incorrect diagnoses equally as numerous, the physician caring for a child with evidence of leukemia would be prudent to talk little and to search thoroughly.

REFERENCES

1. Adamson, J. W., and Finch, C. A.: Erythropoietin and the regulation of erythropoiesis in Di Guglielmo's syndrome, Blood 36:590-597, 1970.
2. Beaven, G. H., Ellis, M. J., and White, J. C.: Studies on human foetal haemoglobin. II. Foetal haemoglobin levels in healthy children and adults and in certain haematologic disorders, Br. J. Haematol. 6:201-222, 1960.
3. Bloom, G. E., Gerald, P. S., and Diamond, L. K.: Chronic myelogenous leukemia in an infant: Serial cytogenetic and fetal hemoglobin studies, Pediatrics 38:295-299, 1966.
4. Goh, K. O., and Swisher, S. N.: Identical twins and chronic myelocytic leukemia: Chromosomal studies of a patient with chronic myelocytic leukemia and his normal identical twin, Arch. Intern. Med. 115:475-578, 1965.
5. Hardisty, R. M., Speed, D. E., and Till, M.: Granulocytic leukemia in childhood, Br. J. Haematol. 10:551-566, 1964.
6. Hayhoe, F. G. J., Quaglino, D., and Doll, R.: The cytology and cytochemistry of acute leukemias. A study of 140 cases, London, 1964, Her Majesty's Stationery Office.
7. Holton, C. P., and Johnson, W. W.: Chronic myelocytic leukemia in infant siblings, J. Pediatr. 72:377-383, 1968.
8. Lane, D. M.: Chronic myelocytic leukemia (letter to the editor), J. Pediatr. 73:298-299, 1968.
9. Morrow, G. W., Jr., Pease, G. L., Stroebel, C. F., and Bennett, W. A.: Terminal phase of chronic myelogenous leukemia, Cancer 18:369-374, 1965.
10. Natelson, E. A., Lynch, E. C., Britton, H. A., and Alfrey, C. P.: Polycythemia vera in childhood, Am. J. Dis. Child. 122:241-244, 1971.
11. Perillie, P. E., and Finch, S. C.: Muramidase studies in Philadelphia chromosome-positive and chromosome-negative chronic granulocytic leukemia, N. Engl. J. Med. 283:456-459, 1971.
12. Scott, R. B., Ellison, R. R., and Ley, A. B.: A clinical study of twenty cases of erythro-leukemia (Di Guglielmo's syndrome), Am. J. Med. 37:162-171, 1964.
13. Seeler, R. A., and Hahn, K. O.: Chronic granulocytic leukemia responding to melphalan, Cancer 27:284-287, 1971.

CHAPTER 13

Hodgkin's disease in children

MARGARET P. SULLIVAN
LILLIAN M. FULLER
JAMES J. BUTLER

The historical review of Hodgkin's disease by Hoster and co-workers[26b] credits the earliest gross description of the postmortem findings to Malpighi in 1661. The first clinical and pathologic description of the disease entity was published by Thomas Hodgkin in 1832. Subsequent reevaluation of the 7 cases reported by Hodgkin has supported the diagnosis of Hodgkin's disease in 3 persons, including 1 child, with more probable diagnoses of lymphosarcoma, tuberculosis, syphilis, and "systemic lymphomatosis" in the 4 remaining patients.[20a] Early efforts to employ radiotherapy in the treatment of this disease resulted in 5-year survival rates of 5% to 10%.

In 1950 Peters[49] astounded the medical profession by demonstrating in a large series of patients that Hodgkin's disease was potentially curable. At that time and in the ensuing 5 to 10 years Hodgkin's disease and the other lymphomas were considered to be closely related clinical entities on the basis of clinical presentation, histologic similarities, and response to treatment with radiation or nitrogen mustard. Since 1960 the concept of lymphomatous diseases has been refined by (1) staging procedures employing lymphangiography, (2) the demonstration of disease specificity of various chemotherapeutic agents, and (3) the outcome of systematic approaches to management. Today, Hodgkin's disease is recognized as a separate and distinct clinical entity differing in clinical behavior and prognosis from other lymphomatous diseases.

The occurrence of Hodgkin's disease in children is of sufficient frequency to merit special consideration of disease characteristics in that segment of the population in which growth and maturation are still in progress. The availability of an unusually large number of children with Hodgkin's disease, managed by the same team of physicians at the M. D. Anderson Hospital (MDAH) clinics, represents a unique opportunity for the study of the disease in children and for assessment of the response to the treatment regimens that have evolved over the years. Since no larger experience has been reported, this group of children has been considered an important source material. Conclusions derived from these data should be more meaningful than observations based on a heterogeneous collection of published reports of small series.

The number of children living with Hodgkin's disease is uncertain; estimates of the percent of cases occurring in children range from 4% to 19%.[13, 41] Since 1949, 72 children with Hodgkin's disease have been studied histologically, staged, treated, and systematically followed up at the MDAH (Appendixes I and III, pp. 297 and 306). Four other children, previously treated, were unstageable at diagnosis

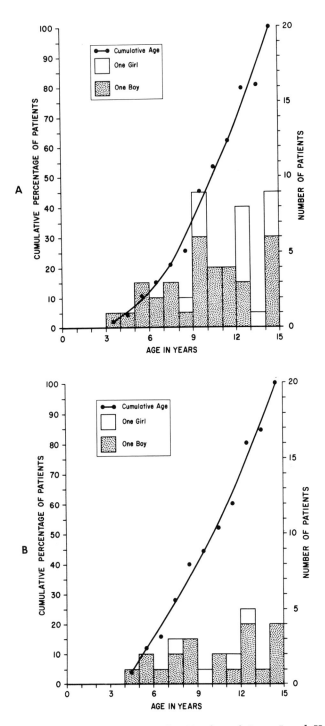

Fig. 13-1. **A**, MDAH Hodgkin's disease study. Number of Stage I and II patients by age and sex. Cumulative age incidence. **B**, MDAH Hodgkin's disease study. Number of Stage III and IV patients by age and sex. Cumulative age incidence. (Courtesy Medical Communications, The University of Texas at Houston, M. D. Anderson Hospital and Tumor Institute.)

(Appendix III). These 76 children constitute about 20% of the entire group of Hodgkin's disease patients seen at the MDAH during this study period.

Hodgkin's disease is exceedingly rare before 5 years of age, but case reports attest to its occurrence in infancy. Both the Mayo Clinic and the Institute Gustave-Roussy-Hospital Saint Louis series contain a 2-year-old child,[4, 62] and several series, including our own, contain 3-year-old children.[26, 31, 60] Other sizable series show no cases of Hodgkin's disease in children less than 4 years of age. In Lebanon, one third of all Hodgkin's disease cases are children, and 20% of these children are under 7 years of age.[3] The distribution of cases within the 5- to 15-year age range has varied among the reported series; peak incidence, however, has usually fallen within the 5- to 9-year age group.[4, 17, 51] The peak incidence occurred later in our children just as in children reported from the University of Chicago[50] (Fig. 13-1). Fifty-five of the 72 stageable patients were boys, and 17 were girls, giving a sex ratio of 3.2:1 in favor of boys. The decreasing number of boys among the older children and the concentration of girls in the older group deserves mention. In the University of Chicago group, preteen and teen-age girls outnumbered boys 2:1.[50] The changing sex ratio after 12 years of age has also been noted by Fraumeni.[21] In the MDAH series of 47 Stage I and II patients, this reversal of sex distribution only occurred in one clinical situation: nodular sclerosing Hodgkin's disease involving the mediastinum (Fig. 13-2).

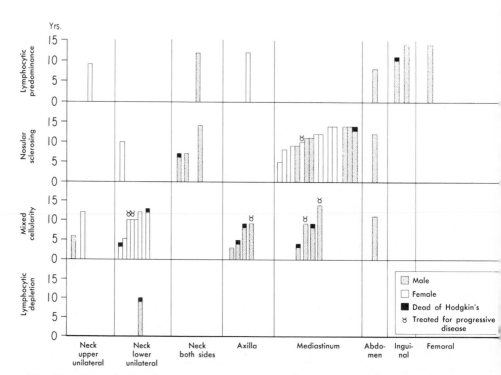

Fig. 13-2. Interrelation of age, sex, presentation, and specific histology in Stages I and II. (Courtesy Medical Communications, The University of Texas at Houston, M. D. Anderson Hospital and Tumor Institute.)

A racial predilection has not been suggested in Hodgkin's disease. However, East African children with Hodgkin's disease have a higher proportion of unfavorable histologic types than a comparable group of English children.[9] Among the MDAH children, 4 were of Negro descent, and each of these children had an unfavorable clinical course. Eleven of our children were of Spanish or mixed Spanish-Indian descent. Only 1 of these children had nonprogressive Stage I disease (patient 24 [DG], Appendix I); 10 had Stage III or IV disease at diagnosis or progressive Stage I or II disease.

PATHOLOGY

Prerequisites for the histologic diagnosis of Hodgkin's disease include (1) adequate biopsy and (2) technical excellence in the preparation of tissue slides. Without benefit of the normal architecture of an intact lymph node, the pathologist frequently cannot differentiate a malignant lymphoma from a benign process. Needle biopsies and frozen sections that distort the normal architecture are contraindicated in patients suspected of having Hodgkin's disease. The surgeon's responsibility to provide the pathologist with a specimen that is likely to contain tumor cannot be overemphasized. The best possibility for obtaining a representative biopsy is to select a well-established prominent node that has been increasing in size. Pathologic changes in very small satellite nodes are likely to be secondary to a reactive hyperplasia rather than tumor. In suspect cases, rebiopsy is indicated if necessary to establish diagnosis. When generalized adenopathy is present, biopsy of inguinal and submaxillary lymph nodes should be avoided, since changes secondary to repeated chronic infections may mask a malignant process.

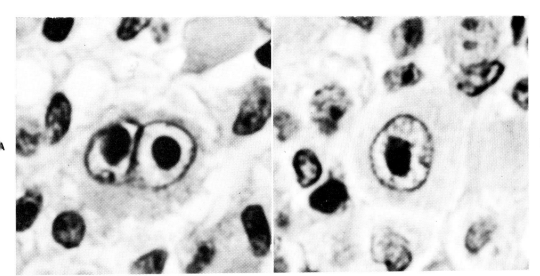

Fig. 13-3. A, Diagnostic Reed-Sternberg cell (H and E ×400). **B,** Atypical histiocyte with large nucleolus (H and E ×400). (Courtesy Medical Communications, The University of Texas at Houston, M. D. Anderson Hospital and Tumor Institute.)

The histologic diagnosis of Hodgkin's disease can be established only when Reed-Sternberg cells are present in the polymorphic inflammatory infiltrate of one of the histologic types of the disease. The diagnostic Reed-Sternberg cell has a lobulated nucleus or is multinucleated; at least one lobe or nucleus contains a nucleolus, which is at least one-fourth the size of the nucleus or of the nuclear lobe in question (Fig. 13-3, A). Mononuclear histiocytic cells with large nucleoli (Fig. 13-3, B) are also present in Hodgkin's disease, but these atypical histiocytes may also be found in reactive processes.[11] Cells resembling the Reed-Sternberg cell have been described in the infectious mononucleosis and other reactive processes of lymphoid tissue and in other neoplastic processes.[59] The correct histologic setting for the Reed-Sternberg cell is therefore essential for the diagnosis of Hodgkin's disease.[59]

The MDAH histologic classification of Hodgkin's disease given here follows that of Lukes and Butler,[44] as modified at the 1965 symposium on Hodgkin's disease held at Rye, New York.[45]

Lymphocytic predominance	Mixed cellularity
Nodular sclerosis	Lymphocytic depletion

The relationship between these two classifications and that of Jackson and Parker[29] is shown in Fig. 13-4. Basically, the classification of Lukes and Butler reflects the inverse relationship that exists between lymphocytes and Reed-Sternberg cells in Hodgkin's disease. Since the classification depends on the number of lymphocytes present, lymph nodes usually cannot be subclassified if the patient has received chemotherapy or radiotherapy to the area of biopsy.

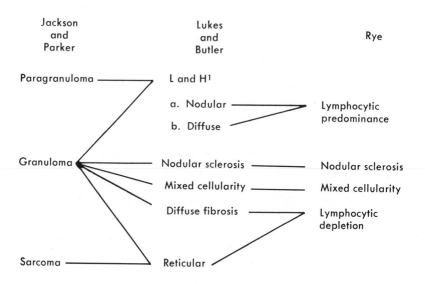

¹Lymphocytic and/or histiocytic

Fig. 13-4. Comparison of the Jackson and Parker,[29] Lukes and Butler,[44] and Rye symposium (Lukes and co-workers[45]) classifications of Hodgkin's disease. (Courtesy Medical Communications, The University of Texas at Houston, M. D. Anderson Hospital and Tumor Institute.)

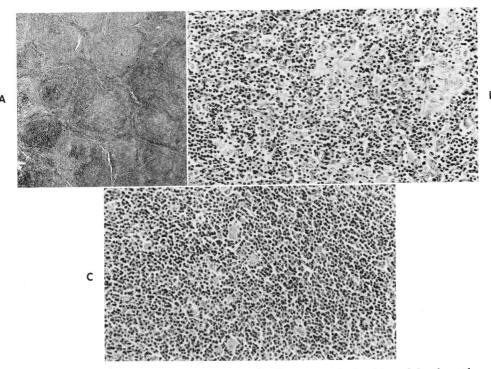

Fig. 13-5. Hodgkin's disease with lymphocytic predominance. **A,** In this nodular form the nodules are best seen under the scanning power of the microscope (H and E ×10). **B,** Histiocytes are prominent in this example (H and E ×100). **C,** Lymphocytes predominate in this example (H and E ×100). (Courtesy Medical Communications, The University of Texas at Houston, M. D. Anderson Hospital and Tumor Institute.)

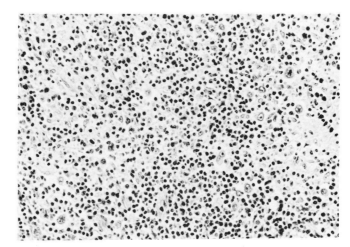

Fig. 13-6. Hodgkin's disease with mixed cellularity; lymphocytes are decreased in number, and Reed-Sternberg cells are easily found. Eosinophils, histiocytes, and plasma cells are also present (H and E ×200). (Courtesy Medical Communications, The University of Texas at Houston, M. D. Anderson Hospital and Tumor Institute.)

The nodular sclerosis type is a common exception to this rule, since its recognition does not depend on the relative number of lymphocytes and Reed-Sternberg cells present.

The Rye classification, which is widely accepted, is useful in management. However, pathologists continue to think in terms of the six histologic types of the disease originally described by Lukes and Butler as shown in Fig. 13-4, which are more descriptive of the histologic findings.

The lymphocytic predominance type of Hodgkin's disease may exhibit a nodular or diffuse pattern. The nodular pattern (Fig. 13-5, A) was first described as the nodular form of Hodgkin's disease by Rappaport, Winter, and Hicks.[52] As in nodular lymphoma, reticulin stains show the nodule to be outlined by reticulin. The nodules, which vary in size, are composed of a diverse mixture of lymphocytes, benign histiocytes, and atypical histiocytes (Fig. 13-5, B). The diffuse form of the disease may be composed solely of lymphocytes and atypical histiocytes (Fig. 13-5, C) or of a mixture of lymphocytes, benign histiocytes, and atypical histiocytes, as seen in the nodular form. At times the arrangement of reactive histiocytes may resemble granulomas. Necrosis does not occur in this form of the disease. Reed-Sternberg cells are difficult to find in both the nodular and the diffuse lymphocytic predominance types. When diagnostic Reed-Sternberg cells are found with ease, the process is not the lymphocytic predominance type of Hodgkin's disease. If the histologic sections being studied are not technically excellent, the diffuse lymphocytic predominance type of Hodgkin's disease may be misinterpreted as well-differentiated lymphocytic lymphoma.[10] Rarely, the nodular form may be misinterpreted as nodular lymphoma.

The mixed cellularity type of Hodgkin's disease is characterized by a decrease in the number of lymphocytes and an increase in the number of Reed-Sternberg cells (Fig. 13-6). Although eosinophils are seen in most cases, their presence is not essential. Necrosis may or may not be present. As in other forms of the disease, the areas of necrosis may be surrounded by reactive histiocytes and Langhans' type giant cells. This type of Hodgkin's disease most closely corresponds to the textbook descriptions of Hodgkin's granuloma.[29] As the name implies, this type of Hodgkin's disease is usually composed of all the types of cells found in lymph nodes of patients with the disease.

The lymphocytic depletion type of Hodgkin's disease has two histologic patterns; in both lymphocytes are decreased in number. In the form designated *diffuse fibrosis* by Lukes and Butler[44] a decrease in lymphocytes and, to a lesser extent, in all other cells is exhibited. In the end stage acellular or almost acellular lymph nodes show only rare Reed-Sternberg cells against a background of proteinaceous material deposited on the connective tissue framework of the lymph node (Fig. 13-7, A). This histologic type, which may develop spontaneously or may be produced by previous local radiotherapy or systemic chemotherapy, is the type most often found at autopsy in previously treated patients. The second form of Hodgkin's disease included in the lymphocytic depletion type was described by Lukes and Butler[44] as the *reticular type;* atypical histiocytes and Reed-Sternberg cells are markedly increased (Fig. 13-7, B).

Diagnosis of the nodular sclerosis type of Hodgkin's disease is based on the presence of collagen septa in various stages of development, which tends to subdivide the lymphoid tissue into nodules containing atypical histiocytic cells lying in spaces or lacunae (Fig. 13-8). The fibrous septa vary in thickness from thin strands that project into the lymphoid tissue from the capsule without producing distinct nodules to the classic thick bands of collagen that surround well-defined islands of lymphoid tissue (Fig. 13-8, *A* and *B*). Atypical histiocytic cells in lacunae are numerous in the nodular sclerosis form of the disease; lobulations of their nuclei are prominent (Fig. 13-8, *C*). However, diagnostic Reed-Sternberg cells are frequently difficult to identify. At times the atypical reticulum cells in lacunae are so numerous and so closely packed that the disease may be misinterpreted as metastatic seminoma or carcinoma, unless the reviewer is familiar with this variant of the disease. Eosinophils are usually numerous in the nodular sclerosis form of the disease; necrosis is frequently present.

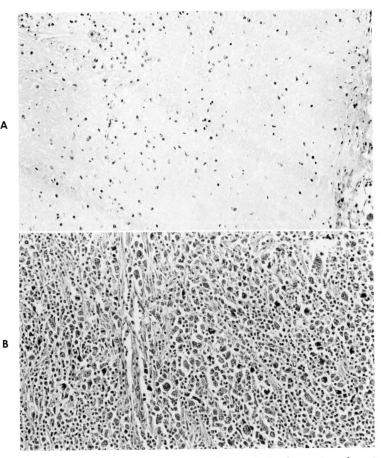

Fig. 13-7. Hodgkin's disease with lymphocytic depletion. **A,** In this variant there is a marked decrease in all cells, with the background appearing to represent proteinaceous material deposited on the connective tissue framework of the lymph node (H and E ×100). **B,** In this example there is a marked increase in the number of Reed-Sternberg cells (H and E ×100). (Courtesy Medical Communications, The University of Texas at Houston, M. D. Anderson Hospital and Tumor Institute.)

The separation of cases of Hodgkin's disease into the various histologic types is subjective; no hard-and-fast rules exist that permit unquestionable classification of every case into one of the described categories. In a small number of cases, differentiation between the mixed cellularity type and the lymphocytic predominance group, the mixed cellularity and lymphocytic depletion group, and the mixed cellularity and nodular sclerosis group is most difficult. An attempt is made to keep the prognostically significant groups, that is, the lymphocytic predominance, nodular sclerosis, and lymphocytic depletion groups, as pure as possible, as illustrated by the triangle in Fig. 13-9, A. Admittedly, the mixed

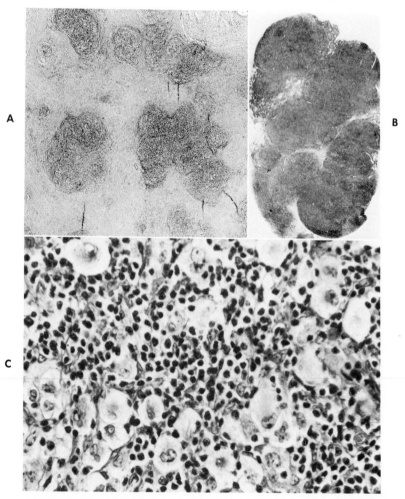

Fig. 13-8. Hodgkin's disease with nodular sclerosis. **A,** Nodules of lymphoid tissue circumscribed by dense collagen (H and E ×10). **B,** In this example there is only a single, thin, well-developed collagen septum (H and E ×3). **C,** The characteristic lacunar cells of nodular sclerosis are atypical histiocytes that frequently exhibit pronounced lobulations of their nuclei and lie in sharply delineated spaces (H and E ×250). (Courtesy Medical Communications, The University of Texas at Houston, M. D. Anderson Hospital and Tumor Institute.)

cellularity group is a less clearly defined group and includes a range of cases, from those closely resembling the lymphocytic predominance group to those closely related to the lymphocytic depletion group, as well as those cases of the nodular sclerosis type in which the changes in the lymph nodes are equivocal.

The evolution of the histologic process in Hodgkin's disease is presented in Fig. 13-9, *B*. The lymphocytic predominance, mixed cellularity, and lymphocytic depletion types of the disease are related in that they represent histologic stages based on the inverse relationship between lymphocytes and Reed-Sternberg cells, through which the disease may theoretically progress. The study of Strum and Rappaport[60a] in which two or more sequential biopsies were performed in patients with Hodgkin's disease has shown that on rebiopsy the lymphocytic predominance type may not change, may change to the mixed cellularity form, or may change to the lymphocytic depletion variety. They also showed that the mixed cellularity form may remain constant or may change to the lymphocytic depletion type. The initial biopsy may of course show the lymphocytic depletion variety and remain the same. The nodular sclerosis type is a distinctive one that does not appear to enter into this orderly progression.

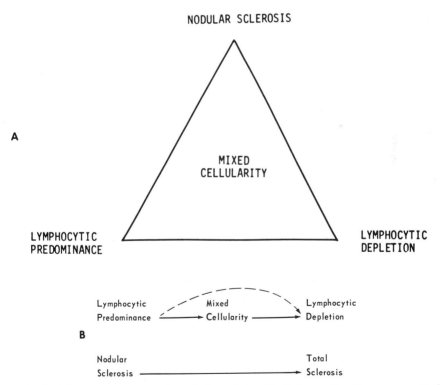

Fig. 13-9. **A**, Schematic representation of the relationship between the three prognostically more significant and histologically more distinct groups and the histologically less well-defined mixed cellularity form of Hodgkin's disease. **B**, Evolution of the histologic process in Hodgkin's disease. (Courtesy Medical Communications, The University of Texas at Houston, M. D. Anderson Hospital and Tumor Institute.)

There is a suggestion[34, 60a] that the progression is from the more cellular forms to ones showing more sclerosis. Total sclerosis in a substantial portion of a lymph node may occasionally be seen spontaneously or after therapy. In nodular sclerosing Hodgkin's disease, however, it has not been possible to establish a definite relationship between any histologic features and the differences in the clinical stages of disease and prognosis.[38]

CLINICAL MANIFESTATIONS

Sites of primary involvement. Painless adenopathy in the lower cervical region, with or without associated fever, is the most common presenting complaint in children with Hodgkin's disease and has been reported as the presenting sign in 60% to 90% of cases.[17, 47, 55] Approximately half the cases with cervical adenopathy have associated involvement of the mediastinum. Hodgkin's disease limited to the mediastinum is rare. Both axillary and inguinal adenopathy are unusual presenting signs except as part of a generalized disease process. Sites of primary involvement in the MDAH series are shown in Fig. 13-2. Splenomegaly has been noted as an initial finding in 10% to 48% of cases and hepatomegaly in 10% to 39%, both of these findings indicating advanced disease.[17, 47]

Symptoms. The common presenting symptom complex seen in approximately half the children with Hodgkin's disease is that of anorexia, malaise, and lassitude.[17] Weight loss is frequently associated with these symptoms. Fever has been noted in 25% to 50% of the children at the time of diagnosis, often in association with this symptom complex. Symptoms were present in 9 of 47 (19%) of our Stage I and II patients and in 18 of 25 (72%) of our Stage III and IV patients. The usual fever pattern shows intermittent elevations of 2° or 3° above normal. Less common are daily, remittent, "picket fence" type fevers with sharp afternoon or evening elevations to 104° F or more, often accompanied by a chill. The well-known Pel-Ebstein recurrent and relapsing fever pattern is rare in children. Pruritus, a very infrequent symptom, was noted in only two of our children. Night sweats are seldom mentioned as a presenting complaint.

Physical findings. Clinical investigations to determine the extent of involvement in a child with Hodgkin's disease begin with the initial physical examination. A careful evaluation of the peripheral node-bearing areas and the abdomen is essential to accurate staging. In children the presence of shotty lymph nodes in one or more of the peripheral lymph node–bearing areas may be difficult to evaluate. In the axilla normal structures may be mistaken for enlarged lymph nodes. Physicians who are inexperienced in evaluating Hodgkin's disease in children have a tendency to overestimate the extent of involvement. In general, this error can be avoided if only those lymph nodes that have been increasing in size are considered significant. When lymph nodes on both sides of the diaphragm are suspect, a second biopsy is indicated to differentiate between localized and generalized disease. Since normal children less than 2 years of age may have palpable livers and, less often, palpable spleens, evaluation of palpable organs in children of this age with Hodgkin's disease is most difficult. Fortunately, the problem is infrequent, since the occurrence of Hodgkin's disease in infancy is rare. Retroperitoneal disease is usually not palpable.

Roentgenographic studies. Radiographic examination of the chest is mandatory for evaluation of mediastinal and hilar nodes. Tomography may yield additional information in selected cases. Oblique views should be obtained if there is a question of parenchymal lung disease.

The development of lymphangiogram techniques constituted a major advance in the diagnosis of retroperitoneal nodal disease. In our hospital, children over 2 years of age may be given intravenous Innovar anesthetic to expedite the procedure. Children less than 2 years of age are given ketamine supplemented with nitrous oxide and oxygen or a general anesthetic using halothane. The diagnostic reliability of lymphangiography was at first thought to exceed 90%.[32] Lymphangiogram interpretation, however, has been more difficult than anticipated, since the findings may be negative or equivocal when there is clinical certainty of involvement of the liver and spleen. In addition, the lymphangiogram does not visualize the high para-aortic nodes, an area likely to be involved. In addition to its value as a staging procedure, the lymphangiogram is essential for designing the radiotherapy treatment fields. Radiopaque media may be retained in nodes

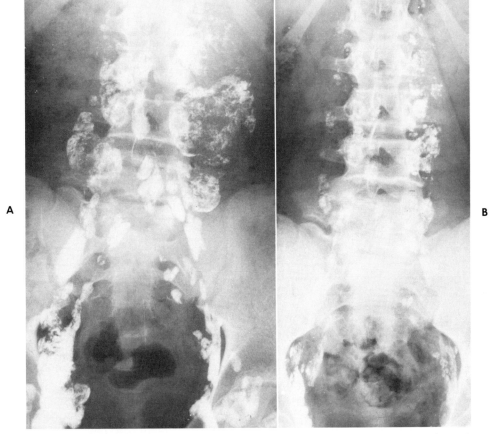

A   B

Fig. 13-10. Lymphangiogram radiographs. **A,** Pretreatment study. **B,** Follow-up film after total abdominal irradiation with a tumor dose of 4000 rads (Appendix III, patient 75 [JT]). (Courtesy Medical Communications, The University of Texas at Houston, M. D. Anderson Hospital and Tumor Institute.)

for 6 months or longer. The follow-up plain films of the abdomen, when compared with the pretreatment study, are helpful in detecting new areas of involvement and in assessing response to both radiotherapy and chemotherapy (Fig. 13-10).

Inferior venacavography may have value in assessing that portion of the retroperitoneal space cephalad to celiac nodes. Occasionally indirect evidence of para-aortic nodal involvement may be obtained by demonstrating renal or ureteral displacement with intravenous pyelography. In children cavography and pyelography can be combined by obtaining properly timed films after rapid injection of the radiopaque medium into a leg vein. In clinical practice, lymphangiography has proved more useful than either of these studies. Today the major use of pyelography is for accurate localization of the kidneys prior to instituting radiotherapy.

Intrinsic involvement of the gastrointestinal tract is rare in children. Radiographic evaluation of the gastrointestinal tract has been recommended as a part of the initial work-up that would aid in the detection of an enlarged spleen or extrinsic masses in the retrogastric and pelvic areas.[26] In our experience, radiographic studies of the gastrointestinal tract have only been positive in occasional symptomatic patients.

The presence of osseous lesions at the time of diagnosis is of such rarity that skeletal survey is usually not included in the routine initial evaluation of the child with Hodgkin's disease. Organ scans with radionuclides are seldom useful in delineating the extent of involvement in Hodgkin's disease.

Hematologic studies. Although not specifically considered in the staging procedure; the presence of anemia is usually an indication of more than localized disease, which calls for further hematologic study. The two known mechanisms of anemia in Hodgkin's disease, hemolysis and impaired mobilization of iron stores, may operate singly or concurrently. Hemolysis may be present shortly after the onset of symptoms or may be delayed until the patient has developed clinical evidence of generalized disease.[12] Once established, hemolysis tends to persist. The Coombs test is seldom positive, but reticulocytosis and normoblastic hyperplasia of the bone marrow will be demonstrable. The diagnosis of hemolysis is dependent on the presence of shortened erythrocyte survival. Hypersplenism with leukopenia, thrombocytopenia, and hemolysis is usually a late occurrence. Hypoferremia, explained only in terms of defective mobilization, occurs in the presence of excessive iron stores in liver and spleen.[24, 64]

Occasionally patients show marked leukocytosis or marked leukopenia. The reasons for these abnormalities in white blood cell counts are not apparent, but in either case the abnormality is associated with an unfavorable course. At onset of disease the absolute lymphocyte count is usually normal or only slightly depressed; in advanced disease the lymphocyte count is markedly reduced.[1a]

Aspirates of bone marrow are unsatisfactory specimens for demonstrating Hodgkin's disease.[64] Failure is related to the fibrous and granulomatous nature of Hodgkin's disease, which prevents aspiration of marrow particles, as well as to the disruption of marrow architecture by the aspiration procedure. Silverman needle biopsies of the posterior iliac crest have provided more satisfactory specimens.[37] For maximum reliability a bone marrow wedge should be obtained by open biopsy for histologic study. Autopsy studies have indicated that during life marrow specimens lacking Reed-Sternberg cells but showing sheets of reticulum cells, plasma cells, eosinophils, and fibrous tissue can be considered positive in known cases of Hodgkin's disease. The absence of Reed-Sternberg cells in marrow biopsies and their presence at autopsy is thought to reflect difference in sample size.[64] Somewhat lower values for hematocrit, white blood cell count, platelet count, and alkaline phosphatase have been found among patients with positive marrow biopsies, when compared with patients with negative marrow biopsies. Differences, however, were not at a level of statistical significance,[64] and no change in a specific parameter has consistently been associated with marrow involvement.

Biochemical studies. Needle and open biopsies of the liver have correlated poorly with biochemical profiles of liver function. In our children, abnormal tests presaged eventual hepatic involvement by Hodgkin's disease. In a battery that included BSP retention, total bilirubin, alkaline phosphatase, SGOT, SGPT, and prothrombin time tests, hepatic involvement did not correlate well with any single test. However, the combination of increased BSP retention and alkaline phosphatase elevation usually proved to be of prognostic significance.[25] Among patients with elevated alkaline phosphatase levels, BSP retention is more frequently abnormal than are 5'-nucleotidase levels.[1b] In adults with Hodgkin's disease elevated serum alkaline phosphatase levels are related primarily to elevated hepatic phosphatase levels.[1b] In children the additive effect of the bone isoenzyme, which may show physiologic elevation, must always be considered. Osseous Hodgkin's disease at the time of diagnosis is rare and would be a most uncommon cause of alkaline phosphatase elevation.

Elevated serum copper levels have been demonstrated in active Hodgkin's disease, and this parameter has been found useful in monitoring disease activity and in detecting recurrence before it is demonstrable by other means.[27, 48] This test, although nonspecific, has shown a high degree of reliability in our patients, and serial determinations showed excellent correlation between the serum copper level and disease activity in 26 of the 27 children studied. It is anticipated that this test will be useful in the early detection of intra-abdominal nodal disease and diffuse Stage IV disease.

Immunologic survey. Patients with active Hodgkin's disease have impaired cellular immunity measurable in terms of loss of delayed skin hypersensitivity to a group of allergens, including tuberculin (PPD), diphtheria toxoid, streptokinase-streptodornase, mumps, and *Trichophyton* and *Candida* species. Anergy also prevents sensitization to dinitrochlorobenzene (DNCB)[1] and keyhole limpet hemocyanin (KLH).[26a] After lymphocyte stimulation with phytohemagglutinin (PHA) and other mitogenic agents, blastogenesis and mitogenesis are reduced in patients with active Hodgkin's disease. Homograft rejection, which involves delayed hypersensitivity, is also prolonged during periods of disease activity. Recovery of skin reactivity follows subsidence of Hodgkin's activity.

Antibody formation in Hodgkin's disease is also abnormal under certain circumstances. Depressed responses to pneumococcal polysaccharide, *Brucella* antigen, and tetanus toxoid (primary exposure) have been described. Normal antibody responses have been reported with typhoid-paratyphoid, mumps, tularemia, blood group substances, and secondary tetanus toxoid immunizations. The primary antibody response to KLH is both delayed and reduced.[26a] As deter-

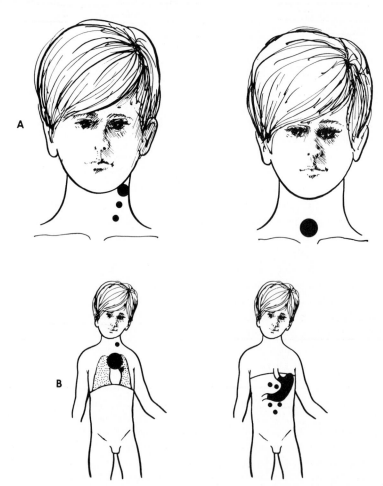

Fig. 13-11. A, *Stage I.* The disease is limited to one lymphatic region or one extranodal site exclusive of the liver, bone marrow, or diffuse involvement of the skin, lung, etc. Stages I through IV were further subdivided according to constitutional symptoms, for example, Stage IA, no constitutional symptoms, and Stage IB, constitutional symptoms such as fever, night sweats, or pruritus. Left, one lymph node region in left side of neck. Right, one extranodal site as thyroid (rare). **B,** *Stage II.* The disease is limited to one side of the diaphragm (i.e., two or more lymphatic regions). Associated involvement of extranodal sites such as the gastrointestinal tract was considered part of Stage II disease. Direct invasion of adjacent structures such as lung, potentially curable with radiotherapy (as opposed to diffuse involvement), was considered as Stage II, not Stage IV. Left, two or more lymph node regions on one side of the diaphragm, for example, supraclavicular and mediastinal lymph nodes with or without direct invasion of the lung. Right, one extranodal site and lymph nodes on one side of the diaphragm (stomach and para-aortic lymph nodes). **C,** *Stage III.* The disease progressed beyond Stage II to involve the lymphatic systems on both sides of the diaphragm. Left, lymph nodes on both sides of the diaphragm (mediastinal, para-aortic, and supraclavicular nodes). Right, one extranodal site and lymph nodes on both sides of the diaphragm (cecum and para-aortic and supraclavicular nodes). **D,** *Stage IV.* The disease has disseminated beyond Stage III to diffusely involve the lung, liver, bone marrow, skin, central nervous system, etc. (Courtesy Medical Communications, The University of Texas at Houston, M. D. Anderson Hospital and Tumor Institute.)

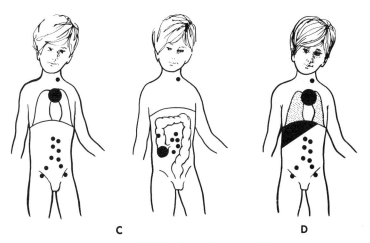

Fig. 13-11, cont'd. For legend see opposite page.

mined by the blastogenic response of the patient's lymphocytes to KLH antigen, the appearance of antigen-reactive lymphocytes is very slow, although continuous for at least 49 days, in patients with untreated Hodgkin's disease.

The demonstration of defective primary antibody formation makes untenable the previously held concept that thymic deficiency might be an etiologic factor in Hodgkin's disease. The subsidence of demonstrable immunologic deficiencies during periods of disease inactivity suggests that immunologic impairment is not the basic cause of Hodgkin's disease but rather a manifestation of advanced or active disease.

Staging. Proper staging, or precise determination of the extent of disease, is of utmost importance in Hodgkin's disease; it has been the cornerstone of therapy since the late 1940's. In general, patients who present with localized manifestations receive intensive radiotherapy. More advanced disease is managed with chemotherapy or radiotherapy or both. Our method of staging Hodgkin's disease and the other lymphomas, which conforms to that of the Ann Arbor Conference on Hodgkin's Disease held in 1971, is a four-stage system that provides for both nodal and extranodal presentations in localized and generalized disease. The system is described in detail in Fig. 13-11. Illustrations of both nodal and extranodal presentations are provided for each stage.

Staging celiotomy. Celiotomy with splenectomy was used initially as an investigative procedure to (1) clarify equivocal lymphangiogram findings, (2) seek occult disease of the spleen, liver, and bone marrow, and (3) detect occult disease of the nodes beyond the scope of the lymphangiogram (celiac axis, mesenteric or retrogastric).[2, 25, 43] On the basis of pilot study findings, celiotomy with splenectomy has become a routine staging procedure at many institutions.[34] Node biopsies are obtained from each iliac chain, two para-aortic sites, the mesentery of the superior mesenteric artery, and the celiac, splenic, and portal areas. Duplicate needle biopsies are obtained from the right and left lobes of the liver; a wedge biopsy is also taken from the right lobe of the liver. A wedge bone marrow biopsy is obtained from the right iliac crest. Accessory spleens are of course removed when splenectomy is performed. Laparotomy also provides an opportunity to reposition the ovaries in the midline or laterally to the iliac crests so that they are excluded from the radiotherapy field.[18] In addition, the removal of the spleen has been reported to alleviate cytopenias in patients tending to have low white blood cell or platelet counts and improve the tolerance of these patients for chemotherapy and radiation therapy.[42]

In an effort to assess the extent of disease at time of diagnosis so that appropriate definitive therapy could be administered, 11 children at the MDAH underwent staging laparotomy and splenectomy as a pilot study after clinical staging, including lymphangiography, had been completed.[23] Eight children presented with clinically localized disease, Stages I and II; 3 of the group were found to have unsuspected splenic involvement at laparotomy. One of these 3 patients also had positive nodes in the celiac axis and splenic hilus. Three children with extensive nodal disease, Stage III, underwent staging laparotomy to rule out extensions to nonnodal sites. One of this group, known to have involvement of the spleen and para-aortic nodes, was found to have Hodgkin's disease of the liver despite normal liver function tests. Among the children undergoing staging laparotomy at the time of initial diagnosis, the procedure significantly changed the staging in 4 of the 11, or more than one third of the patients. In very young children, splenectomy appears to carry an increased risk of fulminating infection, often due to *Diplococcus pneumoniae*. None of the children in our group, however, has experienced a serious postsplenectomy bacterial infection. In our entire group of 18 splenectomized patients with Hodgkin's disease, which includes 7 patients having splenectomy during follow-up care, subsequent laparotomy has been required in three instances for lysis of adhesions and relief of small bowel obstruction.

Clinical behavior. Subsequent spread of Hodgkin's disease initially classed as Stage I or II is dependent on both the clinical presentation and the specific histology.[22] In some centers, regions immediately adjacent to the primary site continue to be considered at greater risk for direct extension. A study of patterns of spread, as related to clinical presentation and specific histology, demonstrates that the lymphatic pathways frequently bypass immediately adjacent regions, as exemplified by the high incidence of occult abdominal involvement in relation to lower neck presentations (Table 13-1).

Nodular sclerosing Hodgkin's disease differs from the other three types in clinical presentation and patterns of spread. The association of supraclavicular and mediastinal involvement in nodular sclerosing Hodgkin's disease suggests that occult involvement in the mediastinum may be prevalent in presentations clinically limited to the lower neck. By contrast, mixed cellularity, lymphocytic predominance, and lymphocytic depletion varieties seldom involve the mediastinum, either primarily or secondarily. When mixed cellularity presents in the mediastinum, generalization eventually occurs. The relation of age, sex, and specific histology is presented in Fig. 13-2.

Differential diagnosis. Many of the children in our series were at first presumed to have adenitis related to infection and were given one or more courses of antibiotics prior to the establishment of the diagnosis of Hodgkin's disease by biopsy. Infectious mononucleosis, tuberculosis, cat-scratch disease, tularemia, and adenitis related to smallpox vaccination may be confused clinically with

Table 13-1. Hodgkin's disease neck presentations (Stages I and II): patterns of subsequent new disease

| | No significant spread | First major site of extension | | |
		Mediastinum	Abdomen (including liver §)	Diffuse dissemination
Clinical staging*				
A 3 (3 alive)	3 (2, 7, 18 yr)	1	3 (§ 1)	
B 6 (3 alive)	2 (8, 14 yr)			
C 3 (2 alive)	2 (7, 10 yr)			1
Lymphangiogram staging				
A 0				
B 3 (3 alive)	1 (3 yr)		2 (§ 1)	
C 1 (1 alive)	1 (2 yr)			
16 (12 alive)	9	1	5 (§ 2)	1

Key: A = upper unilateral; B = lower unilateral; C = both sides of neck.
*Five patients staged during the prelymphangiogram era are deceased. Four died within 3 years. One who survived 8 years was maintained on chemotherapy for 6 years after a diagnosis of hepatic involvement (patient 12 [CS], Appendix I).

one of the lymphomatous diseases; biopsy or repeated biopsies may be required for diagnosis.

SURGICAL THERAPY

The usefulness of surgery in treating Hodgkin's disease in children is confined primarily to the biopsy procedure. Adequate surgical treatment would require en bloc resection of the involved nodal region. The resultant disfigurement and interference with lymphatic drainage would exceed that which follows properly administered radiotherapy. In most instances laminectomy for removal of compressive extradural masses is no longer indicated, since better results can be anticipated from combined therapy with prednisone and radiation.

RADIATION THERAPY FOR STAGES I AND II

Current concepts of treatment for Stage I and II Hodgkin's disease are based on the results of previous treatment programs for both adults and children analyzed in terms of (1) local response in irradiated areas and (2) subsequent new manifestations related to major sites of primary involvement as shown in Tables 13-1 to 13-4.[22] Since 1947, treatment policy for Stage I and II Hodgkin's disease involving the upper torso has dictated relatively high-dose irradiation to the involved regions. In earlier years, treatment of Hodgkin's disease presenting in the lower torso was dependent on the site of origin. Pelvic adenopathy was treated radically after 1947. Intensive irradiation for abdominal presentations was not attempted until 1956. The decision to irradiate the entire abdomen and pelvis for abdominal presentations rather than restrict treatment to an inverted Y-shaped field was influenced by the desire to treat the liver and spleen prophylactically. Although no consistent policy for administering prophylactic

Table 13-2. Hodgkin's disease mediastinal presentations (Stages I and II): patterns of subsequent new disease

| | | First major site of extension | | |
	No significant spread	Lung (direct extension)	Abdomen (including liver§)	Diffuse dissemination
Clinical staging*				
7 (3 alive)	2 (16 and 17 yr)		5 (§ 3)	
Lymphangiogram staging				
12 (11 alive)	9 (2, 7, 8, 8 yr)†	1	2	
19 (14 alive)	11	1	7 (§ 3)	

*Four patients staged prior to lymphangiography are deceased: 1 at 9 years and 3 at 2 years. The fifth patient, who had extension to the liver, is surviving in remission at 7 years (patient 9 [RM], Appendix I).
†Included two cases with subsequent spread limited to one axilla considered of no significance in relation to survival.

Table 13-3. Hodgkin's disease axillary presentations (Stages I and II): patterns of subsequent new disease

	No significant spread	Opposite neck or axilla	Mediastinum	Abdomen	Diffuse dissemination
Clinical staging					
5 (4 alive)	2 (10, 12 yr)				3*
Lymphangiogram staging					
1 (0 alive)				1	
6 (4 alive)	2			1	3

*Of three patients with diffuse dissemination, 2 are surviving at 2 and 6 years in remission on chemotherapy. The third died at 1 year.

Table 13-4. Hodgkin's disease lower torso presentations (Stages I and II): patterns of subsequent new disease

| | | First major site of extension | |
	No significant spread	Upper torso	Abdomen including liver
Clinical staging*			
3 (2 alive)	2 (4, 17 yr)	0	1
Lymphangiogram staging			
3 (3 alive)	3 (4, 4, 5 yr)		
6 (5 alive)	5		1

*Two patients presented with unilateral inguinal adenopathy; one had an associated iliac mass. One patient developed spread to the upper abdomen and liver 7 years after initial treatment (patient 44 [GK], Appendix I).

irradiation was established, the mediastinum was irradiated prophylactically in more than 50% of adults and children with disease clinically limited to the neck. For axillary presentations the associated supraclavicular fossa was included prophylactically in the irradiated area. In the past, prophylactic treatment of the para-aortic area was rarely administered in conjunction with definitive treatment to the mediastinum or the ilioinguinal region.

Tumor dose. Permanent local control has been reported for 80% of cases treated with a tumor dose of 3000 rads.[35] Although not suitable for routine use, tumor doses of 3000 rads delivered in approximately 3 weeks can be administered with confidence to selected patients, that is, patients whose diagnosis was established by excisional biopsy of a single peripheral lymph node and patients with minimal adenopathy that responds rapidly to radiation.

Three thousand rads delivered in 3 to 4 weeks is a critical tumor dose for Hodgkin's disease. The incidence of local recurrence rises with each significant decrease in the tumor dose below 3000 rads.[35] Notable exceptions are exemplified by 2 of our 5 children, treated for mediastinal adenopathy with tumor doses of 2000 to 2500 rads, who are surviving free of disease at 15 and 16 years of age (patients 17 [JK] and 18 [MB], Appendix I). One other child treated with a tumor dose of 2500 rads developed a local recurrence in the mediastinum in 1 year (patient 33 [HC], Appendix I). Local response to low-dose irradiation was not evaluable in 2 patients who died in 1 to 2 years after repeated courses of nitrogen mustard for generalized Hodgkin's disease (patients 32 [BM] and 34 [KC], Appendix I). Although seldom stressed, tumor doses of 2000 to 2500 rads administered for palliation of local symptoms may result in long-term local control, especially when chemotherapy is continued.

The majority of patients with Stage I or II disease present with moderate to massive adenopathy. More extensive disease has a tendency to recur locally if treatment is limited to a minimum tumor dose of 3000 rads.[35] The optimum tumor dose for Hodgkin's disease is partially dependent on the extent of adenopathy and the tolerance of the normal structures. The critical weekly dosage rate is in the range of 750 to 1000 rads. Weekly dosage rates of 500 to 600 rads are apt to result in local failure, regardless of the ultimate tumor dose. Dosage rate depends on tolerance of the normal structures included in the treated area. For the upper abdomen or pelvis, local and systemic tolerance permits a weekly tumor dosage rate of 750 rads. Although some latitude in the dosage rate is permissible for the peripheral node-bearing areas and the mediastinum, response during treatment can best be evaluated when policy is consistent. At the MDAH, experience dictates a preference for a tumor dosage of 1000 rads/wk with few exceptions.

As the total tumor dose cannot be compromised, treatment fields must be designed to exclude all possible normal tissue to minimize the incidence of deformity. Failure to grow to a socially acceptable adult height is seldom a problem after treatment to a short segment of the vertebral column. Insufficient time has elapsed to determine whether short stature will eventually be a problem for very young Stage I and II patients treated prophylactically to the entire spinal axis and pelvis with tumor doses of 4500 rads in 4 weeks as performed in some institutions.

Prophylactic radiation. Studies of subsequent manifestations of Hodgkin's disease indicate that benefit from prophylactic irradiation of anatomically adjacent areas is dependent on the clinical presentation or on the combination of the clinical presentation and specific histology.[22] Since simultaneous presentations in mediastinum and neck are almost always the nodular sclerosing type, it follows that prophylactic irradiation of the mediastinum could be of value in patients with nodular sclerosing supraclavicular presentations. Direct extension from neck to mediastinum would appear unlikely for other varieties of Hodgkin's disease. If prophylaxis is desired in nodular sclerosing disease, the tumor dose should not exceed 3000 rads (Table 13-5). The demonstration of "skip" patterns in the progression of Hodgkin's disease initially staged as I or II after lymphangiography resulted in a new concept of prophylactic irradiation popularly known as "total nodal".[33] As anticipated, "total nodal" irradiation for Stages I and II resulted in an increase in the number of patients surviving 2 and 3 years free of subsequent spread to lymph nodes. Whether the incidence of manifestations that generally occur somewhat later (i.e., involvement of liver or bone marrow) will be correspondingly decreased remains to be determined, as does the incidence of late complications. In view of the findings from surgical staging procedures, the continued use of "total nodal" irradiation for Stages I and II may not be justified. New randomized clinical trials to determine the value of prophylactic irradiation in patients staged with celiotomy and splenectomy appear to be indicated.[46]

Specific sites

The neck. Treatment for Hodgkin's disease originating in the neck is governed by the location of palpable adenopathy. Stage IA presentations in the upper neck seldom metastasize; treatment is limited to the affected side of the neck using cobalt 60 or other appropriate megavoltage equipment. Intense reaction in the skin and mucous membranes contraindicates the use of orthovoltage. To avoid late complications, the spinal cord, larynx, and major salivary glands are excluded from the field of irradiation. Because of numerous lymphatic connections between the right and left sides of the lower neck, both sides of the neck are treated for unilateral lower neck and supraclavicular presentations (Fig. 13-12). In the past the mediastinum was included prophylactically (Fig. 13-13) for all histologic types. Currently our opinion is that prophylaxis is probably of value only in nodular sclerosing Hodgkin's disease.

Table 13-5. Local control in prophylactically treated areas (Stages I and II)

	Depth dose to prophylactically treated areas						
	1000	1500	2000	2500	3000	3500	4000
Neck	1				5 C, 2 R*	2 C	7 C, 1 R
Mediastinum				6 C	4 C		
Axilla					2 C		
Para-aortic nodes					1 C		

Key: C = controlled; R = recurrent.

*One patient who received a prophylactic dose of 3000 rads to one side of the neck and the mediastinum developed subsequent disease in the neck. However, the mediastinum remained free of disease.

Regardless of whether or not the mediastinum is included, treatment is administered at a dosage rate of 1000 rads/wk. This dosage rate is well tolerated, provided midline structures in the neck are shielded and nausea and dysphagia are treated promptly with appropriate antiemetics and analgesics. Preference for a tumor dosage rate of 1000 rads/wk is based on our experience with this dosage range in assessing relative tumor sensitivity. In the majority of patients the main bulk of the tumor responds to 4000 rads delivered in 4 weeks. Usually residual masses disappear with an additional 1000 to 1500 rads (Table 13-6).

The mediastinum. Hodgkin's disease presenting in the mediastinum as an isolated lesion is rare. Generally, a thoracotomy or mediastinoscopy can be avoided if a blind scalene node biopsy is performed in suspected cases. The

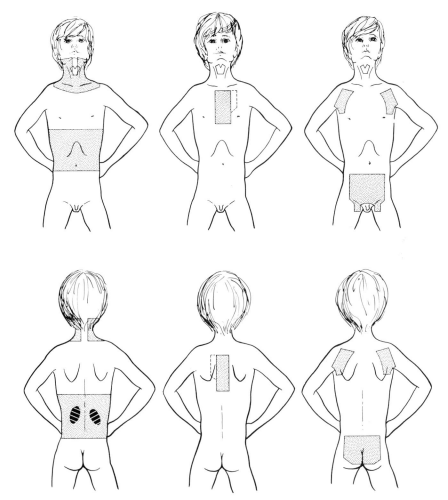

Fig. 13-12. Illustrations of specific fields for localized disease (Stage I). Combinations can be used sequentially to treat generalized disease. Note stylized extension of the mediastinal field to cover involvement in the left hilum. (Courtesy Medical Communications, The University of Texas at Houston, M. D. Anderson Hospital and Tumor Institute.)

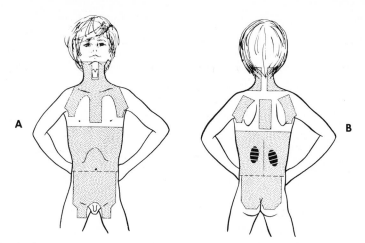

Fig. 13-13. A, *Upper torso.* In general an anterior "mantle" supplemented by posterior mediastinal, axillary, and cervical fields is employed for combinations of definitive and prophylactic treatment. **B,** *Lower torso.* The abdomen and pelvis are frequently treated sequentially. For cobalt 60, two half-value layers of lead are placed over the kidney posteriorly from the beginning of treatment. An alternate approach would be to treat the major regions separately in any desired combination, depending on the local and the systemic tolerance. (Courtesy Medical Communications, The University of Texas at Houston, M. D. Anderson Hospital and Tumor Institute.)

Table 13-6. Local control in Hodgkin's disease involving the neck on admission* (Stages I and II); relation to tumor dose

Dose to neck (rads) Number of patients	Supplemental treatment to residual disease						Controlled	Recurrent	Not evaluable (dead under 2 years of generalized disease)
	None	500	750	1000	1500	2000			
2000 2	2						1		1
2500 2	2								2
3000 8	8						7	1	
3500 2		2					1	1	
4000 16	7	5	1	2		1	14	2 (1†)	
4500 5	3	1			1		5		
5000 0									
35	22	8	1	2	1	1	28	4	3

*In 16 cases of Hodgkin's disease, involvement was limited to the neck. In the remaining patients, the mediastinum or the axilla or both was involved in addition to the neck.
†Neck was difficult to assess initially because of infected and ulcerated biopsy sites.

majority of patients with Hodgkin's disease of the mediastinum have associated adenopathy in the neck; a few have axillary disease in addition to cervical involvement. Rarely, the axilla is the only metastatic site. Changes visualized on the chest film are usually limited to the anterosuperior mediastinum. Associated hilar adenopathy is relatively uncommon. Rarely, the disease may extend into the adjacent bronchus or lung. In such cases hemoptysis may be a presenting symptom (patient 25 [JS], Appendix I).

The radiotherapy fields must include the entire mediastinum and neck. Although Hodgkin's disease tends to spread directly to the axilla, prophylactic treatment of the axilla is avoided in small children because of the effects of radiation on subsequent growth. Whether the involved regions are treated individually (Fig. 13-12) or in continuity with an "extended field" or "mantle" (Fig. 13-13) depends on available equipment and personnel.

The anterior "extended" or "mantle" field extends from a line joining the point of the chin and the tip of the mastoid processes to the crura of the diaphragm (Fig. 13-13). Midline cervical structures are shielded as previously described. The lateral borders of the mediastinal extension are drawn through the hila for minimal adenopathy limited to the upper mediastinum. When the mediastinal involvement is massive, the treatment fields are shaped to exclude as much normal lung as possible. With shrinkage of the mass, the lateral borders are gradually reduced. Axillary extensions of the mantle field are shaped to barely include the rib cage. Humeral heads are excluded insofar as possible. To ensure accuracy, the treatment fields are checked radiographically before treatment is instituted and with each field reduction. A posterior "mantle" or "extended" field is seldom used. Since the supraclavicular nodes are anterior, the dose to the trapezius muscle is limited by using separate mediastinal, neck, and axillary fields. A uniform tumor dose of 4000 to 4500 rads delivered in 4

Table 13-7. Local control in Hodgkin's disease involving the mediastinum on admission (Stages I and II)

Tumor dose (rads)	Supplemental treatment of 500 rads	Controlled	Recurrent	Not evaluable (dead under 1 year of generalized disease)
2000 2		1	1	
2500 3		1		2*
3000 2		2		
3500 3		2	1	
4000 9	1	9		
19	1	15	2	2

*Both patients were placed on a regimen of chemotherapy for diffuse generalized disease during the first year. Both died under 2 years.

weeks to the entire mediastinum may result in serious complications, including pericarditis, myocarditis, and paramediastinal fibrosis.[54, 58] By weighing the treatment in favor of the anterior "extended" or mantle field, a dose gradient is achieved with a maximum of 4500 rads in the anterosuperior mediastinum and a minimum of 3500 rads in the midplane of the lower mediastinum (Table 13-7).

With few exceptions, a tumor dose of 1000 rads a week (calculated at the midplane of the upper mediastinum) is well tolerated, provided a total dose of 4000 rads is not exceeded. Potential damage to the spinal cord precludes additional treatment for residual disease in the midline. Occasionally a residual hilar mass is treated with an additional 500 to 1000 rads. Since complications with the described dosage schedule have been negligible, lower weekly dosage rates are only used when the tumor almost fills the left hemithorax.

The axilla. Because the ipsilateral supraclavicular fossa is commonly involved in association with the axilla, this region is treated prophylactically for Stage I presentations. A satisfactory dose distribution can be achieved in the supraclavicular fossa and the axilla by administering a given dose of 4000 rads to an anterior field covering both regions. The midline tumor dose to the axilla is supplemented with a posterior axillary field. Additional treatment is administered for residual adenopathy through reduced anterior and posterior fields or through an appositional field.

Inguinal area. Inguinal adenopathy may occur as an isolated manifestation or may be associated with para-aortic lymph node involvement. Patients with inguinal adenopathy who have a negative lymphangiogram should undergo exploratory laparotomy. If the results of the exploration are negative, treatment is limited to the involved region.

The abdomen. At the MDAH, total abdominal irradiation is administered for Hodgkin's disease involving the para-aortic lymph nodes, regardless of whether the disease appears minimal or extensive. The extent of the disease, the initial white blood cell and platelet counts, and the age and size of the child determine whether the abdominal irradiation is to be administered to the entire abdomen in a single course or whether the upper abdomen and pelvis are to be treated in sequence with an intervening rest period of 4 to 8 weeks.

When the entire abdomen, including the pelvis, is treated in one course, the anterior and posterior fields are drawn from the dome of the diaphragm to the midsymphyis. Anteriorly, femoral extensions are added to cover the underlying nodes. Laterally, the beam is allowed to fall off over the flank. Posteriorly, two half-value layers of lead are placed over the kidneys to reduce the dose to these organs from the beginning of treatment to 2000 rads in 4 weeks.[20] When the abdomen and pelvis are treated in sequence, the dividing line is usually placed at the iliac crest.

The local and systemic tolerance for abdominal irradiation is approximately 150 rads tumor dose a day (i.e., 750 rads tumor dose a week). Tolerance for treatment is better if both the anterior and posterior fields are treated each day. The total tumor dose that can be tolerated is on the order of 3000 rads. However, additional treatment (i.e., 1000 to 1500 rads tumor dose) can frequently be administered through reduced fields for residual disease, provided the liver and kidneys are excluded. Tumor doses above 3000 rads in 4 weeks have been reported to induce radiation hepatitis.[28] Because the systemic tolerance is limited, the white blood cell and platelet counts should be obtained twice a week. Treatment seldom has to be interrupted unless the white blood cell count falls below 2000 mm[3] and the platelet count below 60,000 mm[3]. Abdominal irradiation is always associated with radiation sickness. To minimize nausea and prevent vomiting, antiemetics should be given on a regular schedule, including Saturdays and Sundays, when radiation therapy is not being given. Chlorpromazine (Thorazine), 25 mg by mouth three times daily may be effective in older children. If not, the morning and afternoon doses should be supplemented with 12.5 mg of promethazine (Phenergan) by mouth. Should the combination be unsuccessful, 25 mg of chlorpromazine should be given by injection 30 minutes before radiotherapy and 4 hours later. Younger children are of course given proportionally smaller doses.

Both the child and the parent should be questioned repeatedly regarding diarrhea, since this symptom must be controlled to maintain body weight and to prevent dehydration. After each loose stool, older children should be given 1 tablespoon of Donnagel-PG by mouth. Younger children are given proportionately smaller doses. Even minimal dehydration should be corrected promptly with intravenous fluids.

CHEMOTHERAPY

At present, supravoltage use is probably near optimal in treating Hodgkin's disease, and future improvements in survival and cure rates for all stages of the disease will be dependent on chemotherapeutic innovations. Until recently, chemotherapy was reserved for Stage III patients unsuitable for radiotherapy and Stage IV patients. When conventional chemotherapy was no longer effective, newer agents were investigated. Limited experience in the chemotherapy of Hodgkin's disease in children makes the comparison of treatment data from the two population groups most difficult. Furthermore, the variability among regimens employed in childhood precludes pooling of data from various series. A systematic method of data acquisition in the MDAH group of children enhances the value of the results obtained, and these data are used frequently in the following discussions of the more important single agents and combination therapy regimens used in treating Hodgkin's disease.

Alkylating agents

Cyclophosphamide and nitrogen mustard. In studies of the Pediatric Division of the Southwest Cancer Chemotherapy Study Group, cyclophosphamide was found to be somewhat more effective than nitrogen mustard (HN_2) in treating children with Hodgkin's disease. Of 12 children who received HN_2 as initial therapy, 75% achieved partial to complete remission, which ranged in duration from 31 to 98 days (median 54 days).[61] Subsequent relapses treated with HN_2 responded less satisfactorily. Of the children treated with cyclophosphamide (5 mg/kg/day, IV × 5, followed by 2.5 mg/kg/day, PO), 5 of 8 responded to treatment from 35 to 666 days (median 190 days). In 22 MDAH patients the response rate was identical to that of the SWCCSG study; however, the median length of complete remission was 26 months and of partial remission 9 months. Hematologic tolerance for the daily cyclophosphamide schedule is excellent, but hemorrhagic cystitis is a limiting factor in long-term therapy. A psychologically disturbing disadvantage of cyclophosphamide is the frequency of alopecia.

Other alkylating agents. Clinical trials with numerous alkylating agents have been conducted in patients with Hodgkin's disease. Triethylenemelamine (TEM), which had the advantage of both oral and intravenous routes of administration, was introduced in 1951.[36] This agent has now been supplanted by more efficacious and less toxic agents and can only be obtained from the manufacturer by special arrangement.

The response rate of 62% for chlorambucil appears similar to that of HN_2, but drug effect is achieved more slowly, and marrow tolerance is better.[7] Additional advantages are the oral route of administration and freedom from nausea and other significant side effects. In 2 of our children (patients 69 [DD] and 75 [JT]) chlorambucil has maintained remissions for remarkable lengths of time when cyclophosphamide was discontinued because of hemorrhagic cystitis.

Thio-TEPA became available in 1954 but showed less activity in Hodgkin's disease than did HN_2.[67]

In trials with uracil mustard, one complete and one partial response occurred among 8 children. Fifty percent of adults have responded for approximately 6 months, and a remission of 3½ years has been recorded.[65] Intermittent courses of this drug are usually recommended.

Vinca alkaloids

Vinblastine (Velban, VLB). This periwinkle product has not been systematically studied in children with Hodgkin's disease, but response rates of 60% to 85% have been reported in adults. In some series, VLB remissions were similar in duration to HN_2 and cyclophosphamide remissions; other investigators report remissions of approximately 300 days.[19, 30, 39, 56] In our experience, VLB was superior to cyclophosphamide in complete response rate (47% of 15 children vs. 32% of 22 children), but remissions were similar in duration with the two agents. Increasing hematologic intolerance characterizes long-term therapy, necessitating dosage reductions and lengthened treatment intervals. The dosage schedule for a patient who has been receiving VLB for several years may be as low as 0.08 mg/kg administered at intervals of 4 weeks (patient 9 [RM], Appendix II).

Vincristine sulfate (Oncovin). The vincristine (VCR) response rate in Hodgkin's disease has been reported as 39%, with remissions lasting 30 days or longer.[6] Although MDAH children showed somewhat longer remissions, the overall performance for VCR, one complete response in 7 patients, was inferior to VLB. Disturbed gastrointestinal motility is a complication of VCR therapy, which may result in severe constipation with symptoms suggesting a surgical abdomen. Constipation must be treated promptly with laxatives or enemas or both. Milk and molasses, used in equal parts as an enema, seems particularly effective in helping to reestablish normal bowel motility. Alopecia should be expected in the majority of patients.

Miscellaneous agents

In a limited study the use of procarbazine hydrochloride (Natulan) in 7 children with Hodgkin's disease resulted in objective improvement in 79%, with a median duration of response of 90 days[5] as compared with 180 days in adults.[8, 14, 63] Nausea and vomiting are troublesome side effects, but they may be minimized by gradual dose increases. Bone marrow suppression may be avoided by careful supervision.

In advanced Hodgkin's disease, BCNU (1,3-bis(2-chloroethyl)-1-nitrosourea) has produced responses in 17 of 31 patients, with a median length of remission of 4 months.[40] Bone marrow depression is the limiting toxicity; venous pain at the time of injection may necessitate slow infusion of the drug.

Bleomycin has been reported to produce remissions lasting up to 4 months in 44% of 30 patients with Hodgkin's disease.[66] Marrow depression does not occur. Pulmonary changes, described as pneumonitis followed by fibrosis, necessitate frequent radiographs of the chest, as well as pulmonary function tests. Use of bleomycin as an additive of "MOPP" therapy is now being studied.

The methyl ester of streptonigrin is also effective in producing regression in Hodgkin's disease.[53] Toxic side effects, including nausea, vomiting, hypotension, and marrow suppression, have prevented enthusiastic use of this agent.

Treatment regimens

Nitrogen mustard adjuvant therapy. An expanded concept of the role of chemotherapy was introduced in 1961 when children with Stage I and II disease registered with the SWCCSG were randomly allocated after completion of radiotherapy to adjuvant chemotherapy with HN_2 (single dose) or no chemotherapy. Six patients received HN_2, and 9 patients received "no adjuvant." All patients have now been followed up for more than 4 years. MDAH contributions to the HN_2 group are indicated in Appendix I—patients 13 (MM), 41 (RS), 8 (JM), 5 (ES), 20 (TJ), and 9 (RM). No advantage for adjuvant therapy has been observed. New disease has developed in 3 of 6 children given HN_2 and in 4 of 9 receiving "no adjuvant." Although this study was inconclusive, the principle has merit that contributed to the eventual development of combined chemotherapy-radiotherapy programs.

Cyclic therapy. Cyclic chemotherapy has been associated with increased long-term survival in the acute leukemias of childhood.[67] The potential of cyclic schedules was studied in SWCCSG children with generalized disease by randomizing to (1) continuous cyclophosphamide therapy to relapse followed by vinblastine therapy and (2) monthly alternating courses of cyclophosphamide and vinblastine. Very few patients were entered in this study. One of the 3 children assigned to cyclic therapy who had diffuse Stage IV disease remains in complete remission after 6 years. A nonstudy child (patient 75 [JT], Appendix III) remained in complete remission for 2½ years, when hemorrhagic cystitis necessitated deletion of cyclophosphamide from the treatment regimen. When data from the two treatment groups was pooled, lengths of remission for cyclophosphamide were 0, 0, 17, 32, and 48 months; vinblastine remissions measured 2, 6, 24, and 60+ months.

Combination chemotherapy. The principles of combination chemotherapy, that is, the use of several agents with differing toxicities for additive or even synergistic antitumor effect without prohibitive toxicity, have been employed in treatment programs for Hodgkin's disease with marked improvement in remission and survival times. In 1965 an 80% complete remission rate was reported for a regimen employing cyclophosphamide, vincristine, methotrexate, and prednisone.[15] Eight-day courses of treatment were repeated every 2 weeks; leukopenia was the major toxicity encountered. Subsequent modifications consisting of the substitution of nitrogen mustard for cyclophosphamide and of procarbazine for methotrexate resulted in the regimen popularly known as "MOPP" (Table 13-8). Remission induction therapy consists of six 10-day courses of treatment given at intervals of 28 days. Eighty-one percent of "MOPP"-treated patients have achieved remission.[16] Currently, all patients have been followed up a minimum of 4 years, and life-table analysis indicates a median survival in excess of 60 months.[11a] No superior regimen has been reported, although similar results have been obtained in Great Britain with a four-drug regimen employing vinblastine rather than vincristine. When "MOPP" remission induction therapy is followed by two "consolidation" treatments given at monthly intervals and nine maintenance treatments given bimonthly, the duration of complete remission is lengthened significantly (180 vs. 85 weeks).[43a] Single agents such as vinblastine are also being employed for maintenance. Recovery from "MOPP"-induced myelosuppression is prompt after each course of therapy if dosage adjustments are made for impaired marrow reserve. Nausea and vomiting are troublesome during drug administration. The neuromuscular side effects of vincristine therapy are less prominent in children than in adults.

Table 13-8. "MOPP" chemotherapy*

Drug	1	2	3	8	10	29
Nitrogen mustard	6 mg/M² IV			6 mg/M² IV		Begin second course
Vincristine (Oncovin)	1.4 mg/M² IV; not to exceed 2 mg			1.4 mg/M² IV		
Procarbazine	50 mg PO	100 mg PO	100 mg/M² PO days 3 through 10			
Prednisone	40 mg/M² day PO days 1 through 10				Dose tapered over 3-day period	

*Nitrogen mustard (6 mg/M²) and vincristine not to exceed 2 mg are injected into the tubing of a running intravenous solution of 5% glucose in distilled water on days 1 and 8 of each course. Procarbazine and prednisone are administered orally. The dose of procarbazine is increased gradually to avoid excessive nausea and vomiting. On the first day, the dose is 50 mg; on the second day, 100 mg; and on days 3 through 10, the dose is 100 mg/M². Prednisone is administered at the rate of 40 mg/M² on days 1 through 10. Twenty-nine days from the first day of treatment, the second course of chemotherapy is initiated, provided the white blood cell count has recovered to 4000/mm³ and the platelet count to 100,000/mm³. The patient should be observed for toxicity of vincristine and prednisone, which is infrequently encountered when chemotherapy is limited to two courses.

COMBINATION RADIOTHERAPY-CHEMOTHERAPY

The concept of radiotherapy-chemotherapy has been accepted for some time by internists and pediatricians. On the basis of results obtained with HN_2 and radiotherapy in treating compressive mediastinal and epidural masses, this enthusiasm was perhaps unjustified. Usually radiotherapy could not be completed because of the nitrogen mustard–induced marrow suppression. This therapeutic approach is no longer recommended, since more satisfactory results are obtained using prednisone and radiotherapy in combination. Surgical intervention to relieve spinal cord compression is no longer considered indicated *in the majority of cases.*

Combined treatment programs attracted the attention of radiotherapists as a means of facilitating definitive treatment to all lymph node–bearing areas and the abdomen and pelvis in Stage III. Our approach to the management of Stage III is based on experience in irradiating transdiaphragmatic progression of Hodgkin's disease in patients treated initially for Stage I or II of the upper torso. Initial attempts to treat Stage III disease in this manner failed because of (1) a gradual drop in the peripheral blood counts below acceptable levels and (2) progression of local or systemic symptoms or both. In a select group of Stage IIIA patients with minimal adenopathy the solution to the problem of maintaining the peripheral blood counts was solved by allowing rest intervals of 4 to 8 weeks between courses of radiotherapy to the upper "mantle," abdomen and pelvis. In patients with more extensive evidence of generalized disease the problem was solved by inducing a partial to complete remission with combination chemotherapy prior to instituting radiotherapy.

In the design of the adult pilot radiotherapy-chemotherapy study, preference was given to pulse chemotherapy to permit rapid recovery from myelosuppression. Initial patients were given single doses of 2 mg of vincristine and 20 mg/kg of cyclophosphamide and rested 2 weeks to permit hematologic recovery before initiation of radiotherapy. This program was well tolerated, and the number of doses of each drug was increased to four. When procarbazine became commercially available, chemotherapy was changed to the more effective "MOPP" regimen. At this time the program was expanded to include children (patients 71 [EK] and 72 [EL], Appendix III).

Two courses of "MOPP" preceded radiotherapy. The treatment goal was to administer definitive radiation for local control of Hodgkin's disease to all major areas (i.e., the mediastinum, abdomen, pelvis, and peripheral regions in series). Sequence and scheduling were dependent on the clinical situation. Areas likely to become symptomatic were treated first. When a choice was possible, the larger volume (i.e., the upper two thirds of the abdomen, including the liver) was treated first to capitalize on maximum bone marrow reserve. Because of the large volume of tissue irradiated, the daily tumor dose was 150 rads, rather than 200 rads as usually given for Hodgkin's disease involving the lymph node–bearing areas of the upper torso. The total minimum tumor dose, including the dose to the liver, was set at 3000 rads in 4 weeks, except for the dose to the kidneys, which was limited to 2000 rads. Residual masses received additional treatment when possible.

A rest period of 4 to 8 weeks for hematologic recovery preceded further radiotherapy to the pelvis or the mediastinum. The hematologic status determined whether the mediastinum, neck, and axillae were treated in series or concurrently with the "mantle" technique. The upper torso was given a minimum tumor dose of 3000 rads in 3 weeks, with additional treatment given for residual disease.

The two pediatric patients indicated previously successfully completed the described treatment and are alive with no evidence of recurrent disease at 23 and 21 months. More recently, an additonal pediatric patient has completed therapy and is alive with no evidence of disease 17 months from diagnosis.

RESULTS

Five- and 10-year survival figures for children admitted to MDAH from 1949 to 1969 with Stage I and II Hodgkin's disease and with Stage III and IV disease have been calculated (Fig. 13-14). Stage I and II patients showed 80% 5-year survival and 67% 10-year survival. Five- and 10-year survivals for Stage III and IV patients were 26% and 11%. These survival figures are comparable with the best results reported for adults with Stage I and II disease.[49a] The overall difference in the survival experience of Stage I and II patients versus Stage III and IV patients was highly significant statistically (P < .01).

In contrast to other series, no statistically significant difference was noted between Stage I and II patients with constitutional symptoms and those without constitutional symptoms.

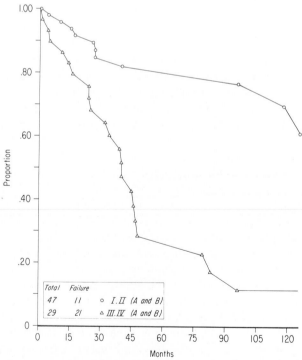

Fig. 13-14. Comparative survival curves for Stages I and II vs. III and IV. (Courtesy Medical Communications, The University of Texas at Houston, M. D. Anderson Hospital and Tumor Institute.)

The incidence of subsequent major new disease for Stage I and II patients was analyzed in relation to clinical presentation and specific histology (Tables 13-1 to 13-4) for patients prior to lymphangiogram versus patients studied by lymphangiography. Abdominal disease occurring as the first manifestation of spread was considered under two categories: (1) without evidence of invasion of the liver and (2) with clinical evidence of involvement of the liver. Spread to the axilla in Stage I and II disease of the upper torso involving the neck or mediastinum was considered of minor importance and was therefore disregarded in this analysis.

The head and neck. Sixteen patients were treated for Hodgkin's disease localized to the neck. Nine have had no subsequent spread. In the remaining 7 children the first site of extension was mediastinum, 1; abdomen, 5 (2 with spread to the liver); and diffuse dissemination, 1.

The mediastinum. Nineteen patients received radiotherapy for mediastinal presentations; 11 had no significant spread of disease. In the remaining 8 patients the major site of extension was lung, 1, and abdomen, 7 (liver 3). Diffuse dissemination did not occur as a first manifestation in this group.

The axilla. Six patients presented with disease in the axilla (Stage I and II). No significant spread was observed in 2 children. In the remaining 4 patients the first major site of extension was abdomen, 1, and diffuse dissemination, 3.

Lower torso. Lower torso presentations occurred in 6 children. Five had no significant spread. In 1 child presenting with an iliac mass the abdomen was the first major site of extension. Para-aortic nodes were involved secondarily in the remaining child, with extension to the liver (patient 44 [GK], Appendix I).

• • •

The effectiveness of various chemotherapy programs, irrespective of radiotherapy, was evaluated by comparing children with Stage III and IV disease at diagnosis who received the following treatments: (1) no chemotherapy, (2) nitrogen mustard only, (3) cyclophosphamide but no vinblastine or combination chemotherapy, (4) cyclophosphamide and vinblastine but no combination chemotherapy, and (5) combination chemotherapy ("MOPP").

No chemotherapy. Three children with Stage III and IV disease at diagnosis did not receive chemotherapy. Survival in these children was as follows: 11 months, "1 to 2 years," and 57+ months. Patient 65 (MM), living with no evidence of disease at 57+ months, is of particular interest, since he is the only Stage III patient successfully completing radiotherapy to all node-bearing areas.

Nitrogen mustard only. Patients 48 (TB) and 50 (JW) received no chemotherapy other than HN_2; survival times were 34 and 46 months. In the case of patient 50 (JW), further therapy was refused.

Cyclophosphamide (no vinblastine or combination chemotherapy). Nine children received cyclophosphamide in addition to other therapy that did not include vinblastine or combination chemotherapy. Survival ranged from 1+ to 81 months (median, 26 months). Patient 63 (PM), expiring at 1 month of *Pseudomonas* septicemia, showed no evidence of viable tumor at postmortem examination. Patient 63 (MC), who has a pericardial window, is living and well at 78 months.

Cyclophosphamide and vinblastine (no combination chemotherapy). Three patients had the opportunity of receiving both cyclophosphamide and vinblastine in addition to other treatments that did not include combination chemotherapy. All 3 children are dead; survival times were 40, 45, and 84 months. The small number of patients in this group makes comparison with the previous group difficult, but the data suggest that the addition of vinblastine contributes significantly to increased survival.

Combination chemotherapy ("MOPP"). Eight children received "MOPP" combination chemotherapy often after treatment with other agents. Survival times range from 21+ to 48 months (median, 35+ months). Five children are living, and 3 (patients 70 [JM], 71 [EK], and 72 [EL]) have not reached the median. Longer follow-up studies are expected to confirm the clinical impression that combination chemotherapy ("MOPP") markedly increases survival in Stage III and IV patients. In addition, morbidity is greatly reduced, and definitive radiotherapy can be administered more easily.

CONCLUSIONS

Successful management of Hodgkin's disease in children requires precise staging using the described procedures, which include lymphangiogram and celiotomy with splenectomy. On the basis of presentation and specific histology, patients with Stage I and II disease can be given definitive radiotherapy with the expectation of 80%, or better, 5-year survival. The routine use of celiotomy and splenectomy may demonstrate occult Stage III disease in as many as one third of the presumptive Stage I and II patients, permitting more appropriate therapy with a potential for significant increase in survival.

The feasibility of combination chemotherapy-radiotherapy regimens for Stage III disease has been demonstrated, and the accumulating data suggest that survival in this group of children will be significantly increased. Search for effective chemotherapeutic agents and combinations must continue.

Stage IV disease can be effectively palliated with drug combinations and radiotherapy. New and innovative approaches to treatment are needed for these children.

Appendixes follow.

Appendix I. Therapy of Hodgkin's disease (Stages I and II at diagnosis)

Patient identity	Age	Race	Sex	Histology	Stage	Class	Lymphogram	Primary radiotherapy (Rads tumor dose/weeks)* and adjuvant chemotherapy	Prophylactic radiotherapy	First manifestation of new disease (XRT, radiotherapy; CRT, chemotherapy)	Current status; survival in years
Major site—unilateral upper neck — No evidence of disease after radiotherapy for presenting involvement (alive)											
1 (WH)	6	W	M	MC	I	A	Not done	Right neck 3000/4 C	None	None	No evidence of disease (18 yr)
2 (ZK)	12	W	F	MC	I	A	Not done	Right neck 4000/4 + boost 500 C	None C	None	No evidence of disease (7 yr)
3 (VE)	9	W	F	LP	I	A	Not done	Left neck 4000/4 C	Right neck 4000/4 C	None	No evidence of disease (2 yr)
Major site—unilateral lower neck — No evidence of disease after radiotherapy for presenting involvement (alive)											
4 (JF)	12	W	F	NS	I	A	Not done	Right neck 3000/4½ C	Left neck 3000/4½ C; Mediastinum 2500/4 C	None	No evidence of disease (14 yr)
5 (ES)	5	W	M	MC	I	A	Not done	Right neck 4000/5½ + boost 500 HN$_2$ 0.4 mg/kg C	Left neck 3000/3 C; Mediastinum 2500/3 C	None	No evidence of disease (8 yr)
6 (RL)	10	W	M	MC	I	A	Negative	Right neck 4500/4½ C	Left neck 3000/3 C	None	No evidence of disease (3 yr)
Adjacent spread to upper torso (dead)											
7 (MV)	4	L	M	MC	I	A	Not done	Left neck 3000/3½ C	None	XRT (1 yr) right neck 3500/6; mediastinum CRT (2 yr) liver and para-aortic nodes	Dead (3 yr)

Key: C = controlled; R = recurrence; SD = new disease in prophylactically treated area; W = white; L = Latin; M = male; F = female; A = no symptoms; B = symptoms; LP = lymphocytic predominance; MC = mixed cellularity; LD = lymphocytic depletion; NS = nodular sclerosing.
*Patients 1, 6, 11, 16, 17, 18, 33, 34, and 35 were treated with kilovoltage. The remainder were treated with cobalt 60 irradiation.
†Bilateral neck dissection for tuberculosis.

Continued.

Appendix I. Therapy of Hodgkin's disease (Stages I and II at diagnosis)—cont'd

Patient identity	Age	Race	Sex	Histology	Stage	Class	Lymphogram	Primary radiotherapy (Rads tumor dose/weeks)* and adjuvant chemotherapy	Prophylactic radiotherapy	First manifestation of new disease (XRT, radiotherapy; CRT, chemotherapy)	Current status; survival in years
Transdiaphragmatic spread (alive)											
8 (JM)	12	L	M	MC	I	A	Not done	Right neck 4500/6 + boost 1500 HN₂ 0.4 mg/kg — C	Mediastinum 2500/2½ C	XRT (8 yr) para-aortic lymph nodes	No evidence of disease (9 yr)
9 (RM)	10	W	M	MC	I	A	Negative	Left neck 4000/4 HN₂ 0.4 mg/kg — R	Left neck 1000/1 SD; Mediastinum 2500/3 C	CRT (2 yr) liver and para-aortic nodes	In remission (9 yr)
10 (BN)	10	W	M	MC	I	A	Negative	Right neck 4000/4 + boost 1000 — R	Left neck 4000/4 SD; Mediastinum 3000/3 C	XRT (< 1 yr) both axillae; CRT (4 yr) abdominal lymph nodes and spleen	In remission (5 yr)
Transdiaphragmatic spread (dead)											
11 (JC)	10	W	M	LD	I	B	Not done	Right neck 2000/4 — C	None	< 1 yr	Dead (< 1 yr)
12 (CS)	13	W	F	MC	I	A	Not done	Right neck 4000/4 + boost 500	Left neck 3000/3 SD; Mediastinum 3000/3 C	XRT (3 yr) liver and para-aortic lymph nodes	Dead (8 yr)
Major site—both sides of neck											
No evidence of disease after radiotherapy for presenting involvement (alive)											
13 (MM)	7	W	M	NS	II	A	Not done	Necks 4000/4 + boost 2000 HN₂ 0.4 mg/kg — C	Mediastinum 2500/3 C	None	No evidence of disease (10 yr)
14 (KC)	12	W	M	LP	II	A	Not done	Necks 4000/4 + boost 500 — C	Mediastinum 2500/3 C	None	No evidence of disease (7 yr)
15 (LB)	14	W	M	NS	II	A	Negative	Necks 4000/4 — C	None	None	No evidence of disease (2 yr)

Transdiaphragmatic spread, etc. (dead)

								Major site—mediastinum	R	None		XRT and CRT (2 yr) diffuse Stage IV disease	Dead (2 yr)
16 (HH)	7	W	M	NS	II	B	Not done	Necks 3000/3½		None		None	

No evidence of disease after radiotherapy for presenting involvement (alive)

17 (JK)	11	W	M	NS	II	B	Not done	Mediastinum 2500/7 including lungs; necks 3000/5	C C	None		None	No evidence of disease (17 yr)
18 (MB)	9	W	F	NS	II	B	Not done	Mediastinum 2000/3½; left neck 2000/3; left axilla 1500/1	C C C	None		None	No evidence of disease (16 yr)
19 (GD)	14	W	M	NS	II	A	Negative	Mediastinum 4000/4; necks 4500/5½ + boost 500	C C	None		None	No evidence of disease (8 yr)
20 (TJ)	9	W	M	NS	II	A	Negative	Mediastinum 3000/3; necks 4500/5; axillae 3000/3; HN_2 0.4 mg/kg	C C	Lungs 1500/3	C	None	No evidence of disease (4 yr)
21 (DW)	14	W	F	NS	II	B	Negative	Mediastinum 4000/4; necks 4000/5 + boost 1000	C	None		None	No evidence of disease (3 yr)
22 (SH)	11	W	M	NS	I	B	Negative	Mediastinum 3500/3½	C	Necks 3500/3½	C	None	No evidence of disease (3 yr)
23 (LC)	12	W	F	NS	II	A	Negative	Mediastinum 4000/4 + boost 500; necks 4000/4 + boost 500	C C	Axilla 3500/3½; para-aortic lymph nodes 3500/3½	C C	None	No evidence of disease (3 yr)
24 (DG)	8	L	F	NS	I	A	Negative	Mediastinum 4000/4	C	Necks 4000/4	C	None	No evidence of disease (3 yr)
25 (JS)	14	W	M	NS	II	A	Negative	Mediastinum 4000/5 + boost 1000; necks 4000/5 + boost 1000	C C	Left neck 4000/C; Right axilla 4000/C	C	None	No evidence of disease (2 yr)

Continued.

Appendix I. Therapy of Hodgkin's disease (Stages I and II at diagnosis)—cont'd

Patient identity	Age	Race	Sex	Histology	Stage	Class	Lymphogram	Primary radiotherapy (Rads tumor dose/weeks)* and adjuvant chemotherapy		Prophylactic radiotherapy		First manifestation of new disease (XRT, radiotherapy; CRT, chemotherapy)	Current status; survival in years
Adjacent spread in upper torso (alive)													
26 (NE)	12	W	F	NS	II	A	Negative	Mediastinum 3000/4; necks 3000/4	C; C	None		XRT (2 yr) axilla	No evidence of disease (8 yr)
27 (MS)	14	W	F	NS	II	A	Negative	Mediastinum 4000/4; left neck 4000/4	C; C	Right neck 4000/4	C	XRT (3 yr) axillae	No evidence of disease (7 yr)
28 (KK)	10	W	F	NS	II	A	Negative	Mediastinum 3500/4; necks 3000/3; left axilla 3500/4	R; C; C	None		XRT (<1 yr) parahilar lung CRT	In remission (2 yr)
Transdiaphragmatic spread (alive)													
29 (RE)	9	L	M	MC	II	A	Not done	Mediastinum 4000/4; left neck 4000/4	C; C	Right neck 4000/4	C	XRT and CRT (3 yr) liver and para-aortic lymph nodes	In remission (7 yr)
30 (MD)	14	W	M	MC	II	A	Negative	Mediastinum 3500/4; left axilla 5000/6	C; C	Necks 3000/3 right axilla 3000/3	C	XRT and CRT para-aortic lymph nodes; diffuse Stage IV disease	In remission (4 yr)
Transdiaphragmatic spread (dead)													
31 (TM)	5	W	F	NS	II	B	Negative	Mediastinum 4000/5; left neck 3500/4 + boost 500	C; C	Right neck 3500/4	C	XRT (<1 yr) para-aortic lymph nodes; CRT diffuse Stage IV	Dead (3 yr)
32 (BM)	9	W	M	MC	II	A	Not done	Mediastinum, necks, axillae approx. 2000; HN_2 0.4 mg/kg		None		CRT (<2 yr) liver and lymph nodes	Dead (2 yr)
33 (HC)	6	C	M	Not available for review	II	A	Not done	Mediastinum necks‡; approx. 2000; unacceptable drop in blood counts		None		CRT (1 yr) para-aortic lymph nodes, etc.	Dead (2 yr)

Transdiaphragmatic spread (dead)—cont'd

No.		Age		Sex	Histology	Stage		Laparotomy	Treatment		Response	Subsequent course	Outcome
34	(KC)	9	W	M	MC	II	A	Not done	Mediastinum 3000/5; necks 3000/5	C C	None	CRT (1 yr) liver and para-aortic lymph nodes	Dead (2 yr)
35	(WB)	14	W	M	NS	II	B	Not done	Mediastinum 4000/5; necks 4000/5	C C	None	XRT (2 yr) para-aortic lymph nodes; CRT (4 yr) diffuse Stage IV	Dead (9 yr)

No evidence of disease after radiotherapy for presenting involvement (alive)

Major site—axilla

No.		Age		Sex	Histology	Stage		Laparotomy	Treatment		Response	Subsequent course	Outcome
36	(RC)	7	W	M	Not available for review	I	A	Not done	Right axilla 3000/3	C	None	None	No evidence of disease (12 yr)
37	(SW)	12	W	F	LP	II	A	Not done	Right axilla 3000/3; right neck 4000/4 + boost 500 / Mediastinum 3000/3	C C	None	None	No evidence of disease (10 yr)

Transdiaphragmatic spread, etc. (alive)

No.		Age		Sex	Histology	Stage		Laparotomy	Treatment		Response	Relapse		Response	Subsequent course	Outcome
38	(RB)	9	W	M	MC	I	A	Not done	Left axilla 4000/4; HN$_2$ 0.4 mg/kg	C	Left neck 3000/3	SD		CRT and XRT (2 yr) diffuse Stage IV	In remission (6 yr)
39	(RY)	3	W	M	MC	II	A	Not done	Right axilla 3500/4; right neck 4000/4 + boost 750	R	Left neck 4000/4	C		CRT (1 yr) diffuse Stage IV	In remission (2 yr)

Transdiaphragmatic spread (dead)

No.		Age		Sex	Histology	Stage		Laparotomy	Treatment		Response	Relapse		Response	Subsequent course	Outcome
40	(TC)	9	W	M	MC	II	B	Not done	Both necks 3000/5; both axillae 2000/3	C C	None	C		CRT (< 1 yr) diffuse Stage IV	Dead (1 yr)
41	(RS)	5	W	M	LD	II	A	Negative	Both necks 3500/4 + boost 500; both axillae 3000/4; HN$_2$ 0.4 mg/kg	C R C	Mediastinum 3000/4	C		XRT and CRT (< 1 yr) para-aortic lymph nodes	Dead (1 yr)

Continued.

Appendix I. Therapy of Hodgkin's disease (Stages I and II at diagnosis)—cont'd

Patient identity	Age	Race	Sex	Histol-ogy	Stage	Class	Lympho-gram	Primary radiotherapy (Rads tumor dose/weeks)* and adjuvant chemotherapy	Prophylactic radiotherapy	First manifestation of new disease (XRT, radiotherapy; CRT, chemotherapy)	Current status; survival in years
Major site—iliac, inguinal, and femoral areas											
No evidence of disease after radiotherapy for presenting involvement (alive)											
42 (MR)	14	W	M	LP	I	A	Not done	Surgery	C	None	None	No evidence of disease (17 yr)
43 (WT)	14	W	M	LP	I	A	Negative	2500/2	C	None	None	No evidence of disease (4 yr)
Adjacent spread in lower torso (dead)											
44 (GK)	11	W	M	LP	I	B	Not done				XRT (7 yr) liver and para-aortic lymph nodes; CRT (9 yr) diffuse dissemination	Dead (10 yr)
Major site—para-aortic lymph nodes											
No evidence of disease after radiotherapy for presenting involvement (alive)											
45 (MC)	8	W	M	LP	II	A	Positive	Total abdomen 3000/4	C	None	None	No evidence of disease (5 yr)
46 (DR)	11	W	M	LP	II	A	Positive	Total abdomen 3000/4 + boost 500	C	None	None	No evidence of disease (5 yr)
47 (RB)	12	W	M	NS	II	A	Positive	Inverted "Y" 3000/3	C	None	None	No evidence of disease (4 yr)

Appendix II. Therapy for extension of Stage I and II Hodgkin's disease

Patient Age-race-sex Yr of diagnosis	Time to extension of disease	Type of extension	Chemotherapy (CRT) Agent	Chemotherapy (CRT) Results	Radiation (XRT)	Survival
11 (JC) 10 W M 1949	< 1 yr	Liver and para-aortic nodes	–	–	–	Dead (6 mo)
16 (HH) 7 W M 1954	2 yr	Diffuse Stage IV disease	HN₂ CB-1348	0 0	Palliative XRT to right infraclav., para-aortic nodes, left neck, left axilla	Dead (27 mo)
44 (GK) 11 W M 1954	7 yr 9 yr	Neck axilla; liver and para-aortic nodes Diffuse Stage IV disease	VLB CYT	CR 0		Dead (126 mo)
34 (CC) 6 W M 1956	1 yr	Liver and para-aortic nodes	HN₂ DAC + HN₂ CB-1348	PR 0 0	–	Dead (29 mo)
33 (HC) 9 C M 1956	< 1 yr	Para-aortic nodes	HN₂ MM HN₂	PR 0 0	–	Dead (28 mo)
32 (BM) 9 W M 1956	< 2 yr	Liver and para-aortic nodes	CB-1348	PR	Axillae	Dead (18 mo)
40 (TC) 9 W M 1957	< 1 yr	Diffuse Stage IV disease	HN₂ CB-1348 HN₂ + DAC	PR S 0	–	Dead (8 mo)
7 (MV) 4 W M 1959	1 yr 2 yr	Neck and mediastinum Liver and para-aortic nodes	HN₂ CYT VCR HU	0 0 S 0	Para-aortic nodes 3500/6; mediastinum—palliative XRT	Dead (40 mo)
35 (WB) 14 W M 1960	2 yr 4 yr	Para-aortic nodes Diffuse Stage IV disease	CYT HN₂ VLB-CYT MOPP	0 0 PR PR	Upper abdomen 4000/4; Pelvis 4000/4; Left axilla 3500/3; left knee 4000/; left axilla 4000/	Dead (107 mo)

Continued.

Appendix II. Therapy for extension of Stage I and II Hodgkin's disease—cont'd

Patient Age-race-sex Yr of diagnosis	Time to extension of disease	Type of extension	Chemotherapy (CRT)		Radiation (XRT)	Survival
			Agent	Results		
8 (JM) 12 W M 1961	8 yr	Para-aortic nodes			Upper abdomen 3000/4; Pelvis 3000/4	No evidence of disease (118 mo)
9 (RM) 10 W M 1961	2 yr	Liver and para-aortic nodes	CYT VLB	CR CR		In remission (118 mo)
12 (CS) 13 W F 1962	3 yr	Left neck, liver, and para-aortic nodes	CYT ⇆ VLB	CR	Para-aortic nodes 4000; total abdomen 3000/4	Dead (96 mo)
26 (NE) 12 W F 1963	2 yr	Right axilla			Right axilla 4000/4	No evidence of disease (95 mo)
27 (MS) 14 W F 1964	3 yr	Left axilla			Left axilla 4000/; right axilla prophylactically	No evidence of disease (85 mo)
29 (RE) 9 W M 1964	3 yr	Liver and para-aortic nodes	VLB	PR	Total abdomen 3000/4 + boost 1000	In remission (83 mo)
38 (RB) 9 W M 1965	2 yr	Diffuse Stage IV disease	CYT ⇆ VLB	CR	Spine 3000/2	In remission (78 mo)
10 (BN) 10 W M 1965	< 1 yr	Both axillae and neck	MOPP	0	Right and left axilla 4000/4; necks 3700/4	In remission (69 mo)
	4 yr	Neck, para-aortic nodes, and spleen (laparotomy)	VLB	CR		
41 (RS) 5 W M 1966	< 1 yr	Para-aortic nodes	VCR VLB	0 0	Total abdomen 3000/4	Dead (10 mo)

Patient	Site	Treatment	Response	Radiation	Outcome
30 (MD) 14 W M 1967	3 yr	Para-aortic nodes; lung and pleura	MOPP	CR	Total abdomen 3000/4 + boost 500 right and left inguinal 3700/4	In remission (51 mo)
31 (TM) 5 W F 1967	< 1 yr	Diffuse Stage IV disease; para-aortic nodes	CYT VLB MOPP IC Bleo CA	? ? ? 0 0 0	Upper abdomen 3000/4; pelvis 3000/4; left scapula 4000/4	Dead (45 mo)
39 (RY) 3 W M 1968	1 yr	Diffuse Stage IV disease (laparotomy)	MOPP (6) VLB	CR CR		In remission (32 mo)
28 (KK) 9 W F 1968	< 1 yr	Para-hilar lung (laparotomy)	MOPP	PR	Right hilum 3500/4	In remission (32 mo)

Appendix III. Therapy of Hodgkin's disease (Stages III and IV at diagnosis)

Patient Age-race-sex Yr of diagnosis	Histologic type	Stage	Chemotherapy		Radiation	Survival
			Agent	Results		
48 (TB) 12 W M 1953	NS	IIIB	HN₂	PR	Palliative XRT to mediastinum, lymph nodes, para-aortic nodes	Dead (34 mo)
49 (JG) 14 W M 1956	LP	IIIB	MM HN₂ CYT	PR S CR	Palliative XRT to total abdomen, mediastinum, lumbar spine, thoracic spine, necks	Dead (81 mo)
50 (JW) 11 W F 1958	NS	IIIA	HN₂	PR	Mediastinum 2000; right axilla 3000; total abdomen 2500	Dead (46 mo)
51 (DM) 7 W M 1958	LP	IVB				12-24 mo
52 (LG) 13 W M 1958	NS	IIIB	CYT VLB MH	PR NR NR	Necks 2400; mediastinum 3500; total abdomen 2750; lymph nodes 5000; left axilla 3000; right axilla 4200	Dead (84 mo)
53 (JC) 8 W M 1959	LD	IIIB			Mediastinum 3000; right neck 3000; right axilla 3000	Dead (11 mo)
54 (CL) 11 W M 1959	NS	IIIA	HN₂ CYT	PR PR	Para-aortic nodes 3000; mediastinum 3360	Dead (14 mo)
55 (PC) 8 W F 1959	MC	IIIB	HN₂ CYT CVR CYT	– CR CR PR	Palliative XRT to mediastinum; right neck; left neck; mediastinum	Dead (47 mo)
56 (ES) 9 W F 1960	NS	IIIA	HN₂ CYT AB-100	PR PR 0	Palliative XRT to left and right neck, left and right axilla, para-aortic lymph nodes	Dead (40 mo)

Case	Histology	Stage	Drugs	Response	Radiation therapy	Outcome
			VCR	0		
			UM	0		
			HU	0		
			NSC 57155			
57 (DT) 10 W M 1960	MC	IIIB	HN₂ / CYT / VCR	PR / PR / PR	Prior therapy to neck and mediastinum; pelvis 3800; left iliac 1150 boost	Dead (26 mo)
58 (CN) 12 C F 1961	NS	IVB	CYT / VCR / UM / HN₂ / AB 100 / Actinogan	PR / PR / PR / PR / 0 / 0	Total abdomen 2745	Dead (45 mo)
59 (TS) 5 W M 1962	NS	IVB	HN₂ / CYT / VLB / MH / trimethyl ammonium chloride	0 / PR / 0 / 0 / 0	Necks 3000; mediastinum 2900; total abdomen	Dead (40 mo)
60 (RJ) 7 C F 1963	MC	IVB	HN₂ / CYT	S / 0		Dead (5 mo)
61 (MR) 7 W M 1963	Unclass.	IIIB	CYT	0		Dead (4 mo)
62 (MC) 14 W M 1963	Unclass.	IIIA	HN₂ / CYT		Necks 3000; mediastinum 3000; neck and mediastinum 3000 (retreatment)	No evidence of disease with pericardial window (78 mo)
63 (PM) 8 W M 1965	MC	IVB	CYT	CR		Expired with septicemia (1 mo)

Continued.

Appendix III. Therapy of Hodgkin's disease (Stages III and IV at diagnosis)—cont'd

Patient Age-race-sex Yr of diagnosis	Histologic type	Stage	Chemotherapy		Radiation	Survival
			Agent	Results		
64 (AH) 14 C M 1966	NS	IVB	CYT VLB MOPP Bleo	0 CR CR ?	Upper abdomen 3000; necks 5000; pelvis 3000	Dead (48 mo)
65 (MM) 12 W M 1966	MC	IIIA			Mantle 3000; lymph nodes 3000 + boost scar 1500; upper abdomen 3000; pelvis 3000	No evidence of disease (57 mo)
66 (MB) 14 W M 1968	NS	IVB	VLB CYT VCR MOPP	S 0 S 0		Dead (44 mo)
67 (DL) 4 W M 1968	LP	IIIA	MOPP VLB IC	CR S Stable	Mantle 3000 + boost neck 800; lymph nodes 4000; retreatment + boost scar 1500	In remission (41 mo)
68 (AR) 10 W M 1968	NS	IIIB	CYT VLB MOPP IC HN$_2$ Bleo	PR S PR 0 0 0		Dead (32 mo)
69 (DD) 5 W M 1968	Unclass.	IIIB	COP MOPP CB-1348	PR PR CR	Abdomen 1640; treatment terminated because of thrombocytopenia	In remission (38 mo)
70 (JM) 6 W M 1968	NS	IIIB	MOPP (6) VLB	CR CR Continues	Mantle 3500; upper abdomen 3000; pelvis 3000	In remission (31 mo)
71 (EK) 12 W M 1969	NS	IIIA (laparotomy)	MOPP (2)	PR	Pelvis 3000; upper abdomen 3000; mantle 3500	No evidence of disease (23 mo)

	NS	IIIB	MOPP (2)	PP		
72 (EL) 12 W M 1969	NS	IIIB	MOPP (2)	PP	Pelvis 3000; upper abdomen 3000; mantle-mediastinum 3500; necks 4000 + boost 1000; axilla 3500	No evidence of disease (21 mo)
Unstageable at diagnosis						
73 (DS) 7 W M 1946	MC	?	HN₂	S	Palliative XRT to multiple sites	Dead (120 mo)
74 (WT) 6 W M 1953	MC	?	HN₂ CB-1348	S	Outside palliative XRT to multiple sites	Dead (39 mo)
75 (JT) 10 W M 1959	MC	?	HN₂ CYT VLB CYT VLB CB-1348	? CR CR CR CR	Outside palliative XRT to multiple sites	In remission (151 mo)
76 (SS) 9 W M 1963	MC	?	HN₂ CYT	? S	Palliative XRT to hilar lymph nodes	Dead (14 mo)

REFERENCES

1. Aisenberg, A. C.: Immunologic aspects of Hodgkin's disease, Medicine 43:189-193, May, 1964.
1a. Aisenberg, A. C.: Lymphocytopenia in Hodgkin's disease, Blood 25:1037-1042, 1965.
1b. Aisenberg, A. C., Kaplan, M. M., Rieder, S. V., and Goldman, J. M.: Serum alkaline phosphatase at the onset of Hodgkin's disease, Cancer 26:318-326, 1970.
2. Allen, L. W., Ultmann, J. E., Ferguson, D. J., and Rappaport, H.: Laparotomy and splenectomy in the staging of Hodgkin's disease, Proceedings of the Society of Laboratory and Clinical Medicine. Forty-second Annual Meeting 74:845, 1969.
3. Azzam, S. A.: High incidence of Hodgkin's disease in children in Lebanon, Cancer Res. 26:1202-1203, 1966.
4. Bailey, R. J., Burgert, E. O., Jr., and Dahlin, D. C.: Malignant lymphoma in children, Pediatrics 28:985-992, 1961.
5. Billmeier, G. J., and Holton, C. P.: Procarbazine hydrochloride in childhood cancer, J. Pediatr. 75:892-895, 1969.
6. Bohannon, R. A., Miller, D. G., and Diamond, H. D.: Vincristine in the treatment of lymphomas and leukemias, Cancer Res. 23:613-621, 1963.
7. Bouroncle, B. A., Doan, C. A., Wiseman, B. K., and Frajola, W. J.: Evaluation of CB 1348 in Hodgkin's disease and allied disorders, Arch. Intern. Med. 97:703-714, 1956.
8. Brunner, K. W., and Young, C. W.: A methylhydrazine derivative in Hodgkin's disease and other malignant neoplasms, Ann. Intern. Med. 63:69-86, July, 1965.
9. Burn, C., Davies, J. N. P., Dodge, O. G., and Nias, B. C.: Hodgkin's disease in English and African children, J. Natl. Cancer Inst. 46:37-41, 1971.
10. Butler, J. J.: Hodgkin's disease in children. In Neoplasia in childhood. A collection of papers presented at the 12th Annual Clinical Conference on Cancer, 1967, at The University of Texas M. D. Anderson Hospital and Tumor Institute at Houston, Chicago, 1969, Year Book Medical Publishers, Inc., pp. 267-279.
11. Butler, J. J.: Non-neoplastic lesions of lymph nodes of man to be differentiated from lymphomas. In Stanton, M. F., editor: Comparative morphology of hematopoietic neoplasms, Natl. Cancer Inst. Monogr. 32:233-255, 1969.
11a. Cannelos, G. P., Young, R. C., Berard, C., and DeVita, V. T.: Effect of combination chemotherapy on survival of patients with advanced Hodgkin's disease, Arch. Intern. Med. 131:388-390, 1973.
12. Cline, M. J., and Berlin, N.: Anemia in Hodgkin's disease, Cancer 16:526-532, 1963.
13. Craver, L. F.: Hodgkin's disease. In Sloan L. H., editor: Tice's practice of medicine, vol. 5, Hagerstown, Md., 1951, W. F. Prior Co., Inc., p. 107.
14. Deconti, R. C.: Procarbazine in the management of late Hodgkin's disease, J.A.M.A. 215:927-930, 1971.
15. DeVita, V. T., Moxley, J. H., III, Brace, K., and Frei, E., III: Intensive combination chemotherapy and x-irradiation in the treatment of Hodgkin's disease, Proc. Am. Assoc. Cancer Res. 6:15, April, 1965.
16. DeVita, V. T., Serpick, A., and Carbone, P. P.: Combination chemotherapy of advanced Hodgkin's disease (HD): The NCI program, a progress report, Proc. Am. Assoc. Cancer Res. 10:19, March, 1969.
17. Evans, H. E., and Nyhan, W. L.: Hodgkin's disease in children, Bull. Johns Hopkins Hosp. 114:237-248, April, 1964.
18. Exelby, P. R.: Method of evaluating children with Hodgkin's disease, CA 21:95-101, March-April, 1971.
19. Ezdinli, E. Z., and Stutzman, L.: Vinblastine vs. nitrogen mustard therapy of Hodgkin's disease, Cancer 22:473-479, 1968.
20. Fairweather, M. J., Fuller, L. M., Gallagher, H. S., and Howe, C. D.: Radiation nephritis: report of a case, J.A.M.W.A. 15:482-485, 1960.
20a. Fox, H., and Farley, D. L.: A discussion on effects of X-ray on adenopathies, J. Cancer Res. 8:162-172, July, 1924.
21. Fraumeni, J. F., Jr., and Li, F. P.: Hodgkin's disease in childhood. An epidemiologic study, J. Natl. Cancer Inst. 42:681-691, 1969.
22. Fuller, L. M., Gamble, J. F., Shullenberger, C. C., Butler, J. J., and Gehan, E. A.:

Prognostic factors in localized Hodgkin's disease treated with regional radiation, Radiology **98**:641-654, 1971.

23. Gamble, J. F.: Personal communication, May, 1971.

24. Giannopoulos, P. P., and Bergsagel, D. E.: The mechanism of the anemia associated with Hodgkin's disease, Blood **14**:856-869, 1959.

25. Glatstein, E., Guernsey, J. M., Rosenberg, S. A., and Kaplan, H. S.: The value of laparotomy and splenectomy in the staging of Hodgkin's disease, Cancer **24**:709-718, 1969.

26. Grossman, H., Winchester, P. H., Bragg, D. G., Tan, C., and Murphy, M. L.: Roentgenographic changes in childhood Hodgkin's disease, Am. J. Roentgenol. Radium Ther. Nucl. Med. **108**:354-364, 1970.

26a. Hersh, E. M., Curtis, J. E., Harris, J. E., McBride, C., Alexanian, R., and Rossen, R.: Host defense mechanisms in lymphoma and leukemia. In Leukemia-lymphoma, a collection of papers presented at the 14th Annual Clinical Conference on Cancer, 1969, at The University of Texas M. D. Anderson Hospital and Tumor Institute at Houston, Houston, Texas, Chicago, 1970, Year Book Medical Publishers, Inc., pp. 149-167.

26b. Hoster, H. A., Dratman, M. B., Craver, L. F., and Rolnick, H. A.: Hodgkin's disease (part I), 1832-1947, Cancer Res. **8**:1-78, 1948.

27. Hrgovcic, M., Tessmer, C. F., Minckler, T. M., Mosier, B., and Taylor, H. G.: Serum copper levels in lymphoma and leukemia: special reference to Hodgkin's disease, Cancer **21**:743-755, 1968.

28. Ingold, J. A., Reed, G. B., Kaplan, H. S., and Bagshaw, M.: Radiation hepatitis, Am. J. Roentgenol. **93**:200-208, 1965.

29. Jackson, H., Jr., and Parker, F., Jr.: Hodgkin's disease and allied disorders, New York, 1947, Oxford University Press.

30. Jelliffe, A. M.: Vinblastine in the treatment of Hodgkin's disease, Br. J. Cancer **23**:44-48, March, 1969.

31. Jenkin, R. D. T., Peters, M. V., and Darte, J. M. M.: Hodgkin's disease in children, Am. J. Roentgenol. **100**:222-226, 1967.

32. Jing, B., and McGrew, J. P.: Lymphangiography in diagnosis and management of malignant lymphomas, Cancer **19**:565-572, 1966.

33. Johnson, R. E., Kagan, A. R., Hafermann, M. D., and Keyes, J. W., Jr.: Patient tolerance to extended irradiation in Hodgkin's disease, Ann. Intern. Med. **70**:1-6, Jan., 1969.

34. Kadin, M. E., Glatstein, E., and Dorfman, R. F.: Clinicopathologic studies of 117 untreated patients subjected to laparotomy for the staging of Hodgkin's disease, Cancer **27**:1277-1293, 1971.

35. Kaplan, H. S.: Role of intensive radiotherapy in the management of Hodgkin's disease, Cancer **19**:356-367, 1966.

36. Karnofsky, D. A., Burchenal, J. H., Armstead, G. C., Jr., Southam, C. M., Bernstein, J. L., Craver, L. F., and Rhoads, C. P.: Triethylene melamine in the treatment of neoplastic disease, Arch. Intern. Med. **87**:477-516, 1951.

37. Karnofsky, D. A., Miller, D. G., and Phillips, R. F.: Role of chemotherapy in the management of early Hodgkin's disease, Am. J. Roentgenol. **90**:968, 1963.

38. Keller, A. R., Kaplan, H. S., Lukes, R. J., and Rappaport, H.: Correlation of histopathology with other prognostic indicators in Hodgkin's disease, Cancer **22**:487-499, 1968.

39. Lacher, M. J.: Vinblastine sulfate in Hodgkin's disease, N Y State J. Med. **69**:808-814, 1969.

40. Lessner, H. E.: BCNU (1,3, bis(β-chloroethyl)-1-nitrosourea). Effects on advanced Hodgkin's disease and other neoplasia, Cancer **22**:451-456, 1968.

41. Longcope, W. T.: On pathological histology of Hodgkin's disease, with report of series of cases, Bull. Ayer Clin. Lab. Pennsylvania Hosp. **1**:1-76, 1903.

42. Lowenbraun, S., Ramsey, H. E., and Serpick, A. A.: Splenectomy in Hodgkin's disease for splenomegaly, cytopenias and intolerance to myelosuppressive chemotherapy, Am. J. Med. **50**:49-55, Jan., 1971.

43. Lowenbraun, S., Ramsey, H., Sutherland, J., and Serpick, A. A.: Diagnostic laparotomy and splenectomy for staging Hodgkin's disease, Ann. Intern. Med. **72**:655-663, 1970.

43a. Luce, J. K.: Personal communication.
44. Lukes, R. J., and Butler, J. J.: The pathology and nomenclature of Hodgkin's disease, Cancer Res. **26:**1063-1081, 1966.
45. Lukes, R. J., Craver, L. F., Hall, T. C., Rappaport, H., and Ruben, P.: Report of the nomenclature committee, Cancer Res. **26:**1311, 1966.
46. Nickson, J. J.: Hodgkin's disease clinical trial, Cancer Res. **26:**1279-1283, 1966.
47. Origenes, M. L., Jr., Need, D. J., and Hartmann, J. R.: Treatment of the malignant lymphomas in children, Pediatr. Clin. North Am. **9:**769-784, 1962.
48. Pagliardi, E., and Giangrandi, E.: Clinical significance of the blood copper in Hodgkin's disease, Acta Haematol. **24:**201-212, 1960.
49. Peters, M. V.: A study of survivals in Hodgkin's disease treated radiologically, Am. J. Roentgenol. **53:**299-311, 1950.
49a. Peters, M. V., Brown, T. C., and Rideout, D. F.: Hodgkin's disease—prognostic influences and radiation therapy according to pattern of disease, J.A.M.A. **223:**53-59, 1973.
50. Pierce, M. I.: Lymphosarcoma and Hodgkin's disease in children, Proceedings of the National Cancer Conference, Sept. 13 to 15, 1960, Philadelphia, 1961, J. B. Lippincott Co.
51. Pitcock, J. A., Bauer, W. C., and McGavran, M. H.: Hodgkin's disease in children, Cancer **12:**1043-1051, 1959.
52. Rappaport, H., Winter, W. J., and Hicks, E. B.: Follicular lymphoma: a re-evaluation of its position in the scheme of malignant lymphoma based on a survey of 253 cases, Cancer **9:**792-821, 1956.
53. Rivers, S., Whittington, R. M., and Medrek, T. J.: Treatment of malignant lymphomas with methyl ester of streptonigrin (NSC 45384), Cancer **19:**1377-1375, 1966.
54. Rosenberg, S. A., and Kaplan, H. S.: Hodgkin's disease and other malignant lymphomas, Calif. Med. **113:**23-38, Oct., 1970.
55. Smith, C. A.: Hodgkin's disease in childhood, J. Pediatr. **4:**12-38, 1934.
56. Sohier, W. D., Jr., Wong, R. K. I., and Aisenberg, A. C.: Vinblastine in the treatment of advanced Hodgkin's disease, Cancer **22:**467-472, 1968.
57. Southwest Cancer Chemotherapy Study Group study: Unpublished data.
58. Stewart, J. R., Cohn, K. E., Fajardo, L. F., Hancock, E. W., and Kaplan, H. S.: Radiation-induced heart disease: a study of twenty-five patients, Radiology **89:**302-310, 1967.
59. Strum, S. B., Park, J. K., and Rappaport, H.: The observation of cells resembling Sternberg-Reed cells in conditions other than Hodgkin's disease, Cancer **26:**176-190, 1970.
60. Strum, S. B., and Rappaport, H.: Hodgkin's disease in the first decade of life, Pediatrics **46:**748-759, 1970.
60a. Strum, S., and Rappaport, H.: Interrelations of the histologic types of Hodgkin's disease, Arch. Pathol. **91:**127-134, 1971.
61. Sullivan, M. P.: Cyclophosphamide (NSC-26271) therapy for children with generalized lymphoma and Hodgkin's disease, Cancer Chemother. Rep. **51:**393-396, 1967.
62. Teillet, F., and Schweisguth, O.: Hodgkin's disease in children. Notes on diagnosis and prognosis based on experiences with 72 cases in children, Clin. Pediatr. **8:**698-704, 1969.
63. Todd, I. D. H.: Natulan in management of late Hodgkin's disease, other lymphoreticular neoplasms, and malignant melanomas, Br. J. Med. **1:**628-631, 1965.
64. Webb, D. I., Ubogy, G., and Silver, R. T.: Importance of bone marrow biopsy in the clinical staging of Hodgkin's disease, Cancer **26:**313-336, 1970.
65. Wilkinson, J. F., Bourne, M. S., and Israëls, M. C. G.: Treatment of leukemia and reticuloses with uracil mustard, Br. Med. J. **5345:**1563-1568, 1963.
66. Yagoda, A., Krakoff, I., LaMonte, C., and Tan, C.: Clinical trial of bleomycin, Proc. Am. Assoc. Cancer Res. **12:**37, April, 1971.
67. Zubrod, C. B., Schneiderman, M., Frei, E., III, Brindley, C., Gold, G. L., Shnider, B., Oviedo, R., Gorman, J., Jones, R., Jr., Jonsson, U., Colsky, J., Chalmers, T., Ferguson, B., Dederick, M., Holland, J., Selawry, O., Regelson, W., Lasagna, L., and Owens, A. H., Jr. (Eastern Cooperative Group in Solid Tumor Chemotherapy): Appraisal of methods for the study of chemotherapy of cancer in man—comparative therapeutic trial of nitrogen mustard and triethylene thiophosphoramide, J. Chronic Dis. **11:**7-33, 1960.
68. Zuelzer, W. W., and Flatz, G.: Acute childhood leukemia: a ten year study, Am. J. Dis. Child. **100:**886-907, 1960.

CHAPTER 14

Non-Hodgkin's lymphoma of childhood

MARGARET P. SULLIVAN

Historical aspects of childhood lymphoma other than Hodgkin's disease are obscured by the variety of diagnostic terms employed and the pooling of patients regardless of age. Only in the Burkitt's type tumor is the historical sequence of events sufficiently clear to merit comment, which is incorporated in that specific section.

Diagnostic, staging, and treatment techniques developed for adults with Hodgkin's disease have been applied to the childhood disease with success equal to that attained in adults; application of the knowledge gained in treating other adult lymphomas to the diseases as seen in childhood has produced dismal results. Whereas 60% to 75% of adults with Stage I lymphoma achieve 5-year survival,[39] the average survival among children is 6 months or less from onset of treatment.[34, 38] Fig. 14-1 illustrates survival curves for children with lymphoma other than Hodgkin's disease seen prior to 1967 at The University of Texas M. D. Anderson Hospital and Tumor Institute at Houston. Hematoxylin and eosin–stained sections were used to determine the type of lymphoma in these children; imprints and special stains were not available.

In lymphoma in children the presence of generalized involvement at the time of diagnosis and the propensity for leukemic transformation are well known. The recognition of distinct histologic entities with characteristic clinical courses has been an event of the past decade. After the delineation of the Burkitt's type of undifferentiated lymphoma in African children, specific effective therapy for this disease was developed. Similarly, the knowledge that leukemic conversion is a frequent phenomenon in the undifferentiated lymphomas of the non-Burkitt's type has resulted in improved therapeutic approaches.[1, 31] Further efforts to characterize specific types of lymphoma in children will hopefully lead to more suitable therapy to replace the traditional adult treatments that have been ineffective in children. Because of its increasing importance, histopathology will be discussed before attention is directed to clinical and therapeutic aspects of the various disease entities.

PATHOLOGY*
General considerations

The many classifications proposed for malignant lymphomas and related diseases reflect the difficulties encountered in the morphologic characterization

---

*Prepared by Dr. James J. Butler.

of these processes. The tendency of different authors to apply the same terms to different entities compounds the problem of communicating the diagnosis and of comparing results of therapy. The chief sources of difficulty in making or communicating the diagnosis of these diseases will therefore be considered briefly, and illustrations of the histopathologic types encountered will be presented.

Problems in establishing histologic diagnoses may be attributable to technical factors or may represent errors in interpretation.[11] One or more of the following technical factors may be responsible:

1. Poor selection of the biopsy site. The lower cervical and axillary lymph nodes should be biopsied if there is a choice of the biopsy site.

2. Poor selection of a lymph node or nodes at the chosen site. If one is to be reasonably certain that the disease process present, whether inflammatory or neoplastic, is represented in the biopsy, the largest node should be removed. Surgeons often remove the most accessible node rather than the largest, if not instructed otherwise.

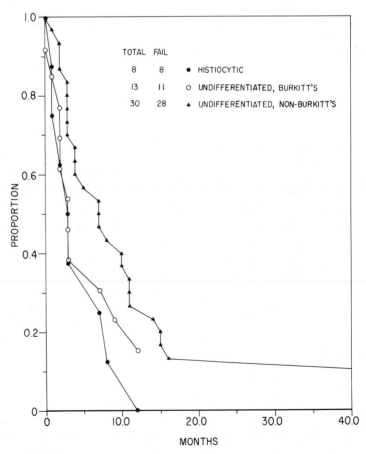

Fig. 14-1. Survival of children with lymphoma. (Courtesy Medical Communications, The University of Texas at Houston, M. D. Anderson Hospital and Tumor Institute.)

3. Improper removal of the lymph node or nodes. It is important that the entire node be removed with the capsule intact, since the pathologist needs to evaluate the relationship of normal anatomic structures to one another and to any disease process present. Although the histologic diagnosis of lymphoma or Hodgkin's disease is primarily a cytologic one, the examiner is encouraged to look for the prerequisite cytologic features by the histologic patterns, which are best seen under low and medium powers of magnification.

4. Frozen section technique or needle biopsy should not be used if lymphoma or Hodgkin's disease is suspected. Technically excellent sections are not possible by the frozen section technique; too little tissue is obtained by needle biopsy to be certain it is representative, and the nature of the technique usually produces distortion.

Recognition of the importance of these technical factors will strikingly reduce the number of cases in which the clinical diagnosis and the initial pathologic diagnosis differ.

Pathologists also must remember the importance of technical factors under their control, since the diagnoses of malignant lymphoma and Hodgkin's disease are primarily cytologic. The detailed discussion of this subject given elsewhere[11] can be summarized by saying that technically excellent sections of lymph nodes and Wright-stained imprints are required to appreciate the cytologic features that are essential in the study of the reticuloendothelial system.

Lymphosarcoma remains the most questionable term still being applied to the lymphomatous diseases because it has been used in so many ways. This term, which has been used as a synonym for malignant lymphoma,[37] may designate the entire group of diffuse lymphocytic lymphomas,[19] may designate a specific cell type,[35] or may indicate a highly malignant solitary tumor composed of

Table 14-1. Comparative classification system for malignant lymphoma

Older diagnostic terms		M. D. Anderson Hospital classification	
Lymphosarcoma	Lymphoblastoma	Malignant lymphoma	
	Brill-Symmers disease	▶ A. Nodular	
	Giant follicle lymphoma	1. Lymphocytic	
		a. Well-differentiated	
		b. Poorly differentiated	
	Follicular lymphoma	2. Mixed	
	Follicular lymphoblastoma	3. Histiocytic (RCS°)	
		4. Undifferentiated (RCS°)	
		B. Diffuse	
	Lymphosarcoma	1. Lymphocytic	
Lymphocytoma	Lymphocytic	a. Well-differentiated	
Lymphoblastoma	Lymphoblastic	b. Poorly differentiated	
Clasmatocytic	RCS°	2. Histiocytic (RCS°)	
		3. Mixed	
Stem cell		4. Undifferentiated (RCS°)	
		a. Burkitt's	
		b. Non-Burkitt's	

°RCS = Reticulum cell sarcoma.

malignant immature lymphocytes.[29] In addition, the terms *lymphoblastic* lymphoma and, less often, *lymphosarcoma* are used to refer to tumors composed of large cells with scant cytoplasm, including poorly differentiated lymphocytic lymphoma, undifferentiated lymphoma, blastic granulocytic leukemia, and undifferentiated (stem cell) leukemia. Both of these terms should be abandoned in favor of the correct cytologic description. If *lymphosarcoma* is used, it should be clearly defined.

In the M. D. Anderson Hospital classification, malignant lymphomas are described as nodular or diffuse (Table 14-1), depending on the low-power growth pattern of the malignant cells. In nodular lymphoma the cells grow in a nodular pattern, which is best appreciated under the scanning power of a microscope. The microscopic picture of a diffuse lymphoma is that of a homogeneous growth of lymphoma cells. This classification differs from that used by Rappaport[35] only in that the nodular and diffuse lymphomas are listed separately to emphasize the nodular group.

When dealing with the pediatric age group, classification is simplified because nodular lymphomas and well-differentiated lymphocytic lymphomas do not occur in children. Additionally, in our experience, poorly differentiated lymphocytic lymphoma does not occur in childhood; those cases so classified are usually undifferentiated lymphoma or undifferentiated (stem cell) leukemia.

Specific histology

The lymphomas that are seen in children are (1) undifferentiated lymphoma, Burkitt's type; (2) undifferentiated lymphoma, non-Burkitt's type; and (3) histiocytic lymphoma. Diagnosis in the pediatric age group is more difficult because of the frequency with which blastic leukemia may present as a lymphoma with either lymph node enlargement or infiltration of soft tissue in the absence of evidence in either the peripheral blood or bone marrow; leukemia may not, in fact, manifest itself for months. Although this presentation also occurs in adults, it is relatively less common. The "starry sky" appearance (Fig. 14-2), which is attributable to benign phagocytic histiocytes scattered throughout the tumor,[4] may be seen in any of these processes.

Undifferentiated lymphoma, Burkitt's type. The cytologic characteristics of undifferentiated lymphoma, Burkitt's type, have been described in detail elsewhere.[4] Briefly, the cells are relatively uniform in size and are no larger than the nucleus of the benign phagocytic histiocyte (Fig. 14-3). The nucleus has a coarsely reticulated chromatin and two to five small nucleoli. The cytoplasm is well defined and stains like that of a plasma cell, that is, it is basophilic with the Giemsa stain and intensely pyroninophilic with the methyl green–pyronin stain. The cytoplasm contains small vacuoles that stain as neutral fat.

Undifferentiated lymphoma, non-Burkitt's type. The cells of undifferentiated lymphoma, non-Burkitt's type, are of two types. Those of the first type are similar in their staining qualities to those of Burkitt's lymphoma. They differ in that the cells of the non-Burkitt's type show much more variation in size and shape of the nucleus and in the amount of cytoplasm (Fig. 14-4, A). In addition, the cytoplasmic vacuolization is much more variable, with some cells containing few if any vacuoles and other cells containing relatively large ones.

The cells of the second type of undifferentiated lymphoma, non-Burkitt's type, have little or no cytoplasm, and the nuclei vary greatly in size and are frequently folded or clefted. The nuclei contain finely distributed chromatin, and the nucleoli are small and seldom prominent (Fig. 14-4, *B*). When this process involves lymph nodes, it appears to begin in the medulla with later extension to the cortex; in the process, islands of normal lymphoid tissue are frequently isolated by islands of tumor cells (Fig. 14-4, *C*). Since this process

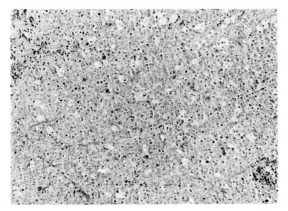

Fig. 14-2. The "starry-sky" appearance is produced by phagocytic histiocytes scattered rather uniformly throughout the tumor (H and E ×100). (Courtesy Medical Communications, The University of Texas at Houston, M. D. Anderson Hospital and Tumor Institute.)

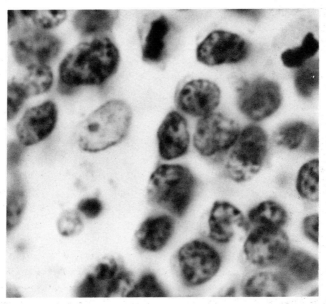

Fig. 14-3. Undifferentiated lymphoma, Burkitt's type. The tumor cells are no larger than the nucleus of the reactive histiocyte; the sharply demarcated cytoplasm contains small vacuoles (H and E ×100). (Courtesy Medical Communications, The University of Texas at Houston, M. D. Anderson Hospital and Tumor Institute.)

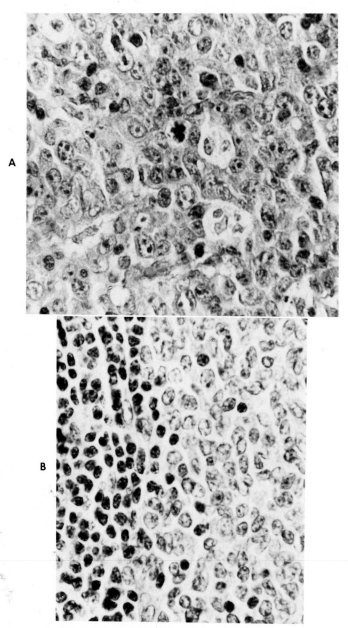

Fig. 14-4. A, Undifferentiated lymphoma, non-Burkitt's type (poorly differentiated histiocytic lymphoma). The cells vary more in size and shape and tend to have more cytoplasm than do the cells of the Burkitt type. The cells are generally larger than the nuclei of the reactive histiocytes (H and E ×400). **B,** Undifferentiated lymphoma, non-Burkitt's type (leukemic). The nuclei vary greatly in size and shape with nuclear folding common; little or no cytoplasm is evident. The tumor cells are generally larger than the normal lymphocytes to the left (H and E ×400). **C,** Undifferentiated lymphoma, non-Burkitt's type (leukemic). Islands of normal lymphoid tissues, some with reactive follicles in the center, are surrounded by the lighter staining tumor cells (H and E ×30). (Courtesy The University of Texas, M. D. Anderson Hospital and Tumor Institute, Houston, Texas.)

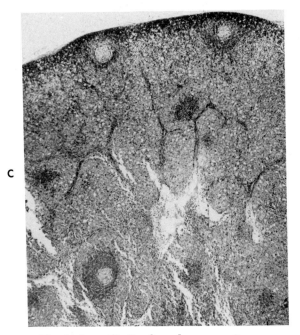

C

Fig. 14-4, cont'd. For legend see opposite page.

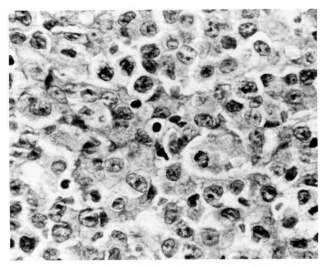

Fig. 14-5. Histiocytic lymphoma. These cells have large nuclei and abundant cytoplasm (H and E ×400). (Courtesy The University of Texas, M. D. Anderson Hospital and Tumor Institute, Houston, Texas.)

frequently begins in the mediastinum, the possibility that this represents a proliferation of thymic lymphocytes must be considered. In a study of lymphomas in children,[12] it was found that leukemic transformation occurred within 2 years after the biopsy in all except 3 of 31 patients with this type of lymphoma. Two of the 3 patients who died before leukemia developed were examined at autopsy; in both children the bone marrow was diffusely involved. Many of the patients who developed leukemia after biopsy initially had normal bone marrow.

Histiocytic lymphoma. The cells of histiocytic lymphoma (histiocytic reticulum cell sarcoma) vary widely from one patient to another and within the same patient with respect to the size of the nucleus as well as the amount of cytoplasm. Typically the cells are large and have a large nucleus and a relatively large eosinophilic nucleolus. Usually the cytoplasm is abundant and not well delineated (Fig. 14-5). The cytoplasm of these cells shows a marked variability in pyroninophilia with the methyl green–pyronin stain; the majority of cells do not stain or are weakly positive.

CLINICAL AND THERAPEUTIC ASPECTS OF CHILDHOOD LYMPHOMA
Undifferentiated lymphoma, Burkitt's type

Population characteristics. Although the entity had been previously described in the Cameroons[13] and in the Congo,[22] attention was not directed to the high frequency of lymphoma occurring in the jaw and abdominal viscera of African children until Burkitt's report appeared in 1958.[6] This lymphomatous tumor constitutes approximately half the malignancies occurring in African children,[33] in contrast to a 6% to 10% incidence of lymphoma among the malignancies of children living elsewhere.[10] Boys are affected far more frequently than girls, with sex ratios as high as 4.7:1 in favor of males being reported.[43] In endemic areas the disease occurs almost exclusively in children, with the peak age incidence of 5 to 9 years[20, 43] coinciding with the time of the second dentition.

Epidemiology. The jaw-abdominal presentation of the African lymphoma occurs primarily in those areas with annual rainfall exceeding 20 inches where the mean temperature of the coolest month remains above 60°.[27] In areas where the incidence of the lymphoma is high the incidence of the jaw, or "African," presentation is high: a low incidence of lymphoma is associated with a low incidence of the "African" presentation.[5] In the absence of the prerequisite climatic conditions the occurrence of the disease is sporadic, and the predilection for involvement of the jaw is not apparent.

Since the incidence of the African presentation is high in areas where *Anopheles* and *Mansonia* mosquitoes are endemic, an arthropod vector has been suggested. These epidemiologic considerations lend support to the concept of a viral etiology.

Virus isolation and serologic studies also support the postulated viral etiology of Burkitt's lymphoma. Members of the herpes group of viruses, as well as the reovirus type 3, have been demonstrated with relative ease in Burkitt's lymphoma.[3, 25, 40] Isolates have been made from minced tissue fragments, ascitic fluid, and tissue cultures of lymphoblasts; similar viruses have been demonstrated by direct electron microscopy.[3] A herpeslike virus, designated the Epstein-Barr

(EB) virus, was first found in the lymphoblastic tumor cells established in continuous tissue culture from Burkitt's lymphoma (African)[25]; subsequently other investigators have found this virus in similar cases. More recently the EB virus has also been implicated in infectious mononucleosis and in nasopharyngeal carcinoma.[24, 26, 28] Antibodies have been demonstrated against four antigenic complexes: the EB virus capsid antigen, the EB virus associated membrane antigen, the "early" EB virus antigen, and the soluble antigen that evokes precipitin. Changes in the various antibody levels during the course of Burkitt's lymphoma and nasopharyngeal carcinoma are not yet fully understood.[23] EB virus DNA has also been demonstrated in Burkitt's tumor and nasopharyngeal carcinoma cells.[46] Strong evidence associates the EB virus and Burkitt's lymphoma, but it is not yet possible to clearly determine whether the virus is a passenger or is directly connected with the etiology of Burkitt's lymphoma.

Clinical manifestations of the African presentation. The striking predilection of Burkitt's tumor (African) for one or more quadrants of the jaw, which is seen in half the patients, supplied the impetus for extensive study of this childhood tumor. The earliest recognizable sign of jaw involvement is loosening of the teeth; at this time tumor is still limited to the marrow cavity of the jaw.[43] The maxilla is involved three times more frequently than the mandible; one to four quadrants of the jaw may be affected. Maxillary involvement is more often manifest as intraoral tumor than as exophthalmos.

Approximately one third of children with the African form of the disease present with abdominal involvement. Ill-defined retroperitoneal masses are frequent.[10] When the primary site is ovarian, involvement is usually symmetrical and often massive.[32] Ovarian deposits are frequently associated with renal involvement. Although solitary tumor masses occur within the bowel wall, intussusception is extremely rare in African children,[17, 43] since the bowel is splinted by tumor involving the mesentery.

Paraplegia as a presenting sign has been reported in 18% of children with the African type of tumor.[10, 43] The lower thoracic spinal region is the most frequent site of involvement.[43] Spinal extradural lesions at several levels are not unusual.[17] Paraplegia is most often attributed to ischemia due to obstruction of radicular arteries by retroperitoneal or retropleural tumor[43]; tumor compressing nerve roots and the spinal cord has also been implicated.[10]

Less frequent primary sites include the long bones, salivary glands, testes, and, very rarely, peripheral nodes.[10] The thyroid gland, although seldom involved primarily, frequently becomes involved as the disease progresses.[10]

Despite the extent of disease seen in the African presentations, symptoms are remarkably few and are usually attributable to tumor bulk. Children with massive jaw tumors have surprisingly little pain and continue to eat until chewing becomes impossible mechanically.[15] Miscellaneous, infrequent presenting complaints include intestinal obstruction, swelling of a limb or bone pain, pathologic fracture, proptosis, and blindness.[17] Constitutional symptoms other than wasting are apparently not prominent even with progressive disease.

Clinical manifestations of the American presentation. As mentioned, involvement of the jaw, typical of the African presentation, is infrequent in nonendemic areas. Fig. 14-6, A, shows a large right cheek soft tissue mass in a girl

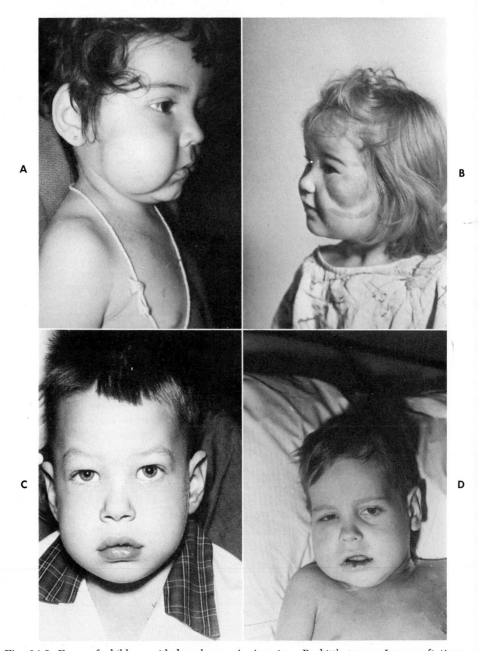

Fig. 14-6. Faces of children with lymphoma. **A,** American Burkitt's tumor. Large soft tissue mass in right cheek associated with minimal destructive changes in right mandible. **B,** Undifferentiated lymphoma, non-Burkitt's type. Primary site in skin of face; patient later developed leukemia. **C,** Undifferentiated lymphoma, non-Burkitt's type. Primary site in mediastinum with early superior vena cava syndrome manifest by fullness of eyelids and lips. Leukemic change not detected during life; autopsy examination not done. **D,** Histiocytic lymphoma. Primary site in abdomen, with metastases to left neck, right mandible, and alveolar ridge. (Courtesy Medical Communications, The University of Texas at Houston, M. D. Anderson Hospital and Tumor Institute.)

with Burkitt's tumor who had only minimal destructive changes in the right mandible. The non-African presentation has been most thoroughly studied in North American children whose mean age at diagnosis, 10.2 to 10.6 years, exceeds that of African children by several years.[14, 18] The male:female sex ratio of 1.3:1 shows an increasing susceptibility in American girls. The occurrence of presenting signs and symptoms in the American disease has been reported as follows: abdominal pain and/or nausea and vomiting, 65%; jaw tumor, 20%; cervical masses, 15%; and effusions, 30%.[18]

The most frequent sites of abdominal disease are (1) the ovaries, with both organs usually being affected, (2) the gastrointestinal tract. Even at diagnosis, abdominal disease is usually extensive and involves adjacent tissues, abdominal nodes, peritoneal surfaces, and, occasionally, the omentum.

Malignant cells are easily demonstrated in the effusions that occur in the American disease.[18] The absence of effusions at the time of diagnosis in the African disease is noteworthy.

Paraplegia has not been noted in the American children at the time of diagnosis. However, cranial nerve palsies, which are apparently infrequent in African children, have been noted in 15% of the American cases.[18]

Constitutional symptoms, including fever, chills, anorexia, and weight loss have been reported in 15 of 20 American children with Burkitt's tumor.[18]

Clinical behavior and metastatic sites. Among African children, Burkitt's tumor shows limited invasiveness, although it does become confluent in bone, where massive destruction of a lytic nature occurs.[43] With jaw involvement there is a singular lack of regional node involvement and tumor-free cervical nodes have been found in direct extensions of tumor.[43]

Among children who initially respond to chemotherapy, new disease usually occurs at a site unrelated anatomically to the primary tumor.[43] Such behavior suggests multicentricity of origin or "reinfection" rather than metastatic disease.

Progression of disease in African children is seldom manifest as leukemic involvement of the bone marrow. Leukemia, as noted in 8% of 50 children in an African autopsy series, was always associated with diffuse periportal and intrasinusoidal liver involvement.[43] In the American material the bone marrow is one of the more frequent sites of new disease, with a half to two thirds of the children eventually showing marrow changes.[14, 18] Two types of marrow involvement have been described in American children: (1) the presence of a small to moderate number of primitive lymphoreticular (LR) cells, which are morphologically identical to cells seen in tumor imprint preparations, and (2) the presence of 5% to 15% lymphoblasts associated with 20% to 60% normal lymphocytes. Progression to complete replacement of the marrow has not been observed with the second type of change, nor has this type of involvement shown a superimposed infiltrate of abnormal primitive lymphoreticular cells.[18] No consistent peripheral blood findings have been associated with the marrow alterations described.

Central nervous system involvement is a prominent feature of the treated African disease; malignant pleocytosis of the cerebrospinal fluid is now found in 45% of patients.[44] In the American disease malignant pleocytosis is apparently less frequent; CNS involvement, described as cranial nerve, meningeal, or both, has ultimately occurred in 25% of patients.[14] Since Burkitt's tumor does not form isolated nodules in brain substance,[43] it must be postulated that malignant cells gain access to the central nervous system through direct extension from involved facial bones or by extension along the course of cranial or peripheral nerves. In addition, the meninges must also be considered as a possible site of multifocal origin.

Understanding of the extent of the African disease may be obtained through study of the autopsy data presented by Wright.[43] All children with any externally visible tumor were found to have intra-abdominal disease at autopsy. Structures involved in over 50% of children studied included the jaw, pancreas, kidneys, ovaries, adrenals, and central lymph nodes. The occurrence of renal involvement in 91% of children is of clinical importance, since early symmetrical involvement may be associated with hyperuricemia and renal failure.

Staging. The diagnostic procedures, both mandatory and optional, for determining the extent of disease in non-Hodgkin's lymphoma are shown in Table 14-2. The staging system described for lymphomatous disease in Chapter 13 is usually employed for all lymphomatous diseases, regardless of the patient's age. This system has been employed in staging the M. D. Anderson material presented in Fig. 14-7. Attention is called to the absence of head and neck presentations. Seven of 13 children had primary abdominal involvement with no spread beyond the regional nodes within the cavity of origin. The remaining children had disease on either side of the diaphragm or involvement of nonnodal sites other than the primary site.

Since the clinical presentation of Burkitt's tumor (African) was indeed unique, a special system was devised to stage the African presentations as follows: Stage I, single facial tumor mass; Stage II, two or more facial tumor masses; Stage III, intrathoracic, intra-abdominal, paraspinal, or osseous tumor (excluding facial bones); and Stage IV, central nervous system (malignant cells in cerebrospinal fluid) or bone marrow involvement.[45] The application of

Table 14-2. Diagnostic procedures for non-Hodgkin's lymphoma

Mandatory	Optional
Biopsy of node or mass	Skeletal survey
Complete blood count, including differential and platelet counts	Serum electrophoresis
Bone marrow aspiration	Prothrombin time
Blood urea nitrogen level	Serum glutamic-oxaloacetic transaminase
Serum uric acid level	Serum glutamic-pyruvic transaminase
Bromsulphalein retention	
Bilirubin level	Liver scan
Alkaline phosphatase level	Serum copper level
Albumin and globulin levels	
Radiograph of chest	Celiotomy and splenectomy
Intravenous pyelogram	
Lymphangiogram	

this staging system to the American disease may be questioned on the basis of the relative infrequency of facial presentations in the American disease. When this staging system is employed, it should be clearly stated lest the reader become confused in not recognizing that Stage II disease in other staging systems is designated Stage III disease. The staging system employed is of particular importance when results of therapy and survival are being evaluated.

Clinical studies employed to determine the extent of disease vary slightly from those described in Chapter 13 for Hodgkin's disease; these differences are briefly discussed. In the American disease the equivalent of a staging laparotomy (without splenectomy) has usually been done as initial therapy for the abdominal presentation. Staging laparotomy and splenectomy are not at present suggested as a part of the routine evaluation of the patient with Burkitt's tumor.

Diagnostic features and accessory clinical findings. The diagnosis of nondifferentiated lymphoma, Burkitt's type, is made on the basis of the specific histologic findings previously described in this chapter. Histochemical and cytochemical characteristics are discussed, and the methyl green–pyronin and oil red O staining reactions are illustrated in the World Health Organization's *Histopathological Definition of Burkitt's Tumor,* published in 1969.

Hematologic findings. Hematologic findings at diagnosis have been reported for 20 patients with Burkitt's tumor (American).[18] Anemia of varying degree was found in fourteen instances. Four of these patients also had leukocytosis with white blood cell counts ranging as high as 12,000 mm³. Differential counts showed no consistent abnormalities. Two of the 20 children showed elevated platelet counts, and thrombocytopenia occurred in one child whose marrow was

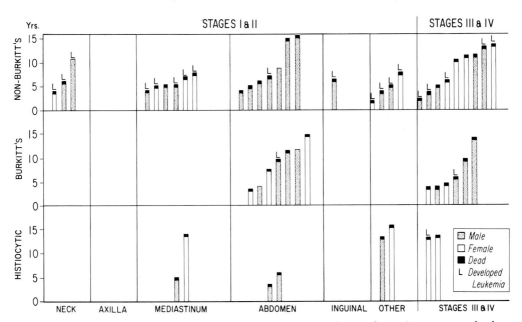

Fig. 14-7. Interrelation of age, sex, presentation, and specific histology. (Courtesy Medical Communications, The University of Texas at Houston, M. D. Anderson Hospital and Tumor Institute.)

replaced by tumor.[18] Six of 17 children who had marrow studies at the time of diagnosis showed normal hematopoiesis. The types of abnormal cells seen in the marrows of the remaining children have been described earlier. It should be noted that bone marrow biopsy is seldom necessary in Burkitt's tumor, since marrow aspiration will usually provide satisfactory specimens.

Radiographic findings. The radiographic aspects of the African tumor have been reported in detail.[17] The radiograph of the chest can be expected to show normal lung fields, since Burkitt's tumor spares the pulmonary parenchyma. The finding of mediastinal masses suggests cardiac involvement, which shows a high incidence at autopsy. Attempts to precisely localize the cardiac deposits by angiography are not thought indicated.[17] Independent involvement of mediastinal nodes is possible although infrequent in the African disease. The rare pleural effusion seen in the African disease appear to be related to cardiac involvement; the easily demonstrated tumor cells of the effusions of American disease suggest pleural involvement.

Intravenous pyelography is indicated because of the high frequency of renal involvement. Both kidneys are usually enlarged by multiple, discrete, rounded nodules that stretch and elongate the calyces in a manner that suggests congenital polycystic disease radiographically. Renal outlines may be difficult to discern in slender patients with little fat or when the tumor involves perinephric soft tissues, the adrenal glands, or the pancreas. Large ovarian or pelvic tumors may displace or compress the ureters sufficiently to produce hydronephrosis.

Bilateral lower extremity lymphangiography should be performed to determine the extent of retroperitoneal disease at diagnosis. Subsequent plain films of the abdomen can be used to monitor the therapeutic response as long as contrast media is retained in the lymph nodes.

The extent of osseous involvement should be determined by radiographic survey of the entire skeleton. The earliest detectable sign of jaw involvement is the presence of minute areas of trabecular bone destruction in the mandible or maxilla.[17] In early stages the lamina dura may be lost around only one tooth. As definite osteolytic lesions become apparent, the laminae dura of many teeth are lost. Subsequently a soft tissue mass becomes apparent, and bone spicules form at right angles to the periosteum. Maxillary tumors rapidly invade the antra and nasal passages.

Most patients with calvarial deposits show suture separation. The deposits are thought to arise in the diploë. As the deposits enlarge, the inner and/or outer tables are eroded, and extracranial and/or extradural and dural plaques are formed. Involvement of the latter sites can be demonstrated by angiography.

If paraplegia occurs, myelography will generally demonstrate an extradural mass or frank block. Localized collapse of a portion of a vertebra is found infrequently. Osteolytic foci in the vertebral bodies are sometimes demonstrable with tomography. Destruction of the intervertebral discs does not occur.

Involvement of the ilium is more frequent than the sternum, and the former site is therefore suggested for marrow aspirations. Of the long bones, the tibiae are most frequently affected, followed by the femora and humeri. Involvement of the tarsal and carpal bones may occur in advanced cases. Radiographically, the destructive process in bone resembles that seen in other small round cell tumors of childhood.

Among African children, lesions of the gastrointestinal tract are usually silent. When found radiographically, intrinsic bowel lesions are shown to be rounded, well demarcated, and suggestive of benign tumors. Primary involvement of the bowel and intussusception are more common in the non-African disease, and radiographic studies of the bowel may show specific diagnostic findings in such cases. Tumor involving other intra-abdominal organs or structures may displace or distort the bowel, but specific characteristic features are lacking.

Renal function. Among 20 patients with the American disease, 3 showed elevated blood urea nitrogen levels at diagnosis; uric acid levels were elevated in eight instances. Precise information as to renal status is essential prior to the onset of therapy. Early deaths during the first week of therapy are usually attributable to renal involvement with subsequent renal failure.[45] Peritoneal dialysis may be necessary in the initial therapy of patients with renal masses.

Profiles of liver function. Among 20 patients studied at the National Cancer Institute, 5 initially showed increased values for SGOT, SGPT, or both, as well as decreased albumin levels. Two of these patients also had prolongation of the prothrombin time, and two others had impairment of bromsulphalein excretion. Four of these 5 patients had enlarged livers and were believed to have tumor invasion of the liver. Serum bilirubin and alkaline phosphatase levels were normal in all patients at time of first study.[18]

Immunologic evaluation. When immunologic studies of 27 patients with the African disease were compared with African and American controls, children with Burkitt's lymphoma showed a low primary antibody response to Vi antigen.[18] Immunoglobulin levels showed IgG values of affected children to be similar to those of African control children but significantly higher than those of American control children. Immunoglobulin IgM values were lower than those found in African control children. Delayed hypersensitivity was intact. Lymphocyte transformation with phytohemagglutinin was comparable to that of control patients; low values were, however, found in several patients with widespread disease.

Results of immunologic surveys among American children with Burkitt's tumor have differed somewhat from those for African children.[18] Response to primary immunization with Vi antigen was normal in 7 of 8 patients studied. Among 10 children, serum IgG levels were normal in 5 and decreased in 5. Four of 5 patients with decreased IgG values also showed decreased IgA concentrations; 2 had low levels of IgM. Low IgA concentrations were also found in 3 patients with normal IgG and IgM levels. Delayed hypersensitivity was intact. In 9 patients tested, lymphocyte transformation to phytohemagglutinin was normal in 6, slightly decreased in 2, and markedly decreased in 2.

Treatment. Surgical removal of tissue for histologic study is indicated for all children with suspected lymphoma. Surgery may also be employed to reduce the bulk of disease requiring treatment when the ovaries are massively involved or when there are other resectable intra-abdominal masses.[9]

Radiotherapy, when applicable, continues to be the recommended treatment for lymphoma of childhood in some centers.[34] Burkitt's lymphoma (African), however, could not be treated successfully with irradiation[15]; this modality has not been employed routinely at the National Cancer Institute, where the American form of the disease has been studied intensively.

Even though Burkitt's lymphoma is sensitive to a number of chemotherapeutic agents as summarized by Oettgen and Murphy,[34] conventional dosage schedules employing these agents have been uniformly unsatisfactory, as demonstrated by a mean survival of 11 weeks among 9 patients at the National Cancer Institute[18] and of 12 weeks among the 13 patients at the M. D. Anderson Hospital and Tumor Institute as shown in Fig. 14-1.

Both methotrexate and cyclophosphamide, when given in high-dosage, intermittent schedules, are capable of producing complete regression in Burkitt's tumor (African)[9]; apparent cures have resulted in some cases from single doses of cyclophosphamide.[8] Early observations equated completeness of response with smallness of tumor size at the time of first therapy; methotrexate and cyclophosphamide were considered to be equally effective in smaller tumors, but cyclophosphamide appeared to be the drug of choice for large tumors.[7] More recently, chemotherapeutic response has been related to stage of disease at the time of diagnosis.[16]

Among Stage I to III African patients who were given 40 mg of cyclophosphamide/kg, single dose or multiple doses (approximately every 2 weeks for a total of six doses), the median duration of remission was about 30 weeks.[45] Multiple-dose therapy did not appear to interfere with host immune responses. In fact, in those children who subsequently developed new diseases the median duration of the initial response was significantly longer in those given multiple-dose therapy. No significant difference was found between response curves of patients with Stage I and II disease and those with Stage III disease.

For 12 Stage I and II African patients, 83% 2-year survival is reported; 55% of Stage III patients achieve 2-year survival.[45] When relapse was in the form of local recurrence after single-dose cyclophosphamide therapy, remission was readily reinduced by reinstitution of cyclophosphamide therapy. Relapse in such instances was attributed to inadequate therapy. When new disease developed at previously uninvolved sites during the course of multiple-dose therapy, persistence of sanctuary disease or acquired resistance to alkylating agents was postulated. Cyclic therapy with vincristine sulfate, methotrexate, and cytosine arabinoside has produced second remissions in 90% of these patients.[45]

Among 12 American patients, Stages I to IV, multiple-dose cyclophosphamide therapy mentioned previously resulted in a median survival of approximately 40 weeks. Actual survivals for patients continuing in remission were 52, 60, 69, 82, 100, and 112 weeks.[14]

The development of malignant pleocytosis of the central nervous system presents a particularly difficult therapeutic problem. Intrathecal methotrexate and cytosine arabinoside appear to have equal therapeutic effectiveness, and no specific treatment schedule has demonstrated superiority.[44] Prophylactic intrathecal therapy has not been successful in preventing the development of malignant pleocytosis.[44]

Undifferentiated lymphoma, non-Burkitt's type

The new histologic classification now being employed at our institution makes comparison with other series most difficult. The 30 children (59% of our series) now classified as having undifferentiated lymphoma, non-Burkitt's type, previously carried a variety of diagnoses that included lymphosarcoma, lymphoblastic lymphosarcoma, lymphocytic lymphosarcoma, malignant lymphoma, unclassified lymphoma, and reticulum cell sarcoma. These cases are the source of the clinical data discussed here.

Population characteristics. The frequency of the common presentations of the study children with undifferentiated lymphoma, non-Burkitt's type, is shown in Fig. 14-7. "Other" Stage I and II presentations included skin (Fig. 14-6, *B*), scalp, jaw, and orbit. Patients with Stage III and IV disease at diagnosis had presumed primary presentations as follows: tonsil, 1; cervical nodes, 1; generalized adenopathy, 1; mediastinum, 3; and abdomen, 3. Thirty percent of patients were thus presumed to have had mediastinal presentations and 30% to have had abdominal presentations. The incidence of bone presentations was much lower than previously reported for children with "lymphosarcoma."[21, 36]

Presenting signs and symptoms relate to site of presentation. The most frequent symptoms related to a mediastinal presentation were respiratory difficulty (7 of 9 patients) and cough (6 of 9). Fever occurred in three instances. Occasional complaints included fatigue, pleuritic pain, poor appetite, weight loss, abdominal pain, substernal pain, nausea, and drowsiness. The superior caval syndrome, depicted in an early stage in Fig. 14-6, *C*, was evident in 4 patients. Extension of disease into the neck had occurred in 4 cases; 4 patients had right pleural effusions.

In our patients with abdominal presentations the specific sites of involvement were as follows: colon, 1; terminal ileum, 2; and small bowel, 4. In two instances the primary sites appeared to be extrinsic to bowel. Fifteen, or 22%, of the children in a gastrointestinal tract "lymphoma" series presented with intussusception; perforation had occurred in one case.[30] The most frequent complaints associated with the abdominal presentation, abdominal pain and vomiting, may be attributed to some degree of intestinal obstruction. Abdominal masses were palpable in over 50% of our children. Occasional complaints included tiredness, diarrhea, constipation, leg pain, fever, and weight loss.

In children with presentations other than mediastinal and abdominal, symptoms were variable and included headache (3 of 12), as well as the previously mentioned constitutional symptoms.

Clinical behavior and metastatic sites. The outstanding clinical feature of undifferentiated lymphoma, non-Burkitt's type, is the propensity for leukemic change. The bone marrow eventually became involved in 21 of our 30 cases. As may be seen in Fig. 14-7, leukemic change occurred in all but one of the children with mediastinal presentations. In contrast, the incidence of leukemic change was very low in children with abdominal presentations. In a more detailed study of our material, Watanabe and co-workers[42] found a 47% incidence of meningeal involvement in patients with leukemic change. Meningeal involvement did not occur without prior or subsequent leukemic change; meningeal changes preceded the development of leukemia in 3 children. Survival was longer in those developing leukemia than in those who did not develop leukemia, suggesting that survival in the latter group may have been too short for leukemic changes to occur. In those not developing leukemia, short survival was attributed to lack of local control, particularly in abdominal presentations, and to metastases in sites other than meninges and marrow.

Staging. The staging system employed for undifferentiated lymphoma, non-Burkitt's type, is that used for Hodgkin's disease, which has been described in Chapter 13. Celiotomy with splenectomy has not yet been advocated as a routine staging procedure for this type of lymphoma.

Diagnostic features and accessory clinical findings. The diagnosis of undifferentiated lymphoma, non-Burkitt's type, is made on the basis of histologic findings as previously described. Even though it is often difficult to make the distinction between the type destined to become leukemic and the nonleukemic variety, this differentiation should be attempted to permit appropriate therapy.

Hematologic findings. Hematologic findings at the time of diagnosis were usually within range of normal for children with undifferentiated lymphoma, non-Burkitt's type. Anemia with a hemoglobin level less than 10 gm/100 ml was noted in only 3 of our patients. Five children had leukocytosis with white blood cell counts above 10,000 mm³, ranging as high as 17,450 mm³. Differential counts were within normal range, and platelet counts were not remarkable at the time of diagnosis. Leukemic marrow changes eventually developed in 70% of patients. The median duration of disease at the time of leukemic transformation has been reported as 27 weeks, range 10 to 60 weeks.[41] Peripheral blood changes associated with the development of a leukemic marrow occurred in the following order of frequency: (1) decrease in percentage of segmented leukocytes, (2) the presence of immature myeloid cells, (3) decrease in platelet count to less than 100,000, and (4) appearance of blast cells.[41]

Radiographic findings. With mediastinal presentations, chest radiographs demonstrate the presence of anterior or anterosuperior mediastinal masses, often of huge proportions, and sometimes extending upward into the root of the neck. Lateral films of the chest are helpful in determining the degree of tracheal compression. Hilar node involvement is not uncommon; parenchymal densities are rare. Pleural effusions are frequent; pleural thickening can be demonstrated occasionally on the chest films.

Intrinsic masses primary in the small bowel, cecal region, or ascending colon can be demonstrated by the appropriate contrast study, an upper gastrointestinal series with small bowel follow-through or barium enema. Intussusception is a relatively common complication, and the initial radiographic studies may show the characteristic radiologic changes. Masses arising outside the bowel may produce extrinsic pressure defects in the barium column during contrast study. With abdominal presentations intravenous pyelography is essential to determine the presence and degree of urinary tract obstruction. Pyelography may also give indirect evidence of retroperitoneal disease through displacement of the ureters. Lateral pyelograph films are especially helpful in demonstrating anterior displacement of the ureters. In contrast to the Burkitt's type tumor, evidence of renal enlargement due to lymphomatous involvement is unusual at the time of diagnosis. Pyelographs of 3 of 14 children in our series showed calyceal distortion suggestive of nodular infiltrates, but renal size was not unusual.

Information is not yet available on pedal lymphangiographic findings in this diagnostic category. Lymphography would appear indicated for accurate staging of upper torso presentations and for determining the degree of retroperitoneal nodal involvement in abdominal presentations.

At the time of diagnosis, radiographs of the skeleton are usually negative.

Symptoms will indicate the site of involvement in those rare children who subsequently develop metastatic bone disease.

Renal function. Screening tests of renal function should include blood urea nitrogen and serum uric acid levels as well as a routine urinalysis. Blood urea nitrogen levels were normal in all 12 children in our series who had this test performed at the time of diagnosis. Four of 12 children tested had uric acid levels that exceeded 7.5 mg/100 ml., but none developed uric acid nephropathy with renal failure. Routine urinalysis showed 4+ albuminuria as an isolated abnormality in 1 of our 30 children.

Profiles of liver function. Liver function tests should be a routine part of the staging procedure for all children with lymphoma. Evaluation of this parameter in 7 of our children showed abnormalities in 3. A serum albumin level of 2.8 gm/100 ml occurred as a single abnormality in 1 child. One child with an abdominal presentation and an enlarged liver showed increased BSP retention, and elevated SGOT level, and prolongation of the prothrombin time; a second child with a similar presentation and an enlarged liver showed increased BSP retention and elevated bilirubin, SGOT, and SGPT levels, whereas the prothrombin time remained normal.

Therapy. Surgical biopsy of abnormal masses is indicated in all cases of suspected lymphoma for the establishment of a specific diagnosis. With abdominal presentations, diagnosis is made at laparotomy. In many instances the preoperative diagnosis is an "acute abdomen," and the malignant tumor is an unexpected finding. In "early stage" bowel presentations with metastases limited to mesenteric nodes, resection of the involved bowel with its mesentery is said to be curative in 10% of cases.[43] Ideally, the liver and representative nodes from various anatomic regions should be biopsied. Nodal biopsy sites and the extent of residual disease should be marked with silver clips. Splenectomy has not been advocated for this diagnostic group.

The relative roles of radiotherapy and chemotherapy in the management of the non-Burkitt's lymphomas are not yet determined; combination radiotherapy-chemotherapy regimens are frequently employed. When the primary disease site is outside the abdomen, local control can be expected after radiotherapy in the 3500 rads tumor-dose range, particularly if histologic features are suggestive of the subtype ultimately developing leukemia. Allopurinol should be given to control hyperuricemia during the period of rapid tumor regression.

When treatment for mediastinal and cervical presentations is restricted to radiotherapy, the development of leukemia can be anticipated in a high proportion of cases. Vincristine sulfate-prednisone therapy during radiation and subsequent maintenance chemotherapy with mercaptopurine-methotrexate-cyclophosphamide in combination, reenforced with vincristine sulfate and prednisone periodically, are reported to delay and hopefully to prevent recurrent or new disease, including leukemic change.[1] The leukemia evolving from non-Burkitt's type lymphoma responds poorly to single-agent chemotherapy,[41] but combination remission induction therapy followed by single-agent maintenance therapy has produced results comparable to those obtained in acute lymphocytic leukemia of childhood.[31] Once leukemia occurs, intensive antileukemic therapy should be given.

Prophylactic central nervous system chemotherapy has no established effectiveness in acute leukemia in children and cannot be recommended for children with lymphoma who develop leukemia. Central nervous system chemotherapy plus cranial irradiation has been effective prophylaxis in childhood acute leukemia,[2] and the usefulness of such combination therapy should be studied in lymphoma patients who are at risk of meningeal involvement. If radiotherapy is contemplated for the entire neuroaxis, this should be included in the original treatment plans because prior therapy to the neck, mediastinum, or both would make subsequent field planning for prophylactic irradiation of the neuroaxis most difficult.

Patients with "early stage" bowel presentations have shown 33% 5-year survival when given postoperative radiation to the entire abdomen in the dose of 2500 rads in 4 weeks.[30] No deaths occurred beyond the first year after therapy. In "late stage" abdominal disease with retroperitoneal involvement, similar therapy resulted in 5% 5-year survival. At the M. D. Anderson Hospital radiation therapy is given to the total abdomen in tumor doses of 3500 rads in an effort to improve the local cure rate. Radiotherapy techniques, including shielding of the kidneys, have been detailed in Chapter 13.

No consistently effective chemotherapy regimen has been devised for the abdominal lesion of undifferentiated lymphoma, non-Burkitt's type, and combination radiotherapy-chemotherapy regimens are usually employed. The combination chemotherapy regimen that was used with success in treating mediastinal and cervical presentations was not effective in treating the only child with primary abdominal tumor in the series of 8 cases.[1] Radiotherapy combined with chemotherapy (vincristine sulfate, prednisone, and 10 mg cyclophosphamide given in pulse doses at intervals of 6 weeks) is under investigation.

Histiocytic lymphoma

The population and clinical characteristics of histiocytic lymphoma have not been defined for the disease in childhood. The findings of our 8 children with this diagnosis will be briefly noted so that they may serve as a base for the accumulation of further data.

Population characteristics. As shown in Fig. 14-7, ages of the 8 children in our group ranged from 3 5/12 years to 15 7/12 years (median, 13 3/12 years), a somewhat older group than that affected by other types of childhood lymphoma.

Clinical manifestations. The variation in presentation in this type of lymphoma is apparent in Fig. 14-7. "Other" Stage I and II presentations occurred in the palate and alveolar ridge of one child and in the ribs of the second child. The two children with Stage III and IV disease both had apparent primary disease in cervical and supraclavicular nodes; in one case metastases were present in skin and subcutaneous tissue, in the other the spleen was involved. On physical examination, the invasive tendencies of the tumor could be recognized in the visible and palpable local extensions beyond the structure of origin.

Clinical behavior and metastatic sites. The first site of new disease activity after initial therapy for primary disease is shown in Table 14-3. The death of 2 children was associated with uncontrolled disease at the primary site despite radiotherapy-chemotherapy. Two children completed planned radiotherapy with apparent good results; 1 showed prompt disease extension from the pri-

Table 14-3. First site of new disease activity after initial therapy for localized histiocytic lymphoma

Presentation (number of patients)	Site of new disease	Survival from diagnosis
Mediastinum (2)	Neck and pleura by direct extension	1 mo
	Uncontrolled primary site with local extension to lung and pericardium	3 mo
Abdomen (2)	Uncontrolled primary site	2 mo
	Left neck, mandible, and alveolar ridge*	8 mo
Alveolar ridge and palate (1)	Local recurrence at primary site	12 mo
Ribs (1)	Retroperitoneal space	1 mo

*See Fig. 14-6, D.

mary site after 3000 rads tumor dose; the second child had local recurrence 12 months after 3600 rads tumor dose. In the remaining 2 children, new disease activity after initial therapy occurred at distant sites. Fig. 14-6, D shows metastatic disease of the head and neck in a child with controlled primary disease in the abdomen.

One of the 8 children in this diagnostic category developed peripheral blood findings suggestive of leukemia; leukemic marrow changes were not documented during life or at postmortem examination. Meningeal involvement did not occur in this group of children; however, this complication has been seen recently in 1 of our children in this diagnostic category.

Staging. The staging procedure for histiocytic lymphoma is that described previously for the other lymphomatous diseases.

Diagnostic features and accessory clinical features. The diagnostic and clinical findings in this type of lymphoma are not yet defined except for (1) the histologic appearance of the tumor and (2) the tendency of the tumor to show local invasiveness that can be recognized microscopically, as well as on physical examination.

Hematologic findings. For staging purposes the peripheral blood and bone marrow of each patient should be studied. Anemia with a hemoglobin level of less than 10 gm/100 ml was found in 1 of our 8 children; blood counts were otherwise within normal limits, as were the initial bone marrow examinations. The child in Fig. 14-7 designated as having leukemia had blast cells in the peripheral blood 2 days prior to death, but the leukemic status of the marrow was not documented. No evidence of leukemia developed in the remaining children with histiocytic lymphoma.

Radiographic findings. Radiographic studies should include those indicated for the other lymphomatous diseases of childhood. Findings of course relate to the presentation. Soft tissue changes associated with nodal and osseous primary sites may be greater than with other types of childhood lymphoma.

One of our 6 children who underwent pyelography had enlarged kidneys, another child showed dilatation of the left pelvis, and 3 showed some abnormality in the position of the ureters, suggesting retroperitoneal disease. In the one instance in which staging might have been altered, these findings were considered "suggestive" only. Unfortunately, lymphography was not performed in any of the children.

Renal function. Blood urea nitrogen levels were normal in the 4 children having this test. Uric acid levels exceeded 7.5 mg/100 ml in 2 of the 3 children tested, but uric acid nephropathy did not occur.

Profiles of liver function. Abnormalities were found in 3 of the 4 children in whom this parameter was evaluated. Increased BSP retention was found as an isolated abnormality in 2 children. One child with an abdominal presentation showed increased BSP retention as well as slight elevation of the bilirubin level.

Treatment. Surgery is of course indicated for biopsy purposes to permit the establishment of a precise histologic diagnosis. Staging celiotomy with splenectomy has not been recommended in this disease category. In institutions studying lymphomas of childhood intensively, this procedure is being employed in pilot investigations.

Successful treatment for this tumor has not yet been devised. The results of treatment at this institution suggest continuing exploration of new agents to be incorporated into energetic radiotherapy-chemotherapy regimens. Combination radiotherapy-chemotherapy with the "pulse" cyclophosphamide regimen previously described is a currently employed, but, again, patient numbers are too small for meaningful conclusions. Results of radiotherapy in the 3000 to 3500 rads tumor-dose range suggest that 4000 to 4500 rads will be required for long-term control or local care.

Leukemic transformation was suspected in only 1 of 8 children; meningeal involvement did not occur. These complications, however, should be expected when more effective therapy prolongs survival. Effective treatment of the disease in this "sanctuary" compartment will probably require intensive combination intrathecal chemotherapy, as well as radiotherapy to the entire neuroaxis in the 4000 rads dose range.

REFERENCES

1. Aur, R. J. A., Hustu, H. O., Pinkel, D., Pratt, C. B., and Simone, J. V.: Therapy of localized and regional lymphosarcoma of childhood, Cancer 27:1328-1331, 1971.
2. Aur, R. J. A., Simone, J., Hustu, H. O., Walters, T., Borella, L., Pratt, C., and Pinkel, D.: Central nervous system therapy and combination chemotherapy of childhood lymphocytic leukemia, Blood 37:272-281, 1971.
3. Bell, T. M.: Review of the evidence for a viral aetiology for Burkitt's lymphoma. In Burchenal, J. H., and Burkitt, D. P., editors: Treatment of Burkitt's tumour, New York, 1967, Springer-Verlag New York, Inc., pp. 52-58.
4. Bennett, J. M., Berard, C., Butler, J. J., Dorfman, R., Gerard-Marchant, R., Hamlin, I., Hartsock, R. J., Lennert, K., Liberman, P. R., Linsell, C. A., Lukes, R. J., O'Conor, G. T., Osunkoya, B. O., Rappaport, H. H., Rebuck, J., Thomas, L. B., Torloni, H., and Wright, D. H.: Histopathological definition of Burkitt's tumour, Bull. W.H.O. 40:601-607, 1969.
5. Burchenal, J. H.: Geographic chemotherapy—Burkitt's tumor as a stalking horse for leukemia: presidential address, Cancer Res. 26:2393-2402, 1966.
6. Burkitt, D.: A sarcoma involving the jaws in African children, Br. J. Surg. 46:218-223, 1958.
7. Burkitt, D.: Malignant lymphomata involving the jaws in Africa, J. Laryngol. Otol. 79:929-939, 1965.
8. Burkitt, D.: Long-term remissions following one and two-dose chemotherapy for African lymphoma, Cancer 20:756-759, 1967.

9. Burkitt, D., Hutt, M. S. R., and Wright, D. H.: The African lymphoma: preliminary observations on response to therapy, Cancer **18**:399-410, 1965.

10. Burkitt, D., and O'Conor, G. T.: Malignant lymphoma in African children. I. A clinical syndrome, Cancer **14**:258-269, 1961.

11. Butler, J. J.: Non-neoplastic lesions of lymph nodes of man to be differentiated from lymphomas. In Comparative morphology of hematopoietic neoplasms, Natl. Cancer Inst. Monogr. **32**:233-255, 1969a.

12. Butler, J. J., and Oates, J.: Unpublished data.

13. Capponi, M.: Note sur le cancer au Cameroun, Bull. Soc. Pathol. Exot. **46**:605-611, 1953.

14. Carbone, P. P., Berard, C. W., Bennett, J. M., Ziegler, J. L., Cohen, M. H., and Gerber, P.: NIH Clinical Staff Conference: Burkitt's tumour, Ann. Intern. Med. **70**:817-832, 1969.

15. Clifford, P.: Personal communication.

16. Clifford, P., Singh, S., Stjernsward, J., and Klein, G.: Long term survival of patients with Burkitt's lymphoma: an assessment of treatment and other factors which may relate to survival, Cancer Res. **27**:2578-2615, 1967.

17. Cockshott, W. P.: Radiological aspects of Burkitt"s tumour, Br. J. Radiol. **38**:172-180, March, 1965.

18. Cohen, M. H., Bennett, J. M., Berard, C. W., Ziegler, J. L., Vogel, C. L., Sheagren, J. N., and Carbone, P. P.: Burkitt's tumor in the United States, Cancer **23**:1259-1272, 1969.

19. Custer, R. P., and Bernhard, W. G.: The interrelationship of Hodgkin's disease and other lymphatic tumors, Am. J. Med. Sci. **216**:625-642, 1948.

20. Dalldorf, G.: Lymphomas of African children with different forms or environmental influences, J.A.M.A. **181**:1026-1028, 1962.

21. Dargeon, H. W.: Lymphosarcoma in childhood, Adv. Pediatr. **6**:13-32, 1953.

22. DeSmet, M. P.: Observations cliniques de tumeurs malignes des tissus reticuloendotheliaux et des tissus hemolymphopoietiques au Congo, Ann. Soc. Belg. Med. Trop. **36**:53-70, Feb. 29, 1956.

23. Editorial: E. B. virus, Burkitt lymphoma, and nasopharyngeal carcinoma, Lancet **1**:218-219, 1971.

24. Einhorn, N., Klein, G., and Clifford, P.: Increase in antibody titer against the EBV-associated membrane antigen complex in Burkitt's lymphoma and nasopharyngeal carcinoma after local irradiation, Cancer **26**:1013-1021, 1970.

25. Epstein, M. A., Achong, B. G., and Barr, Y. M.: Virus particles in cultured lymphoblasts from Burkitt's lymphoma, Lancet **1**:702-703, 1964.

26. Gunvén, P., Klein, G., Henle, W., and Clifford, P.: Epstein-Barr virus in Burkitt's lymphoma and nasopharyngeal carcinoma. Antibodies to EBV associated membrane and viral capsid antigens in Burkitt lymphoma patients, Nature (Lond.) **228**:1053-1056, 1970.

27. Haddow, A. J.: An improved map for the study of Burkitt's lymphoma syndrome in Africa, East Afr. Med. J. **40**:429-432, 1963.

28. Henle, G., Henle, W., and Diehl, V.: Relationship of Burkitt's tumor-associated herpestype virus to infectious mononucleosis, Proc. Natl. Acad. Sci. USA **59**:94-101, Jan., 1968.

29. Jackson, H., Jr., and Parker, F., Jr.: Hodgkin's disease and allied disorders, New York, 1947, Oxford University Press.

30. Jenkin, R. D. T., Sonley, M. J., Stephens, C. A., Darte, J. M. M., and Peters, M. V.: Primary gastrointestinal tract lymphoma in childhood, Radiology **92**:763-767, 1969.

31. Jones, B., Kung, F., Nyhan, W. L., Hananian, J., Blom, J., Burgert, E. O., Jr., Mills, S. D., Treat, C., Wolman, I. J., Chevalier, L., Denton, R., Sheehe, P., Glidewell, O., and Holland, J. F.: Chemotherapy of the leukemic transformation of lymphosarcoma, J. Pediatr. **70**:442-448, Part I, 1967.

32. O'Conor, G. T.: Malignant lymphoma in African children. II. A pathological entity, Cancer **14**:270-283, 1961.

33. O'Conor, G. T., and Davies, J. N. P.: Malignant tumors in African children, J. Pediatr. **56**:526-535, 1960.

34. Oettgen, H. F., and Murphy, M. L.: Malignant lymphoma of childhood in the United States and Burkitt's tumour in Africa: therapeutic results. In Burchenal, J. H., and Burkitt, D. P., editors: Treatment of Burkitt's tumour, New York, 1967, Springer-Verlag New York, Inc., pp. 105-108.

35. Rappaport, H.: Tumors of the hematopoietic system, Washington, D. C., 1966, Armed Forces Institute of Pathology.
36. Rosenberg, S. A., Diamond, H. D., Dargeon, H. W., and Craver, L. F.: Lymphosarcoma in childhood, N. Engl. J. Med. 259:505-512, 1958.
37. Rosenberg, S. A., Diamond, H. D., Jaslowitz, B., and Carver, L. F.: Lymphosarcoma: a review of 1269 cases, Medicine 40:31-84, Feb., 1961.
38. Sagerman, R. H., Wolff, J., Sitarz, A., and Luke, K.: Radiation therapy for lymphoma in children, Radiology 86:1096-1099, 1966.
39. Scheer, A. C.: The course of stage I malignant lymphomas following local treatment, Am. J. Roentgenol. Radium Ther. Nucl. Med. 90:939-943, 1963.
40. Stanley, N. F.: Reovirus type 3 and the etiology of Burkitt's lymphoma. In Treatment of Burkitt's tumor, Burchenal, J. H., and Burkitt, D. P., editors: Treatment of Burkitt's tumour, New York, 1967, Springer-Verlag New York, Inc., pp. 59-63.
41. Sullivan, M. P.: Leukemic transformation in lymphosarcoma of childhood, Pediatrics 29:589-599, 1962.
42. Watanabe, A., Sullivan, M. P., Sutow, W. W., and Wilbur, J. R.: Undifferentiated lymphoma, non-Burkitt's type: Meningeal and bone marrow involvement in children, Am. J. Dis. Child. 125:57-61, 1973.
43. Wright, D. H.: Burkitt's tumour: a post-mortem study of 50 cases, Br. J. Surg. 51:245-251, 1964.
44. Ziegler, J. L., and Bluming, A. Z.: Intrathecal chemotherapy in Burkitt's lymphoma, Br. Med. J. 3:508-512, 1971.
45. Ziegler, J. L., Morrow, R. H., Jr., Fass, L., Kyalwazi, S. K., and Carbone, P. P.: Treatment of Burkitt's tumor with cyclophosphamide, Cancer 26:474-484, 1970.
46. Zur Hausen, H., Schulte-Holthausen, H., Klein, G., Henle, W., Henle, G., Clifford, P., and Santesson, L.: Epstein-Barr virus in Burkitt's lymphoma and nasopharyngeal carcinoma; EBV DNA in biopsies of Burkitt tumours and anaplastic carcinomas of the nasopharynx, Nature (Lond.) 228:1056-1058, 1970.

CHAPTER 15

Histiocytosis[*]

KENNETH A. STARLING
DONALD J. FERNBACH

HISTORICAL ASPECTS

The literature concerning the spectrum of diseases now known as *histiocytosis X*[33] began with the report of a child with "polyuria and tuberculosis" by Hand in 1893. Kay[27] reported a similar case in 1905, which was followed by Schüller's[48] two cases in 1915 and Christian's[13] case in 1920. Although the syndrome later became known as Christian's triad (exophthalmos, membranous bone defects, and diabetes insipidus) or Hand-Schüller-Christian disease, it has been recently pointed out[15] that the "true name" should be Hand-Kay-Schüller-Christian syndrome, or Kay's triad, since he was the first to call it such.

Letterer (1923)[31] and Siwe (1933)[52] are given credit for the classic descriptions of disseminated histiocytosis. However, in a summary of reported cases prior to 1936, Abt and Denenholz[1] pointed out three additional cases that were described prior to Siwe's report.

On reviewing the case reported by Hand, we see that the child had hepatosplenomegaly, petechiae, and a skin eruption similar to scabies, in addition to exophthalmos, polyuria, and bone lesions. It is clear that the child had features that would allow him to be classified as having Hand-Schüller-Christian syndrome, but the other findings would be more consistent with the Letterer-Siwe syndrome.

It is particularly appropriate that the original case report defies classification, since this is still controversial in present-day thinking. The current approach to therapy and evaluation of the results of therapy are generally agreed on, but there is no uniform clinical or histopathologic classification. It seems unlikely that this disagreement will be resolved until the specific etiologic factor or factors are defined.

INCIDENCE

The exact incidence of histiocytosis X is not known, and because this disease covers a broad spectrum from benign to malignant entities, death certificate data are obviously inadequate to determine actual occurrence rates. There is increasing experience of children with this disease responding favorably to therapy, and some appear to have been cured.

---

*Photomicrographs courtesy Dr. Cirilo Sotelo-Avila, Department of Pathology, Texas Children's Hospital, Houston.

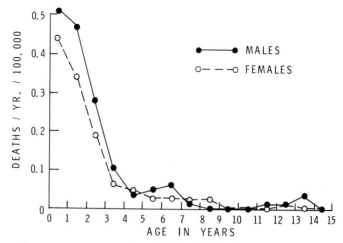

Fig. 15-1. Mortality per year in white children from generalized histiocytosis by age in the United States, 1960-1964. (From Glass, A. G., and Miller, R. W.: Pediatrics **42:**364-367, 1968.)

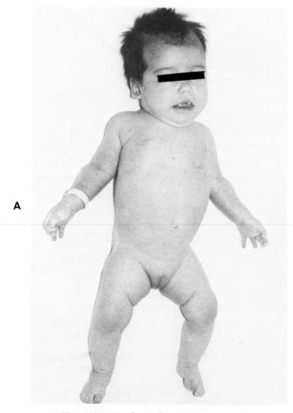

Fig. 15-2. For legend see opposite page.

Glass and Miller[21] reported the United States mortality between 1960 and 1964 for Letterer-Siwe syndrome, reticuloendotheliosis, or disseminated histiocytosis. A summary of the results taken from their study is shown in Fig. 15-1. This disease occurs in all ethnic groups, but its rarity and the lack of data prevent the inclusion of any other incidence data. Assuming a mortality rate of 50%,[30] the annual incidence would be approximately 1 per 100,000 white children under 1 year of age and approximately 0.2 per 100,000 children under 15 years of age. These data do not include children with solitary or disseminated eosinophilic granuloma or children with the Hand-Schüller-Christian syndrome, so that the annual incidence of histiocytosis X is probably greater than 0.5 per 100,000 children a year.

ETIOLOGY

Since no specific etiologic factor is known and because of the peculiar histopathologic features, there is still speculation that these disorders are not true neoplasms. In spite of the many common histologic features, the clinical behavior of the various forms of the disease ranges from totally benign eosino-

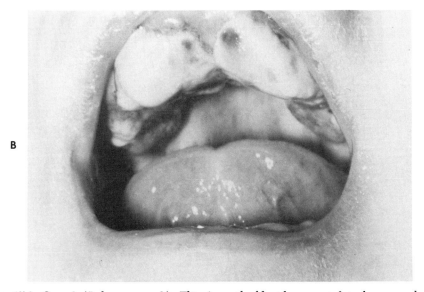

B

Fig. 15-2. Case 1 (Lahey score: 3). This 1-month-old girl was noted to have papular skin lesions scattered over her body at the time of birth. She developed a croupy cough in the neonatal period that persisted until the time of admission. At that time, in addition to the cough and skin lesions, she had a white membrane covering the buccal mucosa and upper gingivae. X-ray films of the chest showed a diffuse infiltrate. A biopsy of the skin and gums was diagnostic of histiocytosis, and she was treated for 4 months with cyclophosphamide. During that time the disease progressed slowly. Therapy was changed to vinblastine and prednisone, but for the next 2 months the disease progressed, and she died at age 7 months. This case is presented to contrast the relentless progression of the disease in some infants with the responsiveness in other infants similarly afflicted. **A,** Appearance of child on admission to the hospital showing the generalized papular rash. **B,** Photograph of the mouth showing the infiltrates of the gums and palate. (Courtesy Department of Medical Photography, St. Luke's Episcopal Hospital and Texas Children's Hospital.)

philic granulomas of bone to highly malignant histiocytic infiltrations of bone and soft tissues. There is no doubt that genetic factors are involved in some cases. Five pairs of siblings, including both of a set of identical twins, died during the 5-year period reported by Glass and Miller. In a summary of the literature by Miller,[41] thirteen instances of familial reticuloendotheliosis were encountered, only six of which were classified as Letterer-Siwe syndrome. Bierman[10] reported the involvement of both of a pair of identical twins. Conversely, Lightwood[36] reported the involvement of only one of a pair of identical twins. There have been no reported cases of isolated eosinophilic granuloma occurring in families, nor have there been any reports of generalized histiocytosis occurring in succeeding generations.

In addition to the familial occurrences of histiocytosis, there are a number of cases that have been diagnosed in the newborn period. Reid and Gottlieb[45]

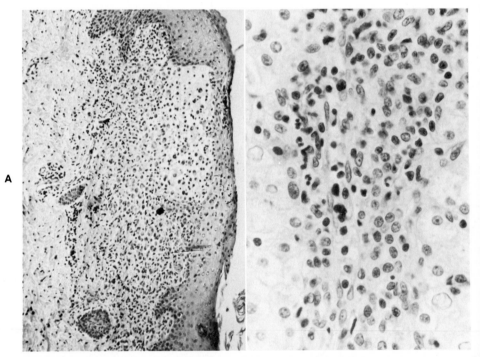

Fig. 15-3. Case 2 (Lahey score: 4). This 2-month-old boy, one of fraternal twins, was noted to have papular skin lesions on the neck, back, groin, and legs at the time of birth. On physical examination at 2 months of age, there were scattered discrete lesions measuring 0.3 to 1 cm on the scalp, face, trunk, and extremities. There was a small white lesion over the buccal mucosa suggestive of candidiasis but unresponsive to nystatin. The liver and spleen were palpable below the costal margins. Biopsy of the liver and of the skin lesions was diagnostic of histiocytosis X. A chest film revealed a pulmonary infiltrate that was consistent with this diagnosis. The patient was treated with cyclophosphamide for 1 year. Regression of all active lesions was complete within 4 months. There has been no evidence of disease in the 32 months since the cyclophosphamide was discontinued. This case is presented to document that early onset and widespread involvement does not necessarily herald a poor prognosis. **A,** Low power view of the skin biopsy. **B,** High power view of the liver biopsy showing histiocytic infiltration in the periportal space.

reported the most recent case and cited fifteen others. We have seen 2 patients who were diagnosed in the neonatal period, both of whom are described in more detail later (Figs. 15-2 and 15-3).

Thus both genetic and congenital or prenatal factors are implicated in the pathogenesis of this disease, since it occurs in familial patterns and in neonates. In most cases, however, no family history of similar disease can be found, nor is there clinical evidence of disease at birth.

Little information is available on the relationship of these diseases to the dysgammaglobulinemias. One case has been observed in which a child who was treated and was otherwise free from any evidence of disseminated disease had a persistant deficiency of IgG. It is not known if the deficiency of IgG preceded the disease.[56]

Intensive efforts to consistently recover an infectious agent, either bacterial or viral, have been futile.

PATHOLOGIC FEATURES AND CLASSIFICATION

Lichtenstein affirmed (1953)[33] and then reaffirmed (1964)[34] the interrelationships of the three syndromes: eosinophilic granuloma, Hand-Schüller-Christian syndrome, and Letterer-Siwe syndrome; he coined the term *histiocytosis X.* Few diseases have created as much controversy regarding classification and prognosis as have the so-called nonlipid reticuloendothelioses. It is our opinion that these syndromes are related entities. If syndrome semantics could be dispelled, it would be easier for the practical student and clinician to understand and manage the variations as they occur, rather than struggle to determine to which syndrome a given case belongs. Lahey,[29] Oberman,[43] Lucaya,[37] and other reviewers have agreed with this concept. According to Lahey, "It hardly seems necessary to belabor further the point made repeatedly that the Letterer-Siwe, Hand-Schüller-Christian and eosinophilic granuloma complex of disorders are intimately related clinically, pathologically, and probably etiologically and as such represent a single nosologic entity with widely variable clinical expression."*

Some authors quoted by Lieberman[35] oppose the use of the term *histiocytosis X* but have suggested nothing to significantly improve the classification or nomenclature. Despite these arguments, the common pathologic feature is characterized by diffuse proliferation of histiocytes, with or without granuloma formation. At some stage masses of eosinophils, lymphocytes, plasma cells, and large histiocytes may accumulate in the lesions. The frequent progression from a solitary eosinophilic granuloma to a disseminated histiocytic infiltrative process makes the term *histiocytosis X* clinically useful. Each patient, or the clinical and pathologic findings for each patient, must be examined separately—not only initially but also as the disease progresses or regresses. The treatment must be directed toward the clinical and pathologic features that the child expresses at a given time. Figs. 15-3 to 15-5 are photomicrographs of typical lesions.

Parasitic eosinophilic granulomas, monocytic leukemia, histiocytic medullary reticulosis,[46] familial lymphohistiocytosis,[38] and sex-linked reticulohistiocytosis

---

*From Lahey, M. E.: Prognosis in reticuloendotheliosis in children, J. Pediatr. **60:**664-671, 1962.

with hypergammaglobulinemia[18] have been separated from the histiocytosis X family of diseases by features that have been recognized as unique. As more specific disease entities of the reticuloendothelial system are identified, the number of patients with the designation histiocytosis X will probably decline. This academic phenomenon has been observed during the past few years with disorders of the immune mechanism and with the nonspherocytic hemolytic anemias.

Familial malignant reticuloendotheliosis with hypergammaglobulinemia is a sex-linked disorder described by Falletta and co-workers.[18] Seventeen boys from eight sibships in two generations were affected and died. The clinical course of the illness is less than 2 months in duration and includes fever, hepatosplenomegaly, lymphadenopathy, purpura, jaundice, and hypergammaglobulinemia. Examination of the tissues reveals reticuloendothelial hyperplasia with widespread infiltration of bizarre mononuclear cells and plasma cells.

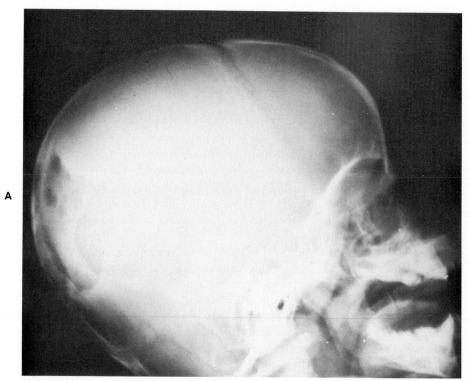

A

Fig. 15-4. Case 7 (Lahey score: 2). This 9-month-old girl was admitted with lumps on the back of her head of 3 months' duration. There was a soft mass 4 by 5 cm in diameter in the area of the right occiput and a similar lesion measuring 5 by 2½ cm in the left occipital region. Two large tender nodes were felt below the right lesion. X-ray films revealed two large and several smaller lytic lesions. Her hemoglobin was 8.6 gm/100 ml. A biopsy revealed eosinophilic granuloma. She was treated with chlorambucil for 2 years with gradual healing of all lesions. Ten years after completion of therapy she is well and has had no further problems. This child is presented to demonstrate the effectiveness of chemotherapy in eosinophilic granuloma. **A,** X-ray film showing the "Swiss cheese" appearance of the skull lesions. **B,** Low power view of the skull biopsy diagnostic of eosinophilic granuloma of bone.

The name *familial erythrophagocytic lymphohistiocytosis* was suggested by MacMahon and associates[38] to describe a group of fatal diseases resembling the Letterer-Siwe syndrome, but whose histopathology is different. Clinically this group of diseases is characterized by fever, weakness, anorexia, and wasting. There is progressive pancytopenia and lymphocytosis with lymphadenopathy and hepatosplenomegaly. Pathologically, erythrophagocytosis is seen throughout the tissues. There is lymphoid depletion in the nodes, with reticulohistiocytic hyperplasia. In other tissues, however, the histiocytic infiltration may be accompanied by lymphoid infiltration. Extramedullary hematopoiesis is also seen.

Unlike familial lymphohistiocytosis and malignant reticuloendotheliosis with hypergammaglobulinemia, histiocytic medullary reticulosis is not a genetically determined disease. It is a rapidly progressive fatal illness that is unresponsive to therapy. Clinical features include fever, hepatosplenomegaly, lymphadenopathy, and pancytopenia. The bone marrow reveals marked erythrophagocytosis.

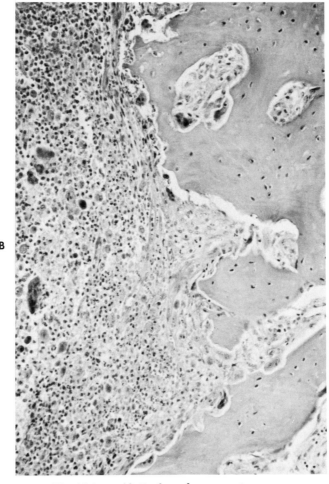

B

Fig. 15-4, cont'd. For legend see opposite page.

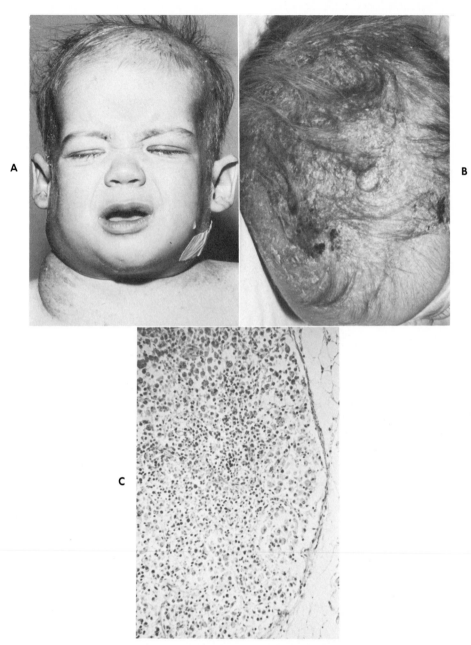

Fig. 15-5. Case 9 (Lahey score: 4). This 11-month-old boy was admitted with seborrhea, draining ears, and enlarged nodes of 6 months' duration. The liver was 8 cm below the right costal margin, and he was anemic. X-ray films revealed a lytic lesion of the left tibia. Skin and node biopsies were diagnostic of histiocytosis X. Therapy was begun with cyclophosphamide, and he received 900 r to the cervical nodes. There was no improvement, and the child died after 3 months of therapy. This case is presented to illustrate the extreme involvement of the most malignant form of the disease. **A,** Appearance of child at diagnosis. **B,** Appearance of scalp at diagnosis. **C,** Low power view of lymph node biopsy with partial obliteration of the subcapsular sinus.

Tissue or postmortem examinations reveal hyperplasia of the histiocytes and reticulum cells with marked erythrophagocytosis.

CLINICAL MANIFESTATIONS

The clinical manifestations or presentations of the child with histiocytosis X are as varied as the pathologic spectrum of this disease itself. Solitary eosinophilic granulomas of bone show predilection for the skull and long bones, with the ribs, pelvis, and vertebrae involved less commonly. Eosinophilic granulomas of the skull generally present as painless swellings (Fig. 15-6). Unilateral proptosis is not uncommonly the first sign of disease. X-ray films of the lesion(s) show sharply demarcated lytic lesions with well-defined borders. The defect may extend through one or both tables of bone (Fig. 15-6, D). Occasionally, large portions of both tables of the skull are missing, creating sizable defects through which the pulsing brain can be palpated. Rarely, there are numerous small lytic lesions, giving a "Swiss cheese" appearance to the skull radiographs (Fig. 15-4, A).

Eosinophilic granulomas elsewhere in the body may present as painful or painless swelling, but the radiographic appearance is the same. Pathologic fractures can occur (case 26, Fig. 15-7; case 29, Table 15-1), and paraplegia from a fractured vertebra has been reported as the presenting complaint.[58]

Eosinophilic granulomas of soft tissue are reported predominantly in the central nervous system[28] and the submucosa of the upper gastrointestinal and respiratory tracts.[17, 40, 55]

Recognition of isolated eosinophilic granulomas of soft tissue is difficult, since they present with symptoms referable to the areas involved. In younger children, chronically draining infected ears are commonly associated with destruction in the mastoid area. Cholesteatomas are common findings in the ear canals. This disease should always be considered in the differential diagnosis of an otherwise healthy child who develops chronic ear or mastoid problems, especially if there is a history of seborrhea or any rashes associated with purpura (Fig. 15-8, A). Fastidious parents sometimes keep the scalp so clean that lesser degrees of skin involvement may be completely concealed by the hair, and an important clue to the diagnosis may be missed.

Polyuria and polydipsia are the symptoms of diabetes insipidus, which may be present at the time of diagnosis or may occur later in the course of progressive disease.

Widely disseminated disease may present with symptoms related to the specific organ involvement. Prominent cervical lymphadenopathy, a rash resistant to conventional therapy, purpura, a pneumonic infiltrate that does not clear, persistent hepatomegaly or splenomegaly, hypersplenism, or a variety of nonspecific complaints such as persistent fever of unknown origin, progressive weight loss, irritability, lethargy, or diarrhea are subtle complaints. These may defy diagnosis until a detailed evaluation is undertaken. In an infant, gingival mucosal lesions that resemble *Candida* infection but resist therapy are strongly suggestive of an infiltrative disease.

DIAGNOSIS

Radiographs of the bony lesions are usually characteristic of the diagnosis, but a biopsy of the lesion, whether bone, skin, liver, lung, or lymph node, is the only definitive diagnostic measure. The site of the skin biopsy can be difficult to choose. What may appear to be an active lesion may reveal only chronic inflammation, whereas a clinically identical lesion may have the typical diagnostic features. For this reason multiple simultaneous biopsies are recommended. Percutaneous liver biopsies are often successful, but an open biopsy may be necessary.

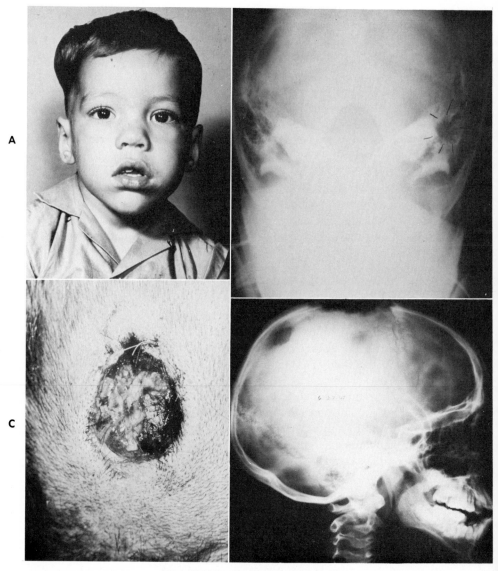

Fig. 15-6. For legend see opposite page.

TREATMENT

Isolated eosinophilic granulomas may resolve and heal spontaneously (cases 18 and 28), or simple biopsy with curettage may be adequate therapy. If there is no evidence of resolution, irradiation to a dosage level of 1000 to 1500 r may be necessary for some bone lesions, but 500 r is often adequate. Alternatively, chemotherapy can be considered if the lesion is not in a critical location such as a weight-bearing bone. In older children with solitary eosinophilic granulomas the choice between radiotherapy and chemotherapy is a matter of judgment, with due consideration of the potential undesirable late effects of radiotherapy (Chapter 4).

Multiple eosinophilic granulomas are more likely to progress to disseminated visceral disease in the younger child. If the evaluation is thorough, many children with multiple eosinophilic granulomas will be found to have evidence of visceral involvement at the onset. These children, as well as those with obvious disseminated disease, are best treated with chemotherapy. Because of the area and volume of tissue to be treated in widespread disease, irradiation is impractical except as supplemental therapy. Occasionally, a more rapid response might be desirable to relieve discomfort or avoid the possibility of spontaneous fractures.

Although spontaneous resolution of generalized histiocytosis has been reported,[36, 39] in most instances the disease progresses inexorably in children who have not been treated.

Antibiotics,[3, 9, 10] corticosteroids,* vinblastine,† vincristine,[25, 54] methotrexate,[16, 20] cyclophosphamide,[54] chlorambucil,[16, 19] nitrogen mustard,[11, 16] 6-mercaptopurine,[16, 30] and daunorubicin[49] have been shown to have beneficial effects, and all have been used successfully in the treatment of children who have been free of disease for years.

---

*References 6, 14, 20, 22, 32, 57.
†References 2, 7, 50, 51, 54, 57.

Fig. 15-6. Case 7 (Lahey score: 2). This 3-year-old boy was well until 3 months prior to his admission when he was noted to have lumps on his head. Two weeks prior to his admission he became excessively thirsty and developed polyuria. On physical examination there were two soft, nonfluctuant scalp masses, one in the right parietal area and one in the right occipital area, measuring 2 by 2 and 4 by 4 cm. The urinary specific gravity was 1.001, and skull films revealed two rounded areas of radiolucency. Therapy was begun with pitressin and chlorambucil. After 2 months a new lytic lesion appeared in the mastoid. The three areas were treated with 1600 r in 5 days, and the chlorambucil was continued for 2 years. At that time all lesions were healed. At 10 years of age he developed a 3 by 4 cm depressed, ulcerated area of the scalp that pulsated with each heartbeat and bulged with increasing intracranial pressure. X-ray films showed a lytic lesion extending through both tables of bone. He received 1500 r in 5 days with complete healing of the lesion. When the patient was 11 years old, a mass in the right posterior parietal area was treated with 1300 r and has subsequently healed completely. He has now been well for 3 years, and his diabetes insipidus is well controlled with pitressin tannate in oil. This case is presented to demonstrate the recurrent nature of the disease in some children and to emphasize the necessity for periodic examination. A, Appearance of child with painless swelling of scalp at the time of diagnosis. B, Lytic lesion in the mastoid area, which appeared while the child was being treated with chemotherapy. C, Depressed ulcerated area of scalp, corresponding to the x-ray film shown in D. D, Lateral view of skull showing the lytic lesion extending through both tables of bone. (Courtesy Department of Medical Photography, St. Luke's Episcopal Hospital and Texas Children's Hospital.)

The Southwest Cancer Chemotherapy Study Group recently evaluated vincristine, vinblastine, and cyclophosphamide in the treatment of histiocytosis. Three of 6 patients treated with vincristine achieved complete remission and had no recurrent disease after the drug was discontinued; 7 of 20 achieved complete remission when vinblastine was used; however, 2 have had recurrent disease. Nine of 20 treated with cyclophosphamide achieved complete remission, but 1 later relapsed.

The ranges of drug dosages that have been commonly used are as follows:

Chlorambucil: 0.1 to 0.2 mg/kg/day PO   Prednisone: 2.2 mg/kg/day PO
Cyclophosphamide: 2.5 to 5 mg/kg/day PO   Vinblastine: 5 to 6.5 mg/M^2/wk IV
Methotrexate: 2.5 to 5 mg/day PO   Vincristine: 1.5 to 2 mg/M^2/wk IV

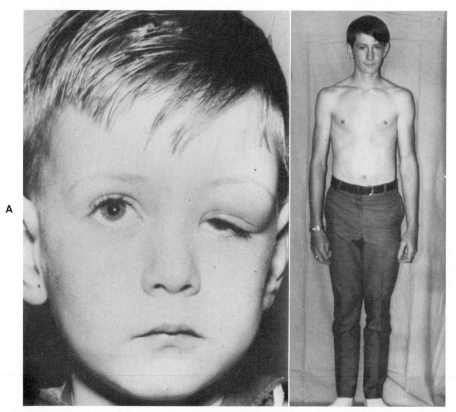

Fig. 15-7. Case 26 (Lahey score: 1). This 3½-year-old boy was admitted with low back pain. There was tenderness over L₁ and a soft tissue mass to the left of L₁. A skeletal survey revealed a compression fracture of L₁. A biopsy was diagnostic of eosinophilic granuloma. He received 1000 r in 1 week to the L₁ area with gradual healing of the lesion and complete remission of pain. Three months later he developed orbital swelling and was found to have two lytic lesions in the frontal area that were treated with 800 r in 2 days. Slow progressive healing occurred during the next year. There was complete healing of all lytic lesions of bone, and there has been no other involvement. This boy is now a 17-year-old "broncobuster" in the rodeo circuit; his case is presented to demonstrate the effectiveness of radiotherapy in localized disease and to show that normal function is returned with healing. **A,** Eosinophilic granuloma of orbit presenting as painless swelling. **B,** Thirteen years after therapy the spine and skull lesions have healed with no residual defects.

The toxicity of these drugs is discussed in Chapter 6.

Cyclophosphamide, vinblastine, and vincristine are generally considered to be the drugs of choice in the treatment of histiocytosis, although the results with chlorambucil have been good. Corticosteroids are particularly useful when there are large areas of skin involvement with secondary infection and inflammation. They may also be particularly helpful with pulmonary disease or in combination with another drug at the onset of therapy when the children may be suffering inanition.

The most important consideration in the treatment of histiocytosis is that the response to therapy may be slow. The gradual improvement that is seen may be marked by episodes of increased disease activity or new areas of involvement. These minor exacerbations should be not considered an indication that the drug has failed, unless there is progressive systemic deterioration or rapid progression of disease in multiple areas of involvement.

If the patient's general condition improves, but a localized soft tissue infiltrate or bone lesion appears to remain active, low-dose, small-field radiation therapy can be of great value, as can a short course of corticosteroids. X-ray

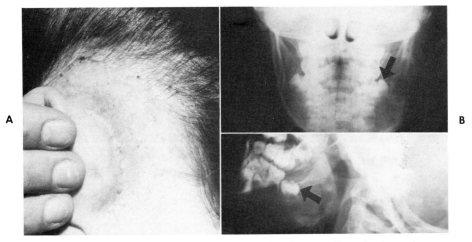

Fig. 15-8. Case 25 (Lahey score: 2). This 3-year-old girl was well until 15 months prior to admission when she had a mastoidectomy for chronic otitis. Twelve months later she was noted to have swelling of the left side of the mandible. The left side of the mandible was more prominent than the right, and a papular rash was noted behind both ears. A skeletal survey showed a smooth lucent defect in the right temporal bone, a defect in the mandible, and an irregular lesion of the left femur. Tissue sections of the original mastoid biopsy were diagnostic of eosinophilic granuloma on reexamination. Therapy with chlorambucil resulted in initial improvement; however, after 1 year of therapy the lesions began expanding rapidly, there was a marked increase in the infiltration of scalp and nodes, and she became anemic and thrombocytopenic. Therapy was changed to vinblastine and prednisone, again with initial improvement, rapidly followed by increasing bone disease, hepatosplenomegaly, and pulmonary infiltrates. She died of sepsis 4 months after the institution of therapy with vinblastine and prednisone. This case is presented to demonstrate progressive disease that was apparently resistant to therapy. A, Papular infiltrative rash behind the ears. B, Destructive lesion on mandible with floating teeth marked by arrows. (Courtesy Department of Medical Photography, St. Luke's Episcopal Hospital and Texas Children's Hospital.)

therapy has been of particular benefit in gingival lesions (case 13 and Fig. 15-9).

Because there has been so much variability in the classifications of these diseases and no less difficulty in staging them within groups, it is virtually impossible to compare the results of therapy from one institution to the next.

In our experience treatment should be continued from 6 months to 1 year after there is no demonstrable disease activity. The child should be examined at frequent intervals for many years after therapy is discontinued.

COMPLICATIONS

Diabetes insipidus is one of the classic complications of histiocytosis X, although it is a clinical impression that the frequency is declining since the advent of chemotherapy.[19] Although this is a serious complication, recognition is not difficult, and it can be controlled in most patients with intramuscular vaso-

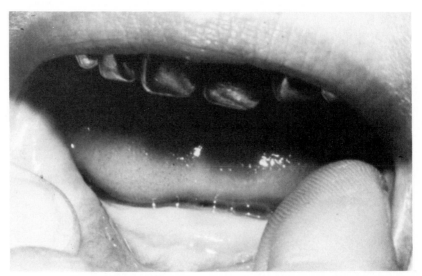

Fig. 15-9. This 15-month-old boy had been well until 2 months prior to referral when his parents noticed that his left ear was displaced. A biopsy of the left mastoid was diagnostic of eosinophilic granuloma. His x-ray films also revealed three radiolucent areas in the parietal bone that were suggestive of additional lesions. He was treated with cyclophosphamide for 10 months with early improvement in the mastoid area, then progression. In addition, soft tissue masses developed in the gingivae. Therapy was changed to vinblastine, and he received 3800 r in four courses to the gums during the next 15 months. During the first year of therapy with vinblastine, his liver became palpable 4 cm below the right costal margin; however, his liver function studies were normal, and the liver gradually returned to normal size. He was entirely asymptomatic for 1 year and had been treated with vinblastine for a total of 27 months when the drug was discontinued. All lower teeth were lost, as were the maxillary molars. His upper teeth were capped, and a prosthesis was made. He has been free from disease for 12 months since the drug was discontinued. This case is presented to demonstrate the conversion of an isolated bone lesion to generalized disease and the response to combined therapy. The photograph shows the absence of lower teeth and steel-capped upper incisors. (Courtesy Department of Medical Photography, St. Luke's Episcopal Hospital and Texas Children's Hospital.)

pressin (Pitressin) tannate in oil or with vasopressin nasal spray. The dose and frequency of administration must be tailored to the child. Irradiation therapy has been given to the hypothalamic area with amelioration of symptoms, but most children will be dependent on vasopressin for life. Growth failure also may result from hypothalamic infiltration.

In children with widespread disease and basilar skull lesions, consideration should be given to x-ray therapy to the area in an attempt to prevent hypothalamic or pituitary involvement. No categoric recommendation can be made because the response to chemotherapy has been prompt in many cases. Unfortunately, statistical data comparing the value of drug therapy versus radiotherapy are not available.

Like diabetes insipidus, other complications arise because of the site of histiocytic infiltration, with resultant bone or soft tissue damage. The damage is permanent if neural or other nonregenerative tissue is involved. Vertebral collapse can cause scoliosis or rarely paraplegia.[58] Chronic infection of the ears accompanying mastoid involvement may result in sclerosis of the auditory mechanism and hearing loss.

Bony involvement will almost invariably heal without residual defect, unless radiation damage is superimposed or a fracture has healed improperly. Surgical prostheses such as tantalum plates are rarely indicated. Damage to the facial and auditory nerves (case 21) resulting from infiltration in the mastoid area or surgical procedures is the exception.

Bony destruction of the mandible and maxilla or soft tissue involvement of the gingivae may result in the loss of or damage to teeth (Fig. 15-8, B). If irradiation therapy is required to control local disease in the mouth, secondary tooth buds may be destroyed. In addition, salivary gland fibrosis may occur after irradiation.[42] With local control of the infiltrates, the remaining teeth can be salvaged by capping (case 13 and Fig. 15-9), and improper growth of the mandible and maxilla can be avoided with the use of properly fitted plates or spacers.

Pulmonary involvement is a grave prognostic sign at any age, and even those children who survive this complication may be faced with chronic pulmonary fibrosis, emphysema, and bronchiectasis.

Other soft tissue infiltration rarely leads to chronic disability. Hepatic, splenic, renal, and marrow involvement are common but rarely lead to dysfunction if the basic process is controlled.

Localized involvement of the brain has been reported[8, 47, 53] and must be considered separately from diabetes insipidus as the only evidence of cerebral involvement. Three patients reported by Rube and co-workers[47] were found to have histiocytic infiltrates in the brain at the time of autopsy.

Other complications occur with relative frequency in children with active disease. Hypersplenism can occur in disseminated disease and unless a bone marrow aspiration is performed, it may be difficult to differentiate the pancytopenia of hypersplenism from pancytopenia due to marrow failure because of histiocytic infiltration or bone marrow depression by drugs.

Secondary infection of the skin and lungs is common, as are bloodstream infections. These must be treated aggressively with bactericidal antibiotics, particularly in those children who may be neutropenic.

Table 15-1. Review of 29 cases of histiocytosis X—Texas Children's Hospital (1957-1970)

Case	Age at diagnosis	Lahey score	Presentation	Diagnosis
1	1 mo	3	Lung, gum, skin	Biopsy:gums, skin
2	2 mo	4	Skin, liver, spleen, lung	Biopsy:skin, liver
3	4 mo	2	Skin, bone: multiple skull	Biopsy
4	6 mo	3	Multiple nodes, liver, spleen, anemia	Biopsy:nodes
5	8 mo	3	Skin, node, bone, anemia	Biopsy:skin, bone
6	8 mo	5	Skin, skull, ileum, ribs, liver, spleen, anemia	
7	9 mo	2	Bone, anemia	Biopsy:bone
8	10 mo	3	Nodes, liver, spleen, skin	Biopsy:nodes
9	11 mo	4	Nodes, skin, bone, liver, anemia	Biopsy:skin, bone
10	1 yr	1	Bone: skull, multiple; spine, multiple; femur, pelvis, nodes	Biopsy:bone
11	1 yr	4	Lung, skin, liver, spleen	Biopsy:skin
12	1 yr	6	Anemia, skin, liver, spleen, lung, bone	Biopsy:skin, liver
13	1 yr, 3 mo	1	Left mastoid Liver, gums	Biopsy:bone
14	1 yr, 4 mo	2	Skin, nodes, bone (humerus)	Biopsy:skin, node, bone
15	1 yr, 4 mo	4	Skin, node, liver, spleen, anemia	Biopsy:skin, bone
16	1 yr, 4 mo	2	Skin, pelvis, rib	Biopsy:ileum
17	1 yr, 9 mo	1	1. Bilateral mastoid 2. Diabetes insipidus, skin, liver, spleen, bone	Biopsy:bone
18	2 yr	1	Fracture of sternum, two skull lesions, pelvis (?)	Biopsy:sternum
19	2 yr, 5 mo	1	Bone: 1. Skull 2. Bilateral mastoid	Biopsy:skull
20	2 yr, 6 mo	5	Skull, mandible, diabetes insipidus, nodes, skin, spleen, liver	Biopsy:nodes
21	2 yr, 6 mo	1	Bone:bilateral mastoid	Biopsy:bone
22	2 yr, 6 mo	1	1. Bone:lytic lesion, right frontal area 2. Recurrent right frontal area 2½ yr later	Biopsy:bone

Treatment	Duration of treatment	Results
yclophosphamide	4 mo	Progressive (died)
inblastine	2 mo	
yclophosphamide	1 yr	Well 26 mo posttherapy
yclophosphamide	1 yr	Well 14 mo after drug discontinued
hlorambucil	2 yr	Well 8 yr after drug discontinued
yclophosphamide	1 yr	Well; off drug 6 mo
rednisone, vinblastine	8 mo	Improved; well on drugs; relapse if tapered
hlorambucil	2 yr	Well 10 yr after therapy stopped
yclophosphamide, prednisone	6 mo	Died (pneumonia)
yclophosphamide, prednisone	3 mo	Died of progressive disease and sepsis
hlorambucil, triamcinolone	5 mo	Progressive disease to involve lung, liver, spleen, kidney; death secondary to sepsis
rednisone, vinblastine	1 mo	Progressive disease and death 2 mo after diagnosis
yclophosphamide	1 mo	
hlorambucil	7 mo	Partial response, then relapse
inblastine, prednisone	15 mo	In partial remission on drugs
yclophosphamide	10 mo	Partial healing, then progression
inblastine, 750 r in 3 days to mastoid, 3100 r in four courses to gingiva	27 mo	Complete remission; off drugs 6 mo
hlorambucil	2 yr	Complete remission; well 6 yr after drug discontinued
yclophosphamide	1 yr	Complete remission; well; off drugs 6 mo
yclophosphamide	1 yr	Healed lesions; well; off drugs 4 mo
yclophosphamide	10 mo	Partial remission; developed hepatitis that resolved when cyclophosphamide discontinued then lost to follow-up study
inblastine, prednisone	18 mo	Good response, then progression; lost to follow-up study
o therapy		All healed; well 11 yr after diagnosis
hlorambucil, 900 r in 5 days to skull	4 mo	Healing of old lesion; relapse with new lesion
yclophosphamide	6 mo	Cyclophosphamide cystitis
hlorambucil	4 yr	Drug change; well; off drugs 5 yr
ultiple courses of x-ray therapy (total unknown), nitrogen mustard		Died 9 mo later with progressive disease
hlorambucil	2 yr	Complete healing; residual facial palsy; residual deafness; well 4 yr after drug discontinued
hlorambucil	3 mo	Complete healing
-ray therapy (1000 r in 9 days)		Complete healing; well 3½ yr after x-ray therapy

Continued.

Table 15-1. Review of 29 cases of histiocytosis X—Texas Children's Hospital

Case	Age at diagnosis	Lahey score	Presentation	Diagnosis
23	3 yr	2	Diabetes insipidus, lytic lesions of skull	X-ray film: multiple skull lesions; diabetes insipidu
			Multiple skull (1967)	
24	3 yr	2	Skull, spleen	Biopsy:skull
25	3 yr	2	Mastoiditis (16 mo), then large nodes, skin Bone:mandible, skull, femur, anemia	Biopsy:bone
26	3 yr, 6 mo	1	1. Fracture, L_1 2. Skull	Biopsy
27	3 yr, 11 mo	1	Bone:solitary skull	Biopsy
28	6 yr, 6 mo	1	Collapsed vertebra	X-ray film
29	7 yr	1	D_8 collapse	Biopsy:bone

PROGNOSIS

The prognosis of this group of diseases has changed greatly since the introduction of chemotherapy. The prognosis of even the disseminated form of the disease is no longer "very grave, if not hopeless."[16] It is still grave, but long-term remission and presumed cures are now possible even with widespread disease. Because late recurrences are occcasionally observed (case 23, Fig. 15-6), the term *cure* is used with reservation.

The prognosis of children with isolated eosinophilic granuloma of bone is excellent, no matter what form of therapy, if any, is used (cases 18 and 28). Serial radiographs of these patients during healing sometimes result in the discovery of one or more bone lesions in other sites that, in retrospect, were present at the time of diagnosis but were too vague to identify.

The prognosis of children with multiple eosinophilic granulomas restricted to bone is also good. In the younger children, however, transition from multiple eosinophilic granulomas to disseminated disease with increased histiocytic infiltration of bone and viscera is not uncommon (case 13, Fig. 15-9).

The prognosis in children with multiple bone and visceral involvement (skin, bone marrow, lymph nodes, liver, spleen, and lungs) is more guarded. The more extensive the visceral involvement, particularly in infants, the worse the prognosis.

The prognosis is extremely unpredictable in those patients with varying degrees of visceral involvement but no bone involvement. Two infants, both of whom had lesions dating to the time of birth, were treated identically (case

1957-1970)—cont'd

Treatment	Duration of treatment	Results
hlorambucil, 1962—booster of x-ray therapy (1600 r in 5 days to skull lesion)	2 yr	
ost to follow-up study for 5 years 500 r in 5 days (healing) 968—right parietal (1300 r in 8 days)		Well 3 yr after last radiation therapy
hlorambucil	2 yr	Well 8 yr after drugs discontinued
hlorambucil	14 mo	Some improvement, then developed hypersplenism
inblastine, prednisone	4 mo	Mixed response, then progression (liver, spleen, lungs, etc.); death secondary to sepsis
-ray therapy (200 × 5), 1000 r in 1 wk mo later 800 r in 2 days		Well 13 yr after radiation
-ray therapy (2500 r in 10 days), chlorambucil	1 yr	Well 2 yr after drug discontinued
ealing when first seen		Not treated; well 3 yr
-ray therapy (2000 r in 7 days)		Well 6 yr after therapy

1, Fig. 15-2; case 2, Fig. 15-3). One is still living and free of disease, whereas the other died of progressive disease within 7 months.

If the classification system originated by Lahey and more recently utilized by Lucaya[37] is applied to the patients reported here (Tables 15-1 and 15-2), the results are similar. In this system, which evaluates the extent of involvement and its relationship to prognosis, a score of 1 was given for involvement of each of the following: (1) skin, (2) liver, (3) spleen, (4) lung, (5) pituitary, (6) skeleton, (7) anemia and/or leukopenia or increased white blood count, and (8) thrombocytopenia or hemorrhagic tendency. The sum can then be related to the question in point (i.e., age at onset, response to therapy, or survival). This also allows comparison of data from different centers as pointed out by Lucaya.

Table 15-1 summarizes the data for 29 patients representing our total experience arranged to illustrate the relationship between increasing age and Lahey scores. The higher Lahey scores are concentrated under 1½ years of age. There were seven deaths in this group. Five occured at 1 year of age or younger; however, four of those five occurred between 10 and 12 months of age.

The Lahey scores of our patients were based on those findings that were present at the time of diagnosis. These scores, although generally lower than those of Lahey and Lucaya, fall into the same age-related pattern.

If Lahey scores are applied to those patients for whom there is sufficient clinical data from several recent series,[4, 5, 24, 26, 44] the pattern of scores with relationship to age remains constant. The cure rate and survival related to age

Table 15-2. Lahey score and survival*

		Status	
Score	Number of patients	Alive	Dead
1	11	10	1
2	7	7	
3	4	2	2
4	4	2	2
5	2	1	1
6	1	1	
	29	23	6

*Survival 2 years with no active disease.

are also constant: the younger the child or the more widespread the disease, the poorer the prognosis (Table 15-2).

In spite of the significance of age and degree of involvement with regard to prognosis, it should be emphasized that remissions or "cures" are possible (case 2, Fig. 15-3; case 4).

SUMMARY

Histiocytosis X is a term used to designate a spectrum of diseases of the reticuloendothelial system whose basic pathology is the infiltration and proliferation of histiocytes in normal tissues. The process may be localized or disseminated, but the natural history of most cases suggests that it is a systemic disease. Thus histiocytosis X is an arbitrary term that is useful to describe a group of patients with interrelated diseases of unknown etiology.

Localized disease, seen more commonly in older children, has had and still has an excellent prognosis. More generalized disease occurs with greater frequency in younger children and has a poorer outlook. The present use of chemotherapeutic agents has greatly improved the overall prognosis.

REFERENCES

1. Abt, A. F., and Denenholz, E. J.: Letterer-Siwe's disease. Splenohepatomegaly associated with widespread hyperplasia of nonlipoid-storing macrophages; discussion of the so-called reticulo-endothelioses, Am. J. Dis. Child. **51**:499-522, 1936.
2. Al-Rashid, R. A.: Successful treatment of an infant with Letterer-Siwe disease with vinblastine sulfate, Clin. Pediatr. **9**:494-496, 1970.
3. Aronson, R. P., and Lond, M. B.: Streptomycin in Letterer-Siwe's disease, Lancet **1**:889-890, 1951.
4. Avery, M. E., McAfee, J. G., and Guild, H. G.: The course and prognosis of reticuloendotheliosis (eosinophilic granuloma, Schüller-Christian disease and Letterer-Siwe disease). A study of forty cases, Am. J. Med. **22**:636-652, 1957.
5. Avioli, L. V., Lasersohn, J. T., and Lopresti, J. M.: Histiocytosis X (Schüller-Christian disease): a clinico-pathological survey, review of ten patients and the results of prednisone therapy, Medicine **42**:119-147, March, 1963.
6. Bass, M. H., Sapin, S. O., and Hodes, H. L.: Use of cortisone and corticotropin (ACTH) in the treatment of reticuloendotheliosis in children, Am. J. Dis. Child. **85**:393-403, 1953.
7. Beier, F. R., Thatcher, L. G., and Lahey, M. E.: Treatment of reticuloendotheliosis with vinblastine sulfate. Preliminary report, J. Pediatr. **63**:1087-1092, 1963.
8. Bernard, J. D., and Aguilar, M. J.: Localized hypothalamic histiocytosis X. Report of a case, Arch. Neurol. **20**:368-372, 1969.

9. Bierman, H. R.: Apparent cure of Letterer-Siwe disease. Seventeen-year survival of identical twins with nonlipoid reticuloendotheliosis, J.A.M.A. 196:156-158, 1966.

10. Bierman, H. R., Lanman, J. T., Dod, K. S., Kelly, K. H., Miller, E. R., and Shimkin, M. B.: The ameliorative effect of antibiotics on nonlipoid reticuloendotheliosis (Letterer-Siwe disease) in identical twins, J. Pediatr. 40:269-284, 1952.

11. Blattner,, R. J.: Reticuloendotheliosis, Postgrad. Med. 12:427-435, 1952.

12. Castleman, B., and McNeely, B. U.: Case records of the Massachusetts General Hospital, case 17-1970, N. Engl. J. Med. 282:917-925, 1970.

13. Christian, H. A.: Defects in membranous bones, exophthalmos and diabetes insipidus; an unusual syndrome of dyspituitarism, Med. Clin. North Am. 3:849-871, 1920.

14. Cox, P. J. N.: A case of Letterer-Siwe disease treated with cortisone, Great Ormond St. J. 19(10):104-111, 1955-1956.

15. Cunningham, J.: Hand-Schüller-Christian disease and Kay's triad, N. Engl. J. Med. 282: 1325-1326, 1970.

16. Dargeon, H. W. K.: Reticuloendothelioses in childhood. A clinical survey, Springfield, Ill., 1966, Charles C Thomas, Publisher.

17. Edwards, W. C., and Reed, R. E.: Chronic disseminated histiocytosis X with involvement of the eyelid, Survey Ophthal. 13:335-344, 1969.

18. Falletta, J .M., Fernbach, D. J., Singer, D. B., South, M. A., Landing, B. H., Heath, C. W., Jr., Shore, N. A., and Barrett, F. F.: A fatal x-linked recessive reticuloendothelial syndrome with hyperglobulinemia; "x-linked recessive reticuloendotheliosis," J. Pediatr. (in press).

19. Fernbach, D. J.: Personal experience.

20. Freud, P.: Treatment of reticuloendotheliosis. Use of corticosteroids and antifolic acid compounds, J.A.M.A. 175:106-109, 1961.

21. Glass, A. G., and Miller, R. W.: U. S. mortality from Letterer-Siwe disease, 1960-1964, Pediatrics 42:364-367, 1968.

22. Goldberg, L. C., and Diamond, A.: Letterer-Siwe disease. Report of a case emphasizing effective corticosteroid therapy, Arch. Dermatol. 92:561-565, 1965.

23. Hand, A., Jr.: Polyuria and tuberculosis, Arch. Pediatr. 10:673-675, 1893.

24. Henderson, J. I.: Histiocytic reticulosis. A review of 20 patients in the paediatric age range, Med. J. Aust. 2:485-488, 1969.

25. Hertz, C. G., and Hambrick, G. W., Jr.: Congenital Letterer-Siwe disease. A case treated with vincristine and corticosteroids, Am. J. Dis. Child. 116:553-556, 1968.

26. Hoh, T. K.: Histiocytosis X in Singapore children, Singapore Med. J. 9:151-160, Sept., 1968.

27. Kay, T. W.: Acquired hydrocephalus with atrophic bone changes, exophthalmos, and polyuria (with presentation of the patient), Pa. Med. J. 9:520-521, 1905-1906.

28. Kepes, J. J., and Kepes, M.: Predominantly cerebral forms of histiocytosis-X. A reappraisal of "Gagel's hypothalamic granuloma," "granuloma infiltrans of the hypothalamus" and "Ayala's disease" with a report of four cases, Acta Neuropathol. (Berl.) 14:77-98, Sept., 1969.

29. Lahey, M. E.: Prognosis in reticuloendotheliosis in children, J. Pediatr. 60:664-671, 1962.

30. Lahey, M. E.: Comparison of three treatment regimens in histicytosis X in children, Proceedings of the International Cancer Congress, Houston, Texas, May, 1970.

31. Letterer, E.: Aleukämische Retikulose. (Ein Beitrag zu den proliferativen Erkrankungen des Retikuloendothelialapparates.), Frankfurt. Z. Pathol. 30:377-394, 1923.

32. Levin, H.: The use of cortisone in the treatment of reticuloendotheliosis. Cases from the pediatric service of the Valley Forge Army Hospital, Phoenixville, Pa., J. Pediatr. 46:531-538, 1955.

33. Lichtenstein, L.: Histiocytosis X. Integration of eosinophilic granuloma of bone, "Letterer-Siwe disease," and "Schüller-Christian disease" as related manifestations of a single nosologic entity, Arch. Pathol. 56:84-102, July, 1953.

34. Lichtenstein, L.: Histiocytosis X (eosinophilic granuloma of bone, Letterer-Siwe disease, and Schüller-Christian disease), J. Bone Joint Surg. 46-A:76-90, 1964.

35. Lieberman, P. H., Jones, C. R., Dargeon, H. W. K., and Begg, C. F.: A reappraisal of

eosinophilic granuloma of bone, Hand-Schüller-Christian syndrome and Letterer-Siwe syndrome, Medicine **48**:375-400, 1969.

36. Lightwood, R., and Tizard, J. P. M.: Recovery from acute infantile non-lipoid reticulo-endotheliosis (?Letterer-Siwe disease), Acta Paediatr. Suppl. **100**:453-468, 1954.

37. Lucaya, J.: Histiocytosis X, Am. J. Dis. Child. **121**:289-295, 1971.

38. MacMahon, H. E., Bedizel, M., and Ellis, C. A.: Familial erythrophagocytic lympho-histiocytosis, Pediatrics **32**:868-879, 1963.

39. Meenan, F. O., and Cahalane, S. F.: Spontaneous resolution of histiocytosis X. Report of a case, Arch. Dermatol. **96**:532-535, 1967.

40. Meranus, H., Carlin, R., Surprenant, P., and Seldin, R.: Histiocytosis X. Problems in diagnosis, Oral Surg. **26**:759-768, 1968.

41. Miller, D. R.: Familial reticuloendotheliosis: concurrence of disease in five siblings, Pediatrics **38**:986-995, 1966.

42. Moss, W. T., and Brand, W. N.: Therapeutic radiology. Rationale, technique, results, ed. 3, Saint Louis, 1969, The C. V. Mosby Co.

43. Oberman, H. A.: Idiopathic histiocytosis. A clinicopathologic study of 40 cases and review of the literature on eosinophilic granuloma of bone, Hand-Schüller-Christian disease and Letterer-Siwe disease, Pediatrics **28**:307-327, 1961.

44. Perttala, Y., Holsti, L. R., and Rissanen, P. M.: Histiocytosis X (reticuloendotheliosis), Radiol. Clin. Biol. **36**:53-64, 1967.

45. Reid, M. J., and Gottlieb, B.: Congenital histiocytosis X, Calif. Med. **111**:275-278, 1969.

46. Rosenstock, H. A., Sandor, I. M., and Hoenecke, H.: Acute histiocytic medullary reticulosis in a pubescent girl, Tex. Med. **65**:56-59, Aug., 1969.

47. Rube, J., Pava, S. D. L., and Pickren, J. W.: Histiocytosis X with involvement of brain, Cancer **20**:486-492, 1967.

48. Schüller, A.: Über eigenartige Schädeldefekte im Jugendalter, Fortschr. Roentgenstr. **23**: 12-18, 1915-1916.

49. Segni, G., Mastrangelo, R., and Tortorolo, G.: Daunomycin in Letterer-Siwe's disease, Lancet **2**:461, 1968.

50. Sharp, H., White, J. G., and Krivit, W.: "Histiocytosis X" treated with vinblastine sulfate (NSC-49842), Cancer Chemother. Rep. **39**:53-59, July, 1964.

51. Siegel, J. S., and Coltman, C. A.: Histiocytosis X: response to vinblastine sulfate, J.A.M.A. **197**:123-126, 1966.

52. Siwe, S. A.: Die Reticuloendotheliose—ein neues Krankheitsbild unter den Hepatospleno-megalien, Z. Kinderheilkd. **55**:212-247, 1933.

53. Smolik, E. A., Devecerski, M., Nelson, J. S., and Smith, K. R.: Histiocytosis X in the optic chiasm of an adult with hypopituitarism. Case report, J. Neurosurg. **29**:217-227, 1969.

54. Starling, K. A., Donaldson, M. H., Haggard, M. E., Vietti, T. J., and Sutow, W. W.: Therapy of histiocytosis X with vincristine, vinblastine, and cyclophosphamide, Am. J. Dis. Child. **123**:105-110, 1972.

55. Tos, M.: A survey of Hand-Schüller-Christian's disease in otolaryngology, Acta Oto-laryngol. **62**:217-227, Sept., 1970.

56. Vietti, T. J.: Personal communication.

57. Winkelmann, R. K., and Burgert, W. R.: Therapy of histiocytosis X, Br. J. Dermatol. **82**:169-175, Feb., 1970.

58. Yabsley, R. H., and Harris, W. R.: Solitary eosinophilic granuloma of a vertebral body causing paraplegia. Report of a case, J. Bone Joint Surg. **48-A**:1570-1574, 1966.

CHAPTER 16

Wilm's tumor

MARGARET P. SULLIVAN

DAVID H. HUSSEY

ALBERTO G. AYALA

The responsiveness of Wilms' tumor (nephroblastoma) to multimodal therapy employing surgery, radiation, and chemotherapy makes it imperative that all pediatricians and general practitioners be alert to this diagnosis and prepared to render optimal therapy either directly or through referral to a treatment center so that children with this tumor will not be denied their chance of cure, which is real. Although the mortality from this malignant renal tumor of childhood is relatively low, an estimated 42 per 100,000 of the population less than 15 years of age,[47] it is the most common intra-abdominal tumor of childhood. Cases of this tumor that had been described earlier were compiled and reported as a clinical entity by Wilms in 1899—hence the eponym "Wilms' tumor."[73] The response of the tumor to multimodal therapy constitutes the first instance of potential cancer cure in children.

POPULATION CHARACTERISTICS OF CHILDREN WITH WILMS' TUMOR

In a period of just over 18 years ending in March, 1970, 77 patients with Wilms' tumor were treated at the University of Texas M. D. Anderson Hospital and Tumor Institute at Houston (MDAH). Forty-seven children were referred for primary therapy. Thirty other patients were referred for treatment of late or massive metastatic disease. The availability of two active antitumor agents, an improved multidisciplinary approach, and the more aggressive attitudes of investigators make it probable, at the present time, that several of the latter patients would be considered candidates for more definitive therapy. The clinical characteristics and results of treatment in this group of children provide the background for the discussions in this chapter. Complementary data from other sources has been used when available to provide a more comprehensive view.

Age. The 77 children in the MDAH study group were similar in age of onset to children reported in other Wilms' tumor series.* The peak age incidence occurred in the third year of life; 50% of the children had not yet passed their third birthday at the time of diagnosis (Fig. 16-1). The youngest child was 4 weeks of age; this tumor, however, has been described at birth.

Sex. As in other series, the number of boys was greater than the number of girls, with a male:female ratio of 1.2:1. No striking differences have been noted between boys and girls in their response to therapy.

---

*References 6, 35, 40, 54, 62, 72.

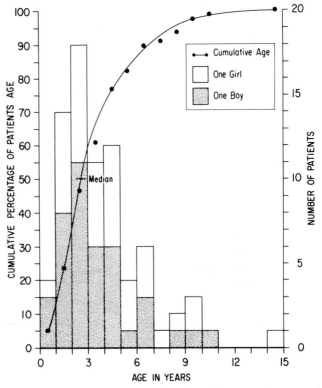

Fig. 16-1. MDAH Wilms' tumor study group: number of patients by age and sex and cumulative age incidence of patients. (Courtesy Medical Communications, The University of Texas at Houston, M. D. Anderson Hospital and Tumor Institute.)

Race. Eight of the 77 children (10%) were of Negro descent. A poor prognosis has been reported for Negro children with acute leukemia,[69] but the influence of race on survival in Wilms' tumor is unknown. It should be noted, however, that 5 of the 8 Negro children had advanced disease, either metastatic or inoperable, at the time of diagnosis.

PATHOLOGIC CHARACTERISTICS

By the end of the nineteenth century the morphologic aspects of nephroblastoma were well recognized; subsequent studies have amplified these early descriptions.[3, 7, 59]

Gross appearance. The tumor may be central or polar in location; the entire renal parenchyma may appear replaced by tumor, with only a rim of compressed normal tissue remaining. On occasion the tumor may appear juxta renal, but these masses are usually attached to the kidney by a small pedicle. The majority of the tumors present as a single, expanding mass surrounded by a pseudocapsule of connective tissue that appears to separate kidney and tumor. Multiple separate nodules are occasionally seen throughout the renal parenchyma.

On section the tumor appears gray-white to gray-pink. Myxomatous areas and patchy hemorrhages are common. Fibrous septa impart a lobular appearance.

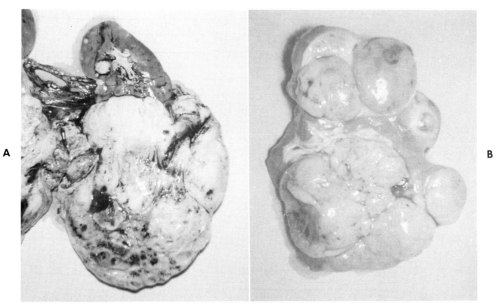

Fig. 16-2. A, Patient 15 (RH): cross section of nephrectomy specimen showing large tumor mass in lower pole of kidney and multiple satellite masses. **B,** Patient 12 (JMcG): cross section of nephrectomy specimen showing bulging nodules throughout kidney with compressed renal parenchyma centrally and at the poles. (Courtesy Medical Communications, The University of Texas at Houston, M. D. Anderson Hospital and Tumor Institute.)

Necrosis, which is a common finding, may lead to cystic degeneration. The cysts may contain either clear fluid or hemorrhagic material. Nephroblastomas may attain very large size, outgrowing the renal capsule and invading the perinephric adipose tissue, the adrenal gland, the diaphragm, the colon, or the liver. Direct extension of the tumor into the calyceal system and renal pelvis, invasion of the renal vein, and metastases to hilar lymph nodes are relatively common.

Extension of the tumor through the renal capsule into surrounding tissues and structures, invasion of the intrarenal vessels, extension into the renal vein and vena cava, and nodal metastases have long been recognized as signs of a poor prognosis. The occurrence of multiple, distinct nodules in the kidney of origin in 8 of the M. D. Anderson Hospital patients would appear to be another ominous finding (Fig. 16-2). Seven of the 8 children in whom this finding was certain have developed metastatic disease, abdominal recurrence, or a second primary tumor. Multimodal therapy was effective in salvaging 2 of these children.

Histologic characteristics. Morphologically, nephroblastomas show varying ratios of mesenchymal to epithelial elements in different stages of maturity. The term *renal blastema* has been used to denote epithelial elements forming abortive or embryonic glomerulotubular structures within nodules of plump hyperchromatic spindle cells. The tubules, when well differentiated, may be lined with low cuboidal or tall columnar epithelium. In some instances the cells show a radial arrangement and appear to form rosettes. Poorly defined masses of epithelial cells may blend imperceptibly with the undifferentiated stroma. Loose spindle myxomatous tissue usually constitutes the major portion of the tumor. In addition, differentiated mesenchymal structures such as striated muscle, cartilage, adipose tissue, and bone may be present singly or in combination.

Tumors with a predominance of epithelial elements, well-formed glomeruloid structures, and tubules appear less prone to metastasize and have been associated with a better prognosis than tumors with a predominance of undifferentiated spindle elements.[59] Data from Roswell Park Memorial Hospital indicates an inverse correlation between favorable prognosis and number of sarcomatous elements.[36] The ratio of epithelial cells to sarcomatous cells could be determined in 26 primary Wilms' tumor specimens from patients in our study group. In these patients improved survival appeared to be related to increasing numbers of epithelial elements. Eleven of our surgical specimens were found to be devoid of glomeruloid bodies. The presence or absence of these structures, however, did not appear to have prognostic significance.

Metastatic tumor has been described as resembling "parent" tumor with greater or lesser differentiation occurring in some cases.[59] Quantitative microscopic comparison of primary and metastatic tumor from the same patient has shown a decrease in undifferentiated and tubular elements in the metastatic deposits and an increase in the fibrous, striated, and smooth muscle components.[4] The influence of abdominal radiotherapy on the histologic appearance of the metastases studied is not fully understood. The effect of chemotherapy on the histologic appearance of metastases has not been reported.

Tumors subjected to radiotherapy generally show a significant decrease in size. Usually necrosis is found to be very extensive, and malignant cytologic characteristics can no longer be distinguished.

From the rather heterogeneous group of tumors known as Wilms' tumor, it is now possible to segregate the mesoblastic nephroma of infancy, which is histologically distinct in its fibroblastic appearance and shows only minimal nuclear pleomorphism and mitotic activity.[5, 8, 18, 55] Although nests of abnormal tubules and glomeruli may be found deep within the tumor, these structures are considered to be normal, trapped elements rather than products of neoplastic proliferation. Even though these tumors may grow to comparatively huge proportions and show evidence of local extension, there is apparently no propensity for metastases, and cure may be achieved with surgery alone. Mesoblastic nephromas may constitute as many as 50% of the renal tumors of early infancy, and the inclusion of these cases in Wilms' tumor series may contribute to the improved survival statistics found in children less than 2 years of age.[8]

SIGNS AND SYMPTOMS OF WILMS' TUMOR

Since early diagnosis is important in determining ultimate outcome, attention has been given to the initial signs and symptoms as reported by the families of our patients. Information was available as to presenting signs and symptoms in 70 patients. An abdominal mass was the first abnormality noted in 29 children, whereas 4 other children were noted to have enlarging abdomens. Only eight of the tumors were discovered by physicians, three apparently during routine examinations. The other 5 children were being examined for other medical reasons. Masses in the other 21 children were usually detected by family members.

Hematuria was the first symptom seen in 19 children, 2 of whom also had fever and 1 of whom had abdominal pain. Eleven of these children are disease free, indicating that hematuria in Wilms' tumor is not a poor prognostic sign as it is in the hypernephroma of adults. Hypertension, which is uncommon, was not seen in our patients. Abdominal pain was the first complaint of 17 children. Pain was precipitated by trauma in two instances. Four of these children also had fever, one complained of headache, and another vomited. Only 7 of the 18 children experiencing abdominal pain as a first symptom are still living. Four children were reported to have anorexia, nausea, vomiting, lethargy, diarrhea and/or fever as initial symptoms.

Laterality. The left kidney was involved in 56% of our 77 cases. More frequent involvement of the left kidney has been noted by other authors, but no explanation is available for this phenomenon.[40, 58, 72] Laterality has important surgical implications, since tumors arising from the left kidney are less difficult to remove because the greater length of the left renal vein facilitates manipulation of the left renal pedicle.

Bilaterality has been reported in as many as 10% to 12% of children in various Wilms' tumor series.[34, 38] Bilateral involvement is detected in approximately two thirds of these children at the time of initial diagnosis[2, 13]; in the remaining third, bilateral involvement usually becomes apparent from 6 to 15 months after diagnosis,[34] although the time interval to involvement of the second kidney may be as long as 10 years.[56]

Associated congenital anomalies. Children with congenital anomalies, particularly hemihypertrophy and aniridia, have been identified as a high-risk population for Wilms' tumor.[25, 26, 48] The frequency of hemihypertrophy was found to be 1:32 among 225 children with Wilms' tumor seen at the Children's Research Foundation in Boston.[26] Hemihypertrophy may not be apparent until several years after the removal of the tumor.[9] One out of 77 in our series had hemihypertrophy.

An excess of congenital aniridia (bilateral) has been found among children with Wilms' tumor; and the converse, an increase of Wilms' tumor, occurs among children with aniridia. In a recent study, 6 of 27 children with aniridia were found to have Wilms' tumor. Aniridia was not present in any of our patients. One had microcephaly, optic atrophy, and mental retardation; another had polydactyly. Although the prenatal mechanism resulting in anomalous development and tumor formation is not understood, clinicians must be aware of this association so that high-risk patients can be observed with special care.

Extent of disease at diagnosis. Clinically evident distant metastases were found at the time of diagnosis in approximately 20% of a group of 168 children with Wilms' tumor.[62] The availability of more intensive and investigative therapy at categoric institutions has been postulated as resulting in a greater incidence of metastases among their referrals. At the M. D. Anderson Hospital the incidence of metastases was 28% in 47 patients referred for primary Wilms' tumor therapy (Table 16-1) and 55% in 77 in the total group. At the Roswell Park Memorial Hospital, 69% of 42 patients with Wilms' tumor had metastases at the time of admission.[36] Among our 13 primary therapy patients with metastatic disease, metastases were restricted to the lungs in 6 children. Three other children had pulmonary metastases as well as metastases to mediastinum[1] and liver (2 patients, 1 with ascites). A fourth child with pulmonary metastases had

Table 16-1. Operability and occurrence of distant metastases in patients receiving primary therapy for Wilms' tumor

	No metastases	Metastatic	Total
Operable	30 (64%)	6 (13%)	36 (77%)
Inoperable	4 (8%)	7 (15%)	11 (23%)
Total	34 (72%)	13 (28%)	47 (100%)

direct extension of the tumor to the subserosa of the colon. A left mediastinal mass of considerable proportion was found in one child with a pleural effusion containing malignant cells. Two additional children had hepatic metastases; 1 of the children had ascites and metastases to the right testicle. In the Roswell Park Memorial Hospital series the lungs and liver were also the most frequent sites of metastatic disease at the time of diagnosis, with lung involved twice as frequently as liver (20 vs. 10 of 29 patients).[36] The mediastinum, extradural space, bone, brain, vagina, soft tissues, and testicles are infrequently noted metastatic sites at diagnosis.

Of our patients, 23% were believed to be inoperable when first seen. The criteria for operability admittedly vary among institutions and even among surgeons at a given institution. At our institution, tumors are considered inoperable when size or fixation makes it reasonably certain that (1) they cannot be delivered surgically without cutting across tumor, in particular when extension across the midline prohibits dissection of the renal pedicle; (2) they cannot be delivered without increased risk of tumor rupture; or (3) the extent of vena caval involvement is such that the affected segment cannot be resected. The availability of chemical methods for preoperative tumor shrinkage that simultaneously treat any known or occult metastatic disease has been enthusiastically accepted by our surgical staff and has perhaps broadened the concept of initial inoperability.[61]

Clinical staging. The great variability in the presenting picture in this tumor has resulted in the formulation of several classification schemes to facilitate the delivery of appropriate therapy to each patient and to permit comparison of data from various institutions. Three of the schemes thus far proposed are shown in Table 16-2 to clarify differences in detail. A fourth classification proposed by Fernbach[19] places emphasis on the presence or absence of tumor emboli in the vasculature of the tumor. The plan devised by the National Wilms' Tumor Study (NWTS) provides for "clinical groups" rather than "stages," with the grouping for each patient to be decided initially by the surgeon.[50] The NWTS groups are similar to the Fleming and Johnson stages with three notable exceptions: (1) NWTS removes liver metastasis from Stage III and includes it with other metastatic disease of hematogenous origin in their Group IV; (2) NWTS removes bilateral renal involvement from Stage III and places it in a new category, Group V; and (3) NWTS includes vena cava involvement in their Group II, along with involvement of renal vessels outside the kidney, whereas Fleming and Johnson place caval involvement in Stage III. On the basis of experiences of this institution, the refinements made by the NWTS seem indicated, but each staging or grouping scheme must further bear the test of time.

Table 16-2. Staging plans for Wilms' tumor

	Garcia and co-workers[28]	Fleming and Johnson[24]	National Wilms' Tumor Study[50]
Stage I	Encapsulated tumor of less than 550 ml in volume; kidney movable; no extra renal spread	Tumor confined to kidney	*Tumor limited to kidney and completely resected;* surface of renal capsule intact; tumor not ruptured during removal; no residual apparent beyond margin of resection
Stage II	No clear demarcation of tumor from renal parenchyma; invasion of collecting system Kidney adherent to adjacent structures without infiltration by tumor Microscopic evidence of tumor thrombi in vessels	Tumor confined to renal fossa Extension beyond renal capsule but no invasion of adjacent viscera or metastases Tumor in renal vessels Positive lymph nodes at renal hilus	*Tumor extends beyond kidney but is completely resected;* Penetration beyond the pseudocapsule into perirenal soft tissue; periaortic lymph node involvement; renal vessels outside kidney substance are infiltrated or contain tumor themselves; no residual tumor apparent beyond the margins of resection
Stage III	Tumor encapsulated but massive (more than 550 ml in volume) Gross or microscopic extension beyond the kidney; complete excision of tumor and its metastases may not be possible Distant metastases present	Tumor confined to abdomen Invasion of adjacent viscera by direct extension Metastases confined to abdomen; tumor rupture; primary tumor not resectable Bilateral Wilms' tumor; involvement of vena cava	Residual nonhematogenous tumor confined to abdomen; tumor biopsied or ruptured before or during surgery; implants on peritoneal surfaces; involved lymphs beyond the abdominal periaortic chains; tumor not completely resectable because of local infiltration into vital structures
Stage IV	—	Metastases outside abdomen (e.g., lung, brain, bone)	Hematogenous metastases; deposits beyond Group III (e.g., lungs, liver, bone, and brain)
Stage V	—	—	Bilateral renal involvement either initially or subsequently

The application of any staging plan calls for the closest cooperation between surgeon and pathologist and a meticulous examination of surgical material. It is noteworthy that age at diagnosis and the histologic type of tumor are omitted from all three staging plans. Data are now being accumulated that indicate that extent of disease at the time of nephrectomy is the most influential factor in determining outcome,[24] and the favorable course in infancy is now attributed to early diagnosis while the tumor remains localized.

PATIENT MANAGEMENT

The palpation of an intra-abdominal mass in a child should result in immediate suspicion of malignant neoplasm, and arrangements should be made for consultation by a team experienced in the management of childhood malignancies. Farber[17] observed that completion of any phase of primary therapy outside the treatment center markedly reduces the child's chances for survival.

Preoperative evaluation and preparation

All efforts should be directed to early surgical removal of the tumor, initiation of systemic chemotherapy using dactinomycin (DAC) or vincristine sulfate (VCR) or both, and radiation therapy to the tumor bed. Surgery is no longer undertaken on an emergency basis as once advocated. A radiograph of the chest and intravenous pyelogram with simultaneous inferior venacavogram should be obtained immediately. Lateral views of the involved kidney should be included in the pyelographic study. The pyelogram is necessary to show the relationship of the tumor to the ipsilateral kidney and to demonstrate the presence of a normal, functioning kidney on the contralateral side. The presence of a renal mass with distortion of the calyceal system is usually evident on the involved side. The inferior venacavogram will be helpful in determining preoperatively whether the tumor has extended retroperitoneally to displace the vena cava or extended into the vessel from the renal vein. Radiographic characteristics of the tumor are clearly described and illustrated in an Eastman Kodak Company publication[33] and in the standard textbook of pediatric radiology.[11] In those cases in which the intravenous pyelogram shows nonfunction, a second dose of dye 30 minutes after the first dose[37] or a "drip infusion pyelogram" may result in demonstration of the tumor. In the few instances when this tactic is unsuccessful, retrograde pyelogram or selective arteriography may be indicated in an effort to rule out cystic disease of the kidney or hydronephrosis.[16, 42, 46] Lymphangiography has not aided in the management of children with this tumor.[29]

Increased diagnostic accuracy has been reported with the simultaneous three-organ scan of liver, spleen, and kidneys.[56a] Developers of the procedure, which requires a single needle stick and 1 hour's time, recommend that it replace pyelography and cavography in the work-up of children with abdominal tumors.

A complete blood count, including platelet count, urinalysis, and blood urea nitrogen level, should be obtained. Right-sided renal tumors will often displace the liver, giving a false impression of size. A liver scan may be helpful in establishing the presence of hepatic metastases. Skeletal survey is optional at this time. Marrow metastases are rare with this tumor; bone marrow examination may be of contributory value in the differential diagnosis.[14, 22, 53] Before surgery is undertaken, any deficits in blood volume and in fluid-electrolyte balance must be corrected. Should severe hypertension exist, medical treatment should be instituted. No attempt should be made to establish a tissue diagnosis preoperatively. Exfoliative cytology of the upper urinary tract is not yet diagnostic. Percutaneous needle biopsy should be avoided due to the propensity of the tumor to seed along needle tracts. No diagnostic laboratory test specific for this tumor is available as yet, but research in this area is encouraging, since hyaluronic acid has been demonstrated in the serum and urine of a patient with Wilms' tumor[49] and an abnormal mucopolysaccharide has been demonstrated in both sera of Wilms' tumor patients and in tumor extracts.[1]

Surgery

If the tumor is deemed operable, a tentative management plan should be formulated so that systemic chemotherapy and radiation to the tumor bed may be initiated without delay. There is a growing belief in some institutions that all children with Wilms' tumor should have two or three doses of VCR pre-operatively.[45] At the present time, however, surgery usually precedes all chemotherapy, and the finalization of the management plan awaits the full surgical report and the evaluation of the gross and histologic findings of the pathologist.

Several surgeons with a large experience in Wilms' tumor have reported their surgical techniques, treatment plans, and results of therapy.[37, 40] From the "team management" point of view, the following aspects of the surgical procedure become important: (1) the transabdominal approach, which may be extended to a combined transabdominal-transthoracic approach, should be used to facilitate inspection of the abdominal contents and clamping of the vessels of the renal pedicle on the involved side prior to dissection of the tumor; (2) the contralateral kidney should be inspected and palpated from both dorsal and ventral surfaces, and suspicious nodules should be biopsied to rule out bilateral disease; (3) the extent of the tumor should be marked with clips so that postoperative radiation therapy fields will be properly designed; (4) the primary tumor should be removed in its entirety if this does not place the patient in jeopardy; (5) any residual tumor should be marked with clips; (6) the abdominal cavity and viscera should be thoroughly inspected for evidence of tumor extension or metastases, any resectable masses should be removed, and the status of the renal vein and vena cava, liver, and nodes of the renal hilus and periaortic region should be clearly documented in the medical record; and (7) rupture and spillage should be reported to the responsible chemotherapist and the radiotherapist.

Routine periaortic node dissection would seem indicated on the basis of the survival rate of 86% obtained after retroperitoneal lymph node dissection in 20 patients, 7 of whom had tumor in one or more nodes.[44] Node dissection would also seem indicated in view of the poor correlation between the gross appearance of the nodes and the histologic demonstration of tumor in the nodes.[32, 44]

Despite the extensive nature of Wilms' tumor surgery, which may include adrenalectomy, partial colectomy, or partial resection of the diaphragm, convalescence is usually rapid and satisfactory. Chemotherapy can usually be started early and continued without interruption during the postoperative period. The prompt initiation of radiation therapy has not significantly complicated wound healing.

Children with Wilms' tumor may have a somewhat increased risk of post-operative intestinal obstruction, and members of the team caring for these children must be alert to (1) signs and symptoms of VCR ileus if that drug is being used, (2) the possibility of radiation-induced edema and obstruction if it is necessary to radiate the entire abdomen, and (3) the possibility of obstruction due to adhesions anytime in the child's future. Among our 47 patients receiving some or all of their primary therapy at this institution, 5 are known to have developed intestinal obstruction that required laparotomy for the following procedures: removal of sutures from abdominal wall to bowel after nephrectomy done elsewhere, lysis of adhesions (2 patients), decompression of ileus, and reduction of jejunal intussusception. Intestinal obstruction due to intussusception has been noted previously in 2 patients, and intestinal obstruction due to adhesions has been reported in 4 children with Wilms' tumor.[30, 39, 43] Since only 1 of the latter group of 4 had obstruction related to tumor recurrence, the authors caution against a presumptive diagnosis of tumor recurrence in patients with malignancies who develop symptoms of intestinal obstruction.

Radiotherapy

Radiotherapy techniques have been developed over a period of time and have been modified with the introduction of each effective chemotherapeutic agent. A variety of treatment methods have been employed, depending on the extent of the disease and the year in which the patient presented. Most patients with apparently localized disease were treated with nephrectomy, postoperative radiotherapy to the renal bed, and chemotherapy. Prior to 1960, preoperative radiation therapy was used to reduce the size of the tumor mass. More recently, chemotherapy has served this function. The current objective of tumor bed or abdominal radiation is eradication of any residual tumor. Presently, M. D. Anderson Hospital patients are treated in accordance with the provisions of the NWTS protocol, as are patients of most all cooperative study group members.

The Stage I patients (Table 16-2) who are randomized to receive postoperative radiotherapy and those showing localized pericapsular extension (Stage II) are treated with cobalt[60] radiotherapy through parallel opposed portals encompassing the renal bed, the entire width of the vertebral bodies, and the top of the ipsilateral iliac crest. The final tumor dose is calculated at the midplane and is related to age as shown here:

Age	Tumor dose
Birth to 18 months	1800 to 2400 rads
19 to 30 months	2400 to 3000 rads
31 to 40 months	3000 to 3500 rads
42 months or older	3500 to 4000 rads

When there is a strong likelihood of intra-abdominal spread (Stage III), part of the irradiation is administered through large portals, usually total abdominal. In total abdominal irradiation the portals extend from the top of the diaphragm to the bottom of the obturator foramina. The femoral heads are shielded. The large portals receive 1500 rads tumor dose in 2 weeks to 3000 rads tumor dose in 4 weeks. The fields are then reduced to the area of apparent disease or to the renal bed for an additional 500 to 1500 rads. The final tumor dose is related to age. The total dose to the remaining kidney is limited to a maximum of 1500 rads. Maximal dose to the liver should not exceed 3000 rads.

Pulmonary metastases are treated with DAC or VCR or both and total thoracic irradiation through parallel opposing cobalt[60] portals. The total thoracic dose is 1250 rads in 2 weeks to 1500 rads in 2½ weeks. An additional 500 to 1000 rads can be delivered to the larger metastatic nodules through small fields. There is no correction for the decreased density of lung. These doses vary in minor respects from those prescribed in the NWTS protocol.

Liver metastases are treated with chemotherapy and with surgery if a limited hepatectomy is feasible. However, if the disease is not resectable because of location or extent, radiotherapy is administered in conjunction with chemotherapy to a dose of 3000 rads in 4 weeks. Smaller volumes can receive additional treatment.

The tumor dose for brain, bone, or lymph nodal metastases is 3000 rads in 3 weeks, with an additional 500 to 1000 rads delivered to reduced portals.

Chemotherapy is of course administered concurrently. For cerebral metastases the entire calvarium is irradiated initially. It is not necessary to irradiate the entire bone for skeletal metastases, but a generous margin is included.

Analysis of radiotherapy data. Between March, 1944, and March, 1970, 77 patients with unilateral Wilms' tumor were treated at the M. D. Anderson Hospital sometime during the evolution of their disease. A 24-month no evidence of disease (NED) rate was used as an indicator of cure. Three of the "cured" patients, however, did develop new disease after this 24-month period. Two of these developed second primary Wilm's tumors 3½ to 4 years after the first diagnosis. The third child, 17 months old at the time of nephrectomy, developed a recurrent tumor in the center of the postoperative radiotherapy treatment field 7 years after nephrectomy, postoperative radiotherapy, and DAC therapy. For the purposes of analysis, all patients free of disease for 2 years have been listed as cured.

In Table 16-3 the 42 patients receiving postoperative abdominal radiotherapy are divided according to the extent of the disease as determined at surgery. In 30 patients there was no evidence of residual abdominal disease after nephrectomy. The remaining 12 patients had known or probable residual tumor. The local control rates and the absolute 24-month NED rates were similar in all groups. Six patients had nephrectomy without postoperative radiotherapy (with or without chemotherapy). Four of these 6 children had positive regional lymph nodes at surgery or other evidence of residual abdominal disease. Three presented with distant metastases initially. In all these cases the extent of the postoperative disease was the factor that resulted in the decision to withhold radiotherapy. Only 1 child had neither intra-abdominal residual disease nor distant metastases at the time of nephrectomy.

An attempt was made to correlate the local control rate with the tumor dose delivered. Since a variety of fractionation schedules were employed, the effective tumor doses have been calculated in terms of the nominal single dose (NSD)[*] as determined by the Ellis formula.[15] This equation relates biologic effectiveness

---

[*]Nominal single dose $= \dfrac{D}{N^{.24} \times t^{.11}}$

Table 16-3. Postoperative radiotherapy in Wilms' tumor (42 patients with 2-year minimal follow-up)[*]

	Percent receiving chemotherapy	Control of abdominal disease[†]	Absolute 24-month NED
No evidence for residual tumor	22/30 (73%)	27/30 (90%)[‡]	19/30 (63%)
Rupture and possible spillage	5/5	4/5	3/5
Local residual tumor[§]	5/7	5/7[‖]	5/7

[*]From Hussey, D. H., Castro, J. R., Sullivan, M. P., and Sutow, W. W.: Radiology 101:663-668, 1971.
[†]Six patients with control of abdominal disease died of distant metastases and had no autopsy.
[‡]Two abdominal recurrences outside the treatment fields.
[§]Includes patients with gross residual tumor, positive regional nodes, or extension to viscera.
[‖]One abdominal recurrence outside the treatment field.

to the total tumor dose and the number of fractions and days in which it is delivered. The units of the nominal single dose are RETs (roentgen equivalent therapy).

In Table 16-4 the 42 patients receiving postoperative abdominal irradiation are divided into four categories of increasing dose. The extent of the abdominal disease and the patient age distribution were similar in all four dose levels. The second column shows the equivalent tumor dose delivered in twenty treatments in 4 weeks. A dose as low as 2000 rads in 4 weeks appears to be sufficient to control abdominal disease if concurrent chemotherapy is administered, since there was control in 14 of 15 patients receiving radiation doses in the range of 801 to 1000 RETs. There was no evidence of an age-tumor response correlation, since the age distribution was the same for all four levels. The abdominal control rate did correlate with field size, since three of the six intra-abdominal failures developed outside the treatment fields.

The importance of field size in thoracic irradiation for pulmonary or mediastinal metastases was also studied. Table 16-5 compares 10 patients treated with total thoracic irradiation to 9 receiving treatment through smaller fields.

Table 16-4. Time-dose relationship for abdominal control with postoperative radiotherapy*

NSD (RETs)	Approximate equivalent dose in 4 weeks (rads)	Receiving chemotherapy	Local control†	Absolute 24-month NED
601- 800	1770-2030	0/3	2/3	1/3
801-1000	2030-2960	10/15	14/15	9/15
1001-1200	2960-3540	13/13	13/13‡	12/13
1201-1400	3540-4130	9/11	10/11§	8/11

*From Hussey, D. H., Castro, J. R., Sullivan, M. P., and Sutow, W. W.: Radiology **101**:663-668, 1971.
†Six patients with control of abdominal disease died of distant metastases and had no autopsy.
‡One patient developed an abdominal recurrence outside the treatment fields.
§Two patients developed an abdominal recurrence outside the treatment fields.

Table 16-5. Thoracic radiation in the treatment of metastatic Wilms' tumor*

Thoracic radiation	Receiving chemotherapy	Control of thoracic disease	Absolute 24-month NED
Total†	9/10	5/10	4/10‡
Less than total†	7/9	2/9	2/9
Unilateral total lung	3/3	0/3	0/3
Small field lung	2/3	1/3	1/3
Mediastinal	2/3	1/3	1/3

*From Hussey, D. H., Castro, J. R., Sullivan, M. P., and Sutow, W. W.: Radiology **101**:663-668, 1971.
†The control of disease at the primary site was similar in both groups: abdominal disease controlled in 6/9 receiving total thoracic radiotherapy and in 4/6 receiving less than total thoracic radiotherapy (4 patients with abdominal status unknown).
‡One patient died of intercurrent disease at 14 months.

The two groups were similar in the extent of abdominal disease, the number of patients receiving concurrent chemotherapy, and the abdominal control rate. In all cases the treatment portals encompassed all known thoracic metastases. The pulmonary disease was more extensive in the patients receiving total thoracic irradiation, since the majority had bilateral pulmonary metastases. The age distribution was slightly older in the group receiving smaller field irradiation. The data suggest that total thoracic irradiation is superior to limited field therapy in the control of known thoracic disease. The metastases were controlled in 5 of the 10 patients in this group. Four of these are alive more than 2 years later. The other child died of intercurrent infection at 14 months and had no evidence of tumor at autopsy. On the other hand, thoracic disease was controlled in only 2 of 9 patients receiving partial thoracic irradiation.

Three patients were treated through unilateral total lung fields to a dose of 1000 to 1650 rads tumor dose in 10 to 15 days. All three received concurrent DAC or VCR. Complete regression of pulmonary disease occurred in each child, but all had metastases in the contralateral lung within 7 months. Similar therapy for the new disease resulted in only temporary control. All died of pulmonary metastases with the primary tumor clinically under control. Postmortem examination in two cases showed no evidence of disease at the primary site.

When total thoracic radiation doses were expressed in terms of the NSD, all patients who received more than 500 RETs (the equivalent of 1150 rads tumor dose in ten treatments in 2 weeks) had complete control of their pulmonary metastases. Nine of these 10 children received concurrent DAC or VCR chemotherapy.

Chemotherapy

Optimal chemotherapy for Wilms' tumor has not yet been defined. At the present time there are no data that would indicate a preference for either DAC or VCR except in preoperative therapy, in which VCR has shown extraordinary antitumor effect in some children. Since firm recommendations cannot be made as to choice of drug and schedule at this time, the attributes and performance of the various agents showing significant antitumor effect in this malignancy will be discussed separately.

Dactinomycin (actinomycin D, DAC). Chemotherapy for Wilms' tumor became a reality in 1954 when Farber and co-workers[17] demonstrated marked regression of pulmonary metastases from a Wilms tumor after treatment with the antibiotic dactinomycin (DAC). The extensive experience of the Boston Children's Hospital with DAC adjuvant therapy in the treatment of Wilms' tumor was summarized 12 years later as follows: (1) 89% of the 53 children with no evidence of metastases at diagnosis who received all therapy at the Boston Children's Hospital had survived 2 years or more with no evidence of disease; (2) 39% of 54 children with no evidence of metastases at diagnosis who received a portion of their primary therapy prior to referral to the Boston Children's Hospital had survived 2 years or more with no evidence of disease; (3) 53% of 15 children with metastatic disease at the time of initial therapy had survived 2 years with no evidence of disease; and (4) 31% of 59 children with late metastatic disease had survived 2 years with no evidence of disease.[17] Meanwhile, DAC had gained widespread acceptance in the multimodal therapy of Wilms' tumor, and improved survival with DAC adjuvant therapy was documented at a number of institutions.[10, 20, 36, 41, 55] The need for long-term DAC therapy was emphasized by a recent study from Children's Cancer Study Group A, which showed that nephrectomy, radiation to the tumor bed, and intermittent courses of DAC over a period of 15 months maintained the disease-free state in 86% of 22 patients.[74] In contrast, only 48% of 23 children receiving a single course of DAC were maintained without evidence of recurrence. The commonly used intermittent schedule calls for DAC, 15 mcg/kg,* intravenously, daily for 5 days, beginning on the day of surgery and repeated at 6 weeks and 3, 6, 9, 12, and 15 months after surgery. Toxicity from this schedule is apparently minimal.

In the treatment of the inoperable Wilms' tumor, DAC alone has not been reported to cause significant tumor regression. Radiotherapy has long been the accepted method of reducing massive tumors to operable proportions. DAC given with radiation doses of 1200 rads to the tumor significantly reduced tumor size in a small series of patients without appreciable morbidity.[68] Surgery after preoperative radiation and chemotherapy was said to be more difficult "due to adhesions between the tumor and surrounding structures, as well as a shortening of the renal pedicle permitting less room for surgical manipulation between the hilus of the kidney and the vena cava."[68]

Attention to the details of DAC administration is necessary to ensure full therapeutic effect and to prevent unfortunate complications. Dactinomycin (Cosmegen) is supplied in 500 mcg vials. The drug is brought into solution by the addition of Sterile Water for Injection, U.S.P. (pyrogen free). Once the drug is reconstituted, it is unstable when exposed to light, and the manufacturer recommends discarding the unused portion of each vial after the dose has been withdrawn. The needle used to withdraw the medication from the vial should not be used for intravenous injection, since minute amounts of extravasated drug may cause marked irritation of the soft tissues. The drug is most safely given to children through "scalp vein" needles that have been inserted into large vein and tested with saline.

The abdominal pain, nausea, and vomiting that occur 4 to 6 hours after DAC injection can be reduced by limiting the daily dose to 200 mcg and extending the time required to administer the total course dose of 75 mcg/kg in older children. Ulcerations of the buccal mucosa usually become apparent after drug administration is complete and heal without incident. Platelet depression may be evident in the 2- to 3-week period after therapy. Thrombocytopenia is more profound when the agent is used in combinations. DAC has the interesting property of increasing the intensity of skin reactions when given simultaneously with radiation or thereafter. On this basis, it is anticipated that the antitumor effect of radiation will also be potentiated by concurrent DAC and radiation therapy. Erythema of the skin of radiation portals has been induced by DAC as late as 7 years after radiation in 1 of our patients. Concurrent DAC and radiation therapy may produce skin reactions of such severity as to interrupt radiation therapy. In teen-aged children intensification of acneiform eruptions is not unusual.

---

*The unit of measure is micrograms, not milligrams, per kilogram of body weight.

Vincristine sulfate (Oncovin, VCR). The antitumor effect of VCR in metastatic Wilms' tumor was demonstrated in December 1961, by the Pediatric Department, MDAH. Through expanded studies conducted by the Pediatric Division, Southwest Cancer Chemotherapy Group, it was possible to demonstrate complete regression of pulmonary metastases from Wilms' tumor in 67% of the patients treated.[64] Regression proved to be temporary in most children unless therapeutic doses of radiation were also given to the areas of involvement. Subsequently, 45% of 22 children receiving combination VCR and radiation therapy for metastatic disease had no evidence of disease 2 years later.[67] These results are similar to or slightly better than results of combination therapy employing DAC in like clinical situations.

In an effort to prevent or successfully manage occult metastases, a pilot study was initiated at the M. D. Anderson Hospital in 1962 incorporating adjuvant VCR therapy into the primary treatment of Wilms' tumor. Early patients received priming doses of VCR, 0.02 mg/kg, intravenously, daily for 5 days, with weekly doses of 0.05 mg/kg for 12 weeks beginning on day 7. Subsequently, the treatment schedule was simplified to the regimen now commonly used, that is, 2 mg/M² (maximum dose, 2 mg), intravenously, weekly for 12 weeks. In 1965, 6 of 7 children who had received multimodal therapy of this type were reported as living and well 11 to 35 months after nephrectomy.[63] By 1969, 11 children had been treated in this fashion with 9 (83%) remaining free of metastatic disease from 4 months to 6¼ years (median, 4½ years).[60] An abdominal recurrence within the radiation field in the child who had remained free of disease over 7¼ years reduced the disease-free survival rate to 73%, with duration of disease-free survival ranging from 3%₁₂ to 8¹¹⁄₁₂ years (median, 6⁸⁄₁₂ years). The unfavorable factors present in each case make the results especially noteworthy.

Striking tumor regression occurring in patients with inoperable tumors who were given VCR in lieu of preoperative radiation was reported in 1967.[61] Fig. 16-3 illustrates such regression. VCR was used in treating seven inoperable tumors occurring in the study group, with the following results: marked tumor regression sufficient to permit nephrectomy, 4 children; regression insufficient to permit nephrectomy, 1 patient (scrotal and liver metastases with ascites); no regression, 2 patients. When the patient with far advanced disease involving liver and scrotum is excluded, regression sufficient to achieve the surgical aim has been achieved in 67% of the children given VCR preoperatively.

Vincristine sulfate (Oncovin) is supplied in 1 mg and 5 mg vials with diluent for reconstitution. If refrigerated, the drug may be kept in the reconstituted state for 2 weeks. The needle used to withdraw the medication from the vial should *not* be used for intravenous injection, since this agent is also irritating to the soft tissues when extravasation occurs. Again, it is recommended that a "scalp vein" needle be used to establish free-flowing venous access prior to injection of the drug. VCR has the unusual attribute among chemotherapeutic agents of producing little myelosuppression. An unusual constellation of neuromuscular disabilities that may occur as toxic side effects include paresthesias in the fingers and toes, jaw or throat pain, weakness and atrophy of the small muscles of the hands and feet, diminution and eventual disappearance of the deep tendon reflexes, particularly in the lower extremities, and wristdrop and

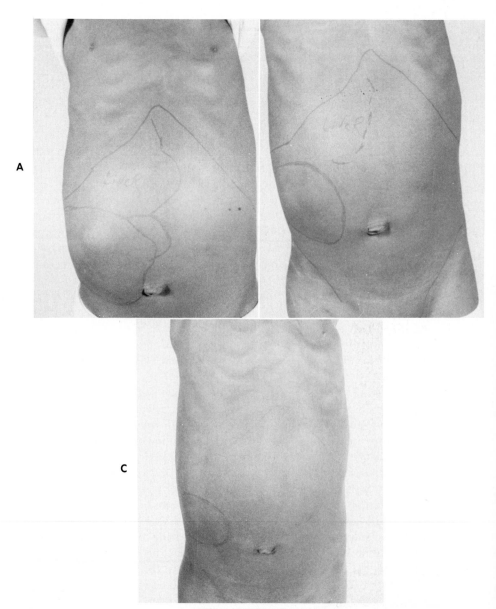

Fig. 16-3. Patient JJ. Serial photographs of abdomen showing outlines of liver and palpable tumor during course of preoperative vincristine sulfate therapy. **A,** October 14, 1970. **B,** October 20, 1970. **C,** October 23, 1970. (Courtesy Medical Communications, The University of Texas at Houston, M. D. Anderson Hospital and Tumor Institute.)

foot drop. These toxic effects are reversible when drug administration is discontinued. Therapy should be withheld as soon as there are indications of wristdrop or foot drop; the other toxicities just listed are not considered indications for cessation of therapy. Constipation and severe abdominal pain occur as VCR side effects somewhat more frequently in older patients than in preschool children. During VCR therapy daily bowel movements must be assured through the use of laxatives and stool softeners. Enemas are indicated if these measures are not successful. Abdominal complaints are also an indication for interruption of drug therapy and downward modification of dosage schedules. Even though the alopecia that occurs in most patients is of no medical significance, the cosmetic implications are enormous at the present time in both girls and boys. A tourniquet may be placed about the head during drug injection and for 10 minutes thereafter in an effort to avert alopecia. Every effort should be made to have an acceptable wig available should the tourniquet technique fail to achieve its purpose.

Cyclophosphamide (Cytoxan). Cyclophosphamide was found to have antitumor effect of low order in Wilms' tumor when first tested using doses of 7.5 mg/kg/day intravenously for 10 to 13 days, followed by daily oral doses of 2.5 mg/kg/day.[31] Data from children given the drug in "pulse" doses (10 mg/kg until the biologic end point of a peripheral absolute granulocyte count of 1000 to 1500/mm³ is achieved) has been more encouraging, and this regimen has had special usefulness prior to radiation therapy.[23] Other cyclophosphamide dosage schedules that have been used include 30 mg/kg intravenously weekly and cyclophosphamide, 30 mg/kg every 2 weeks, alternating with VCR, 2 mg/M² every 2 weeks. Additional data will be required for final assessment of this drug in the treatment of Wilms' tumor; in the meantime the drug may be considered for use in drug combinations as priming therapy for radiation and as an alternate agent in children resistant to VCR and DAC.

Cyclophosphamide has the advantage of various routes of administration—oral, intramuscular, or intravenous. Common toxic side effects include myelosuppression with prompt and predictable recovery, nausea, vomiting, and alopecia. The occurrence of chemical cystitis is an indication for immediate cessation of drug therapy. Fluid intake during cyclophosphamide administration should be more than customary, and an effort should be made to keep the urinary bladder empty by frequent voidings during the day and at least once during the sleeping hours of the night.

Adriamycin. Clinical trials have indicated that adriamycin may have predictable antitumor activity in Wilms' tumor.[70, 75] The manner in which this drug is to be used in treating resistant disease and the ways in which it can be incorporated into combination treatment programs are under investigation. Considerable ingenuity will be required to capitalize on the antitumor potential of the drug while minimizing toxic side effects on the bone marrow and myocardium.

Combination drug therapy. The achievement of additive or even synergistic antitumor effect without prohibitive increase in toxicity through the combined use of antitumor agents of differing toxicities has been a significant advance in the treatment of acute leukemias. The NWTS seeks, through its controlled prospective design, to find which of the two major drugs is the better adjuvant agent in treating Wilm's tumor and to compare combination chemotherapy to either drug alone. The combination treatment program calls for DAC, 75 mcg/kg in 5 days, beginning on the day of nephrectomy, 6 weeks after nephrectomy, and at 3, 6, 9, 12, and 15 months postnephrectomy *and* VCR, 1.5 mg/M^2 weekly for eight doses, beginning on the seventh postnephrectomy day and on the first and last days of each of the DAC courses given 3, 6, 9, 12, and 15 months postnephrectomy.

A second combination adjuvant program that employs repeated courses consisting of DAC, 0.4 mg/M^2/week for 6 weeks, and VCR, 1.5 mg/M^2/week for 6 weeks, followed by VCR every 2 weeks for 6 weeks, has produced encouraging results when tumor had been found to extend beyond the renal fossa but was still confined to the abdomen.[24]

In all combination treatment programs employing DAC + VCR, increased toxicity must be expected, particularly in the postoperative patient receiving radiation. Additive toxicity of VCR + DAC as measured by weight loss was demonstrated in rodents early during the development of VCR.[52] Multimodal treatment programs employing drug combinations call for the closest medical surveillance and individualization of treatment regimens.

Treatment of bilateral Wilms' tumor

The responsible physician must always be alert to the possibility of bilateral involvement in Wilms' tumor. When nephrectomy is performed for presumed unilateral Wilms' tumor, the contralateral kidney should be carefully palpated and, if necessary, freed from its bed for thorough inspection and biopsy of suspicious nodules. In proved unilateral cases the remaining kidney should be monitored by intravenous pyelography at intervals of 3 months for 1 year and at yearly intervals for no less than 5 years.

In assessing the child with bilateral Wilms' tumor the following variables must be considered: (1) volume and geographic location of tumor in each kidney, (2) the apparent discreteness or invasiveness of the tumor nodules, and (3) the mass of conservable, functional renal tissue. Treatment must be individualized in accordance with these variables; all available therapeutic modalities are employed in combination or in sequence as indicated by the clinical findings. When the tumor nodules are discrete and polar in location, partial nephrectomy should be performed and followed by radiotherapy and chemotherapy with DAC or VCR or both. Radiotherapy must be carefully controlled to prevent subsequent radiation nephritis. When diffuse tumor involvement is present, reliance must be placed on radiotherapy and chemotherapy or on bilateral nephrectomy followed by renal transplantation.[13] Despite the enormity of the clinical problems that may present, review of the literature indicates 21 apparent cures among 52 reported cases of bilateral Wilms' tumor.[66]

Treatment of metastatic disease

Successful treatment of metastatic disease can be accomplished by surgical excision when the metastatic disease is limited to a solitary nodule or when multiple nodules are limited to a resectable anatomic segment of an organ.[71]

An unfavorable outcome has been experienced with radiotherapy alone. There is little hope of cure with chemotherapy and radiation unless the latter is

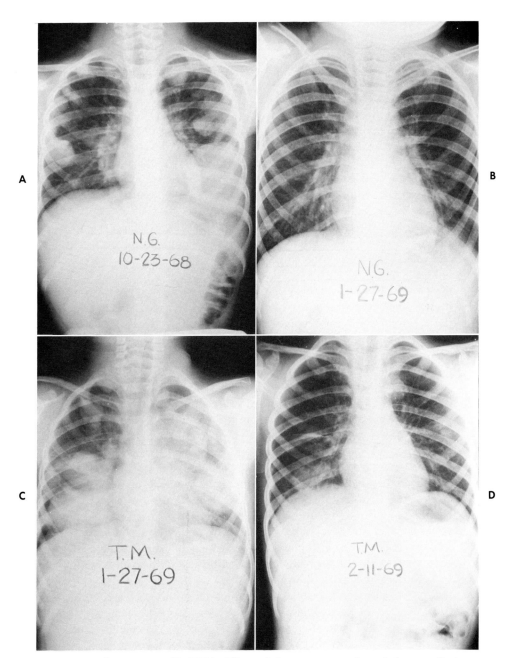

Fig. 16-4. A and **B**, Patient 45 (NG). Effect of dactinomycin and total thorax radiation on pulmonary metastases. Radiograph of chest on October 23, 1968, prior to treatment and on January 27, 1969, prior to second course of dactinomycin. **C** and **D**, Patient 77 (TM). Effect of vincristine sulfate and total thorax radiation on pulmonary metastases. Radiograph of the chest on January 27, 1969, prior to treatment and on February 11, 1969, after completion of radiation therapy as vincristine sulfate therapy continued. (Courtesy Medical Communications, The University of Texas at Houston, M. D. Anderson Hospital and Tumor Institute.)

given to the limit of tolerance to the entire organ of involvement. For example, if pulmonary metastases are present, radiation should be given to "total thorax" fields. If radiation is limited to one lung, an unfavorable outcome may be anticipated.

The evidence supporting adjuvant chemotherapy as a part of the initial therapy for Wilms' tumor is so great that it can be anticipated that children developing late metastatic disease will already have had chemotherapy with DAC or VCR or possibly both drugs. Patients who have had one of the drugs previously should have the alternate drug or both drugs as a part of their therapy for metastatic disease. At present there is insufficient data to recommend either DAC or VCR in preference to the other if the investigator has a choice of agents. Both DAC and VCR, when given in combination with total thorax radiation, are highly effective in producing regression of pulmonary metastases as shown in Fig. 16-4.

Chemotherapy and radiation should be started simultaneously. If DAC is the agent selected, a series of six courses should be given over a period of 12 to 18 months at the same time intervals used in primary therapy. If VCR is to be used, a series of twelve doses should be given at weekly intervals. Some of the poor results obtained at this hospital with the DAC + total thorax radiation regimen may be related to the lack of long-term maintenance therapy in the treatment programs employed in the past. Only 1 of our 8 children given DAC + total thorax radiation survives with no evidence of disease, 2 had complete regression of metastatic nodules with subsequent recurrence, and 5 showed only partial regression of their metastases. All 5 patients treated with VCR + total thorax radiation survive with no evidence of disease, but 1 of this group had a recurrent pulmonary nodule 6 years after initial therapy, which was treated with surgical excision and combination DAC-VCR chemotherapy.

The detection of hepatic or other intra-abdominal metastases shortly after completion of therapy for pulmonary metastases is frequent. At the time pulmonary metastases become evident, the abdomen should be investigated thoroughly with a radiograph of the abdomen (flat plate or plane film), intravenous pyelography, liver function tests, and liver scan. An exploratory laparotomy should be performed if intra-abdominal disease cannot be ruled out at this time.

Liver metastases may be successfully treated in some cases with chemotherapy and radiation, followed by resection of residual tumor. One of our patients had sufficient shrinkage of his solitary liver metastasis with chemotherapy to permit right hepatic lobectomy. Cases with extensive intra-abdominal disease that were apparently cured by sequential, multimodal therapy suggest that greater salvage is possible if there is close cooperation among services in the application of all available treatment modalities. All members of the team caring for these patients should be aware of the poor tolerance for DAC and hepatic radiation after hepatic lobectomy until such time as liver regeneration is complete.[21]

Extradural metastases with spinal cord compression, although infrequent, should be considered in any child with Wilms' tumor who has radicular pain, difficulty emptying the urinary bladder, and/or pain and weakness in the legs. Myelography and prompt laminectomy with removal of the tumor insofar as possible, followed by radiation therapy to demonstrated areas of involvement, can result in full return of function. One of our patients had some return of muscle strength in the legs but no return of bladder function. Another patient whose treatment had been delayed by an erroneous diagnosis of poliomyelitis was not improved by decompressive laminectomy followed by radiation therapy. None of the patients in this series who developed extradural metastases survived.

The treatment of osseous and other rarer, nonresectable metastases is unsatisfactory, and therapy must be individualized in each case. It is of some interest, however, that apparent bone marrow metastases in one of our patients were eradicated as VCR therapy was continued to completion at 12 weeks.

COMPLICATIONS OF THERAPY

Long-term effects of chemotherapy. All side effects of DAC therapy appear to be rapidly reversible, but future use of the drug can be expected to accentuate skin changes and possibly liver changes in previous radiation fields. All side effects of VCR therapy, including severe neuropathy, also appear reversible. Neuropathy is most severe in older children, and full restoration of function may take several years in teen-aged patients. Thus far, no evidence has developed for long-term, latent effects from either DAC or VCR. Even so, these children should be observed closely for unanticipated latent effects as they pass through puberty and begin childbearing.

Growth disturbances after radiation therapy. All children successfully treated for Wilms' tumor can be expected to show some evidence of growth arrest in irradiated areas. Changes increase in severity with increasing dosage and decreasing age of the patient at the time the radiation therapy is given. The orthopedic deformities do not become apparent until some 4 or 5 years after therapy. Inequalities in growth are much more easily appreciated from serial anthropometric photographs of the patient than from physical examination, and photographs should be a routine part of follow-up examinations.

Neuhauser and co-workers[51] have described the following radiographic changes in radiated bone: (1) horizontal transverse lines of increased density, (2) gross irregularity or scalloping of the vertebral epiphyseal cartilage plate, and (3) gross contour abnormalities. Changes were more severe with radiation doses exceeding 2000 r and in children less than 2 years of age when radiated. Vertebral bodies in the radiation field showed a 10% diminution in height; hence the total height of the vertebral column was not significantly diminished.

In an effort to prevent scoliosis the entire width of the vertebral body is irradiated. However, atrophic changes in the irradiated iliac crest, ribs, and soft tissues, including the paraspinal muscles, may result in muscle imbalance and asymmetry. It should be emphasized that the scoliosis occurring with current treatment methods is usually not of clinical significance. In one group of 19 patients surviving 3 to 24 years, curves ranged from 10 to 128 degrees (average, 24 degrees), and surgical correction was required in only three cases.[35]

Radiation-induced neoplasia. Of all children who receive radiation in doses exceeding 1000 rads who survive over 2 years, 5% can be expected to develop a second primary malignant tumor.[65] The incidence of second malignancies has been greatest in children receiving high-dose radiation to fields including bony structures such as that used in treating retinoblastoma. Second malignancies have now been reported in ribs of children treated for Wilms' tumor. In 2 chil-

Table 16-6. Expectations from combination VCR-DAC therapy in multimodal treatment of Wilms' tumor

Chemotherapy	Number and percentage surviving 2 years or more (NED)	
	Primary therapy nonmetastatic disease	Late metastatic disease
Dactinomycin (DAC)	68/107 (63%)	21/59 (31%)
Vincristine sulfate (VCR)	9/11 (73%)	5/13 (38%)
DAC + VCR	90% (calculated*)	57% (calculated*)

$$*RR_{A+B} = RR_A + RR_B \times \frac{(100 - RR_A)}{100}.$$ RR_A = response rate to drug A; RR_B = response rate to drug B; RR_{A+B} = response rate to drug A plus drug B.[27]

dren, retreatment with radiation had been given for recurrent ipsilateral pulmonary nodules.[12, 54] A third child developed an osteoblastoma in a rib that had been included in a previous radiation field, as well as an osteochondroma in the ipsilateral ileum, which was also hypoplastic. Radiation doses for the first 2 children were 4263 and 3168 r; latent periods for 3 children were reported as 3, 8, and 14 years. It is of great interest that the radiation-induced chrondrosarcoma has a basic undifferentiated myxomatous pattern that distinguishes it from the spontaneously occurring chondrosarcoma of childhood.[65]

Long-term follow-up studies for Wilms' tumor patients must be directed to the early detection of second malignancies at a time when treatment by surgical excision may be feasible.

PROGNOSIS

The current prognosis for children with Wilms' tumor would appear to be better than that for any other malignancy of childhood, provided the children receive the benefits of all known effective treatment modalities. The antitumor performances of the two drugs DAC and VCR appear similar, and additive effects in terms of response rate expected might reasonably be anticipated with the use of both drugs in combination (Table 16-6). Based on derived data on DAC from the Boston Children's Hospital[16] and on VCR from the M. D. Anderson Hospital, a survival rate as high as 90% with combination chemotherapy in the primary treatment of Wilms' tumor might be expected.

The NWTS has been organized to provide a mechanism through which combination chemotherapy with DAC + VCR can be compared with either drug alone. It it also hoped that the study will demonstrate whether or not radiation therapy should be given to the tumor bed after complete resection of localized tumors. This question would seem particularly important in view of data from this hospital, which suggest that local control can be obtained with more modest radiation doses than those currently employed.

REFERENCES

1. Allerton, S. E., Beierle, J. W., Powars, D. R., and Bavetta, L. A.: Abnormal extracellular components in Wilms' tumor, Cancer Res. 30:679-683, 1970.
2. Anderson, E. E., Herlong, J. H., Harper, J. M., Small, M. P., and Atwill, W. H.: Bilateral Wilms' tumor: diagnosis and management, Clin. Pediatr. 7:596-599, 1968.

3. Balduin, L., and Schlumberger, H. G.: Tumors of the kidney, renal pelvis and ureter. In Atlas of tumor pathology, Section VIII, vol. 30, Washington, D. C., 1957, American Registry of Pathology, Armed Forces Institute of Pathology, pp. 78-110.

4. Bannayan, G. A., Huvos, A. G., and D'Angio, G. J.: Effect of irradiation on the maturation of Wilms' tumor, Cancer **27**:812-818, 1971.

5. Beckwith, J. R.: Mesenchymal renal neoplasms of infancy, J. Pediatr. Surg. **5**:405-406, 1970.

6. Bjelke, E.: Malignant neoplasms of the kidney in children, Cancer **17**:318-321, 1964.

7. Bodian, M., and Rigby, C. C.: The pathology of nephroblastoma. In Smithers, D. W., and Riches, E., editors: Monographs on neoplastic disease, vol. V, Baltimore, 1964, The Williams & Wilkins Co., pp. 219-234.

8. Bolande, R. P., Brough, A. J., and Izant, R. J., Jr.: Congenital mesoblastic nephroma of infancy, Pediatrics **40**:272-278, 1967.

9. Boxer, L. A., and Smith, D. L.: Wilms' tumor prior to onset of hemihypertrophy, Am. J. Dis. Child. **120**:564-565, 1970.

10. Burgert, E. O., Jr., and Glidewell, O.: Dactinomycin in Wilms' tumor, J.A.M.A. **199**:464-468, 1967.

11. Caffey, J.: Pediatric x-ray diagnosis, ed. 5, Chicago, 1967, Year Book Medical Publishers, Inc., pp. 664-667.

12. Cohen, J., and D'Angio, G. J.: Unusual bone tumors after roentgen therapy of children: two case reports, Am. J. Roentgenol. **86**:502-512, 1961.

13. DeLorimier, A. A., Belzer, F. O., Kounty, S. L., and Kushner, J. H.: Simultaneous bilateral nephrectomy and renal allotransplantation for bilateral Wilms' tumor, Surgery **64**:850-855, 1968.

14. Delta, B. G., and Pinkel, D.: Bone marrow aspiration in children with malignant tumors, J. Pediatr. **64**:542-546, 1964.

15. Ellis, F.: The relationship of biological effect to dose-time-fractionation factors in radiotherapy. In Ebert, M., and Howard, A., editors: Current topics in radiation research, Amsterdam, 1968, North-Holland Publishing Co., p. 382.

16. Farah, J., and Lofstrom, J. E.: Angiography of Wilms' tumor, Radiology **90**:775-777, 1968.

17. Farah, S.: Chemotherapy in the treatment of leukemia and Wilms' tumor, J.A.M.A. **198**:826-836, 1966.

18. Favara, B. E., Johnson, W., and Ito, J.: Renal tumors in the neonatal period, Cancer **22**:845-855, 1968.

19. Fernbach, D. J.: The current therapy of children with Wilms' tumor. In Progress in antimicrobial and anticancer chemotherapy, Proceedings of the Sixth International Congress of Chemotherapy, vol. II, Tokyo, 1970, The University of Tokyo Press, pp. 639-644.

20. Fernbach, D. J., and Martyn, D. T.: Role of dactinomycin in the improved survival of children with Wilms' tumor, J.A.M.A. **195**:1005-1009, 1966.

21. Filler, R. M., Tefft, M., Vawter, G. F., Maddock, C., and Mitus, A.: Hepatic lobectomy in childhood: effects of x-ray and chemotherapy, J. Pediatr. Surg. **4**:31-41, 1966.

22. Finklestein, J. Z., Ekert, H., Isaacs, H., Jr., and Higgins, G.: Bone marrow metastases in children with solid tumors, Am. J. Dis. Child. **119**:49-52, 1970.

23. Finklestein, J. Z., Hittle, R. E., and Hammond, G. D.: Evaluation of a high dose cyclophosphamide regimen in childhood tumors, Cancer **23**:1239-1242, 1969.

24. Fleming, I. D., and Johnson, W. W.: Clinical and pathologic staging as a guide in the management of Wilms' tumor, Cancer **26**:660-665, 1970.

25. Fraumeni, J. F., Jr.: Wilms' tumor and congenital aniridia, J.A.M.A. **206**:825-828, 1968.

26. Fraumeni, J. F., Jr., Geiser, C. F., and Manning, M. D.: Wilms' tumor and congenital hemihypertrophy: report of five new cases and review of literature, Pediatrics **40**:886-889, 1967.

27. Frei, E., III, Freireich, E. J, Gehan, E., Pinkel, D., Holland, J. F., Selawry, O., Haurani, F., Spurr, C. L., Hayes, D. M., James, G. W., Rothberg, H., Sodee, D. B., Rundles, R. W., Schroeder, L. R., Hoogstraten, B., Wolman, I. J., Traggis, D. G., Cooper, T., Gendel, B. R., Ebaugh, F., and Taylor, R.: Studies of sequential and combination antimetabolite therapy in acute leukemia: 6-mercaptopurine and methotrexate, Blood **18**:431-454, 1961.

28. Garcia, M., Douglass, C., and Schlosser, J. V.: Classification and prognosis in Wilms' tumor, Radiology 80:574-580, 1963.
29. Gasquet, C., Schweisguth, O., Debrun, G., Grosdemange, M., and Markovits, P.: Lymphangiography in malignant diseases of childhood, Am. J. Roentgenol. 103:1-12, 1968.
30. Guttman, F. M., Ducharme, J. C., and Collin, P. P.: Intussusception after major abdominal operations in children, Cancer J. Surg. 13:427-433, 1970.
31. Haddy, T. B., Whitaker, J. A., Vietti, T. J., and Riley, H. D., Jr.: Clinical trials with cyclophosphamide (Cytoxan) in children with Wilms' tumor—preliminary report, Cancer Chemother. Rep. 25:81-85, Dec., 1962.
32. Hilton, D., and Keeling, J. W.: Staging in relation to treatment of nephroblastoma with actinomycin D, Br. J. Urol. 42:265-269, 1970.
33. Hope, J. W., and Koop, C. E.: Abdominal tumors in infants and children: embryoma of the kidney (Wilms' tumor), Med. Radiogr. Photogr. 37(1):16-27, 1961.
34. Jagasia, K. H., Thurman, W. G., Pickett, E., and Grabstaldt, H.: Bilateral Wilms' tumors in children, J. Pediatr. 65:371-376, 1964.
35. Katzman, H., Waugh, T., and Berdon, W.: Skeletal changes following irradiation of childhood tumors, J. Bone Joint Surg. 51:825-842, 1969.
36. Kenny, G. M., Webster, J. H., Sinks, L. M., Gaeta, J. F., Staubitz, W. J., and Murphy, G. P.: Results from treatment of Wilms' tumor at Roswell Park 1927-1968, J. Surg. Oncology 1(1):49-61, 1969.
37. Koop, C. E.: Current management of nephroblastoma and neuroblastoma, Am. J. Surg. 107:497-501, 1964.
38. Kretschmer, H. L., and Hibbs, W. G.: Mixed tumors of kidney in infancy and childhood: a study of seventeen cases, Surg. Gynecol. Obstet. 52:1-24, 1931.
39. Kuffer, F., Fortner, J., and Murphy, M. L.: Surgical complications in children undergoing cancer therapy, Ann. Surg. 167:215-219, 1968.
40. Lattimer, J. K., and Conway, G. F.: The place of surgery in Wilms' tumors, J.A.M.A. 204:985-986, 1968.
41. Lemerle, J., Schlinger, M., and Schweisguth, O.: Actinomycin D and radiation therapy in the treatment of Wilms' tumor, Front. Rad. Ther. Oncology 4:181-186, 1969.
42. McDonald, P., and Hiller, H. G.: Angiography in abdominal tumours in childhood with particular reference to neuroblastoma and Wilms' tumour, Clin. Radiol. 19:1-18, 1968.
43. McGovern, J. B., and Gross, R. E.: Intussusception as a postoperative complication, Surgery 63:507-513, 1968.
44. Martin, L. W., and Reyes, P. M.: An evaluation of 10 years' with retroperitoneal lymph node dissection for Wilms' tumor, J. Pediatr. Surg. 4:683-687, 1969.
45. Martin, R. G.: Personal communication.
46. Meng, C. H., and Elkin, M.: Angiographic manifestations of Wilms' tumor, Radiology 105:95-104, 1969.
47. Miller, R. W.: Deaths from childhood cancer in sibs, N. Engl. J. Med. 279:122-126, 1968.
48. Miller, R. W., Fraumeni, J. F., Jr., and Manning, M. D.: Association of Wilms' tumor with aniridia, hemihypertrophy, and other congenital malformations, N. Engl. J. Med. 270:922-927, 1964.
49. Morse, B. S., and Nussbaum, M.: The detection of hyaluronic acid in the serum and urine of a patient with nephroblastoma, Am. J. Med. 42:996-1002, 1967.
50. National Wilms' Tumor Study, D'Angio, G. J., Chairman.
51. Neuhauser, E. B. D., Wittenborg, M. H., Berman, C. Z., and Cohen, J.: Irradiation effects of roentgen therapy on growing spine, Radiology 59:637-650, 1952.
52. Neuss, N., Johnson, I. S., Armstrong, J. G., and Jansen, C. J.: The vinca alkaloids, Adv. Chemother. 1:133-174, 1964.
53. O'Neill, P., and Pinkel, D.: Wilms' tumor in bone marrow aspirate, J. Pediatr. 72:396-398, 1968.
54. Regelson, W., Bross, I. D. J., Hananian, J., and Nigogosyan, G.: Incidence of second primary tumors in chilren with cancer and leukemia: a seven-year survey of 150 consecutive autopsied cases, Cancer 18:58-72, 1965.
55. Richmond, H., and Dougall, A. J.: Neonatal renal tumors, J. Pediatr. Surg. 5:413-418, 1970.

56. Ritter, J. A., and Scott, E. S.: Embryoma of contralateral kidney ten years following nephrectomy for Wilms' tumor, J. Pediatr. **34**:753-757, 1949.

56a. Samuels, L. D.: Organ scan diagnosis of abdominal masses in children, J. Pediatr. Surg. **6**:124-131, 1971.

57. Schneider, B., Sagerman, R. H., Wolff, J. A., and Santulli, T. V.: Wilms' tumor: the evolution of a treatment program, J. Roentgenol. **108**:92-97, 1970.

58. Silva-Sosa, M., and Gonzalez-Cerna, J. L.: Wilms' tumor in children. In Ariel, I. M., editor: Progress in clinical cancer, vol. II, New York, 1966, Grune & Stratton, Inc., pp. 323-337.

59. Stowens, D.: Pediatric pathology, ed. 2, Baltimore, 1966, The Williams & Wilkins Co., pp. 658-664.

60. Sullivan, M. P., and Sutow, W. W.: Successful therapy for Wilms' tumor, Tex. Med. **65**: 46-51, 1969.

61. Sullivan, M. P., Sutow, W. W., Cangir, A., and Taylor, G.: Vincristine sulfate in management of Wilms' tumor, replacement of preoperative irradiation by chemotherapy, J.A.M.A. **202**:381-384, 1967.

62. Sutow, W. W., Gehan, E. A., Heyn, R. M., Kung, F. H., Miller, R. W., Murphy, M. L., and Traggis, D. G.: Comparison of survival curves, 1956 versus 1962, in children with Wilms' tumor and neuroblastoma, Pediatrics **45**:800-811, 1970.

63. Sutow, W. W., and Sullivan, M. P.: Vincristine in primary treatment of Wilms' tumor, Tex. State J. Med. **61**:794-799, 1965.

64. Sutow, W. W., Thurman, W. G., and Windmiller, J.: Vincristine (leurocristine) sulfate in the treatment of children with metastatic Wilms' tumor, Pediatrics **32**:880-887, 1963.

65. Tefft, M., Vawter, G. F., and Mitus, A.: Second primary neoplasms in children, Am. J. Roentgenol. **103**:800-822, 1968.

66. Vietti, T. J.: Personal communication.

67. Vietti, T. J., Sullivan, M. P., Haggard, M. E., Holcomb, T. M., and Berry, D. H.: Vincristine sulfate and radiation therapy in metastatic Wilms' tumor, Cancer **25**:12-20, 1970.

68. Wagget, J., and Koop, C. E.: Wilms' tumor: preoperative radiotherapy and chemotherapy in the management of massive tumors, Cancer **26**:338-340, 1970.

69. Walters, T., Bushore, M., and Pinkel, D.: Identification of black children with acute lymphocytic leukemia (ALL) as high risk patients, Proc. Am. Assoc. Cancer Res. **11**:81, 1970.

70. Wang, J., Cortes, E., Sinks, L., and Holland, J. F.: Therapeutic effect and toxicity of adriamycin in patients with neoplastic disease, Proceedings of the Society of Clinical Oncology, Seventh Annual Scientific Meeting, April 7, 1971 (abs. 54).

71. Wedemeyer, P. P., White, J. G., Nesbit, M. E., Aust, J. B., Leonard, A. S., D'Angio, G. J., and Krivit, W.: Resection of metastases in Wilms' tumor: a report of three cases cured of pulmonary and hepatic metastases, Pediatrics **41**:446-451, 1963.

72. Westra, P., Kieffer, S. A., and Mosser, D. G.: Wilms' tumor: a summary of 25 years of experience before actinomycin-D, Am. J. Roentgenol. **100**:214-221, 1967.

73. Wilms, M.: Die Mischgeschwülste der Niere, Leipzig, 1899, A. Georgi.

74. Wolff, J. A., Krivit, W., Newton, W. A., Jr., and D'Angio, G. J.: Single versus multiple dose Dactinomycin therapy of Wilms' tumor, N. Engl. J. Med. **279**:290-294, 1969.

75. Wollner, N., Tan, C., Ghavimi, F., Rosen, G., Tefft, M., and Murphy, M. L.: Adriamycin in childhood leukemia and solid tumors, Proc. Am. Assoc. Cancer Res. **12**:75, March, 1971.

CHAPTER 17

Neuroblastoma

THOMAS E. WILLIAMS
MILTON H. DONALDSON

Neuroblastoma, ganglioneuroblastoma, and ganglioneuroma are intriguing childhood tumors. Since they develop from neural crest tissue, they may arise from any anatomic site along the craniospinal axis. Their first clinical manifestations often result from metastatic disease and mimic other conditions so well that the diagnosis may be difficult. They may also present as a large, "silent" intra-abdominal mass. Most of these tumors are hormonally active and secrete variable amounts of catecholamines.

The histologic appearance may be extremely variable, and all degrees of cellular maturation can be observed. Neuroblastoma is one of those rare neoplasms in which spontaneous regressions have been reported.[34] Prolonged survival and apparent cure of patients with widespread metastatic disease after seemingly inadequate therapy occasionally occur. Although a favorable prognosis is seen in children under 1 to 2 years of age, in those without metastatic disease, and in those whose primary tumor occurs in certain anatomic sites, the overall mortality is high.

Recent reports have suggested that the unusual biologic behavior of this neoplasm may be influenced by immunologic host defense mechanisms.[51, 52] Other investigations indicate that some poorly understood maturational factor(s)[8] may be operative. These studies emphasize the need to continually adjust therapeutic concepts.[10]

HISTORY

In 1864 Virchow[103] first described neuroblastoma, which he called a *glioma*. Morgan[74] noted microscopically the fibrillated character of an adrenal tumor. In 1891 Marchand[70] noted the similarities between this tumor and the "developing sympathetic ganglia," and Wright[114] showed that the cellular pattern of this tumor was similar to that seen in the embryonic adrenal medulla. Herxheimer,[54] using Bielschowsky's method of silver staining, demonstrated that the fibrils were nerve fibers and further indicated that the neurofibrils arose as outgrowths of nerve cells rather than from sheath cells as noted in the benign ganglioneuroma. Robertson[88] suggested that any large series of these neural crest tumors contained numerous histologic grades and that there could be a transition from highly anaplastic forms to benign tumors with well-differentiated cellular elements. Rinscheid[87] observed fibrils within the tumor cells that were similar to those seen in normal neuroblasts. These findings were later confirmed by Murray and Stout[75] in studies of neuroblastoma cells cultured in vitro. Pepper[80] described an assumed propensity for hepatic metastasis from adrenal neuroblastoma in the young infant (Pepper type*), and Hutchison[57] described a predilection for skeletal (especially skull) metastases from a primary lesion of the adrenal in the older child (Hutchison type†). The correlations among primary sites, ages, and patterns of metastases as suggested by Pepper and Hutchison have since been refuted in experiences with larger numbers of patients.[35, 79]

INCIDENCE

Neuroblastoma is probably the most common malignant solid tumor in childhood.[1, 11, 25] In a review of 1833 cases of childhood malignancies treated during 1926 to 1961 at the Memorial Hospital for Cancer and Allied Disorders, Dargeon[25] found 205 examples of neuroblastoma for an incidence of 11%, whereas Bodian[11] noted 129 (14%) among 907 children with malignancies in England and Wales. From a study of death certificates in the United States during 1960 to 1964, Miller[72] estimated the average annual death rate from neuroblastoma to be 10 per million for children 0 to 4 years of age and 4 per million for those 5 to 9 years of age. Among 1535 neuroblastoma deaths the male:female ratio was 1.1:1.0

Neuroblastoma is a tumor of early childhood. Analyses of composite data[3, 82] from the literature indicate that half the cases occur in children 2 years of age and younger. About three fourths of all cases occur during the first 4 years of life. It is possible that the true incidence of neuroblastoma is greater than that reported. Based on studies of random sections of the adrenal glands of autopsied infants under 3 months of age, the incidence of neuroblastoma in situ was reported to range between 1:179 and 1:259.[5] When deliberate serial sections of the adrenals were obtained,[47] the incidence was reported to be 1:39. The most important implication of this is that some infants may have an innate ability to induce spontaneous regression in a large percentage of such "in situ" tumors.[93]

ETIOLOGY

The etiology of neuroblastoma is unknown. Lee[65] noted an increased incidence of neuroblastoma deaths in England during the summer months and suggested that the seasonal variation might be associated with a specific etiology, perhaps viral. Miller,[72] however, found no seasonal variation in deaths occurring in the United States but "a statistically significant year-to-year variation" in three of nine geographic subdivisions and suggested that there might be a common etiologic agent. One analysis of 28 neuroblastomas yielded no viruses, although human adenovirus type 1 was found in 4 of 145 other tumor types studied.[76]

The concomitant occurrence of neuroblastoma with congenital anomalies of other organ systems has been described,[100] but probably no specific defect exceeds the normal expectation of incidence in neuroblastoma patients.[72] From studying 504 childhood neuroblastoma patients with 59 congenital defects, Miller[72] stated that the exception to this may be the frequency of skull and brain defects in children with neuroblastoma, which approach 2%, a higher incidence

---

*In his original paper Pepper reported 5 infants ranging in age from birth to 5 weeks, 2 with right-sided adrenal neuroblastoma and 3 with left-sided tumors.

†In his original report Hutchison noted that in 10 patients with neuroblastoma, ranging in age from 9 months to 9 years, six tumors arose from the left adrenal and four from the right.

than expected for the general childhood population. The association of neurofibromatosis with neuroblastoma has been reported by Knudson and Amromin.[61]

There have been no unequivocal reports of neuroblastoma in parent and child to date. Chatten and Voorhess'[18] review of the literature yielded five families with more than one sibling with neuroblastoma. The mother of one of these families, in which 3 of the 4 children developed neuroblastoma, had elevated catecholamine excretion during a pregnancy. The infant she was delivered of developed neuroblastoma at 5 months of age. The mother continued to excrete excessive catecholamines and was later found to have a thoracic tumor that did not change during periodic examinations thereafter.[17]

In four families, each of whom had a child with neuroblastoma, Helson[53] found 5 siblings with increased catecholamine levels but without symptoms. These reports support the contention that all members of a family in which a neuroblastoma is diagnosed should be investigated for possible abnormal excretion of catecholamines and for their metabolic products.

PATHOLOGY

The tumors discussed here are derived from cells of the neural crest that form the sympathetic ganglia and adrenal medulla. The most primitive cells, the sympathogonia, can differentiate along two lines: the pheochromocytic line, which will not be considered, and the sympathoblastic line. Three tumor types are generally recognized as arising from the latter: neuroblastoma, ganglioneuroblastoma, and ganglioneuroma.

Neuroblastoma

Small tumors, especially those that are well encapsulated, are usually moderately firm, and the cut surface is gray to pink. Once the tumor breaks through its capsule and begins to infiltrate the surrounding tissues, it becomes very soft and friable, with areas of hemorrhage and necrosis; the cut surface may appear dark red. Calcific foci, hemorrhage, and occasionally cystic areas may be observed in the well-encapsulated and highly invasive tumors.

This tumor is densely cellular and is composed of small round cells with little cytoplasm and darkly staining nuclei. The highly undifferentiated tumor often does not have true rosette formation, and the characteristic neurofibrils may be absent or barely discernible. Development of the rosette pattern with fibrillar material emerging from the cells to occupy the center of the configuration is perhaps the earliest sign of differentiation. The cells of the rosette may be early nerve cells forming nerve fibers; however, no sheath cells are present. Hemorrhage is common, and mitotic figures usually are not present in large numbers.

Ganglioneuroblastoma

Ganglioneuroblastoma is intermediate in its degree of cellular differentiation between the neuroblastoma and the ganglioneuroma. Grossly, the tumor may be smooth or lobulated; it is moderately firm and well encapsulated. Hemorrhage and calcification are not uncommon. This tumor may infiltrate locally, as well as metastasize via hematogenous and lymphatic channels. Microscopically, it may be composed of a sea of undifferentiated neuroblasts surrounding only occasional mature ganglion cells. Areas that have undergone a considerable degree of maturation will look strikingly different from the neuroblastoma. Mature ganglion cells, comparatively much larger and with enlarged nuclei, are surrounded by abundant cytoplasm. The ganglion cells are set in a background of rich collagen tissue surrounded by tangled or parallel bundles of neurofibrils. Occasionally, abundant Schwann cells surround the neurofibrils. Because the histologic pattern may vary from one portion of the tumor to the other, one must examine several areas thoroughly to avoid erroneously labeling a tumor with malignant elements as a benign ganglioneuroma.

Metastatic tumor

Metastatic lesions may be more or less differentiated than the primary tumor. It is well known that occasional tumors, both residual primary and metastatic deposits, have undergone maturation from a very undifferentiated histologic picture to one of benign ganglioneuroma.[111]

Ganglioneuroma

Ganglioneuroma, described by Loretz[68] in 1870, is the benign member of this group of neural crest neoplasms. Ganglioneuromas are very firm and encapsulated and appear yellowish gray on cut surface. By definition they do not metastasize; however, they frequently develop projections that may intimately circumscribe proximate structures or occasionally extend through intervertebral foramina to produce neurologic symptoms. On microscopic examination the mature ganglion cells are large, with a large nuclei surrounded by abundant cytoplasm. These cells are scattered sporadically through a collagen-rich background laced with bundles of neurofibrils.

Ultrastructure

Study of the ultrastructure of neuroblastoma and ganglioneuroblastoma cells by electron microscopy appears to correlate with urinary catecholamine excretion. Misugi and co-workers[73] demonstrated a correlation between increased excretion of vanillylmandelic acid (VMA) and the cytoplasmic concentration of membrane-bound granules approximately 100 mμ in size. These were labeled "catechol" granules because of their similarity to the catecholamine granules seen in the ultrastructure of the adrenal medulla. Similar but larger electron-dense granules 500 mμ in size were thought to be derived from these smaller granules.[44] Such granules were observed in bone marrow and lymph node metastases from a ganglioneuroblastoma, and histochemical studies were consistent with the presence of catecholamines in those tumor cells.[7] The various investigators suggest that these granules may be storage sites for catecholamines, but conclusive proof is lacking.

Histologic grading

Attempts have been made to correlate histologic grading of the neural crest tumor with biologic behavior. It has been noted that vesicular nuclei, cytoplasm and cytoplasmic processes, presence of mature ganglion cells, and probably rosette formation indicate increasing maturity and portend a favorable prognosis.[69]

Beckwith and Martin[4] noted that the prognosis appeared to be more favorable if at least 5% of the cellular elements contained large nuclei, abundant eosinophilic cytoplasm, or nerve processes or were identified as sheath cells. In addition, it should be noted that the histologic gradation of the tumor does not explain the better prognosis in children under 1 year of age but may correlate with the outcome in many older children with primary adrenal neuroblastomas.

CLINICAL MANIFESTATIONS

Signs and symptoms produced by neuroblastoma are largely attributable to compression of other structures by the primary tumor or by metastatic deposits. The most common initial evidence of disease is usually a mass. In approximately half the patients the tumor arises in the abdomen (Fig. 17-1). One third of all neuroblastomas arise from an adrenal gland, and an additional 18% arise from nonadrenal intra-abdominal sites. The mass is usually firm, irregular, and nontender and frequently crosses the midline of the abdomen. Extrinsic pressure by the tumor on the kidney, ureter, or bladder may cause urinary frequency or partial obstruction to the normal flow of urine, especially if the tumor arises in the lumbosacral area. A tumor in this site rarely may extend through the sacrosciatic notch and present as a mass in the buttock even before the abdominal portion is detected.

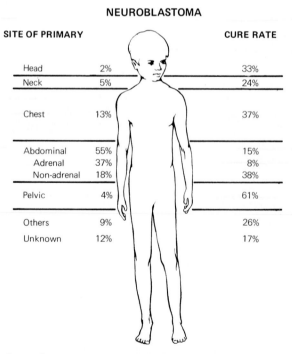

NEUROBLASTOMA

SITE OF PRIMARY		CURE RATE
Head	2%	33%
Neck	5%	24%
Chest	13%	37%
Abdominal	55%	15%
Adrenal	37%	8%
Non-adrenal	18%	38%
Pelvic	4%	61%
Others	9%	26%
Unknown	12%	17%

Fig. 17-1. An analysis of composite data from the literature. See references 3, 11, 25, 28, 40, 46, 67, 91. The cure rate is the percentage of children with neuroblastoma of the corresponding primary site who are said by the authors to be alive and free of neuroblastoma at least 14 months and usually greater than 2 years after diagnosis.

The rare primary intracranial neuroblastoma may cause intracranial hypertension and other neurologic abnormalities, depending on the site and extent of the tumor. Primary tumor arising from the olfactory bulb (esthesioneuroblastoma) produces a mass in the nasal cavity, causing obstructive nasal symptoms. Origin in a cervical sympathetic ganglion can give rise to a neck mass anywhere from the supraclavicular fossa to the angle of the mandible. The tumor may extend through the intervertebral foramina to cause compression of the spinal cord or may extend to the base of the skull. Horner's syndrome may develop early in such patients, or hoarseness may signify compression of the recurrent laryngeal nerve by the tumor.

Thoracic tumor may become massive before causing enough tracheal or bronchial compression to result in respiratory tract symptoms or obstruction of the superior vena cava. Paresis of an upper extremity may herald brachial plexus involvement. Complaints of pain in the neck, back, abdomen, pelvis, or legs may

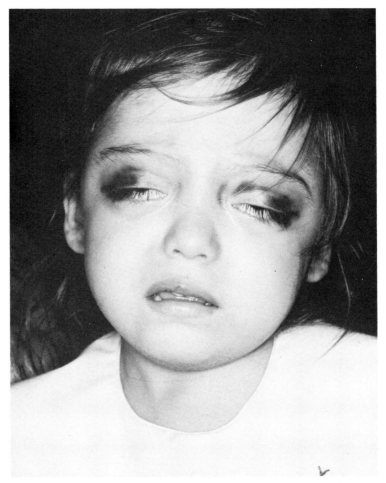

Fig. 17-2. Supraorbital ecchymoses associated with periorbital metastases. (Courtesy Howard A. Britton.)

be caused by tumor pressure, infiltration of dorsal nerve roots, or the "dumb-bell"-shaped projection of the tumor through an intervertebral foramen to compress the spinal cord. This may be followed by progressive signs of urinary tract or bowel dysfunction or both, as well as loss of motor function in the lower extremities, ultimately resulting in complete paraplegia.

Neuroblastoma is typically a silent tumor in its early stages and unfortunately metastasizes rapidly. Up to 70% of patients have metastasis at the time of diagnosis,[46] and in many cases the first signs and symptoms are due to metastatic involvement. Irritability, anorexia, weight loss, and pallor due to anemia are usually manifestations of widespread disease but occasionally are noted first without other evidence of dissemination. Unexplained fever is a common presenting complaint. Skeletal lesions in spite of extensive destruction may or may not result in bone pain. Bone pain may also occur in the absence of demonstrable skeletal lesions. Invasion of the retrobulbar soft tissues causes proptosis of the eye, as well as periorbital swelling and ecchymosis. These are frequently the first signs of this tumor. The ecchymosis characteristically occurs in the upper eyelid, rather than in the lower lid as it does more commonly when due to trauma (Fig. 17-2). Lymphadenopathy may be the first physical abnormality. The most common sites are the cervical and supraclavicular areas. Other nodal groups are less often involved, but generalized adenopathy may occur. One or more subcutaneous nodules may be the primary complaint. In the very young

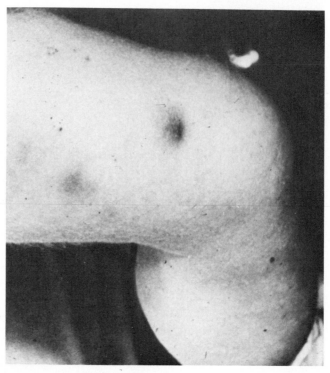

Fig. 17-3. Subcutaneous metastatic nodules with blue or purplish discoloration likened to a blueberry muffin. (Courtesy William G. Thurman.)

child, particularly during the neonatal period, subcutaneous nodules may precede other complaints. Skin involvement has been noted in one third of the cases.[92] These nodules frequently have a bluish discoloration that has resulted in an appearance likened to a blueberry muffin (Fig. 17-3).

Infrequently the initial signs and symptoms are related to the catecholamine production of the tumor; skin flushing, increased perspiration, tachycardia, hypertension, and headaches may occur in paroxysms, simulating manifestations of pheochromocytoma. Hypertension may be found in up to half the cases, but only seldom do the other signs of pressor amine production occur, despite the elevated catecholamine excretion noted in the majority of subjects. The classic syndrome of chronic diarrhea unresponsive to medical therapy, usually accompanied by skin rash and flushing, hypokalemia, abdominal distention, and failure to thrive, is rarely observed. Removal of the tumor results in prompt disappearance of the diarrhea and other manifestations of this syndrome.

Another uncommon manifestation of this tumor is its association with acute cerebellar encephalopathy, which is marked by truncal ataxia, extremity weakness, and oculogyric crisis. Even though the encephalopathy may resolve prior to removal of the tumor, residual mental retardation may occur.[14] The pattern of metastatic spread may be one of the first diagnostic features. Unlike Wilms' tumor, rhabdomyosarcoma, or other soft tissue sarcomas, neuroblastoma does not metastasize to lung parenchyma except in the late stages. This tumor has a predilection for skeletal metastasis, especially to the skull, and lytic skull lesions or orbital metastasis with proptosis may suggest eosinophilic granuloma.

DIAGNOSTIC FEATURES
Laboratory findings

Hematologic studies

Blood. A child with localized neuroblastoma will present with normal peripheral blood counts unless he coincidentally has a concomitant hematologic disorder such as iron-deficiency anemia. Once the disease becomes disseminated, however, anemia and thrombocytopenia are often noted. This is particularly true when bone marrow metastases exist, but in some patients with late-stage disease, anemia may occur without definitely demonstrable tumor cells in the marrow. On occasion the neuroblasts can be seen in the peripheral blood on direct smear or after "buffy coat" preparations of peripheral leukocytes. In the rare patient with virtually complete replacement of the normal marrow elements by metastatic neuroblastoma, the peripheral blood and bone marrow pictures may strongly resemble acute lymphoblastic leukemia.

Bone marrow. Aspiration of the bone marrow in every suspected case of neuroblastoma is important. Particles squeezed between glass cover slips probably allow better preservation of clumps of tumor cells than does the method of making glass slide smears, thus producing a greater opportunity to demonstrate marrow metastasis. As high as 70% of marrows of neuroblastoma patients have been reported to demonstrate metastatic involvement.[29, 39] It is not uncommon to find tumor cells in the marrow when there is no evidence of skeletal metastases, although both may be found simultaneously. Uncommonly, a patient may demonstrate widespread bony involvement with no tumor cells demonstrable in marrow specimens. Neuroblastoma cells in the marrow can be difficult to distinguish from leukemia and from other metastatic cells such as lympho-sarcoma, retinoblastoma, Ewing's sarcoma, or any other small round cell tumor that may metastasize to bone. Nonetheless, their presence in the marrow may be the only clue in a diagnostic dilemma that will lead one to perform those studies necessary to discover neuroblastoma. Neuroblasts will frequently form clumps or "pseudorosettes" in the bone marrow (Fig. 17-4). Occasionally neuro-fibrils can be seen, a feature best demonstrated by phase microscopy (Fig. 17-5). The observation of neuroblasts attempting to differentiate into mature ganglion cells (Fig. 17-6) will sometimes be very helpful in differentiating neuroblastoma from other tumor metastases in the marrow.

Coagulation. In a study of 22 patients with metastatic neuroblastoma, Giro-lami[42] noted that although most patients bled due to thrombocytopenia, some had coagulation studies that suggested that hyperfibrinolysis rather than con-sumptive coagulopathy was the primary mechanism responsible for their bleed-ing diathesis. McMillan and associates[78] reported a neuroblastoma patient with evidence of progressive depletion of coagulation factors suggestive of intravascu-lar coagulation. However, study of the effect of anticoagulation was not possible in that patient. Intravascular coagulation is a well-known phenomenon in patients with cancer. It is probably precipitated, at least in part, by release of tissue thromboplastin from necrosing tumor tissue. The consumptive process may be adequately treated with intravenous heparin. In view of the paucity of informa-tion regarding such coagulopathies in neuroblastoma, it would seem advisable to carefully study all patients with this neoplasm for any evidence of abnormalities of the coagulation system.

Biochemical studies

Catecholamines. A significant advance in the understanding of neuroblastoma was the elucidation of the metabolic pathway of the catecholamines (Fig. 17-7)

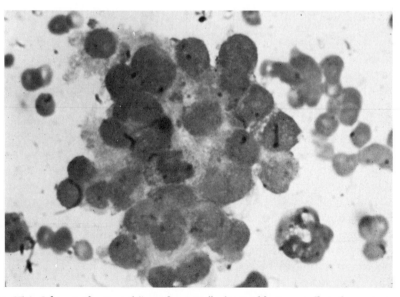

Fig. 17-4. Oil magnification of "pseudorosette" of neuroblastoma cells in bone marrow.

and the discovery of the increased excretion of urinary metabolites of the catecholamines in patients with tumors of the neural crest. The determination of vanillylmandelic acid (VMA), homovanillic acid (HVA), norepinephrine (NE), and dopamine not only has improved the ability of the clinician to diagnose the disease but also has proved of value in judging the therapeutic effect of surgery, radiotherapy, and chemotherapy. Quantitative determination of the entire

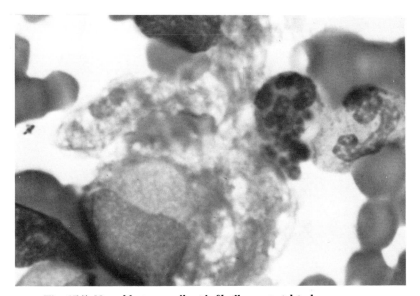

Fig. 17-5. Neuroblastoma cell with fibrillar material in bone marrow.

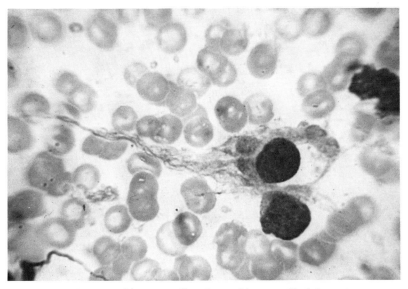

Fig. 17-6. Neuroblastoma cell with axonlike neurofibril formation.

spectrum of catecholamines and their metabolites on 24-hour urine collections is the most accurate approach to biochemical diagnosis, since tumors secrete the substances inconsistently in a variety of patterns. Additional factors to consider are that (1) urinary excretion has a diurnal variation, being decreased at night, and (2) excretion increases gradually with age through adolescence and thus must be correlated with proper normal values for age.

Development of rapid methods of screening for urinary VMA has made practical its determination in the initial investigations of a suspected neuroblastoma and in the follow-up studies of patients known to have the tumor. A simple rapid test has been proposed as a tool for screening patients to detect

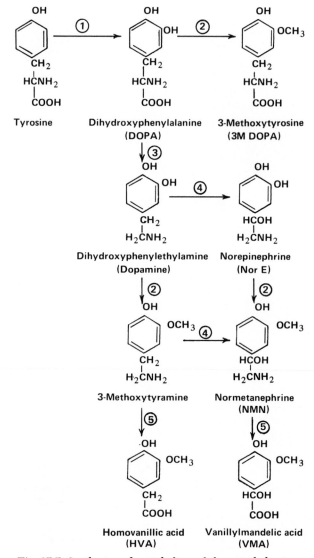

Fig. 17-7. Synthesis and metabolism of the catecholamines.

excessive urinary excretion of VMA.[31] It can be performed on a few drops of urine and does not require a period of dietary restriction. The screening test can be repeated easily to ascertain quickly if it has again reverted to positive. This will allow the clinician to proceed with other diagnostic investigations and an immediate change in therapy rather than await results of the quantitative test, which may not be available for several days. Such a reversion from negative to positive may be noted prior to other evidence of recurrence or progression of the disease.

Although there is no uniform excretion pattern of urinary catecholamines and their metabolic by-products in patients with neuroblastoma, the finding of an elevation of at least one of these products is present in nearly all patients prior to therapy. In tumors that may have arisen from spinal nerve roots and ganglia, urinary levels of these substances may be normal because such neuroblastomas probably are nonsecretors of catecholamines.[106] Table 17-1 includes representative series demonstrating the variability of urinary excretion of catecholamines and their by-products. It would appear that those studies most likely to be positive in neuroblastoma are the urinary Dopa, dopamine, norepinephrine, VMA, and HVA, as determinations of single substances, and the collective assessment of dopamine + norepinephrine + epinephrine. The variability of the urinary excretion of the catecholamines and their by-products has suggested certain groupings of patients and the possibility that differences among neuroblastomas might be inferred.[108] However, no general agreement has been reached. A similar inability to correlate tumor content of catecholamines and their metabolites with urinary excretion patterns of these substances has been noted.[105] This is exemplified by low concentrations of epinephrine, norepinephrine, and dopamine in neuroblastoma tissue, in contrast to elevated urinary excretion of these substances. This suggests abnormal production, storage, and/or release of catecholamines in the tumor. Another paradox is the lack of correlation between patients' blood pressures, which are usually normal, and the excretions of catecholamines and their metabolites, which are usually excessive.[62] The value of serial measurements of the basic catecholamines HVA and VMA in assessing the effectiveness of therapy is well known. de Gutierrez Moyano and associates[27] illustrated this in 13 of 14 children whose norepinephrine and VMA levels returned to normal after therapy; they were free of disease from 14 to 52 months afterward. One had died from an intercurrent disease and not from the neoplasm. All children who did not achieve normal urinary norepinephrine and VMA levels either died of neuroblastoma or were living with evidence of disease at the time of the report.

General findings. Cystathionine is not normally detectable in urine. It has been noted in very rare patients with congenital cystathioninuria and in patients with primary liver tumors.[43] Geiser and Efron[41] found it in the urine of 50% of 28 neuroblastoma patients but not in a variety of other childhood tumors nor in any patients who had responded to treatment for ganglioneuroblastoma or neuroblastoma. Differential diagnosis between hepatic metastases of neuroblastoma and primary liver tumor would be important in children with hepatomegaly and cystathioninuria. Presence of this substance in the urine is frequent enough to justify its use as an aid to diagnosis similar to determination of vanillylmandelic acid. Its presence is indicative of active disease; conversely, lack of it in the

Table 17-1. Incidence of the elevation of urinary catecholamines and their metabolic products in patients with neuroblastoma and ganglioneuroblastoma*

Author(s)	Year	Dopa	Dopamine	NE	E	Dopamine + NE + E	NE + E	NMA	NMA + MA	HVA	VMA (HMMA)
Voorhess and Gardner[107]	1961			5/6							5/6
Stickler and co-workers[94]	1962	3/3				12/12				18/26	43/49
Kontras[62]	1962										5/10
Voorhess[105]	1968		9/9	10/10						10/10	7/10
von Studnitz and co-workers[104]	1963		18/18	21/21						12/18	21/21
Williams and Greer[110]	1963	2/2	16/22	18/23				12/19		32/43	58/75
Voorhess and co-workers[109]	1963		20/26	20/26							15/26
Sunderman[96]	1964								15/26		4/4
Brett and co-workers[16]	1964									1/1	1/1
McKendrick and Edwards[77]	1965										10/13
Greer and co-workers[45]	1965	10/12	11/12	11/12	6/12					13/14	11/12
Bell[6]	1968					24/26			22/26		24/26
Hinterberger and Bartholomew[55]	1968		19/24				11/23			21/29	19/29
de Gutierrez Moyano and co-workers[26]	1970		25/25	27/31							33/38
Totals		15/17	108/126	112/129	6/12	36/38	11/23	12/19	37/52	107/141	261/320
Percent		88%	86%	87%	50%	95%	48%	63%	71%	76%	82%

*Key: NE = norepinephrine; E = epinephrine; NMA = normetanephrine; MA = metanephrine; HVA = homovanillic acid; VMA = vanillylmandelic acid (hydroxymethoxymandelic acid).

urine may occur even in patients with tumor progression. Such paradox obviously limits the usefulness of this test.

Chromosome abnormality. Various investigators have reported abnormalities of chromosomal composition in studies of karyotypes of neuroblastoma cells, but no specific pattern has been consistently detected. Metaphase figures revealed the presence of minute chromatin bodies, marked aneuploidy, endoreduplication, and chromosomal breaks among three cases of neuroblastoma and one each of medulloblastoma and rhabdomyosarcoma.[21] Levan and co-workers[66] noted the minute chromosomes in one case of neuroblastoma as well as aneuploidy in 5 of 73 mitotic figures counted. In addition, they found that one of the chromosomes of the C group was probably derived from a chromosome missing from the D group. Two more cases of neuroblastoma with similar chromosomal aberrations were reported later.[20] The exact implication of these findings is presently unclear, and it is obvious that more such investigations must be conducted.

Roentgenographic findings

A child suspected of having a neuroblastoma should have a complete radiographic survey of the skeleton, chest x-ray examination, and inferior venacavogram with an intravenous urogram as a minimum roentgenographic evaluation. Although anterior and lateral displacement of the inferior vena cava is common, complete obstruction due either to extrinsic pressure or intraluminal tumor thrombus is unusual. The urogram may reveal the kidney to be displaced caudally and laterally without intrinsic distortion of the renal calyces or pelvis (Fig. 17-8). Acute angulation at the ureteropelvic junction is also suggestive that the lesion is extrarenal in origin. This is compatible with an adrenal neuroblastoma but must be differentiated from other entities such as adrenal hematoma or cyst, mesenteric cyst, cortical tumors of the adrenal gland, neurofibroma, pheochromocytoma, and ganglioneuroma. Rarely the tumor may invade the kidney, producing distortion of the pelvis and calyces similar to that produced by Wilms' tumor. Hydronephrosis and nonvisualization of the kidney may occur if the neoplasm develops in such a location as to produce ureteral obstruction. Calcification is present in about half these tumors, showing a diffuse, speckled appearance (Fig. 17-8). Wilms' tumor less often contains calcium and usually shows it as one or more solid amorphous calcific densities, or it may assume a curvilinear shape.

Aortography is abnormal in more than 80% of cases in which intravenous urogram or cavogram-urogram studies suggest an adrenal or renal mass. The displacement of the kidney and other predominantly vascular structures is in proportion to the size of the tumor. In nearly half, the abnormal circulation within the tumor can be seen and may indicate that the renal structures are otherwise intact. Although this may not necessarily rule out a Wilms' tumor, information from this study often is sufficient to suggest the correct diagnosis preoperatively. This is especially true if selective arteriography of the renal and adrenal vessels is carried out to demonstrate presence of the "tumor blush" of neovascularity in the adrenal area.

Radioisotopic studies may also be informative. Liver scan may demonstrate filling defects or "cold spots" in areas involved by metastases. A renal scan would demonstrate a displaced but otherwise normal kidney, thus ruling out tumor intrinsic to that organ.

The next most common site for primary neuroblastoma beyond the abdomen is the chest, usually the posterior mediastinum, although neuroblastoma of the anterior mediastinum has been reported. The distribution is equal for both sides of the thorax, and calcification is seen in about half the cases. In addition to the soft tissue masses, the posterior portions of the ribs may be separated, with some narrowing and erosion often detectable. Eklof and Gooding[30] found that 27% of their patients with intrathoracic neuroblastoma had associated widening of the paravertebral region. This was associated with a poor prognosis, with only 2 of 27 patients surviving more than 6 months.

Metastatic involvement of the skeleton varies from virtually imperceptible to gross destruction of the bone (Fig. 17-9). Most of these lesions are primarily

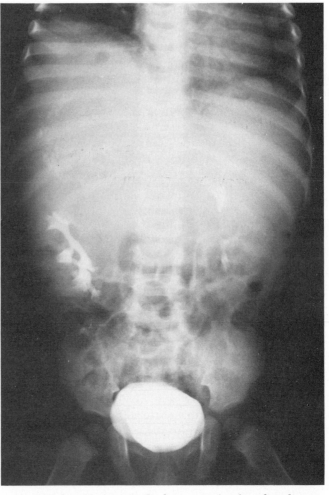

Fig. 17-8. Intravenous pyelogram showing displacement of right calyceal system laterally and caudally by diffusely calcified right-sided neuroblastoma.

lytic and irregular. They occur predominantly in the skull and diaphyses of the distal femora and humeri, rarely being noted distal to the elbows and knees. Other bones, namely the pelvis, vertebrae, ribs, scapula, and tibia, may be involved. Distribution of skeletal metastases is generally bilateral and often symmetrical. Periosteal reaction is common, and occasionally a pathologic fracture occurs. Seldom is epiphyseal involvement encountered except in advanced cases. Bony neuroblastoma metastases may be difficult to distinguish radiographically from Ewing's tumor, osteomyelitis, reticuloendothelioma, reticulum cell sarcoma, tuberculosis, and leukemia. Selenomethionine (^{75}Se) has been used to identify neuroblastoma metastases to the skeleton.[24] The tumor becomes labeled with the radioisotope as it metabolizes the methionine to cystathionine. Marrow involvement may not be detected, but skeletal lesions may be revealed by this procedure even though the conventional radiographic skeletal survery appears normal.

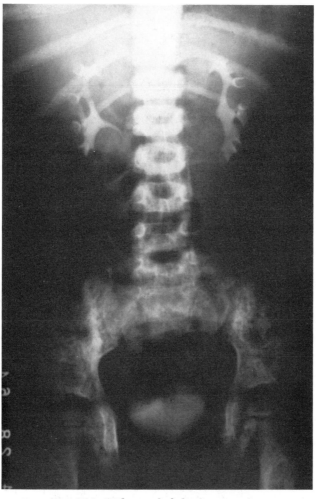

Fig. 17-9. Widespread skeletal metastases.

CLINICAL STAGING AND PROGNOSIS
(see Appendix, p. 405)

Factors such as age of patient and extent of disease at the time of diagnosis, location of the primary tumor, extirpability, presence of bone and/or bone marrow metastases, and degree of cellular differentiation of the tumor are known to influence prognosis, and most have been considered in the various staging systems proposed. In 1967 James[58] suggested a simple classification based on extent of disease and its degree of resectability and assumed involvement of bone and bone marrow to be equivalent. One year later Pinkel and co-workers[85] distinguished between tumors that were totally or partially resectable or totally unresectable but did not consider the implication of bony involvement. Thurman and Donaldson[101] designed a four-stage classification that considered extent of disease, resectability of tumor, and degree of cellular differentiation, distinguished between spread to bone and to bone marrow, and acknowledged the gravity of persistent excretion of elevated catecholamine levels. The schema excluded all patients under 1 year of age because of their highly variable disease courses and occasional tumor regression after insufficient therapy. By implication, then, they consider age to be a critical prognostic factor.

That prognosis is influenced by the degree of histologic differentiation was substantiated by Beckwith and Martin's pathologic study.[4] They noted that lymphocytic infiltration of neuroblastoma was associated with a better prognosis. Since these infiltrates are found primarily in the more differentiated neoplasms that have more favorable outcomes, it is presently impossible to ascertain whether lymphocytic infiltration or cellular differentiation of the tumor is of greater importance to tumor staging and thus to patient survival. Knowledge of the immunologic functions of the lymphocytes serves to stimulate speculation that the lymphocytes are engaged in some immunologic activity that results in destruction and removal of malignant cells (tumor antigen). The prognostic importance of serial catecholamine determinations has already been referred to earlier in this chapter.

Evans and associates[32] proposed another method of clinical staging based on extent of disease without specific reference to age at time of diagnosis, tumor resectability, histologic appearance, biochemical activity, or location of the primary tumor. These parameters were considered in analysis of the patient data but were not incorporated into the actual staging in an effort to prevent the schema from becoming unwieldy and impractical for clinical use. The unique aspect of this classification is that a special group of patients is acknowledged (Stage IV-S) in which the tumor is localized to one side of the midline and, although not necessarily confined to the organ of origin, has remote spread that involves liver, skin, and/or bone marrow without roentgenographic evidence of bony metastasis. The survival rates for the entire IV-S group and for all patients with neuroblastoma under 1 year of age were virtually identical to the rates for patients with Stage I tumors (i.e., those confined to the organ of origin). In the other three groups with progressively more extensive disease (Stages II, III, and IV) survival rates were increasingly poor. It is apparent from these and other data that although primary site, extent of disease, and histologic maturation are important, the age of the patient at the time of diagnosis is probably the most crucial factor in the ultimate prognosis, as was pointed out by Sutow in 1958[97] and again in 1970.[99] However, a statistical analysis by Breslow and

McCann[15] of 234 patients shows that *age* and *clinical stage* of disease at the time of diagnosis each play strong but independent roles in prognosticating survival.

A factor that was generally conceded to indicate a fatal prognosis is radiographically demonstrable bony metastases. However, survival of patients with skeletal metastases has been reported. Reilly[86] has reported 3 infants under 1 year of age who were apparently cured of skeletal lesions by treatment with nitrogen mustard and radiotherapy. Review of the literature by Reilly and his associates yielded only 8 other patients surviving 2 to 20 years from diagnosis. Evans and co-workers[32] have now added 4 more patients, 2 of whom were over 2 years of age at the time of diagnosis. It would appear that current therapeutic approaches of combinations of surgery, radiation, and chemotherapy might change patterns of survival of such patients.

The site of development of the primary tumor is *significantly* related to survival and cure rates. Tumors arising in the thorax and neck have a better prognosis than those arising in the abdomen (Fig. 17-1), presumably because the number who have established metastatic disease when first seen is much less. However, when only patients with localized or regional disease are considered, there is no apparent difference in the survival rate. Although Sutow[97] noted no significant difference in survival when abdominal and extra-abdominal primary tumor sites were compared, the more recent reports[19, 32] suggest that the apparently better prognosis for those children with cervical, thoracic, and pelvic tumors is probably related to earlier diagnosis, occasioned by the production of early symptoms in the sites of origin. Certainly this would appear to explain the favorable prognosis in those dumbbell-shaped tumors with an intraspinal projection that produces early signs of spinal cord compression, thus leading to early diagnosis and treatment.

DIFFERENTIAL DIAGNOSIS
Clinical manifestations

Since the symptoms caused by this tumor and its metabolically active products are variable, the differential diagnosis suggested by the early manifestations of the tumor is necessarily a broad one. The presence of an abdominal mass may suggest other diagnoses such as Wilms' tumor, hydronephrotic kidney, enlarged spleen, lymphomas, and mesenteric cysts. Compression of vital structures in the neck and mediastinum may cause the superior vena caval syndrome or mediastinal syndrome indistinguishable from that caused by other tumors. Occasionally a mediastinal neuroblastoma may be confused with a thymoma. Persistent diarrhea may suggest malabsorption states. Hypertension might be attributed to intrinsic renal pathology or pheochromocytoma or dismissed as "essential." Failure to thrive may be associated with opsoclonus. Bone pain may simulate rheumatic fever, rheumatoid arthritis, or osteomyelitis. If marrow involvement is extensive, the blood picture may suggest nutritional deficiencies, aplastic anemia, or leukemia. When the initial signs are attributable to metastases throughout the reticuloendothelial system, lymphadenopathy, hepatomegaly, or splenomegaly in all possible combinations could be encountered. This then would suggest a broad differential diagnosis that includes primary tumors of the reticuloendothelial system, allergic diseases, storage diseases, acute infections, granulomatous diseases, or primary hematologic disorders.

Pathology

In its highly undifferentiated form the neuroblastoma may be exceedingly difficult to identify histologically. Osteomyelitis, reticulum cell sarcoma, lymphocytic lymphoma, metastatic retinoblastoma, Ewing's sarcoma, and lymphocytic leukemia may resemble neuroblastoma. However, biochemical studies of urinary catecholamines and their metabolic products, tissue culture, electron microscopy, and special histochemical techniques will aid the pathologist in making an accurate diagnosis.

TREATMENT AND PROGNOSIS
Surgery

As is true for most malignant tumors, the most effective therapy is complete surgical removal. Koop[63] has reported a 2-year survival rate of 84% using surgical therapy alone. He believed that no significant improvement was achieved by the addition of irradiation or chemotherapy or both. The adjunctive use of 3600 to 4000 rads over a 4-week period after total excision of the tumor increased gross survival rate only to 88%.[46] Hinton and Buschke[56] also reported no increase in survival rate for patients treated with partial excision of the tumor followed by irradiation as compared to those treated with partial tumor excision and no radiotherapy. Koop[64] advocates an approach of creating a "major surgical insult" by ligating as much of the tumor's blood supply as possible and removing all the tumor tissue feasible even though complete resection obviously cannot be accomplished. Some patients have brisk bleeding. This technique certainly requires considerable experience and sound clinical judgment on the part of the surgeon.

Radiotherapy

Neuroblastoma is considered to be radiosensitive, and most radiotherapists believe that irradiation therapy is indicated if there is a possibility of residual disease after surgical resection. Perez and co-workers[81] obtained 2-year survival in 56% of 36 patients. Thirty-four received radiation and some degree of surgical resection (total, partial, or biopsy); 19 (56%) survived for 2 years or longer. He also noted that other factors influenced survival. Fourteen of the 17 patients less than 2 years of age survived 2 or more years, whereas only 6 of 19 (32%) of those over 2 years old did so. Lingley and associates[67] noted a 65% 3-year survival among 17 patients who were evaluable for radiotherapy, 13 of whom had only biopsy or partial excision of their tumor prior to irradiation. However, 13 of the 17 were younger than 1 year of age at diagnosis.

The dose of radiation used generally ranges from 2000 to 3600 rads. However, in patients being irradiated in the renal or hepatic areas, the usual dose is 1200 rads to avoid radiation nephritis or hepatitis. It is worth noting that patients with metastases confined to the liver have a peculiarly good response after treatment with the modest radiation dose. There has been speculation that radiation may either destroy neuroblastoma or cause its maturation to ganglioneuroma.[22]

Chemotherapy

Although the addition of chemotherapy to surgery and radiotherapy has significantly improved the prognosis for Wilms' tumor, similar results have not been attained for neuroblastoma. Sutow[99] has reported no significant increase in survival among children treated in 1962 compared to those treated in 1956, although the proportion receiving chemotherapy rose from 57% to 80%. The use of adjunctive chemotherapeutic regimens rose only from 12% to 25%, whereas the use of drugs in metastatic disease increased from 59% to 90%. It is apparent then that the chemotherapeutic agents in use thus far have not been successful in improving the survival rate.

In 1959 Bodian[11] reported that vitamin B_{12} was useful in the treatment of neuroblastoma. This could not be confirmed in subsequent survey.[91]

The only conventional chemotherapeutic agents that have been found to cause significant and consistent tumor regression are cyclophosphamide and vincristine. In 1964 the Southwest Cancer Chemotherapy Study Group (SCCSG) administered cyclophosphamide intravenously to 24 patients for 10 days (10 mg/kg/day), then continued it orally (2.5 mg/kg/day) for maintenance therapy.[102] On this regimen 79% responded from 1 to more than 20 months (median, 7.6 months). No previous agent had achieved such a high degree of response. Vincristine was initially noted to be an effective agent in treating acute leukemia in children. Subsequently, a few responses in neuroblastoma and other solid tumors were reported.[92b] However, use of vincristine in 13 patients by the SCCSG resulted in only two partial remissons and one apparent cure (32 months with no evidence of tumor) of an infant diagnosed at 4 months of age.[112]

Use of the combination of vincristine and cyclophosphamide was suggested by James and co-workers[60] to result in more extensive and more frequent regressions of neuroblastoma than did either agent alone. Nine consecutive children with unresectable neuroblastomas were treated. Two sustained complete remissions with drug therapy alone. Local radiation was added for 4 others, and 3 of them had complete regressions. The other 3 patients had objective regressions with the drug combination, and 2 of them had long complete remissions after further treatment with radiation and surgery. Four of this group of 9 patients were less than 1 year of age, whereas another was only 14 months old. Three of the 4 older patients (3 to 11 years) were treated with irradiation as well as the medications. Interpretation and long-term prognostication of such mixed therapy are difficult.

A later report from the same institution[85] reveals that 5 of 18 patients treated with vincristine and cyclophosphamide were living 12 to 55 months with no evidence of disease. All 5 were less than 2 years of age, whereas only 1 of the over 2-year age group was alive and that child had active disease. Other investigators' reports have failed to confirm the long-term effectiveness of these two agents in combination. Overall response rate in a group of 38 children of all ages with metastatic neuroblastoma was 32%, and of the 8 patients alive without disease, 5 were under 1 year of age.[33] The SCCSG study of cyclic vincristine and cyclophosphamide resulted in only two complete and six partial responses among 21 children; all 8 suffered progression of disease in less than 10 months, despite the fact that 5 of them were less than 2 years of age at the time of diagnosis.[95] Sawitsky[90] reported that results of therapy with vincristine and cyclophosphamide were similar whether the drugs were used sequentially, concurrently, or on an alternate-week schedule. He noted a 55% objective tumor response, with 25% achieving complete remission. Duration of survival (median, 245 days) was perhaps increased, even in patients with marrow and skeletal metastases; however, of the 48 patients, only 1 of the 3 alive at the time of the report was in complete remission, and the 3 survivors were each less than 2 years of age at the time of diagnosis.

It seems apparent that these two agents can cause objective tumor regressions, but determining the extent of effectiveness is exceedingly difficult in view of the unique and unpredictable biologic variability of this particular tumor. The reports referred to do not utilize the same staging criteria to allow comparison of results of therapy among various patient groups, nor do they divide the patients into comparable age groups or have other similarities needed for comparative analysis.

Several other chemotherapeutic agents have been shown to have some antitumor effect on neuroblastoma. In a study by Cancer Group A, daunomycin therapy resulted in a 40% partial response rate when given daily but in only an 11% response rate when administered every other day.[89] Among 29 patients with metastatic neuroblastoma treated with daunomycin by members of the SCCSG, however, only 3 achieved transient partial remissions.[98] Severe toxicity in the form of leukopenia and thrombocytopenia limits the usefulness of this agent. The variable response rate with different administration schedules points out the need for better definition of the most appropriate method of using this drug. Adriamycin, a hydroxy analog of daunomycin, has also been noted to cause objective regressions of neuroblastomas.[13] Its toxicities are similar to those of daunomycin. Other agents that have been found not to be significantly effective are uracil mustard,[37] L-sarcolysine,[38] and hydroxyurea.[36]

In the studies just referred to no consideration is given to the possible immunosuppressive effects of the chemotherapy, that is, whether the drugs might actually interfere with the patients' inherent immunologic mechanisms and abilities to control the tumor. At present there are no accurate methods by which to assess these factors, although considerations are of growing importance in view of the recent research by Hellström and associates[48, 49] and Bill.[8-10] Perhaps such investigations will provide information that will allow selection of therapeutic regimens individually tailored to the patient. This may involve combinations or deletions of immunotherapy, chemotherapy, radiotherapy, or surgery in the manner appropriately advantageous to the affected host.

REPRESENTATIVE CASE SUMMARIES

Case 1. F. H. was admitted to the hospital at 12 weeks of age with anemia and hepatomegaly. Bone marrow aspiration revealed clumps of neoplastic cells consistent with rosette formation in neuroblastoma. VMA, HVA, and free catecholamine excretion were all elevated. No metastases were seen on x-ray examination of the entire skeleton. At surgery a retroperitoneal neuroblastoma extending into the posterior portion of the liver was found and was considered not resectable; metallic clips were placed to outline the extent of the tumor. Postoperatively the patient received 2200 rads to the abdomen over a 6-week interval, followed by alternating therapy with vincristine and cyclophosphamide according to the regimen of James and co-workers[60] for 4 months. The decision to stop chemotherapy was made when monthly determinations of VMA, HMA, and free catecholamines returned to normal and no further neoplastic cells were found in the marrow. The child is free of neuroblastoma 32 months after diagnosis. This case illustrates the favorable prognosis for infants in spite of widely disseminated disease.

Case 2. L. F. was admitted to the hospital at 18 months of age with a mass in the left lower quadrant of the abdomen. The liver was displaced 3 cm below the right costal margin, there was left inguinal lymphadenopathy, and both nodes and tumor mass appeared to be fixed to deeper structures. Both VMA and HVA were elevated. An anterior mediastinal mass was noted on chest x-ray examination, and the IVP revealed displacement of the bladder. A roentgenographic survey of the skeleton demonstrated osteolytic lesions of the pelvis, tibia, skull, and sternum. Bone marrow aspiration revealed cells consistent with neuroblastoma, and an inguinal biopsy also revealed a pattern consistent with neuroblastoma. The patient was treated with 1600 rads to the mediastinum and 700 rads to the pelvis. This was followed by alternating weekly therapy with cyclophosphamide and vincristine. Mediastinal and pelvic masses regressed approximately 75%, but new metastases appeared to compress the spinal cord at the T_1-T_2 level. The patients parents refused further therapy, and the child died at 23 months. This case illustrates the pattern commonly seen in children with disseminated disease diagnosed over 1 year of age.

Case 3. D. M. was admitted to the hospital at 9 years of age with progressive paraplegia, and a lesion compressing the spinal cord at T_1-T_2 was subtotally resected at surgery. She was then given cyclophosphamide for 10 weeks while she regained complete recovery of motor function of the lower extremities. Thereafter she was given 1800 rads to the tumor site over a 4-week period, then continued receiving cyclophosphamide. The patient is without evidence of recurrence 37 months after diagnosis. The diagnosis of this tumor pathologically was not clear until the typical "catecholamine granules" were demonstrated by electron microscopy. This case illustrates the favorable response seen in many children with extra-abdominal tumors, although further observation is indicated.

APPENDIX
Classification by James [58]

Stage   I—localized, resectable
Stage   II—regional, unresectable
Stage III—generalized, but without bone or marrow involvement
Stage IV—generalized and with bone or marrow involvement

Classification by Pinkel and co-workers[85]

Stage   I—local, completely resectable
Stage   II—regional
      (A) partly resectable
      (B) not resectable
Stage III—systemic
      (A) no marrow involvement
      (B) tumor cells in marrow

Classification by Thurman and Donaldson[101] (excludes all children under 1 year of age)

Stage   I—localized and totally resectable*
      (A) well-differentiated
      (B) undifferentiated
Stage   II—regional, nonresectable
      (A) well-differentiated
      (B) undifferentiated
Stage III—generalized, with bone involvement

Classification by Evans and associates[32]

Stage   I—tumor confined to organ or structure of origin
Stage   II—tumors extending in continuity beyond the organ or structure of origin but

---

*Automatically reclassified to Stage II if catecholamine excretion remains high 3 months after removal.

not crossing the midline; regional lymph nodes on the homolateral side may be involved*

Stage III—tumors extending in continuity beyond the midline; regional lymph nodes may be involved bilaterally

Stage IV—remote disease involving skeleton, organs, soft tissues, or distant lymph node groups, etc.

Stage IV-S—patients who would otherwise be Stage I or II, but who have remote disease confined only to one or more of the following sites: liver, skin, or bone marrow (without radiographic evidence of metastases on complete skeletal survey)

---

*For tumors arising in midline structures (e.g., the organs of Zuckerkandl), penetration beyond the capsule and involvement of lymph nodes on the same side shall be considered Stage II. Bilateral extension of any type shall be considered Stage III.

REFERENCES

1. Adams, L. T.: Neuroblastoma. Review of literature and report of eighteen cases, North Carolina Med. J. 27:113-125, March, 1966.
2. Allen, J. E., Morse, T. S., Frye, T. R., and Clatworthy, H. W.: Vena cavograms in infants and children, Ann. Surg. 160:568-574, 1960.
3. Bachmann, K. D.: Das neuroblastoma sympathicum. Klinik und prognose von 1030 Fallen, Kinderheilk. 86:710-724, 1962.
4. Beckwith, J. B., and Martin, R. F.: Observations on the histopathology of neuroblastomas, J. Pediatr. Surg. 3:106-110, 1968.
5. Beckwith, J. B., and Perrin, E. V.: In situ neuroblastomas: a contribution to the natural history of neural crest tumors, Am. J. Pathol. 43:1089-1104, 1963.
6. Bell, M.: Neuroblastoma; newer chemical diagnostic tests, J.A.M.A. 205:155-156, 1968.
7. Beltran, G., Leiderman, E., Stuckey, W. J., Ferrans, V. J., and Mogabgad, W. J.: Metastatic ganglioneuroblastoma. Ultrastructural, histochemical, and virological studies in a case, Cancer 24:552-559, 1969.
8. Bill, A. H.: A study of nerve growth factor in the serum of neuroblastoma patients, J. Pediatr. Surg. 3:171-177, 1968.
9. Bill, A. H.: Studies of the mechanism of reggression of human neuroblastoma, J. Pediatr. Surg. 3:727-734, 1968.
10. Bill, A. H.: The implications of immune reactions to neuroblastoma, Surgery 66:415-418, 1969.
11. Bodian, M.: Neuroblastoma, Pediatr. Clin. North Am. 6:449-472, 1959.
12. Bodian, M.: Neuroblastoma. An evaluation of its natural history and the effects of therapy, with particular reference to treatment by massive doses of Vitamin B$_{12}$, Arch. Dis. Child. 38:606-619, 1963.
13. Bonadonna, G., and Monfardini, S.: Therapeutic effects of adriamycin in the neoplastic disease of children and adults (abstract), Proc. Am. Assoc. Cancer Res. 11:10, 1970.
14. Bray, P. F., Ziter, F. A., Lahey, M. E., and Myers, G. G.: The coincidence of neuroblastoma and acute cerebellar encephalopathy, J. Pediatr. 75:983-990, 1969.
15. Breslow, N., and McCann, B.: Statistical estimation of prognosis for children with neuroblastoma, Cancer Res. 31:2098-2103, 1971.
16. Brett, E. M., Oppe, T. E., Ruthven, C. R. J., and Sandler, M.: Congenital dopamine-secreting neuroblastoma with clinical and biochemical remission, Arch. Dis. Child. 39:403-405, 1964.
17. Chatten, J.: Personal communication, July, 1971.
18. Chatten, J., and Voorhess, M. L.: Familial neuroblasoma. Report of a kindred with multiple disorders, including neuroblastomas in four siblings, N. Engl. J. Med. 277:1230-1236, 1967.
19. Clatworthy, H. W., Jr.: The treatment of neuroblastoma, Ca 18:146-150, May-June, 1968.
20. Cox, D.: Chromosome studies in 12 solid tumors from children, Br. J. Cancer 22:402-414, 1968.

21. Cox, D., Yuncken, C., and Spriggs, A. I.: Minute chromatin bodies in malignant tumors of childhood, Lancet **2**:55-58, 1965.

22. D'Angio, G. J.: Effects of radiation on the neuroblastoma, J. Pediatr. Surg. **3**:179-181, 1968.

23. D'Angio, G. J., Evans, A. E., and Koop, C. E.: Special pattern of widespread neuroblastoma with a favorable prognosis, Lancet **1**:1046-1049, 1971.

24. D'Angio, G. J., Loken, M., and Nesbit, M.: Radionuclear (75 Se) identification of tumor in children with neuroblastoma, Radiology **93**:615-617, 1969.

25. Dargeon, H. W.: Neuroblastoma, J. Pediatr. **61**:456-471, 1962.

26. de Gutierrez Moyano, M. B., Bergada, C., and Becu, L.: Catecholamine excretion in forty children with sympathoblastoma, J. Pediatr. **77**:239-244, 1970.

27. de Gutierrez Moyano, M. B., Bergada, C., and Becu, L.: Significance of catecholamine excretion in the follow-up of sympathoblastomas, Cancer **27**:228-232, 1971.

28. deLorimer, A. A., Bragg, K. U., and Linden, G.: Neuroblastoma in childhood, Am. J. Dis. Child. **118**:441-450, 1969.

29. Delta, B. G., and Pinkel, D.: Bone marrow aspiration in children with malignant tumors, J. Pediatr. **64**:542-546, 1964.

30. Eklof, O., and Gooding, A.: Paravertebral widening in cases of neuroblastoma, Br. J. Radiol. **40**:358-365, 1967.

31. Evans, A. E., Blore, J., Hadley, R., and Tanindi, S.: The LaBrosse spot test: A practical aid in the diagnosis and management of children with neuroblastoma, Pediatrics **47**:913-915, 1971.

32. Evans, A. E., D'Angio, G. J., and Randolph, J.: A proposed staging for children with neuroblastoma, Cancer **27**:374-378, 1971.

33. Evans, A. E., Heyn, R. M., Newton, W. A., and Leikin, S. L.: Vincristine sulfate and cyclophosphamide for children with metastatic neuroblastoma, J.A.M.A. **207**:1325-1327, 1969.

34. Everson, T. C., and Cole, W. H.: Spontaneous regression of cancer, Philadelphia, 1966, W. B. Saunders Co. pp. 11-87.

35. Farber, S.: Neuroblastoma, Am. J. Dis. Child. **60**:749-751, 1940.

36. Fernbach, D. J.: Pediatric clinical trials with hydroxyurea (NSC 32065), Cancer Chemother. Rep. **40**:37-38, 1964.

37. Fernbach, D. J., Haddy, T. B., Holcomb, T. M., Lusher, J., Sutow, W. W., and Vietti, T. J.: Uracil mustard (NSC 34462) therapy for children with metastatic neuroblastoma, Cancer Chemother. Rep. **52**:287-291, 1968.

38. Fernbach, D. J., Haddy, T. B., Holcomb, T. M., Stuckey, W. J., Sullivan, M. P., and Watkins, W. L.: L-Sarcolysin (NSC 8806) therapy for children with metastatic neuroblastoma, Cancer Chemother. Rep. **52**:293-296, 1968.

39. Finklestein, J. Z., Eckert, H., Isaacs, H., and Higgens, G.: Bone marrow metastases in children with solid tumors, Am. J. Dis. Child. **119**:49-52, 1970.

40. Fortner, J., Nicastri, A., and Murphy, L. M.: Neuroblastoma: natural history and results of treating 138 cases, Ann. Surg. **167**:132-142, 1968.

41. Geiser, C. F., and Efron, M. L.: Cystathioninuria in patients with neuroblastoma or ganglioneuroblastoma. Its correlation to vanilmandelic acid excretion and its value in diagnosis and therapy, Cancer **22**:856-860, 1968.

42. Girolami, A.: A coagulation study in patients with neuroblastoma, Tumori **53**:495-502, 1967.

43. Gjessing, L. R., and Mauritzen, K.: Cystathioninuria in hepatoblastoma, Scand. J. Clin. Lab. Invest. **17**:513-514, 1965.

44. Greenberg, R., Rosenthal, I., and Falk, G. S.: Electron microscopy of human tumors secreting catecholamines; correlation with biochemical data, J. Neuropathol. Exp. Neurol. **28**:475-500, 1969.

45. Greer, M., Anton, A. H., Williams, C. M., and Echevarria, R. A.: Tumors of neural crest origin, Arch. Neurol. (Chicago) **13**:139-148, Aug., 1965.

46. Gross, R. E., Farber, S., and Martin, L. W.: Neuroblastoma sympatheticum; a study and report of 217 cases, Pediatrics **23**:1179-1191, 1959.

47. Guin, G. H., Gilbert, E. F., and Jones, B.: Incidental neuroblastoma in infants, Am. J. Clin. Pathol. **51**:126-136, 1969.

48. Hellström, I. E.: A colony inhibition (CI) technique for demonstration of tumor cell destruction by lymphoid cells in vitro, Int. J. Cancer. **2**:265-268, 1967.

49. Hellström, I., Hellström, K. E., Evans, A., Heppener, G. H., Pierce, G. E., and Yang, J. P. S.: Serum-mediated protection of neoplastic cells from inhibition by lymphocytes immune to their tumor-specific antigens, Proc. Natl. Acad. Sci. USA **62**:362-368, 1969.

50. Hellström, I., Hellström, K. E., and Pierce, G. E.: Cell-bound immune reactions against tumor specific transplantation antigens, Can. Cancer Conf. **8**:425-442, 1969.

51. Hellström, I. E., Hellström, K. E., Pierce, G. E., and Bill, A. H.: Demonstration of cell-bound and humoral immunity against neuroblastoma cells, Proc. Natl. Acad. Sci. USA **60**:1231-1238, 1968.

52. Hellström, K. E., Hellström, I. E., Bill, A. H., Pierce, G. E., and Yang, J. P. S.: Studies on cellular immunity to human neuroblastoma cells, Int. J. Cancer **6**:172-188, 1970.

53. Helson, L., Blasco, P., and Murphy, M. L.: Familial neuroblastoma (abstract), Clin. Res. **17**:614, 1969.

54. Herxheimer, G.: Uber Tumoren des Nebennierenmarkes, insbesondere das Neuroblastoma sympaticum, Beitr. Pathol. Anat. **57**:112, 1914.

55. Hinterberger, M., and Bartholomew, R. J.: Catecholamines and their acidic metabolites in urine and in tumor tissue in neuroblastoma, ganglioneuroma and phaeochromocytoma, Clin. Chim. Acta **23**:169-175, 1969.

56. Hinton, P., and Buschke, F.: Neuroblastoma in children, 42 cases, Radiol. Clin. Biol. **37**:19-28, 1968.

57. Hutchison, R.: On suprarenal sarcoma in children with metastases in the skull, Q. J. Med. **1**:33-38, 1907.

58. James, D. H., Jr.: Proposed classification of neuroblastoma, J. Pediatr. **71**:764, 1967.

59. James, D. H., Jr., and George, P.: Vincristine in children with malignant solid tumors, J. Pediatr. **64**:534-542, 1964.

60. James, D. H., Jr., Hustu, O., Wrenn, E. L., Jr., and Pinkel, D.: Combination chemotherapy of childhood neuroblastoma, J.A.M.A. **194**:123-126, 1965.

61. Knudson, A. G., and Amromin, G. D.: Neuroblastoma and ganglioneuroma in a child with multiple neurofibromatosis, Cancer **19**:1032-1037, 1966.

62. Kontras, S. B.: Urinary excretion of 3-methoxy-4-hydroxymandelic acid in children with neuroblastoma, Cancer **15**:978-986, 1962.

62a. Kontras, S. B., and Newton, W. A.: Cyclophosphamide (cytoxan) therapy of childhood neuroblastoma. Preliminary report, Cancer Chemother. Rep. **12**:39-50, 1961.

63. Koop, C. E.: Neuroblastoma: two year survival and treatment correlations, J. Pediatr. Surg. **3**:178-179, 1968.

64. Koop, C. E., Kiesewetter, W. B., and Horn, R. C.: Neuroblastoma in childhood. Survival after major surgical insult to the tumor, Surgery **38**:272-278, 1955.

65. Lee, J. A. H.: Summer and death from neuroblastoma, Br. Med. J. **2**:404-407, 1967.

66. Levan, A., Manolov, G., and Clifford, P.: Chromosomes of a human neuroblastoma: a new case with accessory minute chromosomes, J. Natl. Cancer Inst. **41**:1377-1387, 1968.

67. Lingley, J. F., Sagerman, R. H., Santulli, T. V., and Wolff, J. A.: Neuroblastoma. Management and survival, N. Engl. J. Med. **227**:1227-1230, 1967.

68. Loretz, W.: Virchow's Arch. **49**:435, 1870. Cited by Willis, R. A.: Pathology of tumours, ed. 4, New York, 1967, Appleton-Century-Crofts, pp. 857-885.

69. Mäkinen, J.: Microscopic patterns as a guide to prognosis of neuroblastoma in childhood, Cancer **29**:1637-1646, 1972.

70. Marchand, F.: Beitrage zur Kenntniss der normalen und pathologischen Anatomie der Glandula carotica und der Nebennieren, Festschrift für Rudolph, Virchows Arch. **5**:578, 1891.

71. Martin, R. F., and Beckwith, J. B.: Lymphoid infiltrates in neuroblastomas: their occurrence and prognostic significance, J. Pediatr. Surg. **3**:161-164, 1968.

72. Miller, R. W., Fraumeni, J. F., and Hill, J. A.: Neuroblastoma: epidemiologic approach to its origin, Am. J. Dis. Child. **115**:253-261, 1968.

73. Misugi, K., Misugi, N., and Newton, W. A.: Fine structural study of neuroblastoma, ganglioneuroblastoma, and pheochromocytoma, Arch. Pathol. **86**:160-170, Aug., 1968.

74. Morgan, J. H.: Trans. Path. Soc. Lond. **30**:399, 1879. Cited by Willis, R. A.: Pathology of tumours, ed. 4, New York, 1967, Appleton-Century-Crofts, pp. 857-885.

75. Murray, M. R., and Stout, A. P.: Distinctive characteristics of the sympathicoblastoma cultivated *in vitro*. A method for prompt diagnosis, Am. J. Pathol. **23**:429-441, 1947.

76. McAllister, R. M.: Neuroblastoma: A viral etiology? J. Pediatr. Surg. **3**:138-141, 1968.

77. McKendrick, T., and Edwards, R. W. H.: The excretion of 4-hydroxy-3-methoxy-mandelic acid by children, Arch. Dis. Child. **41**:418-425, 1965.

78. McMillan, C. W., Gaudry, C. L., Jr., and Holemans, R.: Coagulation defects and metastatic neuroblastoma, J. Pediatr. **72**:347-350, 1968.

79. Onuigbo, W. I. B.: Cephalic spread of neuroblastoma in children, Arch. Dis. Child. **36**: 526-529, 1961.

80. Pepper, W.: A study of congenital sarcoma of the liver and suprarenal, Am. J. Med. Sci. **121**:287-298, 1901.

81. Perez, C. A., Vietti, T., Ackerman, L. V., Eagleton, M. D., and Powers, W. E.: Tumors of the sympathetic nervous system in childhood. An appraisal of treatment and results, Radiology **88**:750-760, 1967.

82. Peterson, D. R., Bill, A. H., Jr., and Kirkland, I. S.: Neuroblastoma trends in time, J. Pediatr. Surg. **4**:244-249, 1969.

83. Peterson, H. D., and Collins, O. D.: Chronic diarrhea and failure to thrive secondary to ganglioneuroma, Arch. Surg. **95**:934-936, 1967.

84. Pinkel, D., Dowd, J. E., and Bross, I. D. J.: Some epidemiological features of malignant solid tumors of children in the Buffalo, N. Y. area, Cancer **16**:28-33, 1963.

85. Pinkel, D., Pratt, C., Holton, C., James, D., Wrenn, E., and Hustu, O.: Survival of children with neuroblastoma treated with combination chemotherapy, J. Pediatr. **73**: 928-931, 1968.

86. Reilly, D., Nesbit, M. E., and Krivit, W.: Cure of three patients who had skeletal metastases in disseminated neuroblastoma, Pediatrics **41**:47-51, 1968.

87. Rinscheid, J.: Virchow's Arch. **297**:508, 1936. Cited by Willis, R. A.: Pathology of tumours, ed. 4, New York, 1967, Appleton-Century-Crofts, pp. 857-885.

88. Robertson, H. E.: Virchow's Arch. **220**:147, 1915, Cited by Willis, R. A.: Pathology of tumours, ed. 4, New York, 1967, Appleton-Century-Crofts, pp. 857-885.

89. Samuels, L. D., Newton, W. A., Jr., and Heyn, R.: Daunorubicin therapy in advanced neuroblastoma, Cancer **27**:831-834, 1971.

90. Sawitsky, A.: Vincristine and cyclophosphamide therapy in generalized neuroblastoma. A collaborative study, Am. J. Dis. Child. **119**:308-313, 1970.

91. Sawitsky, A., and Desposito, F.: A survey of American experience with vitamin B$_{12}$ therapy of neuroblastoma, J. Pediatr. **67**:99-103, 1965.

92. Schneider, K. M., Becker, J. M., and Krasna, I. H.: Neonatal neuroblastoma, Pediatrics **36**:359-366, 1965.

92b. Selawry, O. S., and Hananian, J.: Vincristine treatment of cancer in children, J.A.M.A. **183**:741-746, 1963.

93. Shanklin, D. R., and Sotelo-Avila, C.: In-situ tumors in fetuses, newborns, and young infants, Biol. Neonate **14**:286-316, 1969.

94. Stickler, G. B., and Flock, E. V.: Neuroblastoma and ganglioneuroblastoma: Associated increased urinary excretion of catecholamines, Cancer Chemother. Rep. **16**:439-442, 1962.

95. Sullivan, M. P., Nora, A. H., Kulapongs, P., Lane, D. M., Windmiller, J., and Thurman, W. G.: Evaluation of vincristine sulfate and cyclophosphamide chemotherapy for metastatic neuroblastoma, Pediatrics **44**:685-694, 1969.

96. Sunderman, F. W.: Measurements of vanilmandelic acid for the diagnosis of pheochromocytoma and neuroblastoma, Am. J. Clin. Pathol. **42**:481-497, 1964.

97. Sutow, W. W.: Prognosis in neuroblastoma of childhood, Am. J. Dis. Child. **96**:299-305, 1958.

98. Sutow, W. W., Fernbach, D. J., Thurman, W. G., Holton, C. P., and Watkins, W. L.: Daunomycin in the treatment of metastatic neuroblastoma, Part I, Cancer Chemother. Rep. **54**:283-289, 1970.

99. Sutow, W. W., Gehan, E. A., Heyn, R. M., Kung, F. H., Miller, R. W., Murphy, M. L., and Traggis, D. G.: Comparison of survival curves, 1956 versus 1962, in children with Wilms' tumor and neuroblastoma. Report of the Subcommittee on Childhood Solid Tumors, Solid Tumor Task Force, National Cancer Institute, Pediatrics 48:800-811, 1970.

100. Sy, W. M., and Edmondson, J. H.: The developmental defects associated with neuroblastoma-etiologic implications, Cancer 22:234-238, 1968.

101. Thurman, W. G., and Donaldson, M. H.: Current concepts in the management of neuroblastoma. In Neoplasia of childhood, Chicago, 1967, Year Book Medical Publishers, Inc., pp. 175-181.

102. Thurman, W. G., Fernbach, D. J., Sullivan, M. P.: Cyclophosphamide therapy in childhood neuroblastoma, N. Engl. J. Med. 270:1336-1340, 1964.

103. Virchow, R.: Hyperplasie der Zirbel und der Nebennieren. In Die krankhaften Geschwülste, vol. 2, Berlin, 1864-1865, A. Hirschwald.

104. von Studnitz, W., Kaser, H., and Sjoerdsma, A.: Spectrum of catecholamine biochemistry in patients with neuroblastoma, N. Engl. J. Med. 269:232-235, 1963.

105. Voorhess, M. L.: The catecholamines in tumor and urine from patients with neuroblastoma, ganglioneuroblastoma and pheochromocytoma, J. Pediatr. Surg. 3:146-148, 1968.

106. Voorhess, M. L.: Neuroblastoma with normal urinary catecholamine excretion, J. Pediatr. 78:680-683, 1971.

107. Voorhess, M. L., and Gardner, L. I.: Urinary excretion of norepinephrine, epinephrine, and 3-methoxy, 4-hydroxy mandelic acid by children with neuroblastoma, J. Clin. Endocrinol. 21:321-335, 1961.

108. Voorhess, M. L., and Gardner, L. I.: Studies of catecholamine excretion by children with neural tumors, J. Clin. Endocrinol. 22:126-133, 1962.

109. Voorhess, M. L., Pickett, L. K., and Gardner, L. I.: Functioning tumors of neural crest origin in childhood. Follow-up report, Am. J. Surg. 106:33-35, July, 1963.

110. Williams, C. M., and Greer, M.: Homovanillic acid and vanilmandelic acid in diagnosis of neuroblastoma, J.A.M.A. 183:134-138, 1963.

111. Willis, R. A.: Pathology of tumours, ed. 4, New York, 1967, Appleton-Century-Crofts, pp. 857-885.

112. Windmiller, J., Berry, D. H., Haddy, T. B., Vietti, T. J., and Sutow, W. W.: Vincristine sulfate in the treatment of neuroblastoma in children, Am. J. Dis. Child. 111:75-78, 1966.

113. Wong, K. Y., Hanenson, I. B., and Lampkin, B. C.: Familial neuroblastoma, Am. J. Dis. Child. 121:415-416, 1971.

114. Wright, J. H.: Neurocytoma or neuroblastoma, a kind of tumor not generally recognized, J. Exp. Med. 12:556-561, 1910.

CHAPTER 18

Retinoblastoma

NORAH ᴅᴜV. TAPLEY

PATRICIA TRETTER

Retinoblastoma, a malignant congenital tumor, arises in the retina of one or both eyes and is frequently multicentric. Its successful treatment results from its tendency to grow inside the globe before involving the periglobal structures or spreading into the intracranial space.

The following discussion utilizes published reports of large series of retinoblastoma patients as well as personal experience in the treatment of retinoblastoma at the Columbia-Presbyterian Medical Center in New York. Carefully documented case histories of 900 patients treated by the Retinoblastoma Team at the Columbia-Presbyterian Medical Center from 1938 through 1968 have provided much of the data reviewed in these pages.

INCIDENCE

Retinoblastoma is a relatively rare tumor in the United States. In 1964 Francois[5] reported an incidence varying from one case in 34,000 births to one case in 14,000 births. Additionally he described a persistent increase in the frequency of occurrence of the disease from 1927 to 1960 based on published series of other authors. This increase could be due to more frequent reporting of retinoblastoma but may also represent greater opportunity for genetic transmission of the disease as a result of a higher survival rate of patients.

Retinoblastoma is usually diagnosed prior to 2 years of age, the average age being 18 months. It has been discovered within the first 6 weeks of life as a result of careful evaluation of a child with a history of a parent or a sibling having had retinoblastoma.

Approximately two thirds of all retinoblastoma cases are unilateral. In selected series bilaterality has been reported to be as low as 20%. According to Ellsworth,[3] probably 5% of his patients who initially present with unilateral disease will eventually show separate tumor foci in the opposite retina.

HEREDITY

Genetic studies by many investigators have suggested that retinoblastoma is produced by either transmission of a defective gene or a spontaneous somatic cell mutation.[4, 5, 7,10, 22] The initial presentation in a given family line, the "sporadic" patient, may have unilateral or bilateral disease. On pedigree analysis, unilateral sporadic cases have been proved to be germinal mutations. Although it has been suggested that somatic mutations[7, 22] may produce retinoblastoma, Ellsworth[2] considers that it is more logical that all retinoblastomas are the result

411

of germinal mutations. A varying rate of penetrance for this mutation is supported by familial occurrence of cases varying from 20% to almost 100%.[4]

Careful analysis of retinoblastoma family pedigrees suggests that the mode of inheritance is by an autosomal dominant gene,[5] although it is evident that some individuals can carry the defective gene without tumor occurrence. Four percent of normal parents of an affected child have produced more than one offspring with retinoblastoma. Macklin[10] found a 6.8% incidence of more than one affected child in a normal family line when a retinoblastoma offspring had been produced. Since the possibility of spontaneous mutation in more than one sibling is astronomically low, the probability of a carrier state for the gene in a parent with ensuing disease in the offspring must be recognized.

When the disease is bilateral, there is frequently a family history of retinoblastoma. Francois[5] reports an increasing occurrence of bilateral disease in the offspring of succeeding generations of retinoblastoma families. When the disease is unilateral and has first appeared in a family, there is an 8% to 25% chance that the offspring of the patient will have retinoblastoma.

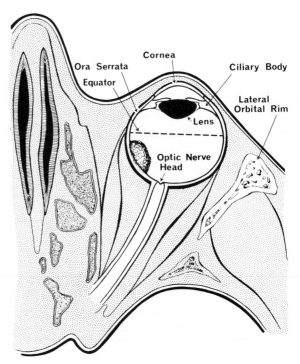

Fig. 18-1. Diagram of horizontal section through an eye that contains a tumor mass. The equator, the midplane of the eye, is used as a reference line in staging the extent of disease for prognosis. The location of the tumor posterior to the equator and its size approximately four times larger than the optic disc places this eye in Group IA. The lateral radiation treatment portal, if placed slightly anterior to the lateral orbital rim and angled 3 degrees posteriorly, will spare the posterior pole of the lens and will encompass most of the retina in the radiation beam. (Courtesy Medical Communications, The University of Texas at Houston, M. D. Anderson Hospital and Tumor Institute.)

PATHOLOGY AND ROUTES OF SPREAD

The glial elements in the spongeoblastic series have been considered the cells of origin for retinoblastoma, although there are preliminary reports that it may arise from the receptor cells.[24] Popoff, working with the Retinoblastoma Team in electron microscopy studies of retinoblastoma cells, found similarities with the outer retinal cells in the normal human embryo. The microscopic picture of retinoblastoma is one of undifferentiated and small cells with deeply staining nuclei and scant cytoplasm or one of larger cells that form rosettes around a central cavity.

Retinoblastoma may present as a single tumor in the retina (Fig. 18-1) but typically arises in multiple foci. Ellsworth[2] reported two or more retinal tumors in 84% of a consecutive series. Spread of tumor in the retinal layers and eruption through the retina at a distance from the original site, as well as separate tumor foci, are the sources of the multiple tumors. Multicentric tumor development is the basis for bilateral disease rather than spread of tumor from one retina to the other by growth along the optic nerves and through the optic chiasm.

Retinoblastoma, when it arises in the internal nuclear layers of the retina, grows forward into the vitreous cavity. This more common type of growth, termed *endophytic*, is easily seen with the ophthalmoscope. If the tumor is *exophytic*, arising in the external nuclear layer and growing into the subretinal space with detachment of the retina (Fig. 18-2, *A*) in the process, diagnosis is more difficult because the tumor itself is not seen.

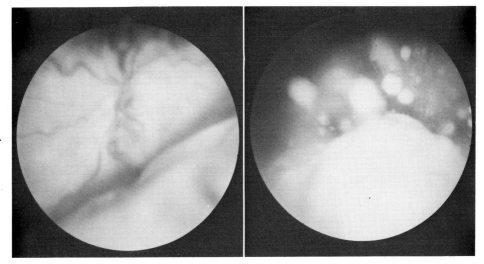

Fig. 18-2. Photograph of retina taken through indirect ophthalmoscope during examination of retinoblastoma patient prior to any treatment being given. **A,** Retinal detachment. A tumor mass arising in the deeper layers of the retina has pushed forward into the posterior chamber of the eye and produced retinal detachment. Tortuous and enlarged vessels can be seen leading toward the tumor. **B,** Vitreous seeds. A large tumor mass projects into the vitreous with numerous vitreous floaters or seeds. Some of the seeds may contain calcium. Vitreous seeds indicate extensive tumor and a poor prognosis for salvaging vision. (Courtesy Medical Communications, The University of Texas at Houston, M. D. Anderson Hospital and Tumor Institute.)

Endophytic tumors may produce seeds in the vitreous (Fig. 18-2, *B*). Tumor fragments break away from the main tumor mass and float in the vitreous cavity. Vitreous seeds are a bad prognostic sign and are associated with large tumors (usually more than 5 disc diameters in size). They are possible sources of new tumor growth if they remain viable, settle out on unaffected parts of the retina, and establish a blood supply.

Extension of retinoblastoma into the choroid, the vascular layer between the retina and sclera, usually occurs with massive tumors and may indicate a poor prognosis for tumor control. However, invasion of the choroid does not necessarily result in hematogenous metastases. The majority of children with choroidal involvement have survived.

Invasion of the sclera has serious prognostic significance. It may occur by either direct extension from the choroid or, less usually, spread along the emissary vessels. Involvement of the periglobal tissues results, and hematogenous spread of tumor may occur. Retinoblastoma cells that enter the general circulation commonly metastasize to the bone marrow, the skeleton, the lymph nodes, and the liver, whereas pulmonary metastases are unusual.

The optic nerve may be directly invaded by growth of tumor into the nerve head and through the lamina cribrosa. If tumor extends 10 to 12 mm along the nerve to the point where the central retinal artery and vein enter and leave the nerve, it will almost certainly gain access to the subarachnoid space, with dissemination of tumor cells into the spinal fluid and seeding along the base of the brain.

In a review of autopsies of retinoblastoma patients, Merriam[11] noted that distant metastases were the cause of death in slightly more than half the patients, with intracranial extension the only site of tumor dissemination in 47%. In every patient with orbital recurrence the cervical lymph nodes were also involved.

DIAGNOSIS

Unilateral and small tumors are rarely diagnosed early because signs and symptoms are not obvious in the young patient. Only 3% of retinoblastoma patients have been identified on routine ocular examination. Half these patients had a known family history of retinoblastoma that prompted early eye examinations.

Usually the parents are first to notice an eye abnormality in the child. A whitish appearance of the pupil seen briefly when the eye is turned, called the *cat's eye reflex*, represents visualization of tumor through the lens (Fig. 18-3) and is the most common presenting sign of retinoblastoma. Strabismus is the next commonest sign and, if the tumor develops in the macula, it can occur early. A red and painful eye with or without glaucoma indicates extensive disease, frequently with widespread choroidal involvement. Limited vision or loss of vision usually occurs with massive bilateral tumor and is a late sign.

Examination for tumor requires meticulous inspection of the entire retina of both eyes with the indirect ophthalmoscope. Maximum dilatation of the pupils is essential, and the patient must be under general anesthesia. The tumor may be obvious, but it can be obscured by retinal detachment (Fig. 18-2, *A*), vitreous hemorrhage, or an opaque anterior chamber. A mass of creamy pink color pro-

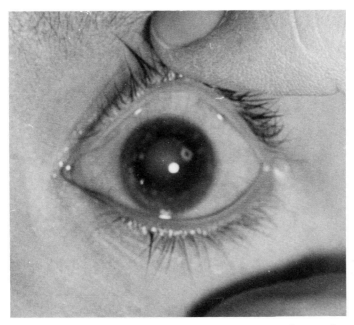

Fig. 18-3. "Cat's eye" reflex, most often observed by the parents as the initial sign of retino-blastoma, is tumor visualized through the lens. A whitish appearance of the lens is produced as the eye moves and light falls on the tumor mass. (Courtesy Medical Communications, The University of Texas at Houston, M. D. Anderson Hospital and Tumor Institute.)

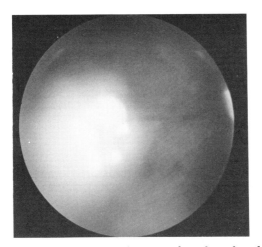

Fig. 18-4. Tumor calcification. Photograph of retina taken through indirect ophthalmoscope during examination of the eye of a patient with retinoblastoma. The ophthalmologist de-scribed this lesion to be 4 disc diameters in size on the nasal side of the retina, behind the equator, and to be partially calcified. In this photograph the optic nerve head can be glimpsed at the far right edge of the field. (Courtesy Medical Communications, The University of Texas at Houston, M. D. Anderson Hospital and Tumor Institute.)

jecting into the vitreous with extensive surface vascularization suggests retinoblastoma. A snow-white mass that is completely avascular is more frequently seen in older children. This type of tumor develops in the retinal periphery and presumably grows slowly over a long period of time, causing progressive loss of vision. The ora serrata is a frequent location for retinoblastoma and in Ellsworth' series[2] occurred in over 75% of the patients. This may result from spread of tumor cells through the subretinal space with mechanical trapping at the ora serrata and formation of a mass.

Typical features of retinoblastoma are vitreous seeding (Fig. 18-2, *B*) and tumor calcification (Fig. 18-4). Calcium can be seen with the ophthalmoscope in over 50% of the lesions. It has been reported[13] that calcium can be identified in as many as 75% on x-ray examination if special roentgenographic techniques are used. Vitreous floaters may be clumps of active tumors cells or calcified tumor masses. If the tumor is not well visualized on funduscopic examination, radiophosphate (^{32}P) sodium localization in the tumor or x-ray studies may assist diagnosis. Fiberoptic transilluminators occasionally aid in evaluating detachments and solid lesions.

In a review of 825 histologically proved retinoblastomas in the files of the Registry of Ophthalmic Pathology of the Armed Forces Institute of Pathology, Stafford[18] reported that 14.9% of the patients were initially misdiagnosed. Almost half these cases had been diagnosed clinically as ocular inflammation. Stafford also observed that a delay in therapy in correctly diagnosed patients or misdiagnosis leading to inappropriate therapy resulted in significantly increased mortality rates when compared with mortality rates in diagnosed patients who received prompt treatment for retinoblastoma.

A potentially useful biochemical approach to the initial diagnosis of retinoblastoma and determination of whether the disease has been controlled by treatment has been the assay of urine of retinoblastoma patients for vanilmandelic acid (VMA) and homovanillic acid (HVA). This approach was suggested by observed similarities between retinoblastoma and neuroblastoma and the presence of VMA and HVA in neuroblastoma patients. Brown,[1] studying retinoblastoma patients at Columbia-Presbyterian Medical Center, reported that these children excreted VMA and HVA in elevated amounts. After successful treatment these substances were excreted in almost normal amounts. Brown pointed out that the number of patients studied was insufficient for the results to be significant but that this suggests an approach of potential advantage both for diagnosis and testing response to treatment.

A number of eye conditions must be differentiated from retinoblastoma, ranging from parasitic infestation and infection to congenital defects, retinal hemorrhage and detachment, and vascular malformation of retinal vessels. The term *leukokoria* means white pupil, and an assortment of eye lesions will present this sign. In these eyes, both the cornea and lens are clear. Any suggestion of an eye abnormality requires careful examination by an experienced ophthalmologist. Unless well-qualified professional personnel and facilities for proper diagnosis and therapy are available, all suspected cases should be referred to the nearest medical center.

Although the findings in the majority of retinoblastomas are characteristic, the disease is rare in the average practice. Other eye conditions usually have pathognomonic signs that help differentiate them from retinoblastoma.

A trial of radiation therapy purely for diagnosis is never justified. If there is extensive unilateral disease and no involvement of the second eye, the diagnosis is provided by enucleation of an eye that has little chance for useful vision. If both eyes are massively involved, removal of the most extensively involved eye is diagnostic, and treatment is administered to the remaining eye.

TREATMENT POLICIES

Treatment is dependent on the presenting stage of the disease. The initial approach is influenced by whether the tumor is confined to the retina or has extended into the periglobal tissues and whether metastases, either to the central nervous system or distant, have occurred. The majority of patients have disease confined to one or both eyes when first seen. If disease has extended outside the globe, it most often is microscopic, with tumor found on sectioning the cut end of the optic nerve or in the periglobal tissues. Occasionally a patient will be seen with massive orbital disease and proptosis or with distant metastases.

Prior to initiating therapy for the primary disease, careful evaluation for central nervous system extension and distant spread is necessary. Work-up should include x-ray examination of the lungs and skeletal system, with orbital views for optic nerve canal enlargement, bone marrow examination for tumor cells, and spinal fluid analysis for tumor invasion.

Stage of disease

When the patient with retinoblastoma first has both eyes examined with the indirect ophthalmoscope, accurate diagrams of the retina should be made. It is extremely important to chart the number, size and location of the retinal tumors. If the eye is not to be enucleated, it is essential to have the extent of disease clearly depicted so that results of treatment can be assessed. Additionally, the radiation therapist is aided in radiation beam placement by an exact description of tumor location. In using the binocular indirect ophthalmoscope with the large field, the size of the lesion can be estimated by comparison with the optic nerve head diameter. The position of the tumor in the fundus can be related to specific landmarks such as the optic nerve head, the fovea, ora serrata, etc.

To assess and compare treatment results more accurately, Reese[14] and Ellsworth[2] evolved the following system of staging according to extent of disease within the eye:

Group   I.   Very favorable
    1. Solitary tumor, less than 4 disc diameters in size, at or behind the equator
    2. Multiple tumors, none over 4 disc diameters in size, all at or behind the equator

Group II.   Favorable
    1. Solitary lesion, 4 to 10 disc diameters in size, at or behind the equator
    2. Multiple tumors, 4 to 10 disc diameters in size, behind the equator

Group III.   Doubtful
    1. Any lesion anterior to the equator
    2. Solitary tumors larger than 10 disc diameters behind the equator

Group IV.   Unfavorable
    1. Multiple tumors, some larger than 10 disc diameters
    2. Any lesion extending anteriorly to the ora serrata

Group   V.   Very unfavorable
1. Massive tumors involving over half the retina
2. Vitreous seeding

The extent of disease or stage determines the group in which the patient is placed and the treatment he will receive. The prognosis that is associated with a particular stage refers to the probability of preserving useful vision, not to the survival rate.

Group I. The prognosis for useful vision is very favorable when the disease is limited to one or more small tumors in the posterior segment of the globe, behind the equator (Fig. 18-1).

Group II. With more retina involved by tumor, the prognosis is slightly less favorable than in Group I.

Group III. The prognosis is definitely less favorable. Although tumors located anteriorly have been considered difficult to observe because of limited visualization of retina anterior to the equator, especially the nasal half, this problem has been eliminated by the binocular indirect ophthalmoscope. However, in irradiating these lesions, the effort made to avoid the lens can result in a geographic miss of the tumor, wholly or in part. Light coagulation can be more difficult with anteriorly located lesions, but practice largely solves this problem. Finally, more retina is involved by these larger tumors, which affects the prognosis for useful vision.

Group IV. The prognosis is unfavorable because of extent of retinal involvement.

Group V. The prognosis is very unfavorable but not hopeless. The disease is controlled in one third of the patients, and in some, moderately good vision has resulted.

Unilateral disease

When disease is confined to one eye, enucleation has been considered the treatment of choice by the group at Columbia-Presbyterian unless the tumor extent places it in Group I, II, or III. However, it is extremely rare to see unilateral disease with a tumor or tumors sufficiently small to make it likely that useful vision will result from radiation therapy. The patient with favorable unilateral disease is usually asymptomatic and is examined only because of the history of retinoblastoma in a sibling or parent. Occasionally the patient will develop a squint because tumor has involved the macula while the tumor is still relatively small.

Enucleation should not be done if the case can be placed in Group I, II, or III. The eye is treated with irradiation, even though a tissue diagnosis has not been made. Since this situation will occur almost always when there is a family history of retinoblastoma, the risk of treating nonmalignant disease that simulates retinoblastoma is very low. If there is no family history of retinoblastoma, irradiation should be given only if the retinal lesion appears strongly suggestive of retinoblastoma to an experienced observer. If the diagnosis is in doubt, careful and frequent reevaluation of the retinal lesion should eventually provide the answer.

If the eye with unilateral disease is to be irradiated, the treatment technique is the same as that used for the patient with bilateral disease who has had one eye enucleated. The lateral x-ray beam should be angled sufficiently to avoid irradiation of the lens of the opposite eye.

Bilateral disease

The patient with bilateral retinoblastoma usually presents with extensive involvement of one eye and less disease in the other eye. With little hope of preserving useful vision due to the degree of retinal involvement, the extensively diseased eye should be enucleated. Unless disease is massive in both eyes and there is no hope of obtaining useful vision in either eye, the least involved eye is always preserved for treatment and often offers a relatively favorable treatment situation. Even if this eye falls into Group V, an attempt should be made to salvage whatever vision there may be. A portion of the retina may eventually function normally even though it is detached at the time the diagnosis is made.

If bilateral retinoblastoma is diagnosed relatively early because of a family history of the disease, the situation may be favorable in that both eyes may contain relatively small tumors. Neither eye will require enucleation, and both eyes can be irradiated. Again a tissue diagnosis will not be available, but the family history as well as the appearance of the tumors should leave little doubt that retinoblastoma is present.

TREATMENT METHODS
Surgery

The extensively diseased eye is enucleated when there is no hope of achieving useful vision with irradiation. It is essential to remove as long a segment of the optic nerve as can be obtained because of possible tumor extension through the lamina cribrosa and for several millimeters into the nerve. Usually 10 to 14 mm of nerve can be removed, which is sufficient to provide a free margin if minimal nerve invasion has occurred. Since tumor extension beyond the point where the major retinal vessels enter and exit from the nerve means spread into the subarachnoid space beyond the reach of surgery, orbital exenteration is not considered of value.

Radiation therapy

External beam. The megavoltage photon beam provided by an 18 to 22 mev Betatron with its limited side scatter and decreased bone absorption offers desirable features in treating the eye positioned in the bony orbit. The treatment field should include as a minimum the entire retina posterior to the equator of the eye (Fig. 18-1). When tumor involves the retina up to the ora serrata, the anterior edge of the beam must be aligned to pass just posterior to the lens to include the entire retina and tumor in the radiation field. Irradiation of a small portion of the posterior lens may cause a cataract to form. This is a necessary risk, particularly if the tumor is located far forward on the nasal side of the globe.

A single 3 by 4 cm temporal portal (4 cm dimension oriented in the caudad-cephalad direction) ensures a margin of irradiation approximately 1 cm in width around the globe except anteriorly. A D-shaped collimator tailors the beam to the globe (Fig. 18-5). The straight anterior edge of the beam is positioned at or slightly anterior to the lateral orbital rim and is angled 3 degrees posteriorly to avoid the lens (Fig. 18-6). The degree of forward protrusion of the eye can be determined with an exophthalmometer. If the eye is somewhat exophthalmic, the edge of the beam should be positioned 1 or 2 mm anterior to the lateral orbital rim.

It is essential to maintain optimum positioning of the eye with reference to the beam during treatment. Satisfactory immobilization of the patient can be achieved by firm but comfortable swaddling, which, in the infant or young child, usually induces sleep. Sedation may be used for the particularly apprehensive child at the onset of therapy, and in some patients must be continued throughout the course of treatment. Repeated anesthesia is undesirable and in our experience unnecessary. Once the child recovers from his initial anxiety, usually he will sleep or will be kept amused during treatment by a brightly colored mobile suspended overhead. This is particularly useful for gaze fixation if the patient remains awake.

In Groups I, II, and III, the dose to the retina is 3500 rads in 3 weeks calculated at a depth 2.5 cm medial to the lateral orbit. The treatment is given

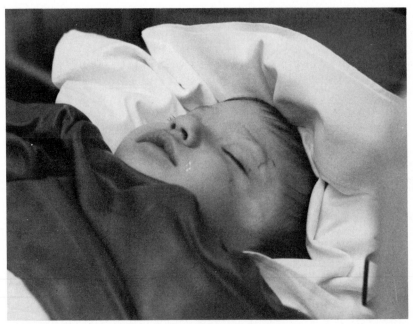

Fig. 18-5. Lateral view of patient in treatment position. The D-shaped treatment field is shown by the light beam on the side of the patient's face. The straight anterior margin of the field crosses the lateral canthus and is dotted on the skin in black marking ink. This 14-month-old boy had enucleation of the right eye for massive retinoblastoma with retinal detachment. The left eye contained one small tumor, 1 disc diameter in size, on the temporal aspect of the retina slightly anterior to the equator. Treatment was given to the left eye with the 18 mev photon beam through a lateral D-shaped portal, 3500 rads in 3 weeks, given in 9 fractions. At follow-up examination 2 years and 10 months after treatment, the patient was doing well with no evidence of disease. Visual acuity is apparently good. (Courtesy Medical Communications, The University of Texas at Houston, M. D. Anderson Hospital and Tumor Institute.)

in 9 fractions, 3 fractions per week, and can be equated with a tumor dose of 4500 rads in 4 weeks or 5000 rads in 5 weeks given in the conventional five times per week fractionation. These are comparable time-dose-fractionation schedules, with NSDs ranging from 1490 to 1570 RETs. With lesions located anterior to the equator, the anesthetized patient is examined at the completion of irradiation, and light coagulation is added if significant tumor regression is not evident. All patients are examined at 4 to 6 weeks after therapy, and if

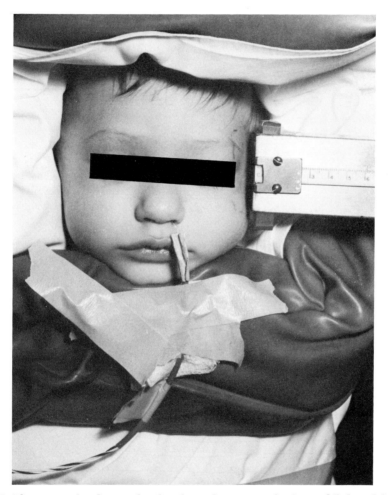

Fig. 18-6. The patient has been sedated and is asleep. He is firmly swaddled, and his head is held in treatment position by a Flexicast.* The lateral portal is angled posteriorly 3 degrees. Lucite bolus is inserted into the end of the treatment portal to provide buildup material so that the highest dose is at 2.5 cm depth from the skin surface. A Thermistor wire is placed at the patient's nostril to monitor breathing during treatment, since the swaddling and restraining coverings make it difficult to observe respiratory movements. (Courtesy Medical Communications, The University of Texas at Houston, M. D. Anderson Hospital and Tumor Institute.)

---

*Developed by Picker X-ray Corporation, White Plains, N. Y.

tumor shrinkage and calicification are not well defined, light coagulation will be used.

In Groups IV and V with large tumors extending to the ora serrata and with vitreous seeding, an anterior 4 cm portal is used to give 1000 to 1500 rads. With the 18 to 22 mev Betatron, the dose to the cornea is very low. A lateral portal provides the major portion of the treatment. The tumor dose to the posterior retina is 4500 rads in 4 weeks administered in 3 fractions per week.

The initial effects from irradiation may be seen at the conclusion of treatment, but the response may not be definite until the third or fourth week after therapy. Examination of the eye with the patient under anesthesia is usually made at 4 to 6 weeks. It is most desirable for the initial and succeeding examination to be made by the same observer for proper evaluation of the degree and rate of tumor regression.

Radioactive applicators. The indications for radioactive surface applicators in the treatment of retinoblastoma include choroidal extension of tumor and recurrence after external beam therapy of tumor too large to be controlled by light coagulation. Additionally, small and solitary tumors located posteriorly or at the ora serrata, especially on the nasal side, are suitable for surface applicators.

The technique of radioactive scleral applicators has been successfully developed by Stallard.[20] Cobalt 60 applicators are made in various sizes and shapes to conform to typical tumor configurations. A dose of 4000 rads is delivered to the surface of the tumor in 7 days, whereas the sclera adjacent to the applicator receives from 40,000 to 55,000 rads, but scleral necrosis does not occur. According to Stallard,[21] cobalt applicators are not satisfactory for the treatment of multiple tumors or neoplasms larger than 10 disc diameters in size, and external beam therapy is indicated. When multiple tumors are present, adequate coverage with applicators overdoses the retina. At the Institute of Ophthalmology over 80% of retinoblastoma eyes contain multiple tumor deposits. Additionally, the incidence of a new tumor appearing in an untreated portion of the retina is high. Stallard,[19] reporting a series of 43 patients, described the occurrence of secondary tumors in 26 patients after treatment of apparently solitary tumors.

Implanting the radioactive applicator requires exposure of the sclera at the tumor site and suture of the applicator to the sclera. The radioactive source remains for 7 days and is removed at a second operation. Possible complications include vascular necrosis with hemorrhage and cataract formation if a high dose is delivered to the lens.

Regression patterns. Three patterns of tumor regression are seen after irradiation of the eye. The most common, "cottage cheese calcium," represents shrunken and necrotic tumor masses that have become white and fluffy in appearance. It has been suggested that this glistening white material may be precipitated DNA.[12] The tumor debris is gradually absorbed, and lesions up to 3 or 4 disc diameters may disappear entirely. Large tumors remain as a white mass for an indefinite period. Calcified seeds may be seen in the vitreous after irradiation. Occasionally an irradiated tumor will break up into noncalcified seeds that, if viable and implanted, produce regrowth of tumor.

A second regression pattern is more difficult to interpret. The tumor shrinks

50% to 85% and loses the pink color of capillary tumor circulation. The surface becomes gray, not white, and the normal retinal vessels may loop over the surface of the tumor. If the tumor remains smaller than the original lesion, control is probable, but careful follow-up observation is necessary.

The third regression pattern has features of the others. There is a glistening white mass in the center of an amorphous translucent gray tumor that may be elevated. A pigment disturbance is often seen around this lesion but usually less than will be seen after light coagulation or diathermy. If there has been tumor shrinkage without evidence of regrowth, the tumor is under control.

Radiation complications. Since the purpose of radiation therapy for retinoblastoma is to eradicate tumor and preserve vision, radiation complications must be avoided. If the total tumor dose does not exceed 5000 rads in 5 weeks, the possibility of radiation injury is kept to a minimum.

Slight vascular injury caused by irradiation produces essentially no impairment of vision. Extensive radiation injury produces retinal hemorrhage leading to secondary glaucoma and eventually requires enucleation. With current radiation techniques and doses, serious radiation sequalae are infrequent. If the tumor mass is relatively small with limited involvement of the retina and the mucula has been spared, vision should be essentially normal after irradiation. If the tumor is massive with extensive retinal destruction or detachment, the probability of obtaining good vision with irradiation is less likely, but useful vision may still be achieved.

The vasculature of the retina and choroid is most sensitive to irradiation. If radiation vasculitis develops, intraretinal and preretinal hemorrhage may occur. If the process is extensive, massive vitreous hemorrhage may develop, which, unless it clears, disturbs vision and can lead to secondary glaucoma. Additionally, an opaque vitreous makes it impossible to assess the status of the irradiated tumor. Ellsworth[2] reports that 85% of patients treated with a second course of irradiation for regrowth of tumor become blind due to radiation complications when the combined tumor doses reach 7000 to 8000 rads. In eyes removed after tumor regrowth and retreatment, 50% have had active residual tumor, and 50% have had hemorrhage and secondary glaucoma although the tumor has been destroyed. The neural elements of the retina are more resistant to radiation than the vasculature, with the macula most sensitive.

In a review of 30 patients with malignancies of the ethmoid sinuses and nasal cavity treated with irradiation at the M. D. Anderson Hospital, Shukovsky[16] described a technique that delivered high radiation doses to the retina and optic nerve while sparing the sensitive cornea and lens. Nine patients lost their sight in twelve eyes as a result of radiation injury to the eye vasculature leading to macular and retinal degeneration in seven eyes, optic nerve atrophy in three eyes, and central retinal artery thrombosis in two eyes. Shukovsky concludes that radiation doses in excess of 6800 rads in 6 weeks (NSD = 2000 RETs) will result in loss of sight within 2 to 5 years.

The doses currently used in the treatment of retinoblastoma confined to the globe have NSDs of 1490 to 1570 RETs. Significant atrophy of the temporal bone does not occur in patients treated with megavoltage radiation. In patients treated in the past with orthovoltage radiation, the deformity has been sufficiently severe to require cosmetic surgery. With megavoltage radiation a decrease in orbital volume occurs, ranging between 10% and 30%, producing some asymmetry that is cosmetically acceptable.

Cataracts rarely occur with proper megavoltage radiation techniques.[9] When the lesion is located close to the ora serrata or is massive, the anterior edge of the beam must pass close to the lens. A small posterior pole cataract may form, with migration of the radiation-damaged cells from the equator of the lens to the posterior pole. These cataracts usually progress very slowly, if at all. They infrequently occur until 2 to 3 years after irradiation and therefore do not interfere with visualization of the fundus during the important early follow-up period.

Secondary tumors arising in the radiated tissues are of concern when treating young children. In a series of 397 patients with retinoblastoma (243 eligible for 5-year analysis) treated at the Columbia-Presbyterian Medical Center, the incidence of radiation-induced tumor or tumors occurring in the irradiated areas was 11.6%.[15] Many of these patients had been treated with high doses of irradiation over long periods of time, some receiving more than 15,000 r in air in 9 to 12 months. Of the twenty-one secondary malignancies, three occurred with doses from 2400 to 4000 r. In the remaining patients the doses ranged from 8000 r to 19,000 r. Of nine osteogenic sarcomas arising in the irradiated area, none occurred with a tumor dose of less than 8000 r. The latent period for the entire group ranged from 4 to 30 years.

If tumor recurs after irradiation, salvage of the eye should be attempted with light coagulation, cryotherapy, or scleral radioactive applicators. With a second course of external beam irradiation, the salvage rate is poor. Frequently the tumor is not controlled, and the risk of radiation damage is high. The possibility of a radiation-induced tumor in later years is added. If a radioactive applicator is used, the high dose of irradiation will be limited to a small portion of the retina.

Light coagulation

Light coagulation is an essential adjunct to the therapy of retinoblastoma, but it should not be selected as the primary treatment for most patients. Its particular value is in the treatment of tumors anterior to the equator that do not show satisfactory regression when the eye is first examined at 4 to 6 weeks after external beam irradiation. Light coagulation of the anterior retina rarely causes hemorrhage or other complications. A second indication for light coagulation is recurrent retinoblastoma after external beam therapy. Tumors up to 4 disc diameters in size and well separated from the optic nerve head are suitable for light coagulation.

The retinal circulation provides nutrition for developing retinoblastomas for a considerable period of time. Light coagulation obliterates the retinal vessels leading to the tumor. When this technique is used, the vasculature of the tumor is destroyed in a series of treatments separated by intervals of 3 to 4 weeks.[6] The resulting tumor necrosis does not produce a large field defect.

Complications of light coagulation, retinal detachment and hemorrhage, rarely become major problems. Retinal detachment, if it occurs, is usually limited and well healed. The most serious complication is the potential dissemination of tumor into the choroid and sclera. The patients in whom this has been demonstrated already have had far advanced tumors with existing choroidal extension.

Light coagulation can be used to treat a small tumor in a patient with unilateral disease, but it is essential that an eye so treated be evaluated at frequent intervals. Light coagulation should not be used for tumors behind the equator because huge field defects will be produced and the danger of hemorrhage is increased. According to Ellsworth,[2] an eye successfully treated by external beam irradiation will show less damage to normal retinal structures than an eye successfully treated by light coagulation, cryotherapy, diathermy, or radioactive applicators.

Chemotherapy

The addition of a chemotherapeutic agent in the treatment of retinoblastoma has been of interest since nitrogen mustard was used in an advanced case of retinoblastoma in the early 1950s.[8] Partial regression of the retinal tumor mass was observed, and the use of alkylating agents in the treatment of retinoblastoma was initiated.

The Retinoblastoma Team at Eye Institute has used triethylene melamine (TEM) in the treatment of retinoblastoma since January, 1953.[14] Initially this agent was administered prior to irradiation in all patients with retinoblastoma confined to the eye or orbit. In 1956 a randomized clinical trial was undertaken to test the premise that the addition of intramuscular TEM would further improve the control of retinoblastoma treated with irradiation. The patients studied had tumor confined to the remaining eye and were in the favorable Groups I and II. A high rate of control with preservation of useful vision was observed in both groups, and it was concluded that the addition of TEM was of no benefit in the treatment of limited disease.[23] A randomized trial of radiation therapy alone versus chemotherapy and irradiations has not been undertaken in patients with extensive localized disease.

It is the current practice of the Retinoblastoma Team to use TEM intraarterially for patients with extensive retinal disease (Groups IV and V) and residual or recurrent orbital disease. The drug is injected into the internal carotid artery under direct exposure 24 hours prior to beginning irradiation, giving 0.08 to 0.1 mg/kg over a period of several minutes. The injection is given on the ipsilateral side, although there is evidence that exchange is good across the circle of Willis.

RESULTS OF TREATMENT

The overall mortality rate in retinoblastoma is approximately 15%, with death due to intracranial spread, distant metastases, or both. Successful treatment requires eradication of disease both for maintenance of life and preservation of useful vision. Useful vision refers to visual acuity ranging from 20/20 to 20/200, recognizing that some benefit to the individual is provided with the lower limit of visual acuity. In Tables 18-1 and 18-2, showing the results of treatment, failure is equated with loss of useful vision and refers to patients who are blind due to uncontrolled tumor or radiation injury or to patients dead with disease. The sharp increase in failure rate in patients with large lesions is in part due to loss of vision because of the large retinal area that is destroyed by tumor.

Up to 1963, 750 cases of retinoblastoma were seen by the Retinoblastoma Team at the Columbia-Presbyterian Medical Center. Table 18-1 provides the overall results of treatment in 391 patients with bilateral disease and 74 patients with orbital disease (residual or recurrent).[2] All patients had received external beam irradiation. Since this series includes patients treated prior to 1953, treatment has included high-dose irradiation alone and after 1953, lower dose irradiation with or without adjunctive chemotherapy and photocoagulation. At the time of review in 1966 all patients had had a follow-up period of at least 40 months. Ninety percent or more of retinoblastoma recurrences will be seen prior to 2 years after the completion of treatment.[23]

Table 18-2 provides the most recently published results of treatment of bilateral retinoblastoma at the Columbia-Presbyterian Medical Center.[2] This is a review of 192 cases treated between 1960 and 1965 according to the policies described in the preceding pages. All patients have received radiation therapy. Intra-arterial TEM has been administered only to patients designated unfavorable (Groups IV and V) and to patients with orbital tumors. Many of these

Table 18-1. Results of treatment in patients with bilateral retinoblastoma or orbital disease (review of 1966)*

Group	Number of patients	Control rate
I	96	77%
II	66	68%
III	67	73%
IV	39	49%
V	123	29%
Orbital disease	74	20%

*This table includes (1) patients treated prior to 1953 with total tumor doses of over 8000 r (in some instances as high as 14,000 r) and (2) patients treated from 1953 to 1963, when the dose of external beam irradiation was sharply decreased and TEM (intramuscular or intra-arterial) was given. This series of patients was treated at the Columbia-Presbyterian Medical Center in New York City.

Table 18-2. Results of treatment in patients with bilateral retinoblastoma or orbital disease (review of 1968)*

Group	Number of patients	Control rate
I	20	95%
II	32	87%
III	24	67%
IV	32	69%
V	74	34%
Orbital disease	10	30%

*These patients were treated between 1960 and 1965, with a minimum follow-up of 3 years. In Groups I and II the failures are frequently deaths due to distant metastases with the treated eye remaining under control and vision maintained. This series of patients was treated at Columbia-Presbyterian Medical Center in New York City.

patients have been followed up for more than 5 years, and the minimum follow-up time for any patient is 3 years. Patients are listed as failures if dead of metastases, even though useful vision had been preserved in the remaining eye up to the time of death.

The mortality rate reported for the retinoblastoma series at the Columbia-Presbyterian Medical Center is 18%.[2] Of the patients dying, 77% have died less than 5 years after diagnosis of retinoblastoma. Ten percent of the patients lived more than 10 years and then died of retinoblastoma or the complications of treatment. In this group of patients dying between 10 and 20 years, 12.5% died of metastatic retinoblastoma, 12.5% died of unrelated intercurrent disease, and 75% died of secondary malignancies. In the large series at Columbia-Presbyterian, 2% of the patients lived more than 20 years before succumbing to the late complications of therapy. The majority of deaths were due to retinoblastoma, with 11.5% caused by secondary malignancies in the radiation field and 3% due to new malignancies outside the treatment field.

ORBITAL TUMOR

Orbital tumor refers to residual disease in the periglobal tissues, tumor in the cut end of the optic nerve, or growth of a tumor mass in the orbit at some time after enucleation (Fig. 18-7). A retroglobal mass can be present prior to enucleation if the tumor has erupted through the retina into the periglobal tissues. With extensive tumor outside the globe there is essentially no possibility for survival, since it is almost certain that there has been spread into the cranium or that

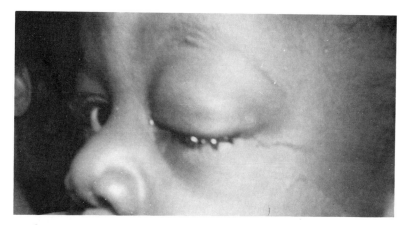

Fig. 18-7. This 2-year, 2-month-old boy was admitted with a history of an injury to the left eye at the age of 11 months. The left eye was enucleated 13 months later because of pain. Pain recurred, and there was proptosis of the left eyelid within 2 months. On admission to M. D. Anderson Hospital, the child had a mass in the left eye socket that was positive for retinoblastoma on biopsy. Treatment to the left orbit was given with lateral and anterior 18 mev electron beam fields, delivering a tumor dose of 5500 rads in 5½ weeks. The patient also received cyclophosphamide (Cytoxan), 2.2 mg/kg daily by mouth. The orbital mass had completely regressed at the conclusion of radiation therapy. The patient died 4½ months later with generalized disease, including metastases to bone marrow, bones, and central nervous system. (Courtesy Medical Communications, The University of Texas at Houston, M. D. Anderson Hospital and Tumor Institute.)

generalized hematogenous metastases have occurred. Exenteration of the eye and mass can be done to relieve pain and as a cleansing procedure.

If the optic nerve is recognizably enlarged at the time of enucleation, there is no rationale for exenteration and removal of the nerve back to the optic chiasm. If tumor extends into the optic nerve to the point where the major retinal vessels enter and exit from the nerve, it invariably gains access to the subarachnoid space, and removal of the remaining proximal portion of the nerve is pointless.

When tumor cells are found in the cut end of the optic nerve at enucleation or outside the globe on histologic section of the enucleated eye or if a mass develops in the orbit after enucleation, the patient must be carefully evaluated both for distant metastases and for intracranial spread of tumor. Orbital films are obtained to evaluate the optic nerve canals and to exclude invasion of the orbital bone. Spinal fluid and bone marrow must be examined for tumor cells.

If residual tumor is suspected in the optic nerve or periglobal tissues after enucleation and the work-up does not reveal central nervous system or distant spread of disease, treatment includes chemotherapy (intra-arterial TEM in the ipsilateral carotid) and irradiation of the entire orbit with an anterior portal, giving 5000 rads in 5 weeks to the depth of the optic chiasm. If orbital recurrence has developed, similar treatment is used.

The results of treatment of orbital tumors are discouraging. No cures have been reported in patients who have massive orbital disease or extensive optic nerve involvement when first seen, since intracranial spread and distant metastases have always occurred. Palliative procedures can prolong life and relieve the patient's discomfort. If microscopic tumor is present in the periglobal tissues or the optic nerve, there is a 30% to 35% possibility of salvaging the patient with irradiation and chemotherapy. Whether the addition of chemotherapy improves the control rate when the disease is localized to the orbit has not been tested by a randomized study.

METASTATIC TUMOR

Metastases include both intracranial and hematogenous spread of retinoblastoma. The presenting symptoms may suggest central nervous system involvement with signs of increased intracranial pressure. If distant metastases have developed, the patient may have bone pain, the liver may be enlarged, lymph nodes may be palpable in the neck, and masses due to metastatic deposits may appear.

If metastasis is suspected, work-up should include a complete skeletal survey, bone marrow aspiration, and examination of the spinal fluid. Death in approximately 50% of the patients is due to central nervous system involvement and in 50% to widespread metastases outside the central nervous system. A histologically abnormal bone marrow will be seen long before there is roentgenographic evidence of bone metastases. The diagnosis of marrow invasion should not be made until many atypical cells and the pattern of clumping are seen.

Retinoblastoma that has extended beyond the orbit may involve the central nervous system or the skeleton and other organs or both. Radiation therapy in palliative doses is used to shrink tumor masses and to alleviate symptoms. In the treatment of distant metastases, triple therapy with actinomycin D, chlorambucil, and methotrexate has been tried with limited response in some patients.[17] The current regimen used at the Columbia-Presbyterian Medical Center utilizes cyclophosphamide, 300 mg/M², and vincristine, 2 mg/M², administered intravenously once a week. One patient with a diseased bone marrow has had a normal marrow for 8 months and has developed no signs of toxicity while receiving this therapy.

If the central nervous system has been invaded, radiation therapy is administered to the base of the brain or the whole head. With tumor cells in the cerebrospinal fluid, irradiation of the spinal cord meninges can be considered. The dose will vary with the age of the patient from 3500 rads in 4 weeks to 5000 rads in 6 weeks. With persistence or recurrence of signs and symptoms after a course of radiation therapy, intrathecal methotrexate is given, 0.5 mg/kg every 2 days, and is repeated until there is clearing of abnormal cells from the spinal fluid and symptoms have improved. Up to eight or nine intrathecal injections may be required.

The results of treatment of both central nervous system spread of tumor and distant metastases have been universally disappointing with no reported cures in proved disease beyond the orbit. Alleviation of symptoms and clearing of signs can be achieved for relatively short periods. With repeated courses of chemotherapy, survival may be prolonged up to 18 months or 2 years.

REFERENCES

1. Brown, D. H.: The urinary excretion of vanilmandelic acid (VMA) and homovanillic acid (HVA) in children with retinoblastoma, Am. J. Ophthalmol. **62:**239-243, 1966.
2. Ellsworth, R. M.: The practical management of retinoblastoma, Trans. Am. Ophthalmol. Soc. **67:**462, 1969.
3. Ellsworth, R. M.: Personal communication.
4. Falls, H. F., and Neel, J. V.: Genetics of retinoblastoma, Arch. Ophthalmol. **46:**367, 1951.
5. Francois, J., and Matton-VanLeuven, M. T.: Recent data on the heredity of retinoblastoma. In Boniuk, M., Editor: Ocular and adnexal tumors, St. Louis, 1964, The C. V. Mosby Co.
6. Hopping, W., and Meyer-Schwickerath, G.: Light coagulation treatment in retinoblastoma. In Boniuk, M., Editor: Ocular and adnexal tumors, St. Louis, 1964, The C. V. Mosby Co.
7. Knudson, A. G.: Mutation and cancer: Statistical study of retinoblastoma, Proc. Natl. Acad. Sci. USA **68:**820-823, 1971.
8. Kupfer, C.: Retinoblastoma treated with intravenous nitrogen mustard, Am, J. Ophthalmol. **36:**1721, 1953.
9. MacFaul, P. A., and Bedford, M. A.: Ocular complications after therapeutic irradiation, Br. J. Ophthalmol. **54:**237-247, 1970.
10. Macklin, M. T.: A study of retinoblastoma in Ohio, Am. J. Hum. Genet. **12:**1-43, March, 1960.
11. Merriam, G. R., Jr.: Retinoblastoma: Analysis of 17 autopsies, Arch. Ophthalmol. **44:**71-108, 1950.
12. Mullaney, J.: Retinoblastomas with DNA precipitation, Arch. Ophthalmol. **82:**454-456, 1969.
13. Pfeiffer, R. L.: Roentgenographic diagnosis of retinoblastoma, Arch. Ophthalmol. **15:**811, 1936.
14. Reese, A. B., Hyman, G. A., Merriam, G. R., Jr., Forrest, A. W., and Kligerman, M. M.: Treatment of retinoblastoma by radiation and triethylenemelamine, Arch. Ophthalmol. **53:**505-513, 1955.
15. Sagerman, R. H., Cassady, J. R., Tretter, P., and Ellsworth, R. M.: Radiation induced neoplasia following external beam therapy for children with retinoblastoma, Am. J. Roentgenol. **105:**529-535, 1969.

16. Shukovsky, L. J., and Fletcher, G. H.: Retinal and optic nerve complications in a high dose technique of ethmoid sinus and nasal cavity irradiation, Radiology **104**:629-634, 1972.

17. Sitarz, A. L., Heyn, R., Murphy, M. L., Origenes, M. L., Jr., and Severo, N. O.: Triple drug therapy with actinomycin D, chlorambucil, and methotrexate in metastatic solid tumors in children, Cancer Chemother. Rep. **45**:45-51, April, 1965.

18. Stafford, W. R., Yanoff, M., and Parnell, B. L.: Retinoblastomas initially misdiagnosed as primary ocular inflammations, Arch. Ophthalmol. **82**:771-773, 1969.

19. Stallard, H. B.: Multiple islands of retinoblastoma: incidence rate and time span of appearance, Br. J. Ophthalmol. **39**:241-243, 1955.

20. Stallard, H. B.: The conservative treatment of retinoblastoma. Doyle Memorial Lecture, Trans. Ophthalmol. Soc. U. K. **82**:473, 1962.

21. Stallard, H. B.: Treatment of retinoblastoma with radioactive applicators. In Fletcher, G. H., editor: Textbook of radiotherapy, Philadelphia, 1966, Lea & Febiger.

22. Stern, C.: In Beadle, G. W., Emerson, R., and Whitaker, D. M., editors: Principles of human genetics, San Francisco, 1960, W. H. Freeman & Co.

23. Tapley, N. duV.: Treatment of retinoblastoma with radiation and chemotherapy. In Boniuk, M., editor: Ocular and adnexal tumors, St. Louis, 1964, The C. V. Mosby Co.

24. Ts'o, M. O., Fine, B. S., Zimmerman, L. E., and Vogel, M. H.: Photoreceptor elements in retinoblastoma, Arch. Ophthalmol. **82**:57-59, 1969.

CHAPTER 19

Malignant tumors of the central nervous system

JORDAN R. WILBUR

BRAIN TUMORS

Tumors of the central nervous system have frequently been regarded with a mixture of fear and hopelessness by both patients and many physicians. The difficulty of successfully removing a brain tumor without causing serious permanent damage to the patient's central nervous system has contributed to this attitude.

However, the expectation of poor results and hopelessness in the treatment of brain tumors is gradually changing. This can be attributed to several factors, including the following:

1. Improvement in surgical techniques and the development of better supportive therapy in the immediate postoperative period
2. Improved diagnostic neuroradiology that allows the physician to determine the extent and operability of the tumor
3. The refinement of techniques of radiotherapy
4. Utilization of chemotherapy for treatment of some brain tumors
5. Development of other scientific techniques in clinical diagnosis, including the use of radioactive isotopes, echoencephalography, and the refinement of electroencephalography
6. Further clarification of the diagnosis, classification, and composition of brain tumors utilizing new techniques of electron microscopy, histochemical analysis, and tissue culture

In addition to these factors that have led to improved results, there has also been a change in the types of intracranial tumors in children. The major change has been a marked decrease in the incidence of intracranial tumors of infectious origin. Forty years ago the most common tumor occurring in children in England was the tuberculoma.[5] More recently, in this country, only one child had a tuberculoma[20] in a large series of 750 children with brain tumors seen over a 30-year period ending in 1966.

Incidence

Central nervous system tumors cause more deaths in children than tumors of any other area, with the exception of leukemia.[24] They may occur at any age, including the newborn period, and reach their peak incidence in childhood between 5 and 10 years of age. The occurrence is more frequent in boys than girls at a ratio of approximately 60%:40%. About 60% of brain tumors in children are infratentorial, whereas in adults about 70% are supratentorial. Brain tumors in children have a tendency to occur along the central neural axis. They most frequently involve the third or fourth ventricle and are within or attached to the brainstem, hypothalamus, or optic pathways. About half of all childhood tumors are connected with the ventricular system. Most of the tumors are classified pathologically in the neuroepithelial tumor group and include medulloblastomas, gliomas, and paragliomas.

Due to some differences in the pathologic classification of tumors as reported by different groups, it is difficult to determine an exact incidence of specific tumor types. However, in the neuroepithelial tumor group the types most frequently seen in children are classified as gliomas. This includes the group called *spongioblastomas* of the cerebellum by some and cerebellar astrocytomas by others. The medulloblastoma occurs next most frequently and is also usually located in the posterior fossa. The glioblastoma (astrocytoma Grades III and IV), which may be located either in the posterior fossa or in the cerebral hemispheres, occurs next most frequently. These tumors have been the most difficult to treat successfully. The ependymomas, which also may develop above or below the tentorium, form the fourth most common group. The only other type of tumor occurring frequently throughout childhood is the craniopharyngioma.

Age

A review of two large series of brain tumors in children indicated that the incidence of brain tumors is about the same in all age groups, including infancy.[12, 20] In infants (0 to 2 years) the tumors that commonly occur with about equal frequency are medulloblastoma, ependymoma, and astrocytoma (cerebellar and cerebral).[6, 19] Choroid plexus papillomas are also common in this age group. These four types of tumors account for about two thirds of those occurring in infancy (Table 19-1).

In preadolescents (3 to 12 years) cerebellar astrocytomas and medulloblastomas each account for about 20% of the tumors. Astrocytomas (Grades III and IV), ependymomas, and craniopharyngiomas each account for about 10%.

In teen-agers (13 to 16 years) cerebellar astrocytoma (spongioblastoma) is the most common tumor and occurs in about 20% of the cases reported. Astrocytoma (Grades III and IV) and craniopharyngioma are next most frequent, each accounting for about 10% to 15%. Medulloblastoma occurs in about 10% of the cases, which is less frequent than in younger children.

Table 19-1. Brain tumors* (frequency of occurrence by age)

Infants (0-2 yr)	Preadolescent (3-12 yr)	Teen-ager (13-16 yr)
Medulloblastoma	Cerebellar astrocytoma	Cerebellar astrocytoma
Ependymoma	Medulloblastoma	Astrocytoma (Grades III and IV)
Astrocytoma	Astrocytoma (Grades III and IV)	Craniopharyngioma
Choroid plexus papilloma	Ependymoma	Medulloblastoma
	Craniopharyngioma	

*In order of frequency of occurrence.

Pathologic characteristics and classifications

One of the major problems in characterizing and analyzing tumors of the central nervous system is the lack of agreement among pathologists in regard to a uniform nomenclature and classification system. A number of detailed classification systems have been described. The most recent one was developed by the Union Internationale Contre le Cancer (UICC) in an attempt to develop a more uniform worldwide system (see the following outline).

Nerve cells
Ganglioneuroma
Gangliocytoma
Ganglioglioma
Ganglioneuroblastoma
Malignant ganglioneuroma
Malignant gangliocytoma
Malignant ganglioglioma
Sympathicoblastoma
Sympathicogonioma
Neuroblastoma
Neuroepithelium
Ependymoma
  Epithelial
  Papillary
  Celullar
Malignant ependymoma
Ependymoblastoma
Plexus papilloma
Olfactory neuroepithelioma
Eye
Medulloepithelioma of ciliary epithelium
Diktyoma
Neuroepithelioma
Retinoblastoma
  With true rosettes
  Without true rosettes
Glia
Astrocytoma
  Fibrillary
  Gemistocytic
  Protoplasmatic
Astrocytoma of nose
Nasal glioma
Oligodendroglioma
Multiform glioblastoma
Polar spongioblastoma
Medulloblastoma

Peripheral and cranial nerves
Neurinoma
Neurilemoma
Schwannoma
Neurofibroma
Malignant neurinoma
Malignant Schwannoma
Malignant neurolemoma
Meninges
Meningioma
  Epithelioid
  Meningotheliomatous
  Endotheliomatous
  Fibroblastic/fibromatous
  Psammomatous
Vascular structures of central nervous system
Hemangioma of cerebellum
von Hippel-Lindau disease
Paraganglia
Carotid body tumor
Nonchromaffin paraganglioma included
Glomus caroticum tumor
Chemodectoma
Pineal gland
Pinealoma
Hypophysis
Chromophobe adenoma
  Diffuse
  Sinusoidal
  Papillary
Oxyphil adenoma
Eosinophil adenoma
  Papillary
Basophil adenoma
Craniopharyngioma
Adamantinoma of ductus
  Craniopharyngeus
Chromophobe carcinoma

The following general grouping based on location and microscopic diagnosis has been simplified to provide a workable classification for the clinician:

I. Infratentorial
    A. Cerebellar astrocytoma (Grade I, spongioblastoma)
    B. Medulloblastoma
    C. Ependymoma
    D. Astrocytoma (Grades III and IV, brainstem glioma)
II. Supratentorial

    A. Astrocytoma (Grades III and IV, glioblastoma)
    B. Astrocytoma (Grades I and II, spongioblastoma)
    C. Ependymoma
    D. Optic nerve glioma
    E. Craniopharyngioma
    F. Choroid plexus papilloma

It includes only the most common tumors in children and does not involve detailed pathologic differentiation. The major pathologic group is the neuroepithelial tumors. The specific subgroups are determined by the basic type of cell present, as well as the extent of tissue differentiation. This group includes the medulloblastomas, gliomas, and paragliomas (ependymoma, pinealoma, choroid plexus papilloma). Tumors originating from mesodermal tissues such as meningiomas, hemangioblastomas, and sarcomas are relatively uncommon. Tumors of ectodermal origin are primarily limited to the craniopharyngioma. Congenital or embryonic tumors, including epidermoids, dermoids, teratomas, and hamartomas, are also rare. More detailed pathologic classification and analysis of other types of tumors occurring rarely in children are reported in further detail by others.[41]

Clinical manifestations

Brain tumors may cause a variety of signs and symptoms, dependent on their location, size, rate of growth, and the age of the patient. The major general manifestations of any brain tumor are caused by brain edema, blockage of cerebrospinal fluid circulation, blood flow disturbances, and direct tumor mass pressure. General effects that may occur include behavioral and intellectual impairment, including changes in personality and impaired consciousness.

Common signs and symptoms include headache, vomiting, visual abnormalities, and ataxia. The specific manifestations depend on both the age of the patient and the site of the primary tumor. The occurrence of headache varies greatly with age and is more frequent in older children. When headache develops, the younger child may be restless and irritable rather than specifically stating that his head hurts. In association with the headache, meningismus may also occur. Vomiting, frequently without preceding nausea, is often a manifestation of increased intracranial pressure. Persistent vomiting may temporarily improve as the skull sutures separate, allowing for expansion of the head. Expansion of the skull sutures occurs most readily in very young children but may occur in children of all ages. The coronal suture is most frequently the site of the earliest and most noticeable separation.

Eye findings frequently denote the presence of intracranial pathology. The presence of diplopia or strabismus may be the first indication of increased intracranial pressure. The most common cranial nerve involvement is that of the sixth nerve. Sixth nerve paralysis is not of particular value in localizing the intracranial pathology, since it usually occurs secondary to increased pressure of the expanding brain on the sixth cranial nerve. The presence of papilledema is a frequent first sign of increased intracranial pressure in the older child. Other eye signs include optic atrophy, visual field defects, and at times proptosis. In the younger child, head enlargement and an associated bulging fontanel indicates the presence of increased intracranial pressure. These signs are not specific for brain tumors and are of no value in localizing the site of the cause of the increased pressure.

Ataxia is a frequent sign of brain tumors in children. This is in part due to the location of the most common tumors in the cerebellar region. However, the presence of ataxia does not in itself confirm the diagnosis of a cerebellar neoplasm because it may also be caused by a tumor in the frontal lobe. Head tilting also often occurs in association with a posterior fossa tumor.

Progressive growth of intracranial tumors, with associated brainstem compression, may cause slowing of the pulse, increase in blood pressure, decrease in pulse pressure, decrease in respiration, instability of body temperature, and vasomotor instability.

In the infratentorial tumors the most common sign of cerebellar involvement is ataxia. Nystagmus, which implies that there is long tract or brainstem involvement, is frequently present in posterior fossa tumors. The absence of nystagmus does not rule out the presence of a cerebellar tumor. The cranial nerves are often involved in the following order of frequency: sixth, seventh, fifth, eighth, ninth, and tenth.

Tumors of the cerebral hemispheres are usually more difficult to diagnose, especially when they occur in the silent brain areas, the frontal and occipital lobes. However, papilledema is present in about 80% of these patients, and headache is a common complaint. Convulsions may occur, especially when the tumor is localized in the temporal lobe.

Tumors of the optic chiasm and sella turcica region frequently cause visual loss or visual field defects and may be associated with unilateral exophthalmus.

The presence of any of these signs or symptoms should suggest the possibility of an intracranial mass and would be an indication for further diagnostic evaluation.

Diagnostic features

After completion of a careful history and physical examination, the physician may turn to a number of diagnostic techniques. These studies are directed toward determining whether or not the patient has a tumor and delineating as accurately as possible the location and extent of the lesion prior to biopsy or attempted removal.

Roentgenographic evaluation includes standard diagnostic films, pneumoencephalography, and angiography. Skull x-ray films may show the presence of split sutures, most commonly the coronal and sagittal sutures, as an indication of increased intracranial pressure. Bony changes may be present at the base of the skull, particularly evidence of pressure at the sella turcica. Specific bony erosion by tumor pressure is most commonly seen in the area of the sella turcica in craniopharyngioma but may occur secondary to chronic increased intracranial pressure due to tumor in other sites. Widening of a bony foramen may indicate the presence of slow-growing tumor, as occurs in the optic foramen secondary to optic nerve glioma. However, in normal individuals bilateral foramina may differ in size by as much as 20%.

Increased digital markings are at times suggestive of the presence of increased intracranial pressure but may be relatively prominent in normal children. The presence of tumor calcification is a more specific diagnostic finding that occurs in about 10% to 20% of tumors in children.

Pneumoencephalography may be helpful in outlining a tumor mass protruding into the ventricular space or causing obstruction to the normal flow of cerebrospinal fluid. When there is evidence of increased intracranial pressure, the air studies are usually done through the lateral ventricle by direct puncture through open sutures or through a burr hole. The introduction of air by lumbar puncture in patients with increased intracranial pressure secondary to a brain tumor is dangerous and may result in herniation of the brain with associated rapid death. Introduction of air by lumbar puncture may be more safely accomplished after ventricular pressure has been reduced.

Angiography is of particular value in localizing and delineating the extent of an intracranial tumor; it may be accomplished by a direct puncture of the appropriate artery or more readily in younger children by percutaneous femoral puncture with retrograde threading of the catheter to the appropriate vessel before injection of the radiopaque dye.

The electroencephalogram (EEG) is often of value in the localization of supratentorial tumors, but it is of little value in the diagnosis of infratentorial tumors. Children with cerebral neoplasms associated with clinical seizures most frequently show high amplitude slow waves on one or more leads of unipolar EEG tracing. This finding can be confirmed further by the presence of phase reversals over the involved area on bipolar tracings. Increased intracranial pressure may cause a diffuse slowing on the tracing that is not diagnostic.

Radioisotope techniques for the diagnosis of brain tumors have become more accepted for general use in children with the availability of technetium 99m as pertechnetate (^{99m}Tc).[25, 31] This short-acting isotope with a half-life of 6 hours can be administered to children suspected of having a brain tumor without significant concern for the low dose of radiation involved. Utilizing gamma-scintigraphy to measure uptake activity, the relative concentration of the radioactive emitter in the tumor versus healthy brain tissue can be measured. This technique is of particular value in the diagnosis of supratentorial tumors. Although technically more difficult to diagnose, posterior fossa tumors can also be detected utilizing ^{99m}Tc scans.

Echoencephalography is a relatively new technique that may have some value in the diagnosis of brain tumors, particularly when the tumor has caused a significant shift in the normal midline structures of the brain. At the present time this technique is still under development, and the information obtained is supplemental to that of the well-known techniques. It is a painless test with no known risk to the patient.

Cerebrospinal fluid evaluation may be an important part of the diagnostic studies. The ventricular fluid may be obtained at the time of ventriculography. The lumbar puncture must be done with great caution in the patient with suspected brain tumor but no clinical evidence of increased intracranial pressure. This means that the patient should be ready for emergency surgery, with a competent neurosurgeon available. A small (No. 22) needle should be utilized, and only the minimal amount of fluid that is necessary for analysis should be removed. If the pressure is elevated, this suggests the presence of an intracranial lesion, and the lumbar puncture site should subsequently be observed closely for significant subcutaneous leakage of spinal fluid. The evaluation of the fluid should include an examination for malignant cells. The presence of malignant cells can be best determined by using the cytocentrifuge or millipore filter to concentrate any cells present. Elevation of the cerebrospinal fluid protein suggests the presence of a malignant neoplasm.

Differential diagnosis

The presence of a space-occupying lesion in the brain does not necessarily indicate that this is a malignant tumor. In many areas of the world infectious organisms are a frequent cause of expanding lesions in the central nervous system. The most common central nervous system bacterial infection in some countries is the tuberculoma. This tumor can frequently be successfully treated if removed in toto surgically. Parasites, including cysticercus and *Echinococcus* tapeworms, may cause space-occupying lesions. The cysticercus usually causes multiple small sites, whereas the *Echinococcus* parasite causes single, large, space-occupying lesions. In this country a brain abscess is most frequently associated with either other evidence of a serious infection elsewhere in the body or the presence of congenital heart disease. The most common organism involved is the anaerobic streptococcus, which occurs in association with congenital heart disease.

Metastatic tumors from a primary site outside the central nervous system should always be considered. Tumors that are associated with brain metastases include soft tissue sarcomas, reticulum cell sarcomas, retinoblastoma, and neuroblastoma. Malignant tumors such as eosinophilic granuloma may extend into the brain from the surrounding bone. Vascular malformation and other nonmalignant congenital lesions may mimic intracranial neoplasms. Cerebral hemorrhage or subdural hematomas may mimic signs and symptoms of a brain tumor and should always be considered in the differential diagnosis.

Pseudotumor cerebri (benign intracranial hypertension) is a clinical syndrome of unknown etiology that occurs occasionally. This syndrome includes increased intracranial pressure with normal cerebrospinal fluid, no structural abnormalities of the ventricular system, and no localizing signs. The diagnosis is made by the exclusion of other possible causes of the increased pressure.

The most important and most common differential diagnosis of brain tumors in children is that of the medulloblastoma versus the cerebellar astrocytoma. These two tumors represent the most common types of malignancies in the posterior fossa in children. The diagnosis can only be finally determined by surgical exploration. This is of the utmost importance because the cystic cerebellar astrocytoma is a benign tumor and, if removed surgically, is curable. In contrast, the medulloblastoma is perhaps the most malignant of the brain tumors of children, rarely if ever can be totally removed surgically, and requires intensive radiotherapy to achieve long-term control.

Tumors of the lateral ventricle require careful study to determine whether they are malignant (ependymoma) or nonmalignant and potentially readily curable (choroid plexus papilloma). The choroid plexus papilloma usually causes a communicating hydrocephalus by overproduction of cerebrospinal fluid.

Treatment

Surgery. Total extirpation of the tumor is the treatment of choice if it does not cause intolerable residual neurologic damage. The feasibility of surgery will depend in part on the exact location and attachment of the tumor. Tumors that have direct attachment to the floor of the fourth ventricle (medulloblastoma, ependymoma) cannot be completely removed without causing life-threatening damage to the vital structures located in that area. However, improved techniques of supportive care during and after surgery now allow the removal of certain intracranial neoplasms that previously were frequently fatal.

Cystic astrocytoma. The cerebellar cystic astrocytoma should be removed surgically.[7] If the tumor nodule itself can be totally removed, then cure can often be achieved even without removal of all protions of the cyst wall. Even incomplete removal of the tumor may result in years of normal life before significant recurrence, and the recurrence may also be surgically treated again. After successful total removal of cerebellar astrocytomas, no other treatment with radiotherapy or chemotherapy is indicated.

Medulloblastoma. Surgical removal of the main bulk of a medulloblastoma or an ependymoma provides the patient with two major benefits. The removal of tumor bulk facilitates the effectiveness of supplemental treatments with radiotherapy and chemotherapy. The reduction of increased pressure and the establishment of normal flow of cerebrospinal fluid improve the likelihood of the patient's survival during treatment with radiotherapy and chemotherapy.

Brainstem glioma. Because of its location, the brainstem glioma cannot be surgically removed and is often not biopsied. This type of tumor has frequently grown to a large size without the development of increased intracranial pressure, and the initial diagnosis is assumed by its location and determined by diagnostic studies. However, surgical exploration can be of value in those cases in which a large neoplastic cyst is present and can be evacuated. In this situation long-term survival is possible.[15]

Supratentorial tumors. Supratentorial tumors may be removed surgically in some instances, depending on their location. Unfortunately, many of them grow to an extremely large size before causing signs or symptoms that indicate the presence of a tumor. Both the glioblastomas and ependymomas have been usually inoperable at the time of diagnosis, although many of the ependymomas are partially resectable. The optic nerve gliomas, however, are frequently operable, particularly those located anteriorly to the optic chiasm.

Craniopharyngioma. The craniopharyngioma, located in the suprasellar region, may be extensive at the time of diagnosis. However, it has at times been possible to totally remove this tumor. At other times it is only possible to temporarily reduce the cystic portion of the tumor. Successful total surgical removal prevents recurrence of the tumor, although the patient frequently has residual endocrine and metabolic deficits.

Choroid plexus papilloma. The papilloma of the choroid plexus may be successfully treated surgically in many instances. This is particularly true when the primary site is in the lateral ventricle. Total surgical removal is associated with long-term survival without recurrence or other problems.

Pineal tumors. Pineal area tumors are usually inoperable because of their location and attachment to surrounding structures. Even biopsy may be associated with increased morbidity and mortality.

Radiotherapy. The utilization of radiation therapy to provide significant treatment for a variety of brain tumors is increasing. With the development of improved radiotherapeutic equipment and techniques, there has been an associated improvement in the results of treatment of brain tumors in children.

Medulloblastoma. The child with medulloblastoma should receive irradiation therapy to the entire cerebrospinal axis even if all the gross tumor has been removed. This tumor notoriously seeds throughout the central nervous system, and radiation therapy may be effective in preventing recurrence or spread of the disease. In recent years there have been several reports of patients surviving many years after treatment with radiotherapy, although many patients still develop recurrence within the first few years.

In several series of children with medulloblastoma, over 30% are alive at 5 years after treatment with radiation therapy.* In many of these series of patients the whole central nervous system received about 3000 to 3500 rads estimated at the posterior fossa and the spinal cord, given over 4 to 5 weeks. A boost is given to the posterior fossa of 1000 to 1500 rads in 7 to 10 days for a total dose to the tumor of about 4500 to 5000 rads. The amount of radiotherapy utilized depends on the age of the child.

Ependymomas and cerebellar sarcomas. Ependymomas and cerebellar sarcomas also may be responsive to radiotherapy. Whether or not the entire central nervous system axis is treated with radiotherapy in these tumors depends in part on the degree of malignancy determined by histologic examination. For patients with ependymomas with particularly malignant appearing cells, prophylactic treatment of the entire central nervous system is indicated. Tumor doses to the primary site of 3000 rads in 3 weeks to 5500 rads in 6 weeks are necessary to achieve significant effect against this tumor.

Astrocytoma (Grades III and IV). Gliomas of the brainstem have often been treated with radiotherapy for temporary palliation, but this usually has had only short-term effectiveness. Glioblastomas of the cerebral hemispheres may also be temporarily responsive to radiotherapy.

Optic glioma. Radiotherapy is of value in the treatment of some optic nerve gliomas. Many of these tumors appear relatively benign histologically and may not be responsive to irradiation. Intraorbital lesions are usually treated by surgical extirpation only. Some intracranial optic nerve gliomas are responsive to irradiation with concomitant improvement in visual acuity.[17]

Craniopharyngioma. Although the tissues of the craniopharyngioma are not usually malignant and the classic treatment has been surgical, there are reports of notably successful treatment of craniopharyngiomas with radiotherapy.[13] Depending on the extent of the tumor and the feasibility of removing it surgically, radiotherapy should be considered for primary or secondary therapy.

Pineal tumors. Tumors of the pineal area, which include pinealomas, pineoblastomas, and teratomas, may be radiosensitive. The 2 patients with pinealomas treated with radiotherapy in our series are both alive without recurrence more than 10 years after radiation therapy.[28]

Choroid plexus papilloma. Although the primary treatment for choroid plexus papilloma is surgical, the presence of significant residual tissue, particularly the papilloma with carcinomatous degeneration noted microscopically, should be treated with radiotherapy. Tumor doses similar to those for ependymoma are necessary to achieve satisfactory results.

---

*References 3, 4, 10, 11, 23, 35.

Chemotherapy. Improved results in the treatment of solid tumors are being achieved with new single agent and combination chemotherapy. This has led to an increased interest in the utilization of chemotherapeutic agents for the treatment of brain tumors. A major theoretic consideration has been the blood-brain barrier and its potential role in preventing drugs from achieving concentrations sufficient to affect tumor growth. Some drugs for study have been selected on the basis of their ability to cross the blood-brain barrier (e.g., BCNU, CCNU), whereas others have been introduced directly into the cerebrospinal fluid (methotrexate, cytosine arabinoside). Other systemic agents (vincristine) have also shown antitumor effects in some instances.

Vincristine. This *Vinca* alkaloid has been shown to be effective against leukemia and a number of solid tumors in children. There have been several case reports of its effectiveness against both medulloblastoma[14, 16] and astrocytoma

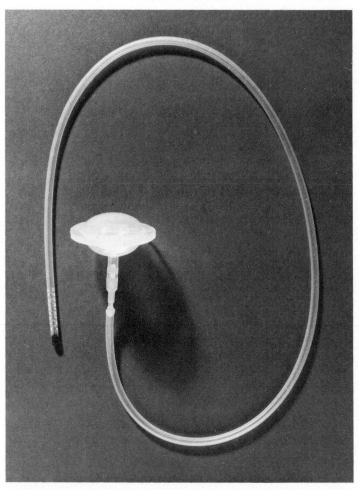

Fig. 19-1. Ommaya reservoir. (Courtesy Medical Communications, The University of Texas at Houston, M. D. Anderson Hospital and Tumor Institute.)

(glioblastoma).[34] It is usually given intravenously weekly at a dosage of 0.05 mg/kg or 2 mg/M[2]. Its major limitation is the development of significant peripheral neurotoxicity with prolonged usage.

Methotrexate. This antimetabolite has been used extensively by direct injection into the cerebrospinal fluid for the treatment of meningeal leukemia. It has been shown to be effective in the treatment of medulloblastoma, ependymoma, and astrocytoma when injected intrathecally.[32, 40] For patients with blockage of the normal cerebrospinal fluid flow, methotrexate has been administered directly into the ventricle. When the drug is to be given on a regular basis intraventricularly, this is usually accomplished through the implantation of a subcutaneous reservoir, such as the one designed by Ommaya (Fig. 19-1)[27] or a Heyer-Pudenz shunt incorporating a Coe-Schulte reservoir.[26] Several schedules of injection of methotrexate have been used, including daily injections of 0.25 mg/kg for 5 to 7 days, or 15 mg/M[2] twice weekly. A newer approach has been the experimental study of cerebrospinal fluid perfusion with methotrexate.[30]

Nitrosoureas. BCNU (1,3-bis(2-chloroethyl)-1-nitrosourea), which crosses the blood-brain barrier well, has previously been shown to have effectiveness against several solid tumors, including glioblastoma (astrocytoma) and ependymoma.[38, 39] In our own series some patients with medulloblastoma have also temporarily responded. Subsequent development of CCNU (1-(2-chloroethyl)-3-cyclohexyl-1-nitrosourea), an analog of BCNU, has resulted in the availability of an oral agent with a spectrum of antitumor effectiveness at least as great as that of BCNU.[9] Early results in the treatment of patients with glioblastoma appear promising. Our own studies with CCNU have also produced a temporary response in some patients with medulloblastoma.

Cytosine arabinoside. This relatively new antitumor agent has been used effectively both systemically in the treatment of leukemia and intrathecally in the treatment of central nervous system leukemia. It is currently being studied experimentally to test its effectiveness in the treatment of brain tumors.

Intra-arterial administration. There have been several studies with adults utilizing intra-arterial chemotherapy with nitrogen mustard, bromouridine, thio-TEPA, and 5-fluorouracil. Although the study of these drugs shows some hope of effectiveness, the results to date have not justified their use in the treatment of cerebral neoplasms in children.

The initial use of chemotherapy in the treatment of brain tumors has been for the treatment of recurrent or gross residual disease after surgery or radiotherapy or both. Studies are currently under way in a few centers to determine if chemotherapy given immediately after surgery and in conjunction with radiotherapy may offer more significant effectiveness against some of the malignant intracranial neoplasms of children.

Supportive care

A number of advances in the supportive care in the preoperative, operative, and postoperative period have resulted in a much higher survival rate after the initial diagnostic and surgical procedures. To ensure that proper supportive medication and fluids can be administered intravenously, a cutdown should always be placed prior to a major neurosurgical procedure. The improved postsurgical survival achieved with better supportive care has allowed an increased opportunity for the application of radiotherapy and in some instances chemotherapy in an attempt to further tumor control or eradication.

Postoperatively, sodium retention secondary to increased levels of adrenal corticosteroids and in some instances inappropriate antidiuretic hormone secretion should be expected. Restriction of intravenous fluids, limitation of sodium intake, and close observation for potassium loss, with supplementation when indicated, are important parts of postoperative care.

Brain edema has always been a major problem, particularly in the immediate postsurgical period. In addition to the techniques of decreased fluid intake, hyperventilation during anesthesia, the administration of intravenous hypertonic solutions such as mannitol or urea, and the administration of corticosteroids, most commonly in the form of dexamethasone, have been significant additions to the treatment of cerebral edema. Dexamethasone is usually given in an initial high dose (4 to 10 mg) intravenously and then 1 to 4 mg every 6 hours, depending on the age of the child and the severity of the problem. Mannitol will produce a rapid osmotic diuresis when given intravenously in a dosage of 1 Gm/kg. A urinary catheter should be in place prior to administration of the mannitol in anticipation of a large urine output.

The development of improved techniques of shunting blocked cerebrospinal fluid with ventriculocardiac or ventriculoperitoneal shunts has also produced more rapid recovery from the effects of increased intracranial pressure. This has helped a greater number of patients to recover sufficiently to receive radiotherapy. In addition, several reservoir-shunt devices have been designed to provide an easy route for the administration of intraventricular chemotherapy.[26]

Particularly in the treatment of craniopharyngioma, the development of the techniques of substitution of glucocorticoids and other substitution hormone therapy made necessary by the absence of normal hypothalamic and pituitary function has improved both the number of survivors and the quality of their survival.[22]

Improved anesthetic techniques, including techniques of cardiorespiratory monitoring and assisted ventilation, have resulted in lower operative and postoperative mortality.

A vigorous rehabilitation program offering physical therapy and occupational therapy is an essential part of the treatment of children with brain tumors. Prompt postoperative physical therapy with the expectation that the patient will do well has resulted in more rapid recovery and a better quality of survival.

Complications

Complications may occur secondary to either the tumor itself or the therapy utilized. Depending on the location of the tumor within the brain, there may be significant residual effect even after successful treatment. These effects may also be secondary to prolonged increased intracranial pressure. Tumors located near the optic chiasm may cause blindness or visual field defects. Tumors in the region of the sella turcica with associated involvement of the pituitary gland and/or hypothalamus may present with a variety of metabolic and endocrine problems associated with disturbances in pituitary and hypothalamic function. Both hyperregulatory or hyporegulatory reactions may occur.

Tumors of the cerebral hemispheres, even when successfully treated, may leave residual foci or scar tissue that results in a subsequent seizure disorder. Tumors of the posterior fossa, with involvement of the cerebellum, may result in residual ataxia and incoordination.

Surgery may cause residual neurologic defects because of the necessity of cutting through or removing tissue in vital areas. It has been possible in many instances to at least partially overcome these deficits with prolonged rehabilitation assistance.

Placement of a shunt to relieve increased intracranial pressure may allow spread of tumor cells to other sites in the body. There have been reports of the development of distant metastases by this mechanism in patients with medulloblastoma[18] and with glioblastoma.[37]

Metastases within the central nervous system have occurred frequently in medulloblastoma when the spinal cord was not treated with radiation therapy as well. A small number of patients with medulloblastoma have developed distant metastases outside the central nervous system not associated with a cerebrospinal fluid shunt.[1] Both bony and lymph node metastases have been described, and they have been responsive to systemic chemotherapy.

Complications secondary to radiotherapy are related to both the location and amount of treatment and the age of the patient. Alopecia usually follows radiation therapy but is generally only temporary. More severe late sequelae include brain necrosis, usually involving the white matter, radiodermatitis, necrosis of skin and bone, and at times malignant degeneration of adjacent tissue.

Long-term complications of chemotherapy are not yet known because of the lack of a significant number of long-term survivors of this form of therapy. Short-term complications include bone marrow toxicity, central nervous system irritation, and alopecia.

Prognosis

The prognosis varies greatly, depending on tumor type, location, and age of the patient. The results in several tumor types are improving significantly.

Cerebellar astrocytoma. The cerebellar astrocytoma can usually be successfully treated by surgical removal. Over 90% of children with this tumor can be expected to survive.[12, 20] With the development of improved techniques of supportive therapy, the number of postoperative deaths has been minimal.

Medulloblastoma. Medulloblastoma has been recognized as a very malignant tumor, frequently associated with death in the first 1 or 2 years. Recent reports from a number of centers indicate that the percentage of patients achieving significant long-term survival is increasing. This can be attributed to improved postoperative supportive techniques and improved radiotherapy. Series of patients with better than 40% 5-year survival and 25% 10-year survival have now been reported.[*] However, in some series as many as 50% of the patients have died within 2 years from diagnosis. Further utilization of multimodal therapy techniques, including chemotherapy, should improve this result in the future.

Ependymoma. Ependymomas vary in their degree of malignancy, as well as

---

[*]References 3, 4, 10, 11, 23, 35.

in their location. Occurrence in the supratentorial region, most commonly in the lateral ventricle, has been associated with prolonged survival in a few cases in which surgical extirpation has been possible. Infratentorial lesions attached to the floor of the fourth ventricle are difficult to completely remove. Results of treatment in one large series indicated 19% 5-year survival rate.[2] However, multimodal therapy with surgery, radiotherapy, and chemotherapy in some instances is producing an increasing number of long-term survivors.

Astrocytoma, Grades III and IV. Brainstem gliomas and supratentorial glioblastomas (astrocytoma, Grades III and IV) continue to represent the most difficult tumor to treat. Surgery is usually impossible, and radiotherapy is only minimally effective. The average survival time is usually less than 1 year. Individual cases, especially those with cystic components to the tumor, may achieve much longer survival.[15] However, the development of chemotherapy, particularly utilizing the nitrosoureas, which have been shown to have a definite effectiveness against some glioblastomas, raises the possibility of at least significant prolongation of good quality survival of some patients with this type of tumor.

Optic nerve glioma. Optic nerve gliomas can often be successfully removed surgically, and when this is impossible, some of them are responsive to radiotherapy with long-term control of disease. In a recent series of 20 patients (many of them children) with glioma of the optic nerve, 85% of the patients were alive 1 to 12 years after surgical and irradiation therapy.[17] For those tumors that are not responsive, the availability of the nitrosoureas (BCNU and CCNU) offers a potential means for improved survival.

Craniopharyngioma. The patient with craniopharyngioma has an excellent chance for long-term survival, as indicated by the surgical results achieved by Matson[22] and the radiotherapeutic results reported by Kramer.[13]

In Matson's series, 76% of the patients are alive, most without significant residual neurologic deficit, and the results of surgery in more recent years have improved this figure. Kramer[13] reported on 10 children with craniopharyngioma who received primary treatment with radiation therapy. Nine of them are alive and well. However, the opportunity for long-term survival with minimal residual defect depends on the skill of the surgeon or radiotherapist and the availability of excellent supportive therapy, particularly in the immediate postoperative period.

Table 19-2. Brain tumors of childhood

Tumor type	Estimated survival (5 yr or longer)
Cerebellar astrocytoma	90%
Medulloblastoma	40%
Ependymoma	30%
Astrocytoma (Grades III and IV)	5%
Optic nerve glioma	50%
Craniopharyngioma	75%

Choroid plexus papilloma. The patient with a choroid plexus papilloma also has an excellent chance for long-term survival, particularly when the tumor is located in the lateral ventricle, which is the most common site. Over 75% of the children in one series achieved long-term survival.[20]

For children with brain tumors the overall prognosis for survival during the immediate surgical and postsurgical period is high. In addition to surgery, the availability of improved techniques of radiotherapy and chemotherapy is helping to produce the increasing numbers of both cures and significant long-term palliation in some of the previously fatal malignant neoplasms of the central nervous system (Table 19-2).

INTRASPINAL TUMORS

Early recognition of the presence of an intraspinal tumor is of particular importance. The tumors are frequently benign, and prompt diagnosis and immediate surgical therapy may prevent severe neurologic damage and allow complete recovery. However, the diagnosis is frequently difficult and often is not apparent for an extended period after the initiation of signs and symptoms.

In 1887 the first intradural tumor of the spinal cord was successfully removed.[8] Subsequently, surgical treatment has been refined, and diagnostic radiologic techniques have been developed. Many intraspinal tumors can now be successfully treated, as indicated by Matson's report[21] of over 50% long-term survival in a large group of patients.[21]

Incidence

Intraspinal tumors are much less common than brain tumors and occur in children at a ratio of one intraspinal tumor for every six brain tumors. However, about 50% of them occur during the first 4 years of life. This is presumably due to the large number of intraspinal tumors that represent a congenital defect such as dermoid cysts and teratomas. They occur more frequently in boys than in girls in a ratio similar to that of brain tumors (60%:40%).

Pathologic characteristics and classifications (Table 19-3)

The most common group of tumors are the intramedullary gliomas. These are more often benign than malignant and include the Grade I and II astrocytomas and, more rarely, glioblastomas or oligodendrogliomas. Other relatively

Table 19-3. Intraspinal tumors in children*

Tumor	Usual location	Usual site	Approximate frequency
Glioma	Intramedullary	Cervical/thoracic	30%
Ependymoma	Intramedullary	Lumbar	10%
Congenital (dermoid, lipoma, teratoma)	Extramedullary or intramedullary	Lumbosacral	10%
Neuroblastoma	Extradural	Any level	20%
Metastatic (Ewing's sarcoma, lymphoma, etc.)	Extradural	Any level	15%

*Data from Matson,[21] Rand,[29] and Slooff.[33]

common intraspinal tumors include ependymomas and dermoid cysts, teratomas, and lipomas. Both neuroblastomas and lymphomas occur as extradural intraspinal tumors usually attached to a mass in the paraspinal tissues. Other primary tumors seen less frequently include meningiomas, ganglioneuromas, nerve sheath tumors (neurilemoma and neurofibromas), and vascular tumors such as the hemangioblastoma. A small group of patients with extradural "round cell" tumors have also been described.[36] These patients had no other known primary site, and specific histologic diagnosis could be determined despite similarities to neuroblastoma and Ewing's sarcoma.

In addition to tumors from the brain that may metastasize to the spinal canal (medulloblastoma, ependymoma), some tumors from elsewhere in the body may also metastasize to the intraspinal area. These include Ewing's sarcoma, soft tissue sarcomas, lymphomas, and leukemia.

Clinical manifestations

The most common initial presentation is that of muscle weakness, which gradually becomes more apparent. This is often associated with muscle spasm, particularly in the muscle group of the neck or back at the level of the tumor. The weakness may be initially subtle and gradually more apparent. Pain is a frequent but not a consistent finding. A more subtle indication of intraspinal tumor is sphincter control abnormality involving bowel, bladder, or both.

Careful physical examination with particular attention to the reflexes may help to make the diagnosis and localize the level of the spinal cord blockage. Sensory abnormalities not previously recognized may often be noted on careful physical examination.

Diagnostic features

Initial diagnostic studies should include careful x-ray examination of the entire spine, regardless of the apparent level of the tumor on physical examination. More definitive information can frequently be obtained by lumbar puncture with analysis of the spinal fluid. Analysis should include evaluation of spinal fluid pressure and spinal fluid manometrics with the Queckenstedt test. When an intraspinal tumor is suspected, it is desirable to be prepared to proceed directly to myelography with injection of the contrast media through the same needle if a spinal cord blockage is apparent. This would be suggested by the presence of xanthochromic fluid and abnormal manometrics. After radiographic determination of the level of the block, the patient should be taken directly to surgery for prompt relief of the obstruction. Laboratory studies include examination of the cerebrospinal fluid for the presence of malignant cells, determination of protein level, and culture. Elevation of the spinal fluid protein is usually present when there is a spinal cord tumor. Elevation may be as little as 50 to 60 mg/100 ml but commonly is greater than 100 mg/100 ml.

Differential diagnosis

Some of the signs and symptoms that may occur secondary to intraspinal tumors can also be caused by a variety of other neurologic diseases, including infection. The major problem is to recognize the possible presence of the intraspinal tumor and then to do the appropriate diagnostic studies to confirm or rule out its presence.

Other pathologic lesions may on occasion cause spinal cord compression, and they also require prompt relief to prevent permanent damage. These other possibilities include primary vertebral tumors, granulomas, vascular malformations, and on occasion a ruptured intervertebral disc. Hydatid cysts may also appear here in patients living in regions where this type of infestation occurs.

Treatment

Surgery. The primary treatment of intraspinal tumors is surgical. The initial main object of surgery is to relieve pressure on the spinal cord. If this can be accomplished with meticulous removal of the tumor without damage to the spinal cord, it is ideal. However, it is often impossible to accomplish total removal of intramedullary tumors without causing significant damage to the spinal cord. The intramedullary gliomas are the most common tumors found in this situation. They vary greatly in their degree of malignancy, and at times long-term improvement can be achieved by removal of cyst fluid without total extirpation of the main tumor mass. Subsequent repeat surgery after decompression often provides a better opportunity for removal of residual tumor without significant spinal cord damage. Extramedullary tumors should have as much of the bulk of the tumor removed as possible without causing damage to the spinal cord. Ependymomas are most frequently located in the lumbar region, usually arise from the filum terminale, and are often wrapped around the roots of the cauda equina. These tumors may frequently be totally removed surgically.

Radiotherapy. Radiotherapy is utilized for treatment of malignant tumors with residual potential for recurrence or spread. These include glioblastomas, ependymomas, neuroblastomas, and lymphomas. In addition, metastatic lesions from malignant tumors inside and outside the central nervous system, including leukemia, sarcomas, and carcinomas, may also be sensitive to radiation therapy. The amount of radiotherapy used depends on the age of the patient and the level of the spinal cord included in the treatment field. Tumor doses in the range of 3500 rads in 3½ weeks to 4500 rads in 4½ weeks are normally utilized.

Chemotherapy. Chemotherapy is utilized in treatment of tumors with potential for systemic spread, particularly neuroblastomas and lymphomas. Many of the medications are the same as those used for systemic treatment. Methotrexate can be used intrathecally for those tumors in which metastatic spread within the spinal canal commonly occurs. In glioblastoma the availability of BCNU and CCNU, which have shown some effectiveness, should be considered for supplementation of surgical and radiotherapeutic treatment of this tumor.

The major supportive and rehabilitative therapy is directed toward recovery of as much function as possible after spinal cord compression. The physical therapy rehabilitation program should be initially undertaken with the expectation of a complete recovery of normal function. Subsequent adjustments in the program can then be made for those patients who are left with a residual deficit.

Complications

The most common complication of spinal cord tumors is the development of paralysis caused either by the disease compression itself or the surgical treatment of the tumor. Patient deaths are usually caused by recurrence and spread of malignant spinal cord tumors or recurrent involvement of tumors in the cervical region, which interferes with vital bodily functions.

The major complications of surgery are those of permanent damage to the spinal cord or nerve roots secondary to the attempted surgical removal of the tumor. Radiotherapy may cause a radiation-induced transverse myelitis, and it must be administered with great care to young children whose normal growing tissues are more sensitive to the radiation therapy. Other potential secondary complications of radiotherapy include radiation inhibition of bone growth and possible induction of secondary neoplasms. Scoliosis is a frequent long-term complication of both surgery and radiotherapy, as well as the direct effect of tumor pressure. Other orthopedic complications may develop subsequently in spite of successful tumor control. All patients with intraspinal tumors should continue to have long-term careful orthopedic follow-up observation.

Prognosis

Because many of the intraspinal tumors are benign, a majority of patients achieve long-term survival. However, the majority of the long-term survivors will have some form of neurologic orthopedic residual defect.

The major means of improvement in the results of treatment of intraspinal tumors will be earlier diagnosis. Improvements in the techniques of radiotherapy and chemotherapy for malignant intraspinal tumors should also help achieve better results in this group of tumors.

REFERENCES

1. Banna, M., Lassman, L. P., and Pearce, G. W.: Radiological study of skeletal metastases from cerebellar medulloblastoma, Br. J. Radiol. **43**:173-179, March, 1970.
2. Barone, B. M., and Elvidge, A. R.: Ependymomas—a clinical survey, J. Neurosurg. **33**: 428-438, 1970.
3. Bloom, H. J. G., Wallace, E. N. K., and Henk, J. M.: The treatment and progress of medulloblastoma in children, Am. J. Roentgenol. **105**:43-62, 1969.
4. Chang, C. H., Housepian, E. M., and Herbert, C., Jr.: An operative staging system and a megavoltage radiotherapeutic technic for cerebellar medulloblastomas, Radiology **93**: 1351-1359, 1969.
5. Critchley, M.: Brain tumors in children: their general symptomatology, Br. J. Child. Dis. **22**:251-264, 1925.
6. Fessard, C.: Cerebral tumors in infancy, Am. J. Dis. Child **115**:302-308, 1968.
7. Geissinger, J. D., and Bucy, P. C.: Astrocytomas of the cerebellum in children, Arch. Neurol. **24**:125-135, 1971.
8. Gowers, W. R., and Horsley, V. A.: A case of tumors of the spinal cord: removal: recovery, Trans. Med. Chir. Soc. Edinburgh **71**:379-430, 1888.
9. Hansen, H. H., Selawry, O. S., Muggia, F. M., and Walker, M. D.: Clinical studies with 1-(2-chloroethyl)-3-cyclohexyl-1-nitrosourea (NSC 79037), Cancer Res. **31**:223-227, 1971.
10. Hope-Stone, H. F.: Results of treatment of medulloblastomas, J. Neurosurg. **32**:83-88, 1970.
11. Jenkin, R. D. T.: Medulloblastoma in childhood: radiation therapy, Can. Med. Assoc. J. **100**:51-53, 1969.
12. Koos, W. Th., and Miller, M. H.: Intracranial tumors of infants and children, St. Louis, 1971, The C. V. Mosby Co.
13. Kramer, S.: Radiation therapy in the management of brain tumors in children, Ann. N. Y. Acad. Sci. **159**:571-584, 1969.

14. Lampkin, B., Mauer, A. M., and McBride, B. H.: Response of medulloblastoma to vincristine sulfate: A case report, Pediatrics **39**:761-763, 1967.

15. Lassiter, K. R. L., Eben, A., Jr., Davis, C. H., Jr., and Kelly, D. L., Jr.: Surgical treatment of brain stem gliomas, J. Neurosurg. **34**:719-725, 1971.

16. Lassman, L. P., Pearce, G. W., and Gang, J.: Sensitivity of intracranial gliomas to vincristine sulphate, Lancet **1**:296-297, 1965.

17. MacCarty, C. S., Boyd, A. S., Jr., and Childs, D. S., Jr.: Tumors of the optic nerve and optic chiasm, J. Neurosurg. **33**:439-444, 1970.

18. Makeever, L. C., and King, J. D.: Medulloblastoma with extracranial metastasis through a ventriculovenous shunt, Am. J. Clin. Pathol. **46**:245-249, Aug., 1966.

19. Matson, D. D.: Intracranial tumors of the first two years of life, West J. Surg. **72**:117-122, May-June, 1964.

20. Matson, D. D.: Neurosurgery of infancy and childhood, Springfield, Ill., 1969, Charles C Thomas, Publisher.

21. Matson, D. D., and Crigler, J. F., Jr.: Management of craniopharyngioma in childhood, J. Neurosurg. **30**:377-390, 1969.

22. Matson, D. D., and Tachdjian, M. O.: Intraspinal tumors in infants and children, Postgrad. Med. **34**:279-285, Sept., 1963.

23. McFarland, D. R., Horwitz, H., Saenger, E. L., and Bahr, G. K.: Medulloblastoma—A review of prognosis and survival, Br. J. Radiol. **42**:198-214, March, 1969.

24. Miller, R. W.: Fifty-two forms of childhood cancer: United States mortality experience, 1960-1966, J. Pediatr. **75**:685-689, 1969.

25. Mussa, G. C., Martini Mauri, M., and Bacolla, D.: Brain scans with 99mTC in the diagnosis of intracranial tumours in children, Panminerva Med. **13**:1-6, Jan.-Feb., 1971.

26. Norrell, H., and Wilson, C.: Brain tumor chemotherapy with methotrexate given intrathecally, J.A.M.A. **201**:93-95, 1967.

27. Ommaya, A. K., Oxon, M. A., and Punjab, M. B.: Subcutaneous reservoir for pump for sterile access to ventricular cerebrospinal fluid, Lancet **2**:983-984, 1963.

28. Pinealoma: Case reports, Cancer Bull. **23**:95-96, Sept.-Oct., 1971.

29. Rand, R. W., and Rand, C. W.: Intraspinal tumors of childhood, Springfield, Ill., 1960, Charles C Thomas, Publisher.

30. Rubin, R. C., Ommaya, A. K., Henderson, E. S., Bering, E. A., and Rall, D. P.: Cerebrospinal fluid perfusion for central nervous system neoplasms, Neurology **16**:680-692, 1966.

31. Samuels, L. D.: 99mTc pertechnetate scans of posterior fossa tumors in children, Clin. Pediatr. **10**:210-217, 1971.

32. Sayers, M. P., Newton, W. A., Jr., and Samuels, L. D.: Intrathecal methotrexate therapy of brain tumors of childhood, Ann. N. Y. Acad. Sci. **159**:608-613, 1969.

33. Slooff, J. L., Kernohan, J. W., and MacCarty, C.: Primary intramedullary tumors of the spinal cord and filum terminale, Philadelphia, 1964, W. B. Saunders Co.

34. Smart, C. R., Ottoman, R. E., Rochlin, D. B., Hornes, J., Silva, A. R., and Goepfert, H.: Clinical experience with vincristine (NSC-67574) in tumors of the central nervous system and other malignant diseases, Cancer Chemother. Rep. **52**:733-741, 1968.

35. Smith, R. A., Lampe, I., and Kahn, E. A.: The prognosis of medulloblastoma in children, J. Neurosurg. **18**:91-97, 1961.

36. Tefft, M., Vawter, G. F., and Mitus, A.: Paravertebral "round cell" tumors in children, Radiology **92**:1501-1509, 1969.

37. Wakamatsu, T., Matsuo, T., Kawano, S., Teramoto, S., and Hidekatsu, M.: Glioblastoma with extracranial metastasis through ventriculopleural shunt, J. Neurosurg. **34**:697-701, 1971.

38. Walker, M. D., and Hurwitz, B. S.: BCNU (1,3-bis(2-chloroethyl)-1-nitrosourea) (NSC-409962) in the treatment of malignant brain tumor—a preliminary report, Cancer Chemother. Rep. **54**:263-271, 1970.

39. Wilson, C. B., Boldrey, E. B., and Enot, K. J.: 1,3-bis(2-chloroethyl)-1-nitrosourea (NSC-409962) in the treatment of brain tumors, Cancer Chemother. Rep. **54**:273-281, 1970.

40. Wilson, C. B., and Norrell, H. A., Jr.: Brain tumor chemotherapy with intrathecal methotrexate, Cancer **23**:1038-1045, 1969.

41. Zulch, K. J.: Brain tumors—their biology and pathology, New York, 1965, Springer Publishing Co., Inc.

CHAPTER 20

Malignant tumors of the soft tissues[*]

ABDELSALAM H. RAGAB

TERESA J. VIETTI

CARLOS A. PEREZ

DAISILEE H. BERRY

The soft tissue sarcomas comprise those malignant neoplastic conditions that originate from undifferentiated mesenchymal cells present in muscle, tendons, bursae, and fascia and in fibrous, connective, lymphatic, and vascular tissue. With the exception of rhabdomyosarcoma, these are rare tumors in children. Andersen,[1] in a review of 116 malignant solid tumors seen at the Babies Hospital in New York in the years 1935 through 1950, recorded only 24 cases of soft tissue sarcoma. Tumors may vary in histologic appearance from one area to another. Many soft tissue sarcomas are so undifferentiated that the cell of origin cannot be determined. All tumors have a tendency to recur locally, and some (especially rhabdomysarcoma) may metastasize early.

Radical surgical excision of the tumor should be performed, followed in most cases by radiation therapy to the primary site and surrounding tissues. Chemotherapy has proved to be of value in the treatment of rhabdomyosarcoma, but its role in the management of other soft tissue sarcomas remains to be established. This chapter will include rhabdomyosarcoma, synovial sarcoma, fibrosarcoma, dermatofibrosarcoma protuberans, liposarcoma, and leiomyosarcoma. The pathologic classification is that listed by the World Health Organization.[29]

RHABDOMYOSARCOMA

Rhabdomyosarcoma is the commonest soft tissue sarcoma in the pediatric age group.[79] Excluding tumors of the central nervous system, it is exceeded in number only by neuroblastoma and Wilms' tumor.[5] Among 1000 children with neoplastic disease seen at the M. D. Anderson Hospital between 1946 and 1966, there were 78 children (8%) with rhabdomyosarcoma. In their series it constituted 13% of 579 children with malignant solid tumor.[93]

Weber (1854), cited by Stout,[85] reported what was probably the first case of rhabdomyosarcoma of the tongue in a 21-year-old man. Rakov (1937) reported the first large series of rhabdomyosarcoma.[69]

---

[*]The data in this chapter were obtained through the support of the following funds: Southwest Cancer Chemotherapy Study (3 R10 CA05587), Clinical Cancer Radiation Therapy Research Center (5 PO2 CA10435), Fern Waldman Memorial Fund, and the Children's Hematology Research Association of St. Louis.

The pleomorphic form of rhabdomyosarcoma, which is rare in children, was thought for many years to be the only existing type.[85] Subsequently the embryonal type, most common in young children, was described by Stobbe and Dargeon[83]; the alveolar form, most common in young adolescents, was described by Riopele and Theriault.[70] Thus a tumor that was thought to be very rare in children has now become one of the more frequent forms.

Clinical features

Age and sex. Rhabdomyosarcoma occurs in all ages. The tumor may be present at birth, and the diagnosis has been made in infants less than 1 month of age in 9 of 280 cases.[47] This suggests that the genesis of these tumors occurs during prenatal life. The peak age of incidence in children is from 2 to 6 years of age,[46, 47, 93, 94] although there seems to be another peak below 1 year of age.[35]

The reported incidence among both sexes varies slightly from one series to another, but it is roughly equal[35, 93] except for sarcoma botryoides, which is more common in girls.

Signs and symptoms. Rhabdomyosarcoma occurs in any anatomic location of the body where there are skeletal muscles. Some cases have been reported in areas where skeletal muscle does not exist such as the distal phalanx. Clinical features and differential diagnosis vary with the sites of origin of the primary lesion.

Site. The most common site of the primary lesion is the head and neck area; 64% (49 of 76 cases) of patients with this tumor seen at the M. D. Anderson Hospital,[93] 50% (38 of 75 cases) seen at the Mayo Clinic,[50] and 31% (13 of 42 cases) seen at the Ohio State University presented with the primary lesion in the head and neck area.[35] The orbital region accounts for 30% of all rhabdomyosarcomas involving the head and neck area.[93] Other sites involved in the head and neck region are the nasopharynx, larynx, maxillary sinus, and middle ear. The next most frequent site is the genitourinary tract and the perineal area.[35, 50, 93] Other sites include the extremities, the retroperitoneal tissues, and body wall. In a small percentage of patients the primary site is unknown, and the patient presents with generalized metastases.

Orbital region. Because of their location, tumors in the orbital region grow rapidly and are detected early after 1 or 2 weeks of symptoms. Generally the tumor is confined to the orbit. The usual history is that the parents have noticed a rapidly developing proptosis of the eye with chemosis of the conjunctiva and loss of extraocular movements. Sometimes the tumor may present as an orbital cellulitis presumably due to necrosis of the tissues. The more common differential diagnoses to be considered are granuloma, hemangioma, optic nerve glioma, metastatic neuroblastoma, histiocytosis X, lymphoma, and retinoblastoma. A complete diagnostic evaluation that includes ophthalmoscopic visualization should be obtained to rule out other possibilities before a biopsy is performed. The clinical appearance of a 7-year-old boy with orbital rhabdomyosarcoma is shown in Fig. 20-1.

Nasopharyngeal and paranasal sinuses. Tumors of the paranasal sinuses usually present with nasal obstruction, discharge, sinusitis, epistaxis, local pain, and swelling. With tumors of the nasopharynx there is usually a nasal voice that may be associated with pain, nasal obstruction, epistaxis, and dysphagia. Occasionally polypoid masses may be seen extending into the nasal or nasopharyngeal passage. Tumors in this area must be differentiated from inflammatory granulomas, juvenile nasopharyngeal angiofibromas, carcinomas, lymphomas, and other soft tissue sarcomas. Radiographic findings in a 12-year-old child with embryonal rhabdomyosarcoma of the oropharynx are illustrated in Fig. 20-2.

Middle ear. Tumors involving the middle ear present with signs and symptoms of chronic otitis media, pain, sanguinopurulent discharge, and sometimes facial nerve palsy. On inspection, granulation tissue or a polyp may be seen protruding from the external auditory canal. Fig. 20-3 shows the microscopic appearance of an embryonal rhabdomyosarcoma of the middle ear in a 2½-year-old girl.

The neck. Tumors in this area present with hoarseness, dysphagia, or a soft tissue mass in the neck. Lymphomas, inflammatory lesions, and branchial cleft cysts must be ruled out.

Retroperitoneal area. Tumors in this anatomic location are generally symptomless until they reach huge proportions. Sometimes patients present with abdominal pain or signs and symptoms of intestinal or genitourinary obstruction. At this time the mother or physician may note a mass. Other tumors to be excluded in the differential diagnosis are Wilms' tumor, neuroblastoma, lymphoma, teratoma, and other soft tissue sarcomas.

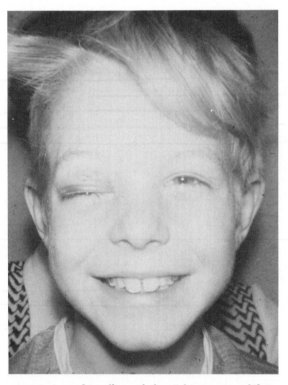

Fig. 20-1. Ecchymosis, ptosis, and swelling of the right upper eyelid in a 7-year-old boy. A firm tumor was noted in the upper nasal quadrant of the orbit, which on biopsy showed embryonal rhabdomyosarcoma. The child was treated with radiation therapy (5000 rads), dactinomycin, vincristine, and cyclophosphamide.

The perineum. Tumors in this area generally present as superficial masses that may extend to interfere with bowel or bladder function. The clinical appearance of a rhabdomyosarcoma of the perianal tissue that was present at birth is shown in Fig. 20-4.

Disseminated disease. Since the tumor metastasizes early and widely, initial symptomatology may be related to the metastases rather than the primary lesion. In a small percentage of the cases the primary lesion is never identified.

Recurrence and metastases. In some cases the initial surgery and radiation therapy is inadequate, leading to local recurrence that may develop years after apparent control of the primary lesion. It is not uncommon to find evidence of widespread metastatic disease at the time of the initial diagnosis. Metastases were noted in one series in 30%[91] and in another series in 40%[46] of the patients at the time of diagnosis.

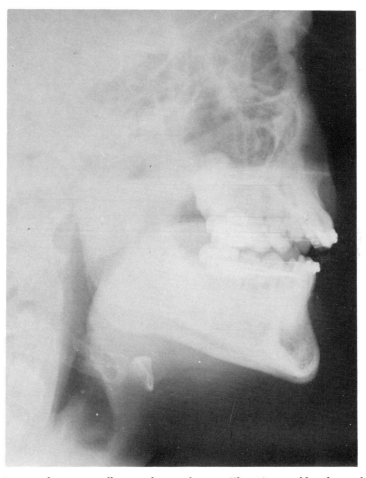

Fig. 20-2. Large soft tissue swelling in the oropharynx. This 12-year-old girl complained of a sore throat and pain in the right ear. Pathologic examination revealed embryonal rhabdomyosarcoma of the oropharynx. She was treated with radiation therapy (6500 rads), dactinomycin, vincristine, and cyclophosphamide. All chemotherapy was stopped after 1 year. Three years after her original diagnosis she is free of disease.

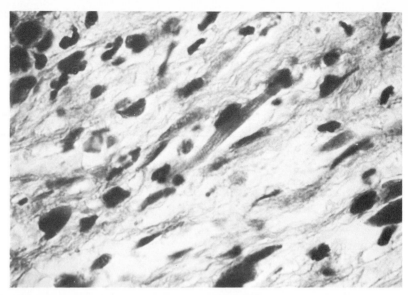

Fig. 20-3. Photomicrograph of embryonal rhabdomyosarcoma showing elongated cells with characteristic cross striations. This 2½-year-old girl complained of earache, a foul-smelling aural discharge, and facial nerve palsy. Biopsy material from the polypoid mass showed embryonal rhabdomyosarcoma. A radical mastoidectomy was performed with incomplete resection of the tumor. She was subsequently treated with radiation therapy (4000 rads over 6 weeks), dactinomycin, vincristine, and cyclophosphamide for 2 years. She is free of disease 4½ years after her original diagnosis. (From Ragab, A. H., Vietti, T. J., Kissane, J. M., and Sessions, D. G.: Cancer 30:648-650, 1972.)

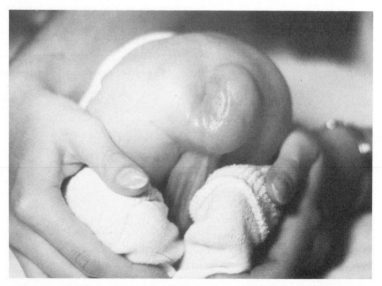

Fig. 20-4. Congenital embryonal rhabdomyosarcoma of the perianal tissue in a 2-week-old infant. An abdominoperineal resection was performed, but there was microscopic evidence of residual tumor. The child was treated with radiation therapy (2500 rads) and only two doses of vincristine. This therapy was not well tolerated, and it was stopped. Despite this presumably inadequate therapy, he remains in good health at 5 years of age and has no evidence of recurrence.

The commonest sites of metastases are the lungs, lymph nodes, bone, bone marrow, liver, brain, and breast.[46, 94]

Pathology

The pathologic diagnosis of rhabdomyosarcoma has been difficult, and in many cases the correct diagnosis was reached only after multiple biopsies. Of 37 cases in one series, the correct diagnosis was made initially in only 4 cases.[53] In another series of 45 cases in the head and neck region, the correct diagnosis was made in the initial microscopic examination in only 10 cases.[7] The tumor often causes a surrounding edematous inflammatory fibrovascular reaction; therefore an inadequate biopsy may be obtained.[61] In doubtful cases electron microscopy may be helpful.[42]

The World Health Organization[29] has divided rhabdomyosarcoma into four categories: embryonal, alveolar, pleomorphic, and mixed varieties.

Patton and Horn[64] correlated the morphology of embryonal rhabdomyosarcoma with skeletal muscle development in the embryo and noted that embryonal rhabdomyosarcoma closely resembled the developing muscle in the 7- to 10-week fetus, whereas alveolar rhabdomyosarcoma resembled the muscle pattern seen at 10 to 12 weeks. They did not find any correlation between embryonal muscle and pleomorphic rhabdomyosarcoma and suggested that this latter tumor represented dedifferentiation of adult skeletal muscle.

Grossly the tumors are usually nodular and vary in consistency from firm to cystic, depending on the amount of collagenous and myxomatous tissue and areas of tissue necrosis. Their gross appearance is not characteristic except for sarcoma botryoides, which appears as multiple grapelike mucinous polyps. There may be ulcerations and secondary infection in the botryoid type if the tumor is exposed to the exterior of the body surface. Some of the tumors appear deceptively circumscribed, but actually none are truly encapsulated. Rhabdomyosarcomas characteristically infiltrate extensively into the surrounding tissue. The cut surface may have some areas of tissue necrosis and hemorrhage, soft mucinous-like areas, and areas of firm pink-white tissue.

Embryonal rhabdomyosarcoma. The basic cell is long, slender, and spindle shaped and tapers to bipolar processes. There is usually a single central nucleus and abundant eosinophilic cytoplasm. Many of these cells do not contain cross striations. Of 48 patients examined, cross striations were found in only 15 of them (31%). Only in an exceptional case were cross striations numerous.[46] Numerous mitotic figures may be seen.

Sarcoma botryoides is a polypoid embryonal rhabdomyosarcoma that develops beneath a mucosal surface. The most common location is the vagina, but other areas include the urinary bladder, biliary tree, larynx, ear, and nasopharynx. Abundant stroma and dilated blood vessels are frequently present so that this tumor may be mistaken for a myxoma or hemangioma on biopsy. In children embryonal rhabdomyosarcoma is the commonest variety, accounting for 50% to 96% of all cases of rhabdomyosarcoma, and is most frequently seen in the head, neck, abdomen, and genitourinary tract.[5, 25, 35, 50, 93]

Alveolar rhabdomyosarcoma. These tumors are generally more firm and less myxoid than the embryonal type. The name is derived from the alveolar pattern produced by the tendency of cells to line connective tissue septa ir-

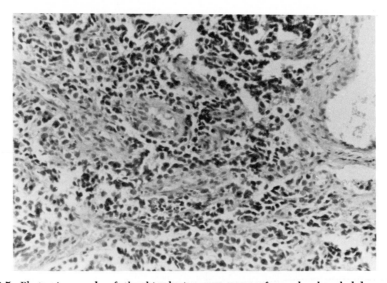

Fig. 20-5. Photomicrograph of the histologic appearance of an alveolar rhabdomyosarcoma that presented as a suprapubic mass in a 2-year-old boy. Laparotomy revealed metastatic disease in the internal iliac lymph nodes. The child was treated with radiation therapy and dactinomycin. Two years later the tumor recurred at the base of the penis, and the child was treated with radium needles followed by dactinomycin and vincristine. The child is now free of disease 6 years after his original diagnosis. (Photomicrograph courtesy Kenneth A. Starling, M.D., and Donald J. Fernbach, M.D., at Texas Children's Hospital, Houston, Texas.)

regularly (Fig. 20-5). The predominant cell is round and has scanty eosinophilic cytoplasm that is occasionally vacuolated. Some of the cells contain glycogen granules, and cross striations can generally be seen. Giant multinucleated cells are seen in the alveolar septa, whereas tadpole and racquet-shaped cells are often found inside the alveoli.

The incidence of the alveolar variety in children varies from 3% to 24%[35, 50, 91] of all cases of rhabdomyosarcoma and is most frequently found in the extremities.

Pleomorphic rhabdomyosarcoma. This type is very rare in the pediatric age group, ranging from 0% to 14% of reported cases of rhabdomyosarcoma.[35, 50, 91] Most of these tumors exhibit extensive hemorrhage; microscopically they are composed of spindle-shaped cells arranged in parallel or interlacing bundles or without any special pattern. Longitudinal myofibrils and cross striations are usually seen. Multinucleated giant cells, strap, and racquet-shaped cells are also seen. The tumors contain numerous mitotic figures.

Mixed rhabdomyosarcoma. In this variety more than one histologic type is seen in the same tumor.

Diagnostic studies

Diagnostic studies should include a chest film, skeletal survey, and bone marrow aspirate for tumor cells. If the child presents with proptosis, an intravenous pyelogram is indicated to rule out metastatic neuroblastoma. Inferior venacavogram, arteriography, urography, and/or gastrointestinal studies may be indicated for intra-abdominal disease. Ideally an excisional biopsy should be done whenever possible.

Treatment

Since rhabdomyosarcoma is very malignant, with a tendency to early local recurrence and generalized metastases, treatment must be aggressive, with an integrated approach utilizing radical surgical excision, radiation therapy, and intensive combination chemotherapy. In the past clinicians believed that the only hope for these patients lay in complete surgical excision of the tumor because of alleged radioresistance[50] and lack of response to chemotherapy.[87] It has now been clearly established that embryonal rhabdomyosarcoma is radiosensitive, alveolar rhabdomyosarcoma is fairly sensitive, and the pleomorphic type is insensitive to radiation therapy. Similar observations, although as yet incomplete, have been made with respect to response to chemotherapeutic agents.

Surgery. For lesions that are in accessible anatomic sites, radical surgical excision is still considered the definitive treatment of choice,[7, 51] although a reevaluation of this approach has been suggested for tumors in special anatomic areas such as the orbit if mutilating surgery is required.[15] The surgical field must include wide margins, despite the fact that the tumor may falsely appear to be well encapsulated and shells out easily, since this tumor infiltrates diffusely into the surrounding tissue and along fascial planes. If the tumor is located in an extremity, surgical removal of the entire muscle mass from origin to insertion or amputation should be performed. If the tumor is unresectable, chemotherapy and radiation therapy may convert an inoperable lesion to an operable one.

Radiation therapy. Radiation therapy has been administered preoperatively in a dose up to 5000 rads tumor dose (in a 5-week period) or after radical resection of the tumor. Patients with tumors in unresectable sites such as the nasopharynx are treated by a combination of chemotherapy and radiation therapy (5000 to 6000 rads tumor dose). Variations in the dose-time relationship may be necessary to minimize injury to normal tissue and systemic toxicity, especially if combination therapy is used.

Cassady[15] treated 5 patients with orbital rhabdomyosarcoma by radiation therapy alone (5000 rads). All were alive 15 months to 5 years later. The disease was controlled by radiation therapy in 3 of 5 patients referred because of recurrence after surgery.[15] Of 15 children treated in a similar manner by Sagerman,[71] 9 are free of tumor 2 years after therapy. Eight of the surviving children developed cataracts, but they still retained reasonable vision in the treated eye. High-energy beams (^{60}Co, linear accelerator, Betatron) are necessary in the treatment of these tumors. In orbital tumors special precautions must be taken to avoid unnecessary radiation of the opposite eye, brainstem, and facial structures.

Chemotherapy. The role of chemotherapy in the primary treatment of non-metastatic rhabdomyosarcoma has been established.[99] Chemotherapy is effective in producing significant, but usually temporary, regression of metastatic lesions. Dactinomycin, methotrexate, vincristine, cyclophosphamide, and daunorubicin have all been shown to have antitumor activity against this tumor when used as single agents or in combination.[5, 68, 92, 94] Dactinomycin in combination with radiation therapy was thought to improve overall survival rates, but the data were inconclusive.[7] In one series there were 24 children with widespread disease at the time of diagnosis. None of these survived 3 years. However, 18 children who received chemotherapy lived longer than 6 who did not (median survival 11 months as compared to 3 months).[91]

Reports of results after the use of triple drug combination in association with radiation therapy have been promising. Wilbur[99] reported on 21 children with inoperable or metastatic rhabdomyosarcomas who were treated with cobalt 60 radiation (5000 to 6000 rads tumor dose), vincristine, 2 mg/M²/wk × 12, dactinomycin, 0.075 mg/kg divided into five to eight daily doses every 3 months for five or six courses, and cyclophosphamide, 2.5 mg/kg/day for 2 years or 10 mg/kg/day for 7 days every 6 weeks for 2 years. Further surgical procedures were undertaken as indicated. Sixteen (76%) of the patients are alive and free of the disease 1 to 4 years after initiation of therapy. This was compared with previous experience at the same institution in children with metastatic disease[91]; the more aggressive regimen has resulted in a significantly improved survival. This therapeutic regimen was associated with considerable toxicity and is best managed under the supervision of experienced oncologists.

Prognostic factors

In a series of 78 children the survival (with and without disease) at 1 year was 68%, at 2 years 47%, at 3 years 40%, and at 5 years 35%.[93] In a series of 42 children, 10 (24%) were living tumor free for more than 2 years.[35] In the Mayo Clinic series of 75 children, only 9 (12%) are alive and free of disease after 5 years.[50] These survival statistics are modified by a number of factors outlined here.

About 70% of all recurrences will occur within the first year and 90% by the end of the second year.[93] Although a child might be considered as a probable "cure" if he has survived 2 years from the original diagnosis with no evidence of local recurrence or metastasis, late recurrences do occur.

Extent of disease. This is the most important factor with regard to the prognosis in a child with this disease. Twenty-four children in one series had extensive local or metastatic disease initially[93]; none of these children survived more than 30 months. Their median duration of survival was 9 months, as compared to 19 months for the entire group (Fig. 20-6). In another series, 9 patients had disseminated disease at the time of their diagnosis[35]; there were no survivals.

Site. Orbital tumors have the best prognosis (Fig. 20-7), probably because diagnosis is made while the tumor is still localized. It is probable that surgical accessibility permits complete removal of the tumor. Of 15 patients with orbital tumors treated, 11 were tumor free for more than 36 months.[93] Other tumors of the head and neck, especially of the nasopharynx, have had the worst prognosis. Recent studies suggest that this is no longer true with the addition of intensive chemotherapy.[99]

Histologic type. The best survival occurred in children with sarcoma botryoides, whereas the prognosis was poorest in those with alveolar rhabdomyosarcoma. Embryonal rhabdomyosarcoma was intermediate[93] (Fig. 20-8). Alveolar rhabdomyosarcoma is generally more extensive at the time of diagnosis and tends to metastasize earlier and more frequently than the embryonal variety. In this study, none of the children with alveolar rhabdomyosarcoma remained tumor free more than 2 years after diagnosis.[93] Pleomorphic rhabdomyosarcoma is extremely rare in the pediatric age group. In a series of 42 children there were 6 cases of the pleomorphic type, with only 1 survivor.[35]

Age. In the M. D. Anderson study younger children (under 7 years) had a significantly better survival rate than older children. The median survival was 78 months for those under 7 years of age compared to 18 months for older children[93] (Fig. 20-9). The younger children had less extensive disease at the time of diagnosis, lower rates of recurrence, and a more favorable tumor type (embryonal) than older children. Grosfeld and co-workers[35] noted that the best survival occurred in the age group from 1 to 3 years. They had no long-term survivals in the 7 infants under 1 year of age.

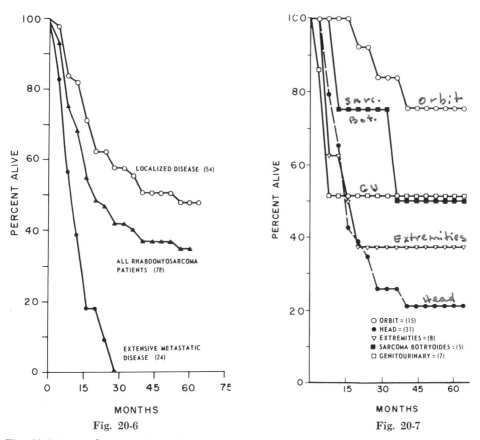

Fig. 20-6. Survival curves for children with localized and disseminated rhabdomyosarcoma. (From Sutow, W. W., Sullivan, M. P., Ried, H. L., Taylor, H. G., and Griffith, K. M.: Cancer 25:1384-1390, 1970.)

Fig. 20-7. Survival curves for children with rhabdomyosarcoma in different anatomic sites. (From Sutow, W. W., Sullivan, M. P., Ried, H. L., Taylor, H. G., and Griffith, K. M.: Cancer 25:1384-1390, 1970.)

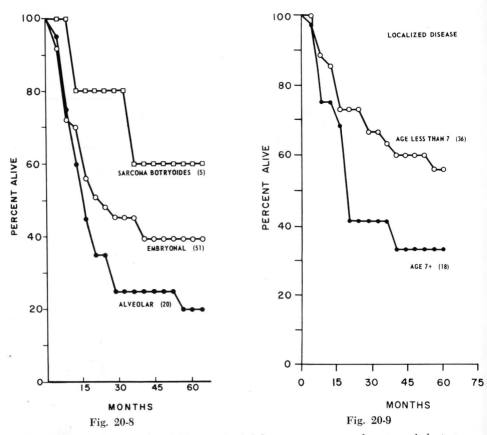

Fig. 20-8

Fig. 20-9

Fig. 20-8. Survival curves for children with rhabdomyosarcoma according to pathologic type. (From Sutow, W. W., Sullivan, M. P., Ried, H. L., Taylor, H. G., and Griffith, K. M.: Cancer **25**:1384-1390, 1970.)

Fig. 20-9. Survival curves for children with rhabdomyosarcoma according to age at time of diagnosis. (From Sutow, W. W., Sullivan, M. P., Ried, H. L., Taylor, H. G., and Griffith, K. M.: Cancer **25**:1384-1390, 1970.)

Summary

Rhabdomyosarcoma is the most common soft tissue sarcoma and one of the frequently occurring tumors in children. It has a poor prognosis, mainly because of its rapid local and generalized spread. The best therapeutic approach is a combination of radical surgery, radiation therapy, and chemotherapy. Most of the recurrences (90%) occur within 2 years of diagnosis. Localized disease, orbital tumors, embryonal type, and young age are favorable prognostic factors. These factors have to be considered in any clinical staging system that may be devised.

SYNOVIAL SARCOMA

Synovial sarcoma is a rare malignant tumor in adults and is even more uncommon in children. In adults it has been found to constitute between 8%[3] and 10%[13] of all malignant soft tissue tumors. Cadman[13] reviewed 134 tumors and found only eight in patients under 9 years of age. Crocker and Stout[18] reviewed the literature and found only 11 well-documented cases of synovial sarcoma in children; to this they added 10 cases of their own. In their experience it accounted for 2% of malignant mesenchymal tumors in children. Recently, in the Mayo Clinic series[77] ten of 135 soft tissue sarcomas in children (7%) were synovial sarcomas.

According to Berger,[8] who reviewed the world literature, the first recorded case of synovial sarcoma was described by Stur in 1893. The first pediatric cases of this tumor were described by Coley and Pierson in 1936.[17] Their patients, a 9-month-old infant and a 12-year-old boy, both had synovial sarcoma in the knee joint that was treated by local excision, radiation therapy, and, in the older boy, amputation. They were both alive and well 3 years and 6 years, respectively, after treatment.

There are no specific etiologic factors, although preceding trauma and malignant transformation of a benign tumor have been noted.[60]

Clinical features

This tumor presented as a painless mass in 58% of patients, a tender mass in 22%, and as pain preceding the development of a mass in 18%.[60] Most lesions (95%) are located in the extremities, and the majority are in the lower limbs.[13, 60] The knee joint, thigh, foot, and hand are the usual sites of involvement. Synovial sarcomas are the commonest malignant soft tissue tumors in the hands and feet.[40]

In adults and children there is no preponderance of either sex.[40, 60] This tumor generally occurs in young adults. Nearly three fourths (73%) of patients were in the third, fourth, or fifth decade.[13] In children more than 50% of cases occurred between the ages of 10 and 14 years.[18] The youngest patient was 2 weeks old at the time of diagnosis.[60]

Local recurrences are very common; 57 of 85 patients (66%) in one series[60] and 103 of 134 patients (77%) in another series[13] developed recurrences. Metastases occurred mainly to the lungs (81%) but also involved the regional lymph nodes (23%) and bone (20%).[13]

There are no diagnostic roentgenographic findings.

Pathology

Grossly the tumor appears as a firm pink or gray lobular mass. Areas of hemorrhage, necrosis, calcification, and cyst formation may be seen. Mucoid or gelatinous material may be present. The tumor often appears to be encapsulated, but there is usually microscopic peripheral invasion and no true encapsulation exists. Invasion of adjacent bone and tissues may occur.

Although the histopathology of the tumor resembles synovial tissue and in some cases it may arise from the synovial membranes of joints, tendons, and bursae, it is almost never directly connected to the joint space. Since it may also arise in areas that are totally devoid of synovial tissue, it is postulated that the cell of origin may be an undifferentiated mesenchymal cell.[13]

In the evolution of synovial tissue the progenitor mesenchymal cell differentiates into two components: an inner synovial layer and an outer connective tissue layer. Electron microscopy demonstrates that the cells of both layers are of the same type without a basement membrane separating them.[48] Murray[54] cultured cells in vitro from three human synovial sarcomas and noted their similarity to normal synovial tissue.

Histologically the tumor has a biphasic component and is composed of two neoplastic cellular elements. The fibrous tissue spindle cells, which resemble fibrosarcoma, are present in whorls or sheets and make up the basic stroma. This stroma surrounds glandlike slits lined by epithelioid cells, which are columnar or cuboidal in shape and one or more layers in thickness. The glandlike spaces may contain a mucinous mucopolysaccharide secretion. Mackenzie[49] believes that this biphasic character is the only histologic criterion by which synovial sarcomas may be diagnosed with certainty.

Treatment and prognosis

The treatment of choice is radical surgical excision followed by radiation therapy. Of 59 patients treated by local excision alone, 54 (91%) developed local recurrences, whereas only 16 of 32 patients (50%) treated by local excision followed by radiation therapy developed local recurrences.[13] When a lesion involves the hand or foot, amputation should be performed; the amputees generally have a more favorable prognosis.[60] The rarity of this tumor in children precludes any statement regarding the value of chemotherapy.

The 5-year survival rate for adults varies from 25%[13, 60] to 44%.[37] Although 25% survived 5 years in one series, only 11% lived beyond 10 years. Six patients developed local recurrences after tumor-free periods of 6 to 11 years, and 3 patients died of tumor 11 to 14 years after treatment.[13] Therefore 5- and 10-year "cure" rates must be accepted with reservation in dealing with this tumor. The prognosis in children is also unfavorable. Twenty-two percent of children were clinically tumor free for more than 5 years.[13] In the Mayo Clinic series of 12 children, 9 died of their tumor, and 3 were tumor free 4, 5, and 28 years later.[13]

FIBROSARCOMA

Fibrosarcoma is a tumor of fibrous tissue that has a tendency to local recurrence and very rarely shows a tendency to widespread metastases. Although common in adults, it is rare in children.

In a review of 120 cases of congenital mesenchymal tumors, fibromas constituted 30% (37 cases) of all tumors. Its incidence was second only to vascular tumors in the neonatal period. In the same series only 4 cases (3%) of fibrosarcoma were documented.[45] Balsaver,[6] after a critical analysis of the world literature, found only 6 cases of congenital fibrosarcoma. To this they added 5 cases of their own. In the Mayo Clinic series[79] only 6 of 135 children (4%) with soft tissue sarcomas had a diagnosis of fibrosarcoma.

This tumor, although common in adults, is rare in the pediatric age group. Of 129 cases of fibrosarcomas reported by Gentele,[32] only 8 (6%) were found in children. Warren and Sommer[97] studied 163 cases of fibrosarcoma of the soft parts, and only 4 (2%) were found in the pediatric age group. Wilson[100] found eight tumors in the first decade and nineteen in the second decade of life out of a total of 111 fibrosarcomas.

There are generally twice as many males as females afflicted with this tumor.[88]

Ionizing radiation may be a predisposing factor in the development of this tumor. Fibrosarcomas have been observed in rats and monkeys after experimental radiation therapy. Goldstein[34] reviewed sixty-five fibrosarcomas of the tongue; approximately half of these followed interstitial radiation therapy (radium needles). Six cases of fibrosarcoma followed irradiation for retinoblastoma,[78] and 7 cases of intracranial fibrosarcomas followed irradiation of gliomas and pituitary adenomas.[56] In the soft tissues, 5 cases of fibrosarcoma have been reported in 32 cases of lupus vulgaris treated by radiation therapy.[23] The time interval between radiation therapy and the appearance of the tumor varies between 3 and 38 years.

Fibrosarcomas have also been noted to follow prolonged implantation of plastic prostheses in rats[58] and in man.[38] They have also been noted to follow smallpox vaccination.[2]

Pathology

Grossly these tumors are generally well circumscribed although not encapsulated. Their consistency varies, but most tumors are firm and rubbery. Soft areas of necrosis may be seen. They are mostly located in the skeletal muscle and tend to infiltrate the surrounding tissues. They rarely extend to the underlying bone and cause pathologic fractures.

Microscopically, these tumors are composed of spindle cells arranged in sinuous interwining bands. They are sometimes arranged in a herringbone pattern. Both ends of the spindle cells are pointed. The nuclei are hyperchromatic with scattered mitotic figures. Reticulin fibers are sometimes found surrounding each cell or group of cells. No giant cells are seen.

Stout[86] noted that the degree of cellularity and differentiation of cells, manner of infiltrative growth, and percentage of mitotic figures were not reliable criteria for predicting the degree of malignancy of this tumor. Many of the mesenchymal tumors may be confused with fibrosarcoma; this is because lipoblasts, synovioblasts, mesothelial cells, and histiocytes can make fibrous tissue.

The tumor is usually located in the muscles of the extremities. It is generally firm and painless, although it may cause some limitation of movement. Fibrosarcomas may also occur in bone.[20] In contrast to osteogenic sarcoma, patients, are predominantly adults, although 13% of the 114 cases reviewed occurred in the first two decades of life. Twenty-three lesions developed in bones that had been subjected to prior radiation. The 5-year survival rate (28%) of patients with this tumor is significantly better than that for osteogenic sarcoma.[20]

Fibrosarcomas may also occur in the brain,[74] orbit,[27] lung,[41] and retroperitoneal tissues.[77]

Treatment and prognosis

This tumor is prone to local recurrences. As many as twenty recurrences have been reported[97] in a single patient. The recurrences may appear as long as 16 years later.[4] However, the incidence of generalized metastases is low. Stout[88] noted that of 54 cases of juvenile fibrosarcoma reported in the literature, only 4 (8%) are known to have metastasized.

The treatment of choice is wide total excision of the tumor, passing well outside its palpable limits. Although this tumor is believed to be radioresistant, cures have been reported with radiation therapy.[74]

It would seem that this tumor has a very good prognosis because of the low incidence of metastases. Wide total excision is the treatment of choice, and amputation is rarely required. If metastases occur, then chemotherapy may be administered. Because of the rarity of this tumor, the role of chemotherapy in its treatment is difficult to evaluate.

DERMATOFIBROSARCOMA PROTUBERANS

Dermatofibrosarcoma protuberans is a slow-growing fibrous tissue tumor of the skin characterized by a high frequency of local recurrence but an extremely low incidence of metastases. According to Binkley,[9] this tumor was first described by Pijjard in 1891. Hoffmann[39] gave the tumor its current name. The clinical and pathologic entity was first discussed in detail by Darier and Ferrand.[21]

Clinical features

The condition usually begins as one or more small firm nodules in the skin. They generally have a bluish or reddish discoloration and are loosely attached to the underlying skin. They then increase in size and form plaques. Subsequently sessile or pedunculated tumors develop in the plaques. The lesions tend to grow very slowly. In the Mayo Clinic series more than 10 years elapsed in 50% of their cases between the time the tumor was noted and the time it was initially excised; however, they can suddenly grow very rapidly. Pain or tenderness was noted by 28% of patients, and ulceration with bleeding occurred in 10%.[11] Trauma was reported as the cause of initial development or sudden enlargement of the tumors by 10% of patients.[76]

These tumors tend to occur in all age groups. In the M.D. Anderson series, cases were evenly distributed from the first to the seventh decade of life.[12] In the Mayo Clinic series, 14 (25%) of their cases occurred in patients under 20 years of age.[11] In all series reviewed there was a slight male preponderance.

Recurrence and metastases. There is a high incidence of local recurrence. Gentele[32] found that thirty-five recurrences occurred in 16 patients (46%) in his review of 38 cases. In the Mayo Clinic series[11] the recurrence rate was 33%. One patient with a neck lesion had ten recurrences in 15 years. Pillsbury[66] believes that occult lateral spread is the cause of local recurrence.

Metastases are very rare. Burkhardt[11] reviewed the literature and found 9 cases of suspected metastases and only 8 cases of histologically proved metastases.

Pathology

The tumor is composed of fibroblasts, and mitotic figures are rarely seen. These spindle cells are arranged about a central area of collagen or a small vascular space. This arrangement gives the appearance of a cartwheel, considered by Taylor and Helwig[95] to be pathognomonic of the tumor. This characteristic appearance is not found in metastatic lesions. The tumor commonly infiltrates the subcutaneous tissue and striated muscle. Because of the fibroblastic nature of the tumor, it is commonly mistaken for fibroma, fibrosarcoma, and neurofibroma. In the Mayo Clinic series[11] the correct pathologic diagnosis was made initially in only 20% of cases.

Treatment and prognosis

Wide local excision is the treatment of choice. Radiation therapy is believed by most investigators to be of limited value. Because of the extreme rarity of metastases, this tumor has a very good prognosis.

LIPOSARCOMA

Liposarcoma is a malignant tumor of adipose tissue derived from lipoblasts. Although this tumor constitutes 15% of all soft tissue sarcomas in adults,[62] it is rarely seen in children.

Virchow[96] reported the first case of liposarcoma in 1857. The following year Senftleben[73] reported the first case of liposarcoma of the left cheek in an 8-year-old child. The first large series of liposarcomas was reported by Pack and Anglem in 1939.[59] Kauffman and Stout[44] reviewed the literature and found 15 documented cases of liposarcoma in children; to this they added 13 cases of their own.

Clinical features

This tumor presents initially as an inconspicuous swelling of the soft tissues. It exhibits progressive growth generally without alarming exacerbations until it reaches such proportions as to demand the attention of the patient. These tumors, like lipomas, can reach enormous sizes. A 7-year-old boy was reported by Pinto[67] who had progressive abdominal enlargement since the age of 18 months. The liposarcoma weighed 13 kg and accounted for half the child's total body weight. It is interesting that although these are tumors of adipose tissue, the body cannot actively metabolize this fat, and the patient becomes emaciated.[24]

Another interesting feature is the variability in the rate of growth of this tumor. The known duration of symptoms varies from a few weeks to 18 years.[81] Pressure symptoms may develop when the tumor reaches a certain size, but pain is rare at the onset. Persistent pyrexia, which usually disappeared with treatment, has been noted in 10% of the patients in one series.[81] Retroperitoneal tumors usually reach huge proportions before they are detected. They generally give rise to a feeling of fullness, vague abdominal pain, and pressure symptoms.

On physical examination, liposarcomas are firmer, less compressible, and more fixed to the underlying tissues than lipomas. The diagnosis is made by pathologic examination of the excised tumor if it is small or by punch biopsy of a larger tumor.

Age and sex. Liposarcoma is predominantly a tumor of late life, occurring in patients in their fifth or sixth decade.[16, 72] In children there seem to be two age peaks: infancy and adolescence.[44] In most series reported in adults the sex distribution is about equal. However, in the 28 pediatric cases reviewed there were 19 boys and 9 girls.[44]

Anatomic distribution. Liposarcomas may occur wherever adipose tissue is found, and by far the commonest single site of involvement is the thigh. Rarely these tumors arise in the pleura,[36] mediastinum,[14, 19] breast,[57] and bone.[33] In the pediatric survey there were four tumors in the thigh and three in the neck. Other sites were the shoulder, chest wall, back, leg, foot, and labium majus.

Relationship to lipoma. Liposarcomas rarely develop in preexisting lipomas. The great frequency of lipomas and rarity of liposarcomas (120:1)[62] would suggest that the percentage of lipomas undergoing malignant transformation is very small and that most liposarcomas arise de novo. Rapid growth of a preexisting lipoma or associated pain should alert the physician to the possibility of malignant transformation. Speed[80] believes that the development of a pressure ulcer over the surface of a large lipoma should suggest sarcomatous change. Trauma rarely predisposes to the development of this tumor,[63, 98] although

Ewing[31] believes that since trauma to adipose tissue is followed by enhanced proliferation, this proliferation in some cases may transform to malignancy.

Recurrence and metastases. Distant metastases occur in one third of adults with liposarcoma.[81] Metastases tend to occur to the lungs, liver, and bone. In the pediatric age group generalized metastases are rare, although local recurrences are very common.

Pathology

Grossly the tumors are multilobed, with a partially defined or totally absent capsule. They have the gross appearance of mature fat with a gelatinous mucoid consistency. Hemorrhagic, fibrous, calcific, or cystic degeneration may be found. Stout[84] proposes the following histologic classification:

1. Well-differentiated myxoid type. This resembles embryonal fat with stellate or spindle-shaped cells containing lipoid material. Mitoses are rare. This is the commonest type seen in children.

2. Poorly differentiated myxoid type. The lipoblasts here are bizarre in shape with misshapen nuclei, often pyknotic and hyperchromatic. Signet ring–form lipoblasts are occasionally seen.

3. Round cell type. The lipoblasts are round cells with centrally placed nuclei and voluminous foamy cytoplasm. The vacuoles are filled with lipoid material. The cells may reach enormous size.

4. Mixed type. These tumors contain two or more elements of the preceding groups.

Treatment

Surgery and radiation therapy play dominant roles in the treatment of this tumor. Surgical excision should be radical, passing well beyond the tumor margin or capsule if it is present. In some huge tumors or those infiltrating the underlying bone, amputation may be required. Del Regato[22] published a case report describing a highly radiosensitive embryonal liposarcoma. Pack and Pierson[62] reported 2 of 12 cases controlled by radiation therapy alone. They noted that 60% of their cases showed definite regression and 15% showed complete clinical regression with radiation therapy. Edland[26] recommends postoperative radiation therapy because of the high incidence of local recurrences after surgical excision. Spittle[81] found that the local recurrence rate in the irradiated group was only 20%, whereas the unirradiated group had a recurrence rate of 73%. Stout[84] and Suit[90] believe that only small tumors should be treated by radiation therapy alone.

The exact role of chemotherapy in the treatment of this tumor is not well established. Significant palliative responses using both chemotherapy and radiation therapy have been reported by Molander[52] and Newton.[55] Stehlin[82] treated 3 cases by perfusion with phenylalanine mustard and dactinomycin. One patient responded, but the other 2 showed no improvement. James[43] reported the case of a 2-year-old child with massive recurrent intra-abdominal liposarcoma treated with a combination of vincristine and cyclophosphamide. The tumor disappeared completely, and the patient was alive and well 18 months later.

Prognosis

The 5-year survival rate in adults is between 36%[62] and 64%.[22, 28] The pathologic type is an important factor influencing the prognosis. Enzinger and Winslow[30] report 70% 5-year survivals with well-differentiated liposarcomas and only 18% with round cell tumors. Retroperitoneal tumors have a poorer prognosis than those occurring in the limbs.

In contrast to adults, the prognosis of liposarcomas in children is much better. This is probably because most of these tumors are of the well-differentiated variety (70%).[44]

LEIOMYOSARCOMA

Leiomyosarcoma is a malignant tumor of smooth muscle. It is a very rare tumor in the pediatric age group; of 116 malignant tumors seen in children at Columbia University from 1935 to 1950, only two were leiomyosarcomas.[1] Similarly, only 2 cases were observed in a series of 135 pediatric tumors reviewed at the Mayo Clinic.[79]

Clinical features

In adults and in children there is no familial, racial, or sex predilection. Of these tumors, 50% to 60% occur in the fifth or sixth decade of life,[75] whereas in children 53% of the tumors were noted in the first 5 years of life.[101] The commonest sites of origin for leiomyosarcomas in children are the gastrointestinal, genitourinary, and respiratory tracts and the soft tissues. It is interesting that although smooth muscle tumors are common in the uterus in adults, Yannopoulos and Stout[101] could not find a single case in children. Patients with these tumors in the gastrointestinal tract generally present with abdominal pain, hemorrhage, and associated anemia. Nausea, vomiting, and weight loss may also occur. Occasionally the tumor may present as an asymptomatic abdominal mass. Intestinal obstruction with or without intussusception may occur, especially in the neonatal period.[65]

Genitourinary leiomyosarcomas (bladder and prostate) generally cause dysuria and urinary retention. Since benign prostatic tumors are rare in children, any mass in the prostate must be regarded with suspicion.

Radiologic investigation in tumors of the gastrointestinal tract frequently shows a soft tissue mass, filling defects, obstruction, ulceration, or the presence of a sinus tract or fistula. Whenever possible the diagnosis is made by radical excision of the tumor and pathologic examination. If the mass is very large, an incisional biopsy may be necessary.

Recurrence and metastases. Leiomyosarcomas in adults have a tendency to local recurrences and metastases. Metastases from tumors of the gastrointestinal tract tend to disseminate via the bloodstream to the liver, lungs, peritoneum, and pancreas.[75] Occasionally the regional lymph nodes may be involved. Metastases from soft tissue leiomyosarcomas tend to lodge in the lungs. Of the 36 cases of soft tissue leiomyosarcoma described by Stout and Hill,[89] 26 (72%) either metastasized or recurred locally. Tumors of the prostate, bladder, and stomach are very malignant in children and show evidence of early metastases.[79]

Pathology

These tumors may appear as small nodules or, more frequently, larger nodular masses. They are usually reddish brown. Their consistency varies; small tumors are usually firm, whereas larger tumors, because they outgrow their blood supply, result in central necrosis and cavitation and are usually soft. There is no capsule, and the tumor infiltrates the surrounding tissues.

Tumors of the gastrointestinal tract are generally divided into (1) submucosal tumors that protrude into the lumen and give rise to bleeding, (2) dumbbell-shaped tumors that have submucosal and subserosal extensions, and (3) extrinsic tumors that arise from the serosal surface.

Histologically these tumors are composed of spindle cells with blunt-ended nuclei that are oval and often contain prominent nucleoli. The cells are generally arranged in intertwining bundles or whorls. Longitudinal myofibrils may be seen in the cytoplasm. The generally accepted criteria of malignancy—size of tumor, increased mitotic figures, anaplasia, and bizarre cell forms—are not reliable in this tumor. Other tumors that may be confused with leiomyosarcoma are leiomyoma, neurofibroma, and fibrosarcoma.

Treatment

Since these tumors are generally considered to be radioresistant, radical surgical excision is the treatment of choice. Surgical aggressiveness in the gastrointestinal tumors is sometimes limited by wide local infiltration of other abdominal organs.

Chemotherapy may be of benefit in cases with metastases.

Prognosis

The prognosis is guarded. Tumors of the prostate, bladder, and stomach are very malignant and show evidence of early metastases. Botting and co-workers[10] described 10 children with soft tissue leiomyosarcomas; only 3 survived 5 years or more.

REFERENCES

1. Andersen, D. H.: Tumors of infancy and childhood. I. A survey of those seen in the pathology laboratory of the Babies Hospital during the years 1935-1950, Cancer 4:890-906, 1951.
2. Archampong, E. Q., and Clark, C. G.: Fibrosarcoma at the site and immediately following small-pox vaccination, Br. J. Surg. 57:937-938, 1970.
3. Ariel, I. M., and Pack, G. T.: Synovial sarcoma, N. Engl. J. Med. 268:1272-1275, 1963.
4. Bahgat, H.: Interesting clinical cases with operations, J. Egypt. Med. Assoc. 16:678-686, 1933.
5. Bailey, W. C., Holaday, W. J., Kontras, S. B., and Clatworthy, W. W., Jr.: Rhabdomyosarcomas in childhood, Arch. Surg. 82:943-949, 1961.
6. Balsaver, A. M., Butler, J. J., and Martin, R. G.: Congenital fibrosarcoma, Cancer 20:1607-1616, 1967.
7. Bardwil, J. M., and MacComb, W. S.: Sarcomas of the head and neck with special references to rhabdomyosarcomas, Am. J. Surg. 108:476-480, 1964.
8. Berger, L.: Synovial sarcomas in serous bursae and tendon sheaths, Am. J. Cancer 34:501, 1938.
9. Binkley, G. W.: Dermatofibrosarcoma protuberans; report of 6 cases, Arch. Dermatol. 40:578-594, 1939.
10. Botting, A. J., Soule, E. H., and Brown, A. L.: Smooth muscle tumors in children, Cancer 18:711-720, 1965.
11. Burkhardt, B. R., Soule, E. H., Winkelmann, R. K., and Ivins, J. C.: Dermatofibrosarcoma protuberans; study of fifty-six cases, Am. J. Surg. 111:638-644, 1966.
12. Butler, J. J.: Fibrous tissue tumors: nodular fasciitis, dermatofibrosarcoma protuberans and fibrosarcoma, grade I, desmoid type. In Tumors of bone and soft tissue, presented at

the Eighth Annual Clinical Conference On Cancer, 1963, at the University of Texas, M. D. Anderson Hospital and Tumor Institute, Houston, Texas, Chicago, 1965, Year Book Medical Publishers, Inc., p. 402.

13. Cadman, N. L., Soule, E. H., and Kelly, P. J.: Synovial sarcoma; an analysis of 134 tumors, Cancer 18:613-627, 1965.

14. Caputo, N. T., and Spalding, E. D.: Mediastinal liposarcoma, Harper Hosp. Bull. 11: 122-127, 1953.

15. Cassady, J. R., Sagerman, R. H., Tretter, P., and Ellsworth, R. M.: Radiation therapy for rhabdomyosarcoma, Radiology 91:116-120, 1968.

16. Cicciarelli, F. E., Soule, E. H., and McGoon, D. C.: Lipoma and liposarcoma of the mediastinum: a report of 14 tumors including one lipoma of the thymus, J. Thorac. Cardiovasc. Surg. 47:411-429, 1964.

17. Coley, B. L., and Pierson, J. C.: Synovioma; report of 15 cases with review of literature, Guthrie Clin. Bull. 6:89-101, 1936.

18. Crocker, D. W., and Stout, A. P.: Synovial sarcoma in children, Cancer 12:1123-1133, 1959.

19. Currie, R. A.: Mediastinal liposarcoma; report of case, Dis. Chest 46:489-491, 1964.

20. Dahlin, D. C., and Ivins, J. C.: Fibrosarcoma of bone; a study of 114 cases, Cancer 23:35-41, 1969.

21. Darier, J., and Ferrand, M.: Dermatofibromes progressifs et recidivants ou fibrosarcomes de la peau, Ann. Dermatol. Syphiligr. 5:545-562, 1924.

22. Del Regato, J. A.: Liposarcoma of thigh, Cancer Semin. 1:12-13, 1950.

23. Deuticke, P.: Über Röntgensarkome, Beitr. Klin. Chir. 169:214-239, 1939.

24. DeWeerd, J. H., and Dockerty, M. B.: Lipomatous retroperitoneal tumors, Am. J. Surg. 84:397-407, 1952.

25. Edland, R. W.: Embryonal rhabdomyosarcoma, Am. J. Roentgenol. Radium Ther. Nucl. Med. 93:671-685, 1965.

26. Edland, R. W.: Liposarcoma. A retrospective study of 15 cases. A review of the literature and a discussion of radiosensitivity, Am. J. Roentgenol. Radium Ther. Nucl. Med. 103:778-791, 1968.

27. Eifrig, D. E., and Foos, R. Y.: Fibrosarcoma of the orbit, Am. J. Ophthal. 67:244-248, 1969.

28. Enterline, H. T., Culberson, J. D., Rochlin, D. B., and Brady, L. W.: Liposarcoma, Cancer 13:932-950, 1960.

29. Enzinger, F. M., Lattes, R., and Torloni, H.: Histological typing of soft tissue tumors, Geneva, 1969, World Health Organization.

30. Enzinger, F. M. and Winslow, D. J.: Liposarcoma; study of 103 cases, Virchow's Arch. [Pathol. Anat.]335:367-388, 1962.

31. Ewing, J.: Fascial sarcoma and intermuscular myxoliposarcoma, Arch. Surg. 31:507-520, 1935.

32. Gentele, H.: Malignant fibroblastic tumor of skin: Clinical and pathological anatomical studies of 129 cases of malignant fibroblastic tumors from cutaneous and subcutaneous layers observed at Radiumhemmet during period 1927-1947, Acta Derm. Venereol. 31(supp. 27):1-180, 1951.

33. Goldman, R. L.: Primary liposarcoma of bones and report of a case, Am. J. Clin. Path. 42:503-508, 1964.

34. Goldstein, H. I.: Sarcoma of the tongue, Med. Times 49:158-160, 1921.

35. Grosfeld, J. L., Clatworthy, H. W., Jr., and Newton, W. A., Jr.: Combined therapy in childhood rhabdomyosarcoma; an analysis of 42 cases, J. Pediatr. Surg. 4:637-645, 1969.

36. Gupta, R. K., and Paolini, F. A.: Liposarcoma of pleura; report of a case with review of literature and views on histiogenesis, Am. Rev. Resp. Dis. 95:298-304, 1967.

37. Hampole, M., and Jackson, B. A.: Analysis of 25 cases of malignant synovioma, Can. Med. Assoc. J. 99:1025-1029, 1968.

38. Herrmann, J. B., Kanhouwa, S., Kelley, R. J., and Burns, W. A.: Fibrosarcoma of the thigh associated with a prosthetic vascular graft, N. Engl. J. Med. 284:91, 1971.

39. Hoffmann, E.: Über das knollentreibende Fibrosarkom der Haut (Dermatofibrosarkoma protuberans), Dermatol. Ztschr. 43:1-28, 1925.

40. Hale, D. E.: Synovioma with special reference to clinical and roentgenologic aspects, Am. J. Roentgenol. Radium Ther. Nucl. Med. **65**:769-777, 1951.

41. Holinger, P. H., Johnston, K. D., Gossweiler, N., and Hirsch, E. C.: Primary fibrosarcoma of bronchus, Dis. Chest **37**:137-143, 1960.

42. Horvat, B. L., Caines, M., and Fisher, E. R.: The ultrastructure of rhabdomyosarcoma, Am. J. Clin. Pathol. **53**:555-564, 1970.

43. James, D. H., Johnson, W. W., and Wrenn, E. L.: Effective chemotherapy of an abdominal liposarcoma, J. Pediat. **68**:311-313, 1966.

44. Kauffman, S. L., and Stout, A. P.: Lipoblastic tumors of children, Cancer **12**:912-925, 1959.

45. Kauffman, S. L., and Stout, A. P.: Congenital mesenchymal tumors, Cancer **18**:460-476, 1965.

46. Lawrence, W., Jr., Jegge, G., and Foote, F. W., Jr.: Embryonal rhabdomyosarcoma: a clinicopathological study, Cancer **17**:361-376, 1964.

47. Li, F. P., and Fraumeni, J. F.: Rhabdomyosarcoma in children: Epidemiologic study and identification of a familial cancer syndrome, J. Natl. Cancer Inst. **43**:1365-1373, 1969.

48. Luse, S. A.: A synovial sarcoma studied by electron microscopy, Cancer **13**:312-322, 1960.

49. Mackenzie, D. H.: Synovial sarcoma: a review of 58 cases, Cancer **19**:169-180, 1966.

50. Mahour, G. H., Soule, E. H., Mills, S. D., and Lynn, H. B.: Rhabdomyosarcoma in infants and children: a clinicopathologic study of 75 cases, J. Pediatr. Surg. **2**:402-409, 1967.

51. Martin, R. G., Butler, J. J., and Albores-Saavedra, J.: Soft tissue tumors: surgical treatment and results. In Tumors of bone and soft tissue; presented at the Eighth Annual Clinical Conference on Cancer, 1963, at the University of Texas, M. D. Anderson Hospital and Tumor Institute, Houston, Texas, Chicago, 1965, Year Book Medical Publishers Inc., pp. 333-347.

52. Molander, D. W.: Palliative treatment of the metastatic tumors of soft somatic tissue with irradiation and chemotherapy, Am. J. Roentgenol. Radium Ther. Nucl. Med. **96**:150-157, 1966.

53. Moore, O., and Grossi, C.: Embryonal rhabdomyosarcoma of the head and neck, Cancer **12**:69-73, 1959.

54. Murray, M. R., Stout, A. P., and Pogogeff, I. A.: Synovial sarcoma and normal synovial tissue cultivated *in vitro*, Ann. J. Surg. **120**:843-851, 1944.

55. Newton, K. A.: Radiotherapy combined with chemotherapy in treatment of selected tumors, Br. J. Radiol. **40**:823-827, 1967.

56. Noetzli, M., and Malamud, N.: Post-irradiation fibrosarcoma of the brain, Cancer **15**:617-622, 1962.

57. Oberman, H. A.: Sarcomas of the breast, Cancer **18**:1233-1243, 1965.

58. Oppenheimer, B. S., Oppenheimer, E. T., Stout, A. P., and Danishefsky, I.: Malignant tumors resulting from embedding plastics in rodents, Science **118**:305-306, 1953.

59. Pack, G. T., and Anglem, T. J.: Tumors of the soft somatic tissues in infancy and childhood, J. Pediatr. **15**:372-400, 1939.

60. Pack, G. T., and Ariel, I. M.: Tumors of the soft somatic tissues and bone. In Treatment of cancer and allied diseases, vol. 8, ed. 2, New York, 1964, Hoeber Medical Division of Harper & Row, Publishers, pp. 184-193.

61. Pack, G. T., and Eberhart, W. F.: Rhabdomyosarcoma of skeletal muscle: Report of 100 cases, Surgery **32**:1023-1064, 1952.

62. Pack, G. T., and Pierson, J. C.: Liposarcoma: a study of 105 cases, Surgery **36**:687-712, 1954.

63. Pack, G. T., and Tabah, E. J.: Primary retroperitoneal tumors; a study of 120 cases, Int. Abstr. Surg. **99**:209-231, 1954.

64. Patton, R. B., and Horn, R. C., Jr.: Rhabdomyosarcoma; clinical and pathological features and comparison with human fetal and embryonal skeletal muscle, Surgery **52**:572-584, 1962.

65. Pennino, J. V., and Abbene, M. M.: Intussusception in an infant due to leiomyosarcoma of the jejunum, Am. J. Surg. **93**:461-465, 1957.

66. Pillsbury, D. M., Shelley, W. E., and Kligman, A. M.: Dermatology, Philadelphia, 1956, W. B. Saunders, Co., p. 1177.

67. Pinto, V. C., Mattos, A. G., Pimenta, E., Moraes, R. V., and Altenfelder, P.: Retroperitoneal myxolipoma; report of a case in child 7 years of age, Pediatrics **14**:11-15, 1954.

68. Pratt, C. B.: Response of childhood rhabdomyosarcoma to combination chemotherapy, J. Pediatr. **74**:791-794, 1969.

69. Rakov, A. I.: Malignant rhabdomyoblastomas of skeletal musculature, Am. J. Cancer **30**:455-476, 1937.

70. Riopele, J. L., and Theriault, J. P.: Sur une forme meconnue de sarcome des parties molles: le rhabdomyosarcoma alveolaire, Ann. Anat. Pathol. **1**:88-111 (1956).

71. Sagerman, R. H., Tretter, P., and Ellsworth, R. M.: The treatment of orbital rhabdomyosarcoma of children with primary radiation therapy, Am. J. Roentgenol. Radium Ther. Nucl. Med. **114**:31-34, 1972.

72. Sawyer, K. C., Sawyer, R. B., Lubchenco, A. E., Bramley, H. F., and Fenton, W. C.: The unpredictable fatty tumor, Arch. Surg. **96**:773-785, 1968.

73. Senftleben, H.: Zur Casuistik seltenerer Geschwülste; 1) Myxoma lipomatodes, 2) Cancroides hodencystoid mit verschiedenartigen Gewebstypen, Virchow's Arch. **15**:336-352, 1858.

74. Senyszyn, J. J., and O'Conor, G.: Fibrosarcoma of the brain. A case report describing response of the primary and metastatic tumors to radiotherapy, Oncology **24**:431-437, 1970.

75. Skandalakis, J. E., Gray, S. W., Shepard, D., and Bourne, G. H.: Smooth muscle tumors of the alimentary tract, Springfield, Ill., 1962, Charles C Thomas, Publisher.

76. Smith, J. L.: Dermatofibrosarcoma protuberans, Cancer Bull. **23**:46-48, 1971.

77. Snyder, W. H. Jr., Kruse, C. A., Greaney, E. M., and Chaffin, L.: Retroperitoneal tumors in infants and children; A report of 88 cases, Arch. Surg. **63**:26-38, 1951.

78. Soloway, H. B.: Radiation-induced neoplasms following curative therapy for retinoblastoma, Cancer **19**:1984-1988, 1966.

79. Soule, E. H., Mahour, G. H., Mills, S. D., and Lynn, H. B.: Soft tissue sarcomas of infants and children, Mayo Clin. Proc. **43**:313-326, 1968.

80. Speed, K.: Lipoma of the thigh, Arch. Surg. **8**:819-826, 1924.

81. Spittle, M. F., Newton, K. A., and MacKenzie, D. H.: Liposarcoma; a review of 60 cases, Brit. J. Cancer **24**:696-704, 1970.

82. Stehlin, J. S.: Regional chemotherapy for soft tissue sarcomas. In Tumors of bone and soft tissues, presented at the Eighth Annual Clinical Conference on Cancer, 1963, at the University of Texas, M. D. Anderson Hospital and Tumor Institute, Houston, Texas, Chicago, 1965 Year Book Medical Publishers, Inc. p. 368.

83. Stobbe, G. D. and Dargeon, H. W.: Embryonal rhabdomyosarcoma of head and neck in children and adolescents, Cancer **3**:826-836, 1950.

84. Stout, A. P.: Liposarcoma, the malignant tumor of lipoblasts, Ann. Surg. **119**:86-107, 1944.

85. Stout, A. P.: Rhabdomyosarcoma of the skeletal muscle, Ann. Surg. **123**:447-472, 1946.

86. Stout, A. P.: Juvenile fibromatosis, Cancer **7**:953-978, 1954.

87. Stout, A. P.: Sarcomas of the soft tissues, CA **2**:210, 1961.

88. Stout, A. P.: Fibrosarcoma in infants and children, Cancer **15**:1028-1040, 1962.

89. Stout, A. P., and Hill, W. T.: Leiomyosarcoma of the superficial soft tissues, Cancer **11**:844-854, 1958.

90. Suit, H. D.: General discussion. In Tumors of bone and soft tissue, presented at the Eighth Annual Clinical Conference on Cancer at the University of Texas, 1963, M. D. Anderson Hospital and Tumor Institute, Houston, Texas, Chicago, 1965, Year Book Medical Publishers, Inc., p. 422.

91. Sutow, W. W.: Chemotherapeutic management of childhood rhabdomyosarcoma in neoplasia in childhood, presented at the Twelfth Annual Clinical Conference on Cancer, 1967, at the University of Texas, M. D. Anderson Hospital and Tumor Institute, Houston, Texas, Chicago, 1969, Year Book Medical Publishers, Inc., pp. 201-208.

92. Sutow, W. W., Berry, D. H., Haddy, T. B., Sullivan, M. P., Watkins, W. L. and Wind-

miller, J.: Vincristine sulfate therapy in children with metastatic soft tissue sarcoma, Pediatrics 38:465-472, 1966.

93. Sutow, W. W., Sullivan, M. P., Ried, H. L., Taylor, H. G., and Griffith, K. M.: Prognosis in childhood rhabdomyosarcoma, Cancer 25:1384-1390, 1970.

94. Tan, C., and Moore, O.: Chemotherapy for malignant tumors in children. In Conley, J., editor: Cancer of the head and neck, Washington, 1967, Butterworth Publishers. Inc., pp. 477-488.

95. Taylor, H. B., and Helwig, E. B.: Dermatofibrosarcoma protuberans; a study of 115 cases, Cancer 15:717-725, 1962.

96. Virchow, R.: Ein Fall von bösartigen, zum Thiel in der Form des Neuroms auftretenden Fettgeschwülstein, Virchow's Arch. 11:281, 1857.

97. Warren, S., and Sommer, G. N. J., Jr.: Fibrosarcoma of the soft parts, with special reference to recurrence and metastases, Arch. Surg. 33:425-450, 1936.

98. Wells, H. G.: Adipose tissue; a neglected subject, J.A.M.A. 114:2177-2183, 1940.

99. Wilbur, J. R., Sutow, W. W., Sullivan, M. P., Castro, J. R., Kaizer, H., Taylor, H. G.: Successful treatment of inoperable embryonal rhabdomyosarcoma, The American Pediatric Society and the Society for Pediatric Research (ABST), Atlantic City, N. J., April 28 to May 1, 1971.

100. Wilson, D. A.: Tumors of the subcutaneous tissue and fascia with special reference to fibrosarcoma—clinical study, Surg. Gynec. Obstet. 80:500-508, 1945.

101. Yannopoulos, K., and Stout, A. P.: Smooth muscle tumors in children, Cancer 15:958-971, 1962.

CHAPTER 21

Primary malignant tumors of the bone

HERMAN D. SUIT
RICHARD G. MARTIN
WATARU W. SUTOW

Primary bone cancers are relatively more common in children than in adults. The incidence of bone sarcoma was reported to be 0.68% of all malignant lesions in all age groups seen at a large cancer center over a 20-year period.[12] The overall frequency of primary malignant bone tumors among a total of 2248 children under 15 years of age with cancer treated at Memorial Hospital (New York) and at the M. D. Anderson Hospital (Houston) was 13% of all malignancies and 21% of the solid tumors.[21, 79] The United States mortality rates (1960 to 1966) from bone cancer of all types were 2.87 and 11.97 per million for children 0 to 14 years and 15 to 19 years old, respectively.[58] Primary malignant tumors of bone in the pediatric age group fall almost exclusively into two histologic categories: osteogenic sarcoma and Ewing's sarcoma.

DIAGNOSTIC EVALUATION

Diagnostic evaluation of a probable primary bone malignancy in a child should include a complete history and physical examination, thorough radiographic study of the site of the primary lesion (this must include films that are of high technical quality and that show the entire affected part on one film), a complete bone survey (long bones, pelvis, spinal axis, and skull), chest film, and biopsy.

Clinical evaluation. In the history and physical examination, notation should be made of these points: antecedent trauma or infection (osteomyelitis may simulate primary bone sarcoma); duration of symptoms and estimate of tumor growth rate; elevation of body temperature, hemogram, sedimentation rate, alkaline phosphatase, and signs of local inflammation (although these signs are often present in patients with osteomyelitis, they may also be present in patients with primary bone sarcoma); size, pattern of growth, local characteristic of primary lesion, and functional status of affected part; and status of regional lymph nodes. Laboratory biochemical tests have not been too helpful in establishing the diagnosis of primary bone cancer except in multiple myeloma. The characteristic protein changes in the urine and serum can be pathognomonic in myeloma.[14] Elevations in the levels of serum alkaline phosphatase have been associated with osteoid-producing tumors.[44] In neuroblastoma the determination of urinary catecholamine excretion may be helpful.[3] In Ewing's sarcoma the presence of glycogen can be demonstrated histochemically, a finding that may be used to differentiate this tumor from reticulum cell sarcoma.[71]

Radiographic evaluation. Tomographic studies assist in estimating the extent of the lesion, detecting presence of fracture, and evaluating the extent of infiltration of soft tissue by tumor.[22, 23, 53] This type of information is of practical value in planning radiation therapy. Often an arteriogram assists in the evaluation of extension of tumor into adjacent soft tissues. Bone scanning techniques by radioisotopes at the present time have only limited usefulness, primarily in the detection of metastatic lesions.[10] If amputation is being considered, full-chest tomograms are mandatory to examine for presence of small metastases in the lungs. Such lesions in the lungs have been detected in patients who had "normal" chest films.

Biopsy. If after these procedures have been completed the clinical impression remains that the lesion represents a primary sarcoma of bone, biopsy should be performed. Some clinicians have recommended that the involved area as shown radiographically be given 1000 rads (in two fractions of 500 rads, the day before and the day of biopsy). This treatment would be expected to inactivate or kill more than 90% of tumor cells and accordingly should reduce the number of viable tumor cells that might establish metastases or "autotransplants" by bloodstream dissemination during the operative procedure.

Biopsy procedures should be performed in the operating room with the patient under general anesthesia. It should be decided before surgery whether amputation, depending on the diagnosis, would follow immediately after frozen section studies. Before biopsy is attempted, the case should be reviewed by the diagnostic radiologist, the pathologist, the surgeon, and the oncologist so that an adequate and proper sample can be obtained. The incision should be small but sufficient to assure a good specimen. Whenever possible, a portion of the bone should be included in the biopsy specimen. The procedure can be bloody, and careful attention to hemostasis is important, especially if immediate amputation is not contemplated and radiotherapy is planned such as in Ewing's sarcoma. Great care should be taken in closing the biopsy site in layers to promote good healing. Drains and packs should not be used. Aspiration biopsies usually are not adequate for the diagnosis of malignant bone lesions when radical treatment may be required.

DIFFERENTIAL DIAGNOSIS

Histologic confirmation is required to establish any diagnosis of a primary bone cancer. However, the clinical picture, as well as the results of radiologic studies, requires the consideration of a great number of conditions, neoplastic and nonneoplastic, in the differential diagnosis. Histiocytosis X, either as a solitary eosinophilic granuloma of bone or as multiple skeletal lesions, is frequently considered in the differential diagnosis. This condition is discussed separately in Chapter 15.

Nonneoplastic conditions (Fig. 21-1). The nonneoplastic conditions that may simulate bone tumors in children and from which the primary bone cancers must be differentiated include the following:

Osteomyelitis	Hypervitaminosis A and D
Osteitis	Hyperparathyroidism
Bone abscess	Pseudohypoparathyroidism
Infantile cortical hyperostosis	Fibrous dysplasia

Bone infarct	Lipid storage diseases
Ossifying (calcifying) hematoma	Myositis ossificans
Heterotopic ossification	Simple cyst
Giant cell reparative granuloma	Aneurysmal bone cyst
Foreign body reaction	Epidermoid cyst
Exuberant callus	Cartilaginous metaplasia of synovium
Avitaminosis C and D	Cortical defects

Benign neoplastic conditions.* Benign bone neoplasms constitute another group of conditions that must be differentiated from primary bone cancers. The clinical importance of recognizing the benign neoplasms is the avoidance of any

---

*References 8, 15, 31, 42, 51, 53.

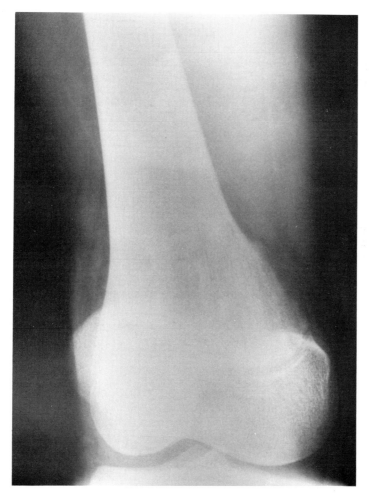

Fig. 21-1. Normal developmental irregularity of the cortex of distal femur in a 13-year-old girl. Such a finding may be misinterpreted as a malignant bone tumor. (Courtesy Medical Communications, The University of Texas at Houston, M. D. Anderson Hospital and Tumor Institute.)

Table 21-1. Benign bone neoplasms

Neoplasm	Predilections	Clinical features	Treatment
Osteocartilaginous exostosis (osteochondroma)	More than half under 20 yr of age; develops in any bone preformed in cartilage; most commonly found in juxtaepiphyseal area in metaphysis of femur, humerus, tibia, ilium, scapula	Most common benign neoplasm of bone; many asymptomatic; history of hard swelling for long period of time; may be solitary or multiple; tumor growth ceases when epiphyses close; solitary lesions become malignant (chondrosarcoma) in less than 1%; multiple (hereditary) osteochondromas undergo malignant transformation (to chondrosarcoma) in over 10%	Surgical extirpation if clinically symptomatic
Enchondroma	About one third under 20 yr of age; develops in bone preformed in cartilage; frequently in hand phalanges, also humerus, femur, feet	Many asymptomatic; slow growing; may be solitary or multiple; pathologic fractures common; solitary lesions occasionally become malignant; multiple enchondromas (Ollier's disease) become malignant in 50% of patients	Curettage or en bloc resection for solitary lesions
Benign chondroblastoma	Rare neoplasm; mostly (60%) in 10- to 20-yr age group; most commonly in epiphyses of femur, tibia, humerus	Persistent local pain of long standing; tumefaction usually absent; no report of malignant change	Thorough curettage
Chondromyxoid fibroma of bone	Rare neoplasm; peak incidence among adolescents and young adults; most commonly involves metaphyses of limb bones of lower extremities	Mild pain; malignant changes reported rarely	Block excision or thorough curettage; no tendency to recur
Osteoma	Rare in infants and children	No malignant changes	Often no treatment required; conservative resection
Osteoid osteoma	More than half under 20 yr of age; lower extremity bones (femur and tibia) most commonly involved, male predilection	Progressively increasing pain; tumor mass usually small	Surgical excision of nidus; recurs if nidus is not completely removed
Benign osteoblastoma (giant osteoid osteoma) (osteogenic fibroma of bone)	Rare neoplasm; half under 20 yr of age; vertebral column most frequently involved	Long-standing back pain; paresthesias or paraplegia from pressure	Conservative local surgical treatment

Table 21-1. Benign bone neoplasms—cont'd

Neoplasm	Predilections	Clinical features	Treatment
Nonosteogenic fibroma of bone (nonossifying fibroma) (metaphyseal fibrous defect)	Almost all in children and young adults; metaphyses of long bones of lower extremities; more common in males	Mostly asymptomatic; pathologic fractures may occur; may develop from fibrous cortical defects	Local curettage or block resection; many undergo spontaneous regression
Hemangioma	All ages; vertebrae and skull involved in 75%; anatomic (symptomless) incidence much higher; female predilection	May be symptomless	Local curettage; laminectomy; irradiation in some instances (e.g., calvarial lesions)
Giant cell tumor of bone (osteoclastoma)	Uncommon under age 20 yr; ends of long bones (femur, tibia, radius) most frequent sites	Solitary; may be asymptomatic for long time; potentially aggressive or malignant in about 10%	Curettage; radical surgery in some; irradiation for surgically inaccessible sites; relationship suggested between irradiation and subsequent sarcomatous changes
Neural tumors Neurilemoma (rare) Glomus tumor (rare) Solitary neurofibroma (rare) Neurofibromatosis of Recklinghausen	May involve bone by propinquity and local pressure or by growth on or in bone		Resection or curettage

erroneous institution of radical treatment required for malignant tumors. The benign neoplasms have been listed in Table 21-1 which gives the apparent incidence in the pediatric age group, some of the clinical features, and the treatment generally used for each condition.

Metastatic cancer. The cancers in children that originate primarily in other parts of the body and only secondarily metastasize to or involve the bone include the following:

Neuroblastoma
Rhabdomyosarcoma
Retinoblastoma
Wilms' tumor

Thyroid cancer
Leukemia
Hodgkin's disease
Malignant lymphoma

Table 21-2. Uncommon primary malignant bone tumors in children

Malignant neoplasm	Frequency in children	Clinical features	Treatment and prognosis
Myeloma[14]	Rare before age 50; almost never occurs in children; M:F ratio about 2.5:1	Bone marrow containing bones involved; pathologic fractures common; protein and hematologic disturbances characteristic	Radiotherapy if localized; chemotherapy if systemic; less than 10% with multiple lesions survive 5 yr
Reticulum cell sarcoma[15, 30, 41, 51, 60, 89]	Uncommon in children; less than 10% of all cases occur under age 20 yr; M:F ratio about 3:2	Femur, tibia, humerus, skull and facial bones, rib, scapula, vertebrae most commonly involved	Generally radiotherapy; amputation in radiotherapy failures or complicated cases; 5-yr survival rate from 33% to 50%
Chondrosarcoma[15, 51, 56, 62]	Rare in children; less than 5% of all cases; M:F ratio about 2:1	Predilection for bones of trunk, shoulder, pelvis, and upper ends of femur and humerus; generally slow growing and metastases occur late; secondary chondrosarcomas occur in enchondromas, juxtacortical chondromas, and cartilage caps of hereditary multiple exostoses	Radical surgery; 5-yr survival rate of 30% to 50%
Malignant giant cell tumor[15, 18, 39, 51]	Probably does not occur in children	Predilection for epiphyses of long bones about the knee; often follows treatment (radiotherapy) for benign giant cell tumor	Radical surgery; prognosis varies with location and type of sarcoma present
Adamantinoma (malignant angioblastoma)[9, 15]	Rare, tumor at all ages; up to one-third occur in older children and adolescents	Tibia most frequently affected; slow-growing tumor; tends to recur locally and eventually metastasize	Amputation; more than one third survive 5 yr
Fibrosarcoma[19, 26, 43]	About 20% of all patients under age 20	Femur, tibia, innominate, maxilla, sacrum most commonly involved; many have preexisting bone disease or previous irradiation	Amputation; 5-yr survival rate 25% to 30%
Desmoplastic fibroma[15, 42]	Extremely rare at any age; majority occur before age 20	Long tubular bones affected most commonly; cells lack nuclear anaplasia and mitotic activity, but tumor is locally infiltrative	Complete resection
Chordoma[15, 34, 49]	Very rare under age 20; M:F ratio 2:1	Characteristically occurs in midline of body; spheno-occipital and sacrococcygeal regions and vertebrae most commonly involved; develops from remnants of notocord; slow growing; rarely metastasizes but is invasive locally	Radical excision Radiotherapy after incomplete resection Palliative radiotherapy for inoperative cases Prognosis grave, but duration of survival may be long

Table 21-2. Uncommon primary malignant bone tumors in children—cont'd

Malignant neoplasm	Frequency in children	Clinical features	Treatment and prognosis
Hemangiosarcoma (angiosarcoma; angioendothelioma; hemangioendothelioma)[6, 51]	Extremely rare at all ages		Amputation; cures reported
Liposarcoma[72, 76]	Extremely rare at any age		Amputation probably

In most cases the clinical findings in the patient will establish the diagnosis of primary source. The carcinomas that frequently spread to the bones in the adult, such as those originating in the breast, lung, prostate, testis, kidney, gastrointestinal tract, cervix, and uterus, are extremely rare or practically nonexistent in children.[13]

Primary malignant bone tumors. Osteogenic sarcoma and Ewing's sarcoma, the two most frequent types of primary bone cancer in children, are discussed in separate sections of this chapter. Table 21-2 lists the other less common primary malignant bone tumors that may develop occasionally in children. The relative incidence in the young age group, sex and site predilections, some of the clinical features, treatments most frequently used, and reported prognosis have been tabulated for each tumor.

EWING'S SARCOMA

In 1921 Ewing described a small-celled malignant tumor of bone that he considered to be distinct from the previously recognized types of primary bone tumors.[25a] Although there has been considerable discussion regarding its pathogenesis, the tumor is known as a clinical entity and bears Ewing's name.

Clinical and diagnostic features

Ewing's sarcoma (Ewing's tumor, diffuse endothelioma of bone, endothelial myeloma, endothelial sarcoma) is accepted as being a primary sarcoma of nonosseous origin involving bone. Histologically the tumor is highly anaplastic; it is composed of solidly packed, uniform, small round cells. There is virtually no stroma, and presence of lymphocytes is uncommon (Fig. 21-2). In most cases special histochemical stains will demonstrate presence of glycogen in tumor cells.[71] No chondroid or osteoid matrix is produced. This tumor occurs mostly in children, adolescents, and young adults; 90% of the patients are under 30 years of age, and 70% are under 20 years of age.[15, 17, 27] The primary lesion arises in the trunk bones or bones of the extremities in the majority of cases. The most frequently involved bones are femur, innominate, rib, tibia, humerus, vertebra, fibula, and scapula.[15, 27] Ewing's sarcoma occurs more frequently in males than in females, with the M:F ratio approximating 1.6.[15, 17, 27]

The roentgenographic features are frequently difficult to differentiate from conditions such as osteomyelitis, reticulum cell sarcoma, and other bone tumors.

The roentgenograms may show a single ill-defined lesion or patchy, multiple, permeative, destructive lesions. Lamellated periosteal reaction may occur sometimes, producing the so-called "onion-peel" or "onionskin" appearance. No tumor ossification occurs in the soft tissue masses associated with Ewing's sarcoma[23, 53] (Fig. 21-3).

From 14% to 28% of these patients have apparent metastases at the time of diagnosis.[2, 90] In most of the remainder, rapid and extensive hematogenous spread of the tumor develops within 12 months. Multiple other bones (especially the skull) and the lungs most commonly are the initial metastatic sites. Metastases may be found also in lymph nodes, liver, spleen, heart, kidney, pancreas, and thyroid.

Prognosis for survival among patients with Ewing's sarcoma has been extremely poor. In a large series involving 210 patients treated at Mayo Clinic, the 5-year survival rate was 15% and the 10-year survival rate 10%.[15] Data from a composite series of 987 cases accumulated from the published literature indicated a 5-year survival rate of 8%.[28] Phillips and Higinbotham[63] reported that among 54 patients with Ewing's sarcoma, all of whom were under 19 years of age, the 5-year survival incidence was 24%.

Treatment

The primary treatment for all patients with Ewing's sarcoma should be radical dose radiation therapy combined with an intensive course of chemotherapy.[4, 45, 47] There are two basic problems in the management of these patients:

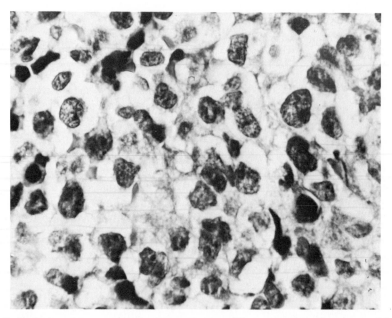

Fig. 21-2. Ewing's sarcoma, microscopic appearance. The paramount features in this tumor are round to oval regular nuclei with occasional inconspicuous nucleoli and coarse chromatin granules (×460).

(1) destruction of the primary lesion with preservation of useful function of the affected part and (2) killing or at least markedly delaying the growth of any subclinical metastatic deposits by the action of the chemotherapy. Thus these two modalities must be integrated on a thoughtful basis to maximize the contribution of each. The primary lesion must be controlled if there is any expectation of cure. Unfortunately, only about 10% of the patients remain free of metastatic tumor if only the primary tumor is treated. Accordingly, serious effort must be directed toward the secondary disease. In this section a description of the treatment policy at the M. D. Anderson Hospital will be given.

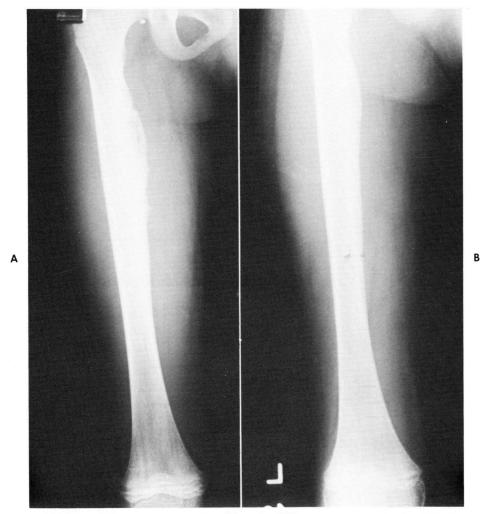

Fig. 21-3. A, Roentgenographic appearance of Ewing's sarcoma involving the distal left femur of an 8-year-old girl. **B,** Appearance of primary lesion 13 months later after radiotherapy (6775 rads tumor dose) and adjuvant chemotherapy. Patient was free of disease 25 months after diagnosis. (Courtesy Medical Communications, The University of Texas at Houston, M. D. Anderson Hospital and Tumor Institute.)

Radiation therapy for the primary lesion. Radiation therapy is almost invariably successful in achieving prompt relief of symptoms, regression of mass of tumor, and improvement of radiographic appearance of the lesion. This can be done with doses from 4000 to 5000 rads. However, the attempt to achieve permanent control or destruction of tumor demands high radiation doses and an elaborate treatment plan.

Effective radiation therapy depends on achieving the following goals:

1. Administration of 4500 rads in 4½ weeks to the entirety of the affected bone, that is, treatment of the entirety of the primary lesion and any intramedullary spread of disease. The treatment fields for those portions not affected by gross disease need cover only the bone and a minimum of normal tissue adjacent to the bone. At the local site of the clinically and radiographically evident primary lesion, fields should be generous, with coverage of all soft tissues likely to be infiltrated by tumor. This means that the fields must be specially shaped and not be simple square or rectangular areas.

2. The second part of treatment should consist of an additional 2000 rads in 2 to 2½ weeks given only to the radiographically evident area of involvement. This is determined by review of plain, tomographic, and soft tissue radiographic studies. The final 1000 rads should be given through conservatively drawn fields. This plan yields a total dose of 6500 rads in 6½ to 7 weeks to the obvious lesion and 4500 rads in 4½ weeks to any intramedullary extension of tumor. Such a schedule provides a high dose to those tissues with the largest number of tumor cells and a moderate dose to tissues containing subclinical extensions of tumor.

3. This treatment should be administered using a cobalt[60] or comparable unit.

4. A narrow (1 cm) strip of bolus (four layers of petrolatum gauze is satisfactory) should be placed over the biopsy scar to give full dose to the scar.

5. In almost all instances the technique should require at least two fields, and each field should be treated each day.

6. Portal localization films are essential.

7. To assure a reproducible setup technique, special immobilization devices should be employed. As a minimum, level points on each field should be used in patient positioning. Since the treatment volume must be large, special effort is expended in design of fields so that only those tissues that are considered to have a reasonable likelihood of being involved are treated.

There are several additional clinical factors to consider in planning treatment. To maximize the return and preservation of function, a program of active (not passive) exercise of all affected joints should be implemented with the start of therapy. Each case should be reviewed with an orthopedic surgeon and a plan for exercise and weight bearing developed. For treatment of lesions in the lower extremities, male patients should be advised to wear loose-fitting trousers. If the ilium is to be treated, girls should wear loose-fitting dresses (no belts), and boys should wear suspenders or a loose belt to avoid a severe reaction along the belt line. Clothing should be modified to reduce chronic irritation of irradiated tissue during treatment and until the acute reaction has subsided. By doing this, an excessive acute reaction may be avoided and severity of late reaction diminished. Another consideration in treatment of a lesion is the upper thigh; do not employ a technique that treats the skin and subcutaneous tissue over the inner aspect of the thigh to full dose, that is avoid the exaggerated skin reaction produced by the rubbing together of the inner aspects of the thighs during walking. Finally, the general rule in radiation therapy that all fields should be kept clean and dry should be strictly followed.

Radiation dose levels recommended here are high, and successful use of such doses requires that extra time be employed in shaping fields to the particular situations, use of high-energy machines, and treatment of all fields each day. Based on data available, there is no established dose-response relationship. At a dose level of 5000 rads delivered over a total time of about 5 weeks, approximately 25% of 29 patients treated similarly in several institutions developed regrowth of tumor.[35] The frequency of local control almost certainly depends on radiation dose. However, assessment of frequency of local control is not easy because many patients die from metastatic lesions before local recurrence is seen. Relevant to this is the fact that during the period that the patient is being managed for gross metastatic disease, attention of the clinician and the patient is directed to this problem; therefore continued observation (clinical and radiographic) of the primary site is often overlooked.

Assessment of successful control of the primary tumor may be overestimated. In a report of results of treatment of Ewing's sarcoma from this institution in 1965,[77] the necessity for high doses to achieve permanent local control was established. This policy has been followed over the last 6 to 7 years. During this period, even with high-dose levels ($\geq$ 6000 rads), local regrowth of tumor occurred in some patients. D'Angio[20] usually administers a dose in excess of 6000 rads; he has seen local failures at 6000 rads but not at 7000 rads. These tumors cannot be categorized as radiosensitive and easily controlled. Aggressive radiation therapy is required if good results are to be obtained consistently.

Chemotherapy. At the M. D. Anderson Hospital vincristine and cyclophosphamide have been administered according to the schedule shown in Fig. 21-4. This adjuvant regimen is tolerated, but the treatment required close medical supervision. In particular, the WBC count must be monitored closely during each cycle of cyclophosphamide so that the drug may be stopped early if indicated. This protocol can be used for the treatment of most patients.

There are situations in which a modification is necessary because of the location of the tumor. Tumors of the pubic ramus (probably also tumors of the ischium or of the lower part of the ilium) will have to be treated in fields that unavoidably include the urinary bladder (Fig. 21-5). Cyclophosphamide has a potent toxic effect on bladder mucosa. For this group of patients cyclophosphamide therapy should be delayed until about 6 weeks after radiation therapy, or another chemotherapeutic agent (e.g., chlorambucil) should be employed. If cyclophosphamide is used at any time during or after irradiation of the urinary bladder, a vigorous effort must be made to effect a high fluid intake with frequent evacuation of bladder contents, particularly for several hours after the drug is taken. Irradiation of lesions in the ilium, pubis, sacrum, or lumbar spine will include a large portion of the intestinal tract in the treatment fields. Because of the toxic effect of radiation, vincristine, and cyclophosphamide on the intestinal mucosa, chemotherapy should be withheld for about 6 weeks after completion of the radiation therapy. In other situations the radiation dose per fraction may have to be reduced and the total treatment time accordingly prolonged. For example, if the mucous membrane reaction is excessively severe in

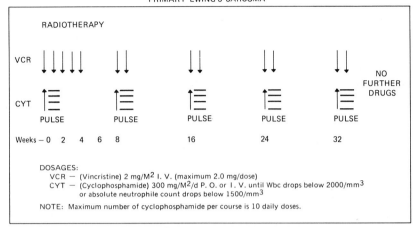

CHEMOTHERAPY SCHEDULE
PRIMARY EWING'S SARCOMA

RADIOTHERAPY

VCR

CYT

PULSE   PULSE   PULSE   PULSE   PULSE

NO
FURTHER
DRUGS

Weeks — 0   2   4   6   8   16   24   32

DOSAGES:
VCR — (Vincristine) 2 mg/M^2 I. V. (maximum 2.0 mg/dose)
CYT — (Cyclophosphamide) 300 mg/M^2/d P. O. or I. V. until Wbc drops below 2000/mm^3
or absolute neutrophile count drops below 1500/mm^3
NOTE: Maximum number of cyclophosphamide per course is 10 daily doses.

Fig. 21-4. Schema of adjuvant chemotherapy regimen for primary treatment of patients with Ewing's sarcoma. (Courtesy Medical Communications, The University of Texas at Houston, M. D. Anderson Hospital and Tumor Institute.)

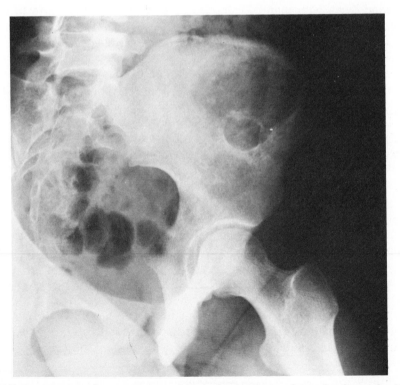

Fig. 21-5. Roentgenographic appearance of Ewing's sarcoma involving the ilium of a 14-year-old girl. Patient was free of disease after radiotherapy (6500 rads tumor dose) and adjuvant chemotherapy (as outlined in text) more than 2 years from diagnosis. (Courtesy Medical Communications, The University of Texas at Houston, M. D. Anderson Hospital and Tumor Institute.)

the treatment of a lesion of the mandible or maxilla, the therapy may have to be interrupted or the dose per fraction decreased. In general, the planned treatment should be administered unless there are strong indications for reducing total dose or lengthening total time. This plan for combining radiation therapy and chemotherapy must be read as a description of the current treatment program, which will be continually altered and hopefully improved.

Results at the M. D. Anderson Hospital. Treatment of patients at the M. D. Anderson Hospital appears to be more effective now that high-dose radiation therapy is being combined with vincristine and cyclophosphamide. This is evident by comparison of median times between initial treatment and the detection of the first metastasis in the 12 patients who received this combined treatment and the 34 "control" patients who were treated by radiation alone or combined with a single chemotherapeutic agent. This makes a total of 46 patients who received treatment for lesions of tubular or flat bones or the vertebral bodies at the time when there was no clinical or radiographic evidence of metastatic disease. The control group of 34 patients is comprised of 25 patients who were treated by radiation therapy alone (Group I) and of 9 patients treated by irradiation plus one of a variety of chemotherapeutic agents (Group II). Two of the patients in Group I are alive and free of disease at 7 and 10 years after radiation therapy alone for lesions in the humerus. The median time for appearance of metastasis in patients in Groups I and II was 8 months, with a range of 1 to 40 months. Of the 32 patients in Groups I and II who have developed distant metastasis, 28 of the 32, or 87%, did so by the fifteenth month after treatment. These results contrast sharply with the experience in the group of 12 patients who were treated by radiation therapy and a combination of vincristine and cyclophosphamide (2 of the patients also received actinomycin D). Metastatic tumor has appeared in 3 of these 12 children. The time of detection of first metastasis in these 3 patients has been 15, 18, and 33 months. The other 9 patients were alive without evidence of disease at 6, 8, 9, 11, 16, 22 (2), and 34 (2) months. Therefore 5 of the patients were apparently free of tumor after more than 15 months. These results demonstrate a definite effect of this multimodal therapy in prolonging the disease-free interval. Control of the primary tumor has been good in this group: one local regrowth appeared at 42 months after treatment of a lesion in the humerus.

Two other patients with tumors of the maxilla have been treated. The first patient received radiation therapy and amethopterin and then had surgery (specimen was negative). The second patient was referred to our institution after incomplete surgery followed by several doses of cyclophosphamide. He was treated by radiation therapy alone. These two patients are alive and well at 8 and 15 years after treatment. In addition, 3 patients with Ewing's sarcoma of the mandible have been seen. One of these is only 9 months after treatment (6000 rads combined with cyclophosphamide and vincristine). The other 2 patients developed local recurrence at 6 and at 27 months after 4000 rads and 5000 rads, respectively; no chemotherapy was given to those patients at the time of their primary therapy.

Metastatic disease. The treatment of patients with a single focus of metastatic disease should be almost as radical as treatment of the primary tumor. For the second or subsequent lesion, a less aggressive course is planned both in terms of total dose and time for treatment. Management of patients with metastatic Ewing's sarcoma should be conducted on the basis that prolonged survival may be achieved by prudent and aggressive combination of radiation therapy and chemotherapeutic agents. Accordingly, for lesions in other bone or soft tissue careful treatment planning and a dose level of $\geq$ 6000 rads in 6 weeks are essential to strive for long-term control of the disease.

The full length of the affected bone need not be included in the treatment field in every instance. For example, a metastatic lesion in the upper end of femur could be treated by fields that provided a margin of 10 cm beyond bone change as determined radiographically. Thus radiation therapy for metastasis to other bone should be administered through rather less generous fields than are used in treatment of the primary lesion, and the dose level should be at least 6000 rads in 6 weeks. If metastasis to bone is detected after metastasis has been detected at other sites (lung, bone, brain, etc.), the dose level is lower (e.g., about 4000 rads in 3 weeks).

The other common site of metastasis is the lung. Here the dose must be lower; even so, marked regression of the small lesions in the lung is often achieved. Our practice has been to administer 2000 rads in 3 weeks (fifteen doses of 135 rads, with an allowance for decreased absorption by the lung, or approximately 1700 rads for 3 weeks if no such allowance is made) to the entirety of both lung fields. During this 3 weeks an additional 1000 rads (200 rads × 5) may be given to the major tumor mass or perhaps cluster of nodules. This yields a dose of 3000 rads in 3 weeks to the main tumor mass; supplemental field(s) should not cover more than 25% of the area of the lung field. A higher dose level to the whole lung field may be followed by a severely symptomatic or even fatal radiation pneumonitis. In almost all instances, palliative radiation therapy will be given in conjunction with some form of chemotherapy, and consideration must be given to the possible enhancement of radiation effect.

Treatment of lesions at other sites is planned on a knowledge of the normal tissue tolerance. This must never be based on the assumption that the patient will not survive long enough to develop a complication. If the patient arrives at a preterminal state and symptomatic lesions require radiation therapy, the treatment plan must consider all the pertinent clinical details of the individual case. As an example, a painful lesion in bone may be relieved for a reasonable period of time by administering 400 rads per fraction for a total of 1600 to 2000 rads. An acceptable response is considered as either regression or cessation of growth. Because of the extensive calcified stroma in some lesions, regression will be slight, regardless of the effect of the treatment on the tumor cell population.

Rarely can surgical excision of pulmonary metastases be accomplished because the nodules are usually multiple. Palliative amputation may become necessary if symptomatic recurrence develops, irrespective of the presence or absence of pulmonary spread. Recurrence in the treated area without other evidence of spread is an indication for amputation. The site of amputation must be proximal to the irradiated field to avoid problems in wound healing.

Chemotherapy is resumed immediately when metastases develop. If the child had been receiving adjunctive chemotherapy, a change in the drug regimen is considered. If the patient has not had any previous chemotherapy, the combination of vincristine, actinomycin D, and cyclophosphamide would appear to be the treatment of choice. If palliative radiotherapy is being given, then the dose and timing of cyclophosphamide administration in the combination will vary with the amount and extent of the radiation. Varying degrees of regression of metastatic Ewing's sarcoma have been produced by vincristine,[73] actinomycin D,[74] and cyclophosphamide[80] used singly and in combination.[48] Temporary responses have been achieved after the use of such drugs as daunomycin,[82] adriamycin,[91] 5-fluorouracil,[52] BCNU,[40] and uracil mustard.[82]

Perspectives

Hustu and co-workers[36, 37] have reported that 3 of 5 patients treated by irradiation and systemic chemotherapy did unexpectedly well, with no evidence of disease at 32, 50, and 58 months. The adjuvant chemotherapy consisted of the administration of cyclophosphamide and vincristine alternately each week for 1 year. Johnson and associates[48, 55] also have indicated that the preliminary results of treatment combining radiotherapy with chemotherapy show an encouraging prolongation of the disease-free interval. Cyclophosphamide, vincristine, and actinomycin D were used. Intrathecal methotrexate and whole brain irradiation have been added to the treatment program in an effort to control further the potential sites of metastatic spread.[65]

Another approach aimed at the destruction of microscopic foci of metastatic disease that has been employed is elective whole body irradiation in combination with radiotherapy of the primary lesion.[46, 57] At Toronto, 300 rads whole body irradiation has been given as a single dose. Early results suggested a slightly better survival curve and a higher rate of subsequent solitary (instead of multiple) lung metastases among patients so studied.[46]

Some of the experiences described in the literature would appear to justify the employment of a radiation dose to the primary site of about 5000 rads. The good results reported by Phillips and Higinbotham[63] by using 3500 to 4000 rads and one of a variety of adjuvant drugs were not repeated here. Slightly less conservatively, Phillips and Sheline[64] conclude that doses in the range of 5500 rads to 6000 rads in 6 to 7 weeks "appear to be adequate." The basis for our recommendation that the dose be 6500 rads in 6½ weeks is that at lower doses recurrences have often been observed and that local regrowth of tumor is a very poor prognostic sign.

The preliminary reports from our studies are interesting. Clearly much additional data have to become available before the real impact of the combined therapy on survival rates can be defined. At this writing, there appear to be generous grounds for encouragement of further work along these lines. The treatment program just described was initiated prior to the recent interest in actinomycin D for the chemotherapy of this tumor.[48, 74] Since cyclophosphamide, vincristine, and actinomycin D have different modes of action, their combined use might exhibit additive antineoplastic activity if the potential bone marrow toxicity can be kept within clinically tolerable limits.

OSTEOGENIC SARCOMA

Osteogenic sarcoma (osteosarcoma) presumably arises from bone-forming mesenchyme and is characterized by the production of malignant osteoid by the sarcomatous stroma.

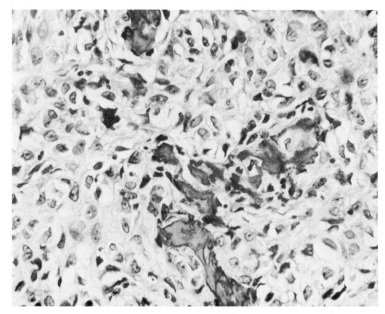

Fig. 21-6. Osteogenic sarcoma, microscopic appearance. Note the moderately pleomorphic spindle cell tumor with production of poorly calcified osteoid (×225). (Courtesy Medical Communications, The University of Texas at Houston, M. D. Anderson Hospital and Tumor Institute.)

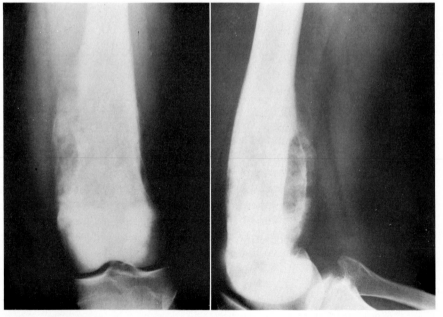

Fig. 21-7. Roentgenographic appearance of osteogenic sarcoma of the distal femur in a 15-year-old girl. (Courtesy Medical Communications, The University of Texas at Houston, M. D. Anderson Hospital and Tumor Institute.)

Multiple sections of the tumor may present histologically different patterns, and the tumor has been subclassified into osteoblastic, chondroblastic, and fibroblastic types[1, 15, 16] (Fig. 21-6).

When all cases are considered, osteogenic sarcoma occurs more frequently in the younger age group (peak range of 10 to 25 years of age), shows a definite male preponderance (M:F ratio around 1.6), and commonly involves extremity bones, especially of the lower extremity.[15, 16, 31] Of 145 patients under 21 years of age with lesions of the extremity long bones in one reported series, 99 were 15 years of age or younger, and 31 were under 10 years of age. The youngest children were 3 years old.[54] In another report from a different institution the records on 129 children less than 16 years of age with osteogenic sarcoma were reviewed. Of this group, 30 (23%) were 10 years of age or younger.[33]

In osteogenic sarcoma the roentgenograms show variable degrees of osteoblastic and osteolytic bone changes. Periosteal response is irregular and interrupted and may show "sunburst" spiculation. Significantly, tumor bone is produced in the parosseous soft tissue components[23, 53] (Fig. 21-7).

Predisposing factors

The conditions that may predispose to the development of osteogenic sarcoma include Paget's disease, giant cell tumor, fibrous dysplasia, osteochondroma, and irradiation.

Although about 0.2% of the patients with Paget's disease (osteitis deformans) will develop sarcomas,[67] this disease does not occur in children. Malignant degeneration of chondromas and exostoses, when it occurs, would appear to be more commonly in the direction of chondrosarcoma.[15] Occasionally, however, osteogenic sarcoma has been reported in solitary enchondroma,[69] multiple enchondromas (Ollier's disease),[5] and osteocartilaginous exostosis.[16, 56] In general, the long natural history of the benign lesions is such that almost invariably the patients are adults by the time the malignant changes are established.

With extremely rare exceptions, giant cell tumors, benign or malignant, do not appear until after epiphyseal closure[18, 39] Fibrous dysplasia has also been associated with the later development of osteogenic sarcoma.[61] Osteogenic sarcoma has been observed in patients 4 to 30 years after bones have received high doses of ionizing irradiation.[56, 68, 75]

Clinical course

In uncontrolled cases osteogenic sarcoma metastasizes principally to the lungs, usually within 6 to 9 months from time of amputation. Metastatic growth is rapid, the lesions increasing in number and size. In advanced disease extensive hematogenous seeding becomes apparent. Other bones may be affected, as well as other organs. Lymph node involvement is uncommon.

Treatment

There appears to be no new treatment method for this group of patients that seems certain to represent a major advance. For lesions appearing in an extremity, two approaches have been used in the treatment of patients who have no clinical evidence of metastatic tumor: immediate amputation or administration of 6000 to 8000 rads over 6 to 9 weeks and amputation 6 to 9 months later, provided metastatic disease is still not detectable. When amputation is indicated, it is done only after a positive diagnosis by biopsy. The entire bone involved is removed; therefore the amputation site is usually above the adjoining joint, above-the-knee amputation for tibia lesions and a hip disarticulation for femur lesions. Lesions of the ilium require hemipelvectomy. Usually a forequarter amputation is needed for tumors of the proximal humerus and the head of the humerus. Whenever possible, an immediate fitting of a prosthetic device is recommended at the time of surgery. However, this is generally done only in cases in which an above-the-knee or an above-the-elbow amputation has been performed. A cast is applied to the stump immediately after the surgery in the operating room, and then a temporary pylon prosthetic device is fitted so that the patient may stand weight bearing within 24 hours. Not only is this a great psychologic boost for the patient, but also the cast prevents swelling and promotes more rapid healing of the stump. Without the swelling the stump is less painful, and this results in a marked reduction in the amount of narcotics necessary to control pain. When immediate fitting devices are used, the patient does not have to be immobilized because of the amputation. Although metastatic lesions usually develop within 6 months to 1½ years after primary surgery, the use of a prosthetic device is urged even for these short periods of time. It aids greatly in the patient's psychologic rehabilitation and facilitates his ability to move around and take care of himself.

Since 1931, Cade[7] has advocated preoperative radiotherapy followed 6 to 9 months later by elective amputation. Such a treatment program would avoid "futile mutilation" in cases in which the development of metastatic disease presages an early death. Others in whom radical ablation of the limb would be withheld include those with "exceptionally good response (to radiotherapy) with good function and no disability." Lee and MacKenzie[50] have reported that, using this approach, the 5-year survival in 92 patients was 21%. Poppe[66] reported 14% 5-year survival among 127 patients. Sweetnam,[84] however, has pointed out that local control is not always achieved by the radiation doses given; thus tumor dissemination definitely remains possible, and the pain and morbidity from local disease before death may be worse than the advantages of limb preservation. In our opinion, this approach is a reasonable alternative to immediate amputation, provided that the primary lesion is not large ($<$ 10 cm in diameter) and that there is reasonable likelihood of obtaining a moderately good functional result. Massive lesions should be treated by amputation.

For lesions located at certain sites in the pelvis, vertebral column, or skull, surgery is not technically feasible. For those situations radical dose radiation therapy should be employed, using a dose of $\geq$ 7000 rads if possible.

Chemotherapy. It has been the general experience that osteogenic sarcoma is resistant to currently available (1972) chemotherapeutic regimens. Therefore the use of drugs as an adjuvant to definitive surgical treatment in patients without any evidence of metastatic disease must be considered an investigative approach at the present time. The administration of melphalan for such adjuvant therapy has not been significantly effective.[81]

Metastatic disease. The treatment program for the child with metastatic osteogenic sarcoma should be directed toward two objectives: first, the symptomatic management of clinical sequelae of progressively growing and spreading tumor masses, and second, the continuing efforts, within reason, to decelerate the growth rate of the cancer, to induce regression of tumor if possible, and to excise surgically the metastatic lesions when indicated.

Among the symptoms that become increasingly more difficult to palliate as the disease progresses are pain, cough, and dyspnea. Neurosurgical blocks or interruption of pain pathways may afford temporary or long-term relief of intractable pain. Careful, sympathetic, and even expectant attention must be paid to a number of complications such as hemothorax, bedsores, infection of open tumor masses, and disuse atrophy of muscles of unaffected body parts. In addition to these medical demands, the morale and attitudes of the patient and the family constellation require full professional support.

Surgical excision of a solitary pulmonary metastasis or even multiple nodules situated in a strategically accessible area is a practical approach, particularly if the number of metastatic lesions has not increased over a period of 2 months or so.[59, 85] The possibility of performing palliative amputation of a second limb should not be peremptorily dismissed as inhumane. If the pattern of metastatic disease is such that early death cannot be anticipated, the patient will face a period of inevitable and prolonged suffering with a useless and incapacitating limb. Removal of such an extremity can provide immediate relief of pain and unfetter the patient.

Radiation treatment of metastatic lesions only occasionally achieves any prolonged control, although short-lived regressions may be observed. The treatment plan for pulmonary lesions is very much the same as that described for Ewing's sarcoma. For metastasis to other bone or to soft tissue, palliation may be attempted if the lesion is not massive, but the dose should be at least 6000 rads in 6 weeks. Likelihood of success in this type of palliation decreases rapidly with increasing size of the lesion. Massive lesions (e.g., $\geq$ 12 cm in diameter) probably should not be treated. Attempts at palliation of lesions at other sites are occasionally justified.

Although chemotherapy has not produced meaningful regression of metastatic lesions in most patients,[25, 82, 83] marked and significant responses have been documented occasionally after treatment with melphalan,[78, 81] Mitomycin C,[24] 5-fluorouracil,[88] high doses of cyclophosphamide,[29] and adriamycin.[13a] Recently, the use of massive doses of methotrexate in conjunction with citrovorum factor "rescue" has produced some significant regression of pulmonary metastases from osteogenic sarcoma.[*] These sporadic beneficial results justify the use of carefully planned chemotherapy trials in a positive effort to help the patients with metastatic disease.

Prognosis

A review of published reports from single institutions provides a basis for evaluation of prognosis in children with osteogenic sarcoma. The Mayo Clinic data indicate a 5-year survival rate of 20% for 408 patients of all ages and a 10-year survival rate of 17%.[15] In an earlier publication[33] the Mayo Clinic ex-

---

[*]Jaffe, N.: Recent advances in the chemotherapy of metastatic osteogenic sarcoma, Cancer 30:1627-1631, 1972.

perience with osteogenic sarcoma in 126 children under 16 years of age demonstrated a 5-year survival rate of 22% and a 10-year survival rate of 19%.

The Memorial Hospital report covering 145 patients under the age of 21 years with operable tumors in the long bones showed a 5-year survival rate of 17%.[54] In this study no age or sex difference in survival was noted. The 5-year survival rate also appeared to be the same in the different age subgroups and for varying primary sites. A trend was noted for the pulmonary metastases to appear earlier in those 10 years of age or younger as compared to older children. In the same institution the 5-year survival rate for osteogenic sarcoma for all ages and all primary sites, which included the group just mentioned under 21 years of age, was 13% of 258 patients.[56]

Variants

Ossifying parosteal sarcoma (juxtacortical osteogenic sarcoma, parosteal osteogenic sarcoma, parosteal osteoma) represents an uncommon (4% of all cases of osteogenic sarcoma), slow-growing variant of osteogenic sarcoma with an exceedingly good prognosis.[11, 32, 70, 87] The lesion originates in the parosteal or periosteal tissues and spreads along and encircles the shaft of bone. It is broadly attached to but generally does not invade the cortex of the underlying bone.

About 20% of patients with this tumor variant are under 20 years of age. The male:female ratio is about 2:3. The metaphyseal region of femur (distal), humerus, or tibia is generally involved. The treatment is amputation; recurrence with increased malignancy has been reported after local excision.[11] Long-term survivals can be expected in 70% to 80% of cases.[11, 32, 70, 87]

The designation *primitive multipotential primary sarcoma of bone* has been applied recently to a group of tumors, each of which was characterized histopathologically by the presence of more than one major type of sarcoma (e.g., mixture of Ewing's sarcoma, chondrosarcoma, and osteogenic sarcoma).[38] In addition to the basic pattern, varying degrees of differentiation occurred in different combination along a number of histologic lines, including vascular, osteoid, chondroid, adamantine, plasmacytoid, and squamous. In several cases the patterns mimicked metastatic adenocarcinoma or neuroblastoma or reticulum cell sarcoma. More than half the cases occurred in patients under 20 years of age. Long tubular bones as well as short or flat bones that included those of the face were involved. The survival rate in this group of patients was approximately 20%.

Multicentric osteogenic sarcoma has been described.[74a] In these cases, which are extremely rare, multiple primary osteogenic sarcomas originate independently in various areas of the skeleton. *Extraosseous osteogenic sarcoma* of soft tissues or viscera has also been reported.[28a]

REFERENCES

1. Ackerman, L. V., and Spjut, H. J.: Tumors of bone and cartilage. In Atlas of tumor pathology, Section II, Fascicle 4, Washington, D. C., 1962, Armed Forces Institute of Pathology.
2. Bhansali, S. K., and Desai, P. B.: Ewing's sarcoma. Observations on 107 cases, J. Bone Joint Surg. 45-A:541-553, 1963.
3. Bohoun, C.: Catecholamine metabolism in neuroblastoma, J. Pediatr. Surg. 3:114-118, 1968.

4. Boyer, C. W., Jr., Brickner, T. J., Jr., and Perry, R. H.: Ewing's sarcoma. Case against surgery, Cancer **20**:1602-1606, 1967.
5. Braddock, G. T. F., and Hadlow, V. D.: Osteosarcoma in enchondromatosis (Ollier's disease). Report of a case, J. Bone Joint Surg. **48-B**:145-149, 1966.
6. Bundens, W. D., Jr., and Brighton, C. T.: Malignant hemangioendothelioma of bone. Report of two cases and review of the literature, J. Bone Joint Surg. **47-A**:762-772, 1965.
7. Cade, S.: Osteogenic sarcoma. A study based on 113 patients, J. Roy. Coll. Surg. Edinb. **1**:79-111, Dec., 1955.
8. Caffey, J.: Pediatric x-ray diagnosis, ed. 4, Chicago, 1961, Year Book Medical Publishers, Inc.
9. Changus, G. W., Speed, J. S., and Stewart, F. W.: Malignant angioblastoma of bone. A reappraisal of adamantinoma of long bone, Cancer **10**:540-559, 1957.
10. Charkes, N. B.: Bone scanning: principles, techniques and interpretation, Radiol. Clin. North Am. **8**:259-270, 1970.
11. Copeland, M. M.: Parosteal osteoma: differential diagnosis and treatment. In Tumors of bone and soft tissue, Chicago, 1965, Year Book Medical Publishers, Inc. pp. 201-218.
12. Copeland, M. M.: Primary malignant tumors of bone. Evaluation of current diagnosis and treatment, Cancer **20**:738-746, 1967.
13. Copeland, M. M.: Metastases to bone from primary tumor in other sites. In Proceedings of the Sixth National Cancer Conference, Philadelphia, 1970, J. B. Lippincott Co., pp. 743-756.
13a. Cortes, E. P., Holland, J. F., Wang, J. J., and Sinks, L. F.: Doxorubicin in disseminated osteosarcoma, J.A.M.A. **221**:1132-1138, 1972.
14. Craver, L. F., and Miller, D. G.: Multiple myeloma, CA **16**:142-155, 1966.
15. Dahlin, D. C.: Bone tumors. General aspects and data on 3987 cases, ed. 2, Springfield, Ill., 1967, Charles C Thomas, Publisher.
16. Dahlin, D. C., and Coventry, M. B.: Osteogenic sarcoma. A study of six hundred cases, J. Bone Joint Surg. **49-A**:101-110, 1967.
17. Dahlin, D. C., Coventry, M. B., and Scanlon, P. W.: Ewing's sarcoma. A critical analysis of 165 cases, J. Bone Joint Surg. **43-A**:185-192, 1961.
18. Dahlin, D. C., Cupps, R. E., and Johnson, E. W., Jr.: Giant-cell tumor: a study of 195 cases, Cancer **25**:1061-1070, 1970.
19. Dahlin, D. C., and Ivins, J. C.: Fibrosarcoma of bone. A study of 114 cases, Cancer **23**:35-41, 1969.
20. D'Angio, G. J.: Personal communication, 1971.
21. Dargeon, H. W.: Tumors of childhood. A clinical treatise, New York, 1960, Paul B. Hoeber, Inc.
22. Diagnostic radiology of bone disease (Symposium), Radiol. Clin. North Am. **8**:171-290, 1970.
23. Edeiken, J., and Hodes, P. J.: Roentgen diagnosis of diseases of bone, Baltimore, 1967, The Williams & Wilkins Co.
24. Evans, A. E.: Mitomycin C., Cancer Chemother. Rep. **14**:1-9, Oct., 1961.
25. Evans, A. E., Heyn, R. M., Nesbit, M. E., and Hartmann, J. R.: Evaluation of Mitomycin C (NSC-26980) in the treatment of metastatic osteogenic sarcoma, Cancer Chemother. Rep. **53**:297-298, Oct., 1969.
25a. Ewing, J.: Diffuse endothelioma of bone, Proc. N. Y. Pathol. Soc. **21**:17-24, 1921.
26. Eyre-Brook, A. L., and Price, C. H. G.: Fibrosarcoma of bone. Review of fifty consecutive cases from the Bristol Tumour Registry, J. Bone Joint Surg. **51-B**:20-37, 1969.
27. Falk, S., and Alpert, M.: The clinical and roentgen aspects of Ewing's sarcoma, Am. J. Med. Sci. **250**:492-508, 1965.
28. Falk, S., and Alpert, M.: Five year survival of patients with Ewing's sarcoma, Surg. Gynecol. Obstet. **124**:319-324, 1967.
28a. Fine, G., and Stout, A. P.: Osteogenic sarcoma of extraskeletal soft tissues, Cancer **9**:1027-1043, 1956.
29. Finkelstein, J. Z., Hittle, R. E., and Hammond, G. D.: Evaluation of a high dose cyclophosphamide regimen in childhood tumors, Cancer **23**:1239-1242, 1969.
30. Francis, K. C., Higinbotham, N. L., and Coley, B. L.: Primary reticulum cell sarcoma of bone. Report of 44 cases, Surg. Gynecol. Obstet. **99**:142-146, 1954.

31. Geschickter, C. F., and Copeland, M. M.: Tumors of bone, ed. 3, Philadelphia, 1949, J. B. Lippincott Co.
32. Geschickter, C. F., and Copeland, M. M.: Parosteal osteoma of bone: a new entity, Ann. Surg. 133:790-807, 1951.
33. Hayles, A. B., Dahlin, D. C., and Coventry, M. B.: Osteogenic sarcoma in children, J.A.M.A. 174:1174-1177, 1960.
34. Higinbotham, N. L., Phillips, R. F., Farr, H. W., and Hustu, H. O.: Chordoma. Thirty-five year study at Memorial Hospital, Cancer 20:1841-1850, 1967.
35. Hittle, R. E.: Personal communication, 1971.
36. Hustu, H. O.: Personal communication, 1969.
37. Hustu, H. O., Holton, C., James, D., Jr., and Pinkel, D.: Treatment of Ewing's sarcoma with concurrent radiotherapy and chemotherapy, J. Pediatr. 73:249-251, 1968.
38. Hutter, R. V. P., Foote, F. W., Jr., Francis, K. C., and Sherman, R. S.: Primitive multi-potential primary sarcoma of bone, Cancer 19:1-25, 1966.
39. Hutter, R. V. P., Worcester, J. N., Jr., Francis, K. C., Foote, F. W., Jr., and Stewart, F. W.: Benign and malignant giant cell tumors of bone, Cancer 15:653-690, 1962.
40. Iriarte, P. V., Hananian, J., and Cortner, J. A.: Central nervous system leukemia and solid tumors of childhood. Treatment with 1,3-bis (2-chloroethyl)-1-nitrosourea (BCNU), Cancer 19:1187-1194, 1966.
41. Ivins, J. C., and Dahlin, D. C.: Malignant lymphoma (reticulum cell sarcoma) of bone, Mayo Clin. Proc. 38:375-385, 1963.
42. Jaffe, H. L.: Tumors and tumorous conditions of the bone and joints, Philadelphia, 1958, Lea & Febiger.
43. Jaffe, H. L.: Fibrosarcoma of bone and bone involvement by direct extension of soft-part sarcoma. In Tumors of bone and soft tissue, Chicago, 1965, Year Book Medical Publishers, Inc., pp. 219-228.
44. Jeffree, G. M., and Price, C. H. G.: Bone tumors and their enzymes. A study of the phosphatases, non-specific esterases and beta-glucuronidase of osteogenic and carti-laginous tumours, fibroblastic and giant-cell lesions, J. Bone Joint Surg. 47-B:120-136, 1965.
45. Jenkin, R. D. T.: Ewing's sarcoma. A study of treatment methods, Clin. Radiol. 17:97-106, April, 1966.
46. Jenkin, R. D. T., Rider, W. D., and Sonley, M. J.: Ewing's sarcoma. A trial of adjuvant total-body irradiation, Radiology 96:151-155, 1970.
47. Johnson, R., and Humphreys, S. R.: Past failures and future possibilities in Ewing's sarcoma, Cancer 23:161-166, 1969.
48. Johnson, R. E., Senyszyn, J. J., Rabson, A. S., and Peterson, K. A.: Treatment of Ewing's sarcoma with local irradiation and systemic chemotherapy—a progress report, Radiology 95:195-197, 1970.
49. Kamrin, R. P., Potanos, J. N., and Pool, J. L.: An evaluation of the diagnosis and treatment of chordoma, J. Neurol. Neurosurg. Psychiatry 27:157-165, 1964.
50. Lee, E. S., and MacKenzie, D. H.: Osteosarcoma. A study of the value of preoperative megavoltage radiotherapy, Br. J. Surg. 51:252-274, 1964.
51. Lichtenstein, L.: Bone tumors, ed. 4, St. Louis, 1972, The C. V. Mosby Co.
52. Livingston, R. B., and Carter, S. K.: Single agents in cancer chemotherapy, New York, 1970, IFI/Plenum Data Corp.
53. Lodwick, G. S.: The bones and joints. In Hodes, P. J., editor: Atlas of tumor radiology, Chicago, 1971, Year Book Medical Publishers, Inc.
54. Marcove, R. C., Miké, V., Hajek, J. V., Levin, A. G., and Hutter, R. V. P.: Osteogenic sarcoma under the age of twenty-one. A review of one hundred and forty-five operative cases, J. Bone Joint Surg. 52-A:411-423, 1970.
55. Marsa, G. W., and Johnson, R. E.: Altered pattern of metastasis following treatment of Ewing's sarcoma with radiotherapy and adjuvant chemotherapy, Cancer 27:1051-1054, 1971.
56. McKenna, R. J., Schwinn, C. P., Soong, K. Y., and Higinbotham, N. L.: Sarcomata of the osteogenic series (osteosarcoma, chondrosarcoma, parosteal osteogenic sarcoma, and sar-comata arising in abnormal bone). An analysis of 552 cases, J. Bone Joint Surg. 48-A:1-26, 1966.

57. Millburn, L. F., O'Grady, L., and Hendrickson, F. R.: Radical radiation therapy and total body irradiation in the treatment of Ewing's sarcoma, Cancer **22**:919-925, 1968.

58. Miller, R. W.: Fifty-two forms of childhood cancer: United States mortality experience, 1960-1966, J. Pediatr. **75**:685-689, 1969.

59. Mountain, C. F.: Surgical management of pulmonary metastases, Postgrad. Med. **48**:128-132, Nov., 1970.

60. Parker, F., Jr., and Jackson, H., Jr.: Primary reticulum cell sarcoma of bone, Surg. Gynecol. Obstet. **68**:45-53, 1939.

61. Perkinson, N. G., and Higinbotham, N. L.: Osteogenic sarcoma arising in polyostotic fibrous dysplasia. Report of a case, Cancer **8**:396-402, 1955.

62. Phemister, D. B.: Chondrosarcoma of bone, Surg. Gynecol. Obstet. **50**:216-233, 1930.

63. Phillips, R. F., and Higinbotham, N. L.: The curability of Ewing's endothelioma of bone in children, J. Pediatr. **70**:391-397, 1967.

64. Phillips, T. L., and Sheline, G. E.: Radiation therapy of malignant bone tumors, Radiology **92**:1537-1545, 1969.

65. Pomeroy, T. C., and Johnson, R. E.: Integrated therapy for Ewing's sarcoma, Proc. Am. Assoc. Cancer Res. **12**:80, March, 1971.

66. Poppe, E., Liverud, K., and Efskind, J.: Osteosarcoma, Acta Chir. Scand. **134**:549-556, 1968.

67. Price, C. H. G., and Goldie, W.: Paget's sarcoma of bone. A study of eighty cases from the Bristol and the Leeds Bone Tumour Registries, J. Bone Joint Surg. **51-B**:205-224, 1969.

68. Radiation carcinogenesis in man. VI. Bone tumours. In Report of the United Nations Scientific Committee on the Effects of Atomic Radiation, Supplement No. 14 (A/5814), New York, 1964, United Nations, pp. 94-95.

69. Rockwell, M. A., and Enneking, W. H.: Osteosarcoma developing in solitary enchondroma of the tibia, J. Bone Joint Surg. **53-A**:341-344, 1971.

70. Scaglietti, O., and Calandriello, B.: Ossifying parosteal sarcoma. Parosteal sarcoma or juxtacortical osteogenic sarcoma, J. Bone Joint Surg. **44-A**:635-647, 1962.

71. Schajowicz, F.: Ewing's sarcoma and reticulum cell sarcoma of bone. With special reference to the histochemical demonstration of glycogen as an aid to differential diagnosis, J. Bone Joint Surg. **41-A**:349-356, 1959.

72. Schwartz, A., Shuster, M., and Becker, S. M.: Liposarcoma of bone. Report of a case and review of the literature, J. Bone Joint Surg. **52-A**:171-177, 1970.

73. Selawry, O. S., Holland, J. F., and Wolman, I. J.: Effect of vincristine (NSC-67574) on malignant solid tumors in children, Cancer Chemother. Rep. **52**:497-500, June, 1968.

74. Senyszyn, J. J., Johnson, R. E., and Curran, R. E.: Treatment of metastatic Ewing's sarcoma with actinomycin D (NSC-3053), Cancer Chemother. Rep. **54**:103-107, April, 1970.

74a. Singleton, E. B., Rosenberg, H. S., Dodd, G. D., and Dolan, P. A.: Sclerosing osteogenic sarcomatosis, Am. J. Roentgenol. Radium Ther. Nucl. Med. **58**:483-490, 1962.

75. Soloway, H. B.: Radiation-induced neoplasms following curative therapy for retinoblastoma, Cancer **19**:1984-1988, 1966.

76. Stewart, F. W.: Primary liposarcoma of bone, Am. J. Pathol. **7**:87-93, March, 1931.

77. Suit, H. D.: Ewing's sarcoma: treatment by radiation therapy. In Tumors of bone and soft tissue, Chicago, 1965, Year Book Medical Publishers, Inc., pp. 191-200.

78. Sullivan, M. P., Sutow, W. W., and Taylor, G.: L-phenylalanine mustard as a treatment for metastatic osteogenic sarcoma in children, J. Pediatr. **63**:227-237, 1963.

79. Sutow, W. W.: Drug therapy and curability of cancer, Postgrad. Med. **48**:173-177, Nov., 1970.

80. Sutow, W. W., and Sullivan, M. P.: Cyclophosphamide therapy in children with Ewing's sarcoma, Cancer Chemother. Rep. **23**:55-60, Oct., 1962.

81. Sutow, W. W., Sullivan, M. P., Wilbur, J. R., Vietti, T. J., Kaizer, H., and Nagamoto, A.: L-phenylalanine mustard (NSC-8806) administration in osteogenic sarcoma: an evaluation of dosage schedules, Cancer Chemotherap. Rep. **55**:151-157, April, 1971.

82. Sutow, W. W., Vietti, T. J., Fernbach, D. J., Lane, D. M., Donaldson, M. H., and Lonsdale, D.: Evaluation of chemotherapy in children with metastatic Ewing's sarcoma and osteogenic sarcoma, Cancer Chemother. Rep. **55**:67-78, Feb., 1971.

83. Sutow, W. W., Wilbur, J. R., Vietti, T. J., Vuthibhagdee, P., Fujimoto, T., and Watanabe,

A.: Evaluation of dosage schedules of Mitomycin C (NSC-26980) in children, Cancer Chemother. Rep. **55**:285-289, June, 1971.

84. Sweetnam, R.: Osteosarcoma, Ann. R. Coll. Surg. Engl. **44**:38-58, Jan., 1969.

85. Sweetnam, R., and Ross, K.: Surgical treatment of pulmonary metastases from primary tumours of bone, J. Bone Joint Surg. **49-B**:74-79, 1967.

86. Tumors of bone and soft tissue, a collection of papers presented at the Eighth Annual Clinical Conference on Cancer, 1963, at The University of Texas M. D. Anderson Hospital and Tumor Institute at Houston, Chicago, 1965, Year Book Medical Publishers, Inc.

87. Van der Heul, R. O., and Von Ronnen, J. R.: Juxtacortical osteosarcoma. Diagnosis, treatment, and an analysis of eighty cases, J. Bone Joint Surg. **49-A**:415-439, 1967.

88. Vietti, T. J.: Personal communication, 1971.

89. Wang, C. C., and Fleischli, D. J.: Primary reticulum cell sarcoma of bone. With emphasis on radiation therapy, Cancer **22**:994-998, 1968.

90. Wang, C. C., and Schulz, M. D.: Ewing's sarcoma—a study of 50 cases treated at the Massachusetts General Hospital, 1930-1952 inclusive, N. Engl. J. Med. **248**:571-576, 1953.

91. Wollner, N., Tan, C., Ghavimi, F., Rosen, G., Tefft, M., and Murphy, M. L.: Adriamycin in childhood leukemia and solid tumors, Proc. Am. Assoc. Cancer Res. **12**:75, March, 1971.

CHAPTER 22

Malignant genitourinary tumors

MILTON H. DONALDSON
JOHN W. DUCKETT
S. GRANT MULHOLLAND

Tumors of the urinary organs account for only 6% of the cancer deaths in children and tumors of the genital organs only 1%.* The group of tumors covered in this chapter excludes Wilms' tumor (Chapter 16) which is the most prevalent genitourinary tumor in childhood.

RENAL CELL CARCINOMA

The vast majority of flank masses involving the kidney are either Wilms' tumors or neuroblastomas. One other renal malignancy that should be considered, especially in the older child, is the renal cell carcinoma.

In 1883 Grawitz proposed the term *hypernephroma* for the tumor that is now known as adenocarcinoma or renal cell carcinoma of the kidney. He believed that the cellular appearance of the neoplasm so resembled the cells of the adrenal gland that it must arise from ectopic nests of adrenal or "hypernephroid" tissue within the confines of the renal capsule and parenchyma. This theory has since been disproved, and the tumor is now known to arise from the epithelial cells of the renal tubules.

Although renal cell carcinoma of the kidney comprises some 85% to 90%[13] of the adult renal tumors, it is rare in children. Riches[74] found none of these tumors in children below 10 years of age and only five among those 11 to 20 years of age in a review of 1735 cases for an incidence of 0.3%. The frequency as compared to that of Wilms' tumor was 2.6% in several studies,[6, 51, 74] which tallied 342 Wilms' tumors and only nine renal cell carcinomas. The exact number of renal cell carcinomas that have been reported in the pediatric age group cannot be determined because adequate documentation is lacking in some of the early cases. Aron and Gross' review in 1969[3] eliminated such cases and reported only those from 1940 to 1966. With the 2 cases of their own, this resulted in a total of 30 cases. Since then, several publications have brought the total reported cases to 54.† One might assume from the increased reporting of cases in recent years that the incidence of this tumor may not be as low as previously thought.

The pathologic findings of renal cell carcinoma do not differ with the age of the patient. The mass may be located in any portion of the kidney. Frequently it is huge, but it may still be small enough to be completely encompassed

---

*From Division of Vital Statistics, National Center for Health Statistics, 1959-1961.
†References 14, 18, 43, 50, 62, 67, 70, 79.

497

by renal parenchymal tissue. The appearance is so distinctive that this tumor can be recognized grossly. The cut surface is variegated, with the predominant color of yellow from its lipid content but with areas of red to brown due to hemorrhage and cysts of varying sizes.

The microscopic picture usually is characteristic. The cells are usually large and round with a strikingly clear or vacuolated cytoplasm due to the presence of lipid, chiefly cholesterol, and glycogen. This is the so-called clear cell type of renal adenocarcinoma. Less often noted is a predominance of darker granular cells; these tumors are labeled the granular type of renal cell carcinoma. The latter is stated to be a more malignant variety.[8] The cellular arrangement varies from a cystic papillary formation to an alveolar arrangement of solid cords and, lastly, to a tubular arrangement that suggests a renal origin. Stroma is scanty, and blood vessels are usually large and numerous (Fig. 22-1).

Spread occurs by direct extension and by metastasis via lymphatics and blood vessels, predominantly the latter. The most frequent sites of metastatic involvement are the lungs and the skeletal system, with liver and brain less commonly involved. Solitary bone metastases occur in 60% of adults; thus a spontaneous fracture may be the first manifestation of the neoplasm. This has not been reported in children.

The manifestations of this neoplasm have been very similar in children and adults. The classic triad of a palpable mass, pain, and gross hematuria occurs in both age groups but is uncommon in children. The mass is usually detected in the flank of the adult but is more often felt in the anterior abdomen of a child. A mass is more frequently palpated in a child than in an adult, probably due to the greater ease with which the abdomen of a child can be examined

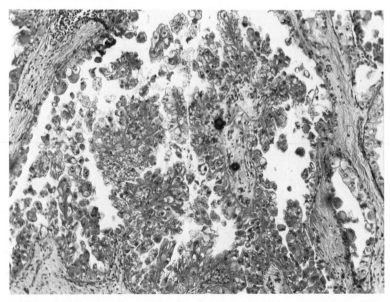

Fig. 22-1. This magnification of a renal cell carcinoma from a 10-year-old boy shows a papillary projection composed of both clear cells and granular cells, with two small calcifications (×130). (Courtesy Maurice Srouji, M.D.)

and is not necessarily related to a more advanced stage of disease resulting in a larger tumor. As in the Wilms' tumor, the mass is usually firm and smooth, and slight tenderness is often present on palpation. In contrast, the neuroblastoma is generally firm, irregular, and nontender. Pain occurs with similar frequency in each age group (i.e., 30% to 50% of cases), but it is more often noted to be abdominal in children while localized to the flank in the adult. Gross hematuria develops in 45% to 60% of cases and is often the manifestation that prompts the patient to seek medical care. Constitutional symptoms such as weight loss, nausea and vomiting, weakness, night sweats, and fever are commonly noted. Fever occasionally is the sole presenting symptom in this neoplasm; the temperature may be high and fluctuating. Extrarenal manifestations such as hepatosplenomegaly, leukemoid reactions, polycythemia, elevated serum haptoglobin, and abnormal liver function tests in the absence of liver metastases are well known in the adult.[25, 89] These abnormalities have rarely been noted in children.[67]

Excretory urography demonstrates an intrarenal mass that causes distortion of the calyces similar to that caused by a Wilms' tumor. Aortography and renal arteriography demonstrate the neoplastic hypervascularity and the "tumor blush" of the arteriolar and capillary phases of the study. Radioisotopic scan reveals renal cell carcinoma as filling defects or "cold spots" on the scintograms. The latter study is a safer one and is comparable to aortography for diagnosis. Angiographic studies may reveal arteriovenous shunts in renal cell carcinomas.[79] This is not seen in Wilms' tumors.

The most effective treatment for renal cell carcinoma is surgical removal. This is true even though part of the primary tumor or distant metastases or both have to be left unresected, since, in a rare patient, partial or complete regression of the remaining neoplastic tissue has occurred.[24] Robson recently has stressed the value of a radical surgical approach by achieving 52% 5-year and 49% 10-year survival rates.[74a] Therefore every reasonable effort should be made to use an aggressive surgical approach even though permanent cure is effected in a minority of patients.

Radiation therapy has been used both prior to and after nephrectomy.[73] Preoperative radiation may change an inoperable tumor into an operable one and appears to increase survival in those patients with renal vein invasion. The value of postoperative radiotherapy is as much debated as that of preoperative radiation, but increases in 5- and 10-year survivals were noted in one study.[74] If perinephric spread or metastasis to regional lymph nodes has occurred or if the renal vein has been invaded, postoperative irradiation should be administered to the primary tumor bed and the surrounding involved areas.

Chemotherapeutic agents of various types have been used to treat residual and metastatic renal cell carcinoma, but with discouraging results. In a review of the literature combined with their own experience, Woodruff and co-workers[96] reported only twenty-seven objective responses among 260 patients treated with thirty-six different drugs. Talley and his associates[84] noted only two objective responses among 57 patients treated with various alkylating agents, antimetabolites, and other drugs. Bloom and Wallace[7] described a 21% objective regression rate in patients given progestins or testosterone, whereas Talley and associates[84] reported that 2 of 16 patients responded to progestins for a 12.5%

regression rate. All these patients were adults. Reports of treatment of children with chemotherapeutic agents and hormones are rare. One child with inoperable hypernephroma was living 8½ years after treatment with the combination of actinomycin D, oral methotrexate, and chlorambucil, along with surgery and irradiation.[18] Another child demonstrated regression of the primary tumor and pulmonary metastases while receiving vincristine and cyclophosphamide preoperatively; however, after nephrectomy the metastases progressed even though the chemotherapy was continued.[62] A solitary pulmonary lesion should be removed surgically, but disseminated metastatic disease is best treated with irradiation. Since the results of hormonal therapy are better than the spontaneous regression rate, a trial of a progestin or testosterone or both would seem worthwhile in a patient with progressive disease.

TUMORS OF THE LOWER URINARY AND GENITAL TRACT
Rhabdomyosarcoma

Rhabdomyosarcoma, probably arising from the urogenital sinus, is the most common cancer involving the bladder, prostate, and vagina in children. The histologic characteristics of rhabdomyosarcomas are classified into three patterns[36]: embryonal (including botryoid), alveolar, and pleomorphic. These histologic characteristics are described in Chapter 20. The majority of urogenital rhabdomyosarcomas are the embryonal type,[48] which has the most favorable prognosis. Varied terminology for this entity has made classifications confusing. MacFarland[54] in 1935 found 119 different terms for dysontogenic tumors arising in the genitourinary system.

Batsakis[5] indicates that pathologic, embryologic, and developmental studies support the conclusion that the source of these urogenital rhabdomyosarcomas is the nonspecific mesenchyme incorporated in mesonephric duct. In children, it is important to note the absence of other heterologous tissue such as cartilage, bone, or epithelium in these tumors. The rarely occurring mixed tumors such as leiomyosarcomas or fibromyxosarcomas do not appear to have the same genesis.

The term *sarcoma botryoides* was originally intended to describe the polypoid, grapelike cluster and therefore characterizes a gross configuration. Sarcoma botryoides is a type of embryonic rhabdomyosarcoma whose growth assumes the pattern of multiple polyps when it involves the mucosal surface of a hollow organ such as the bladder, vagina, bile duct, or larynx. The term is descriptive and should not be used diagnostically for an embryonal rhabdomyosarcoma.

Tumors arising in the bladder, posterior urethra, or vagina cause symptoms sooner than those arising in the prostate. The much graver prognosis for prostatic tumors may relate to their late detection. All tend to remain relatively localized and spread along tissue planes. Without surgical intervention, death results from urinary tract obstruction. Even after active treatment of the primary tumor, widespread metastases are observed. With such a rapidly growing tumor a delay in diagnosis significantly alters survival.[93]

The vagina. "Sarcoma botryoides" was historically described as lobules of tumor arising from the vagina and protruding through the vulva. This tumor usually appears during the first 3 years of life as fleshy polypoid masses that ulcerate, bleed, or cause purulent discharge. There may be a flat, spreading, submucosal element to the tumor as well as the clusters. Biopsy material is easily obtained, but at times it is histologically difficult to interpret and may be misinterpreted as benign (Chapter 23).

The bladder. Rhabdomyosarcoma of the bladder presents a multicentric pattern, causes urinary obstruction, and is more frequently seen in boys before 4 years of age. Strangury (the urgency to pass urine with no success) is characteristic since the bladder contracts on the tumor. Urinary tract infection is frequent, incontinence due to urinary retention is common, and hematuria is unusual. The cystogram phase of the excretory urogram often confirms the diagnosis with lobulated filling defects (Fig. 22-2, *B*). The upper tracts are usually dilated, and the lower ureters may show widening of the trigonal area (Fig. 22-2, *A*). Endoscopic visualization of the lobulated, pearly gray growths and biopsy with the infant resectoscope are not difficult. It is imperative not to biopsy the tumor through a suprapubic approach to avoid leaving a sinus along which the tumor may spread.

The prostate. The exact origin of rhabdomyosarcomas of the perineum may be difficult to determine,[63] but the solid tumors of the prostatic region are clinically separate from tumors arising from the bladder and vagina. There are few long-term survivors from this site of origin. It is still a question whether the neoplasm is indeed more aggressive or detection is delayed. Local spread and distant metastases are usually further advanced, and the average patient at diagnosis is older than the patients with tumors of the bladder or vagina. A large, solid, globular mass fills the pelvis, displacing the bladder upward and stretching the urethra over its surface (Fig. 22-3, *B*). The base of the bladder is infiltrated, and submucosal extension occurs along the urethra.[91] Rectal examination locates the mass anterior to the bowel, distinguishing it from sacral neuroblastoma or teratoma. Symptoms are notably vague until the gradual onset of urinary obstruction leads to infection or urinary retention.

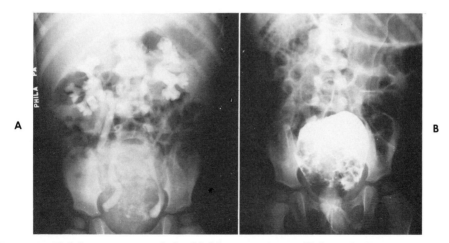

Fig. 22-2. Rhabdomyosarcoma of the bladder in a 3-year-old boy. **A,** Excretory urogram demonstrates widely separated lower ureters with tumor in the base of the bladder causing hydroureteronephrosis. **B,** Cystogram shows polypoid masses within the bladder.

A voiding cystourethrogram showing distortion of the urethra usually confirms the prostatic origin of the tumor. Often there is obstruction and displacement of the ureters (Fig. 22-3, A). Endoscopy is unnecessary and fraught with difficulty. Biopsy of the tumor is best done by needle through the perineum. To detect these tumors early, a rectal examination should be performed on all boys with urinary tract infection.

Treatment of urogenital rhabdomyosarcoma. Although each patient must be evaluated individually, wide local excision usually entails radical pelvic exenteration. Occasionally some of the genital tract can be spared in girls, leaving the rectum in anteriorly situated tumors and saving the bladder in posteriorly located lesions. If possible, one ovary should be spared, bringing it into the abdomen on a pedicle of the ovarian vessels and marking it with a radiopaque clip so that pelvic irradiation can be given without destroying ovarian function. Radiation proctitis is likely to occur if the rectum remains in the irradiated field. In some of these cases a final colostomy and excision of the rectum may be necessary. In others a temporary colostomy may permit recovery from radiation proctitis and eventual reestablishment of intestinal continuity. The same concept may apply for radiation cystitis if the bladder remains. Secondary procedures are advised for metastases and local recurrences if surgically feasible.

There were 21 children living more than 3 years with bladder rhabdomyosarcomas studied by MacKenzie and co-workers,[48] and all but one had radical surgical extirpation. Williams and Young[93] reported the largest single series of 15 infants and children with rhabdomyosarcoma of the bladder and vagina, with 8 of the 15 surviving after extensive surgery. Since three of the fifteen tumors were not considered operable, the data could be interpreted as a 67% survival rate for "operable" rhabdomyosarcomas of the bladder and vagina. Of

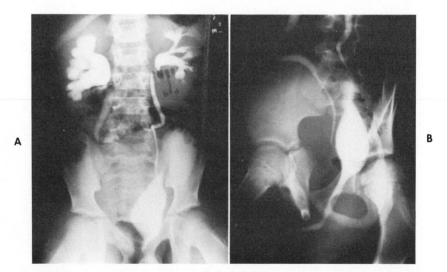

Fig. 22-3. Rhabdomyosarcoma of the prostate in a 9-year-old boy with (**A**) a large mass filling the pelvis, obstructing the ureters, and (**B**) elongating the prostatic urethra.

9 boys with prostatic rhabdomyosarcoma, only 1 is surviving; his lesion arose in the prostatic urethra and was detected early.

Reports over the last 10 years indicate improved survival of patients with embryonal rhabdomyosarcomas in the bladder and vagina treated with radical surgical excision. The responsiveness of soft tissue sarcoma[55] and, more specifically, embryonal rhabdomyosarcoma to radiation therapy[59] is indeed hopeful for the treatment of the more advanced lesions. The combination of chemotherapy and radiotherapy recently reported for rhabdomyosarcomas[28, 83, 90] is exciting. At the M. D. Anderson Tumor Institute over the past 5 years, 21 of 32 children with rhabdomyosarcomas are alive without evidence of disease 1 to 4 years after the initiation of therapy. Twenty-one of the 32 children had inoperable or metastatic disease at the start of therapy. Sixteen of them are alive without evidence of disease.

Other tumors of the lower urinary and genital tract

The bladder. Transitional cell carcinoma occurs in children under 12 years old but is exceedingly rare.[46] It behaves like the adult tumor. Leiomyosarcoma is rare and less aggressive than rhabdomyosarcoma, so that less radical surgery is acceptable.[48] The adenocarcinoma found arising from the urachus occurs in later life, as does the malignant transformation to carcinoma in the exstrophied bladder. Engel and Wilkinson[17] found 3 patients with malignancy (35, 41, and 52 years of age) among 42 patients with exstrophy of the bladder. It is debatable whether this incidence of cancer condemns attempts at reconstruction of the exstrophied bladder. Neurofibroma of the bladder causing bilateral ureteral obstruction may require urinary diversion.[78] Hemangioma of the bladder is usually a hamartomatous mass that involves other organs.

The vagina (see Chapter 23). Squamous cell carcinoma of the cervix is rare in children,[68] and adenocarcinoma of the uterus is exceedingly rare.[45] Adenocarcinoma[61] of the infant vagina is histologically similar to adenocarcinoma of the infant testis and embryonal cell carcinoma, with an "endodermal sinus" pattern. Mesonephric remnants seem the most likely source, with diverticula of yolk sac endoderm or extra embryonic membrane[32] another likely source. Of 6 patients from 8 to 15 months old with vaginal adenocarcinoma, only 2 survived for more than 3 years,[61] and all 4 children in another series died.[91] Mesonephric papilloma of the infant vagina may be the benign counterpart of adenocarcinoma of the vagina.

Herbst and Scully[31] recently reported adolescent adenocarcinoma of the clear cell type in the vagina, which is distinctly different from the infant "endodermal sinus" variety. Because of the clear cell pattern the origin is more likely mullerian rather than mesonephric. Their epidemiologic study strongly implicates the maternal ingestion of stilbestrol during pregancy as the etiology. Of 7 children, 15 to 22 years of age, only 1 has died. This malignancy may become more prevalent in the future as more hormones are utilized to support pregnancies.

The penis and scrotum. Hemangioma and lymphangioma affecting the penis and scrotum are relatively common and may become cavernous and large. However, most of them sclerose spontaneously and require little treatment.[91] Primary sarcoma of the penis involving the corpus cavernosum in two infants, histologically an endothelioma, was reported by Joelson.[39] Priapism in children is usually associated with leukemia or sickle cell disease. A benign pedunculated fibrous polyp of the posterior urethra in males occasionally causes obstruction to bladder outflow, but this is not truly a tumor.[91]

TESTICULAR NEOPLASMS

Testicular tumors in infants and children are rare, and this scarcity of cases has made diagnosis, classification, and treatment of these tumors difficult. Testicular neoplasms can be divided into two large groups, nongerminal and germinal. In the adult, germinal tumors comprise 98% of all testicular tumors,[15] whereas in the child they comprise only 40%.[37] Testicular tumors are seventh in frequency among malignant neoplasms in children[77] and represent 2% to 5% of the total number of testicular tumors occurring at all ages. More than 600 have been reported.[37] Testicular tumors are exceedingly rare in Negroes. In most cases the presenting complaint is a painless scrotal swelling, especially if the tumor is hormonally inactive.[20] In over 50% of cases the duration of symptoms is more than 3 months, and sometimes there is a delay of a year or more before treatment. Generally, a testicular tumor in a child is associated with a better prognosis than in an adult.

The average age at presentation varies in different series. Abell and Holtz[1] noted that two thirds of 100 tumors occurred in children 2 years old or younger. In a series of 100 tumors in infants studied by ReMine and co-workers,[72] 42% were discovered at birth. Mostofi[57] reported 24 cases in children, the majority of which occurred before the third year. A majority of the cases in the series of Young and associates[97] occurred in infants under 2 years of age.

Two classifications of testicular tumors are widely used today. The classification of Collins and Pugh[12] for the Testicular Tumor Panel of Great Britain will not be used in this discussion. Dixon and Moore's[15] classification for germinal tumors, which is most widely accepted in the United States, is based on both the morphology and the clinical course of the tumor. Four main histologic patterns are generally recognized: seminoma, embryonal carcinoma, teratoma, and choriocarcinoma. Their relationship to clinical course is correlated into the following five groups:

1. Seminoma, pure
2. Embryonal carcinoma, pure or with seminoma
3. Teratoma, pure or with seminoma
4. Teratoma with either embryonal carcinoma or choriocarcinoma or both and with or without seminoma
5. Choriocarcinoma, pure or with either seminoma or embryonal carcinoma or both

In a series of in vitro experiments with multipotential embryonal cancer cells, Pierce and Dixon[66] demonstrated the development of more differentiated appearing elements belonging to all three germ layers characteristic of a teratoma. Their results strongly support the theory that embryonal carcinoma of the human testis is a stage in the morphogenesis of teratoma. Dixon and Moore[15] discuss the theoretical development of specific tumor types from embryonal carcinoma, but the maturation or stepwise progression of these tumors is not known. Adult teratoma, the most mature form, has recognizable fetal or adult tissues. Choriocarcinoma shows both cytotrophoblastic and syncytial trophoblastic tissue. Tumors of germinal cell origin are closely related except for seminomas. All appear to have a common germ cell origin. Seminomas are often found intermixed with other types, but histologically they are usually distinct and separate.[15] Embryonal carcinoma, choriocarcinoma, and teratoma are very closely related. Melicow[56] thought that these tumor types represented stages of maturation of adult teratoma, the most immature form being embryonal carcinoma, an intermediate form, teratocarcinoma, and the most mature form, adult teratoma.

Germinal cell tumors

Seminoma and choriocarcinoma so rarely occur in the pediatric age group that they are not included in this discussion (Chapter 24). The management and response of these tumors in children are essentially the same as in adults.

Teratoma. Most authors consider teratoma to be the most common type of testicular tumor in childhood.[77] If the classification of teratoma is as broad as in the Collins and Pugh classification, there is no doubt that it is the most common. When the Dixon and Moore classification is used, embryonal carcinoma may be considered the most common undifferentiated testicular tumor in childhood.[1, 37, 57] The term *embryonal carcinoma* is a poor one. To eliminate confusion, perhaps all tumors previously categorized as embryonal carcinoma or teratoma should be grouped together and classified according to the degree of differentiation, that is, poorly differentiated, partially differentiated, and well-differentiated teratomas.

Teratoma occurring in infancy and childhood is thought to be clinically benign,[20, 65] in contrast to the adult teratomas. Death is uncommon after treatment with orchiectomy. This tumor has been divided into two groups: partially differentiated (occurring in the infant) and differentiated (occurring in the older child).[1] The differentiated types do not metastasize. Pediatric teratomas that do metastasize, which are very rare, are usually undifferentiated and should probably be placed in the embryonal carcinoma group.

In a review[72] of 100 cases of testicular tumors in infants less than 1 year of age, approximately one third were teratomas, and 42% of these were discovered at birth. The average age of patients at surgery in other series was 2½ years[37] and 3½ years.[1] Whether there is a morphologic and prognostic difference between those tumors that occur during the first year of life and those occurring later is debatable.[1, 72] Although the patient's age may affect the selection of treatment, most authors agree that orchiectomy is the treatment of choice in a child under the age of 1 year or in any child with a mature, well-differentiated tumor. If there are areas of undifferentiated cells, one might consider more extensive treatment, that is, retroperitoneal node dissection with or without chemotherapy or radiation or both.

Pathology. These tumors are well circumscribed, confined to the testis, and 3 to 4 cm in diameter.[1] They usually have cysts of varying sizes. The tissue varies in appearance and consistency on cut section. In differentiated tumors there are mature elements representing tissue from the three germ layers. Cysts are commonly lined with epidermis and epithelium from respiratory, neural, and intestinal systems. Mesenchymal tissue is often seen (i.e., muscle, cartilage, and fatty tissue). Representative tissue from the central nervous system, lymphoid tissue, and glandular tissue occur often. In the tumors that tend to be undifferentiated, immature recognizable tissue is present, as are undifferentiated foci of indeterminate origin.

Embryonal carcinoma. This tumor may be regarded as an undifferentiated teratoma and generally is similar to the adult type of embryonal carcinoma. However, some reports[1, 37, 71, 88, 97] have indicated that the prognosis is better when the tumor is discovered in a child. If adenocarcinoma of the testicle and embryonal carcinoma are considered together, the survival statistics are better in children than in embryonal carcinoma in adults because of the relatively high cure rate with adenocarcinoma.

This group of tumors requires a more aggressive treatment regimen than teratoma. Immediate radical orchiectomy followed by a retroperitoneal node dissection is considered the best treatment. Separate or combined chemotherapy and radiation may be considered if metastatic foci are present in the nodes.* In patients with a solitary metastasis, orchiectomy, node dissection, and removal of the metastatic lesion should be attempted with the added protection of chemotherapy or radiation or both. There is no consensus regarding therapy for this tumor in children.

Pathology. This tumor is composed of highly malignant, multipotential anaplastic cells that may be entirely undifferentiated or may show slight differentiation toward somatic or trophoblastic cell form.[71] There is disagreement as to whether embryonal carcinoma and adenocarcinoma are the same tumor. Magner and co-workers[49] used the classification adenocarcinoma with clear cells to designate a separate tumor with a benign clinical course occurring only in infants. Later Teoh and associates[88] also showed that this was a distinct entity peculiar to the infant testis. The origin was thought to be embryonic tubular cells of the testicle; therefore the name orchioblastoma was suggested. Teilum[87] discussed these tumors occurring in both the ovary and the testicle. He believed that the papillary structures were analogous to the endodermal sinus of Duval found in the rat placenta. Embryonal carcinoma and adenocarcinoma with clear cells possess similar cytologic appearance, growth patterns, and histochemical features.[1] It has been suggested that this tumor pattern may be a shift toward a more differentiated teratoma. Perhaps all these tumors should be classified together as undifferentiated teratomas. Two basic patterns of embryonal carcinoma have been suggested: the classic adult and the embryonal adenocarcinoma. The latter occurs in the pediatric age group, does not metastasize as frequently, and is comprised of adenomatous, papillary, or cystic formations of flattened, cuboidal, or columnar cells.[97] Thus there is an adenocarcinoma that occurs in the pediatric age group, has a better prognosis, and presents a different cellular pattern than the adult embryonal carcinoma.

These tumors may be 2 to 12 cm in size. The cut surface often reveals nearly complete replacement of the testicle by firm, light yellow-tan or gray tissue, occasionally cystic, usually solid, and gelatinous or mucoid in appearance. They are ovoid in shape, with occasional lobulation. Areas of yellow necrosis with hemorrhagic or cystic degeneration are often seen.

---

*References 9, 20, 40, 52, 81, 85.

Microscopically,[1, 37, 88, 97] there is usually a monotonous but distinctive pattern of growth composed of a meshwork of medullary masses of undifferentiated cells; these are polygonal, cuboidal, and low columnar cells that form irregular acinar and cystic spaces. Sometimes papillary structures are seen. The cytoplasm is eosinophilic and vacuolated. The cells are rich in glycogen. Necrosis is often seen.[1] Embryonal bodies, which are nests and tufts of small, closely packed, hyperchromatic cells, may be seen as in the adult variety.

Nongerminal cell tumors

These tumors are exceedingly rare and comprise only 3.5% of all testicular tumors.[15] They are relatively more common in patients less than 2 years of age than in older children. The histologic appearance varies considerably. Interstitial cell tumors and gonadal stromal tumors are of the greatest interest. Other tumors arising from the testicle proper (sarcomas, adenocarcinomas of rete testis, lymphoblastomas, hemangiomas, fibromas, etc.) are so rare that they will not be discussed.

Interstitial cell (Leydig cell) tumor. Interstitial cell tumor is the most common nongerminal tumor, with most of the approximately 170 reported cases occurring in adults.[35] This neoplasm comprises 1% of all testicular tumors[15, 69] and is found in all age groups. In the child it usually occurs at 4 to 5 years of age and is generally benign. Sixteen of 170 reported adult cases were malignant histologically.[35] Metastasis has never been reported in the prepubertal male. Endocrinologic abnormalities are variable but occur classically in the child: precocious puberty with macrogenitosomia, growth of pubic hair, voice changes, advanced skeletal and muscle development, and, in approximately 1 out of 19 cases, gynecomastia or feminization. The diagnosis is usually easily made by palpation of a testicular mass in a boy with precocious puberty and elevated 17-ketosteroids. A small testicular tumor may lead to enlargement of both testes and the epididymis on the involved side, which may mask the spreading lesion. This is due to the maturation effects of the tumor on the prepubertal testicle.[22]

Very slow growth of these tumors is classic. The first signs and symptoms are abnormal sexual development; the tumor appears later.

Pathology. This tumor is usually small but ranges in size from 2 to 15 cm. It it spherical, nodular or lobulated, yellowish brown, and usually encapsulated. Histologically, the cells are large, relatively uniform, closely packed, and polyhedral and grow in sheets or cords. The cytoplasm is granular and eosinophilic and contains lipoid vacuoles, crystoids, and brown pigment. It is often difficult to distinguish between hyperplasia and tumor.[53] The histologic appearance of the metastasizing form does not differ from that of the benign tumor.

None of these tumors in the pediatric age group has been malignant. Therefore simple excision of the tumor itself will be sufficient,[37] since the preoperative diagnosis is almost certain in these cases. Orchiectomy is also acceptable.[69]

Androblastoma. Androblastoma, Sertoli cell tumor, granulosa-theca cell tumor of the testis, and gonadal stromal tumor are testicular homologues of ovarian arrhenoblastomas. These rare tumors resemble fetal testes and may be associated with feminizing characteristics in the male.[15] There is considerable speculation regarding the relationship of these tumors to some ovarian stromal tumors. Only a small number of cases have been reported (0.4% of all testicular tumors),[15] but a variety of names have been used to describe them. They have been classified as tubular, mixed, and diffuse stromal. The tubular form occurs in both the ovary and the testis. The mixed and diffuse forms have been reported in the testis by Teilum.[86] The tubular epithelial elements in these growths are analogous to Sertoli's cells and are capable of producing estrogen. The stromal tissue is related to Leydig's cells and produces androgen.[86] Therefore this tumor may be either masculinizing or feminizing. Androblastomas are not malignant, but their ovarian counterparts, arrhenoblastomas, can be malignant. These tumors have a wide range of presentation between 1 and 52 years of age. They develop slowly as a painless testicular enlargement. Reported hormone assays in these patients have shown elevation in only a sparse number of cases.[58]

The ideal treatment for these tumors is not well established due to the infrequency of cases. An inguinal orchiectomy has been used in the majority of cases and appears to be adequate.

Pathology. These tumors vary in size from 1 to 10 cm. They are usually firm, solitary, well-encapsulated, gray-white to yellow, and spherical or ovoid. They are rarely cystic. These tumors may be diffuse stromal, mixed, or tubular. The stromal type is comprised of small, closely packed cells that are round, polygonal, or spindle shaped. The microscopic appearance reveals a tubular orientation of the cells, which have an epithelial characteristic.[58]

Carcinoma in the undescended testicle. Malignant change in an undescended testicle presents only rarely during childhood.[91] The incidence of undescended testicle in military recruits is 0.23%.[10] About 10% of testicular tumors develop in undescended testicles,[10, 12, 21, 41] and the probability of a malignancy developing is twenty to forty-eight times greater in an undescended testicle than in a normal testicle.[10, 21, 41] The bilateral cryptorchid, after developing tumor on one side, has a one in four chance of developing a malignancy in the other testicle.[21] Also, separate tumors may develop on each side, and their presentation may be separated by years.[2, 42]

The development of tumor after orchiopexy has generated a considerable amount of discussion in the literature. Orchiopexy probably does not alter the risk of malignant disease but does make the testicle more accessible to palpation and visualization, thereby allowing for an earlier diagnosis. Testicular atrophy and dysgenesis begin to develop at 10 years of age[11] or even during the preschool age.[2] Therefore orchiopexy has been recommended at the preschool age to preserve spermatogenesis. These changes in the testicle appear to be a possible etiologic factor in the development of carcinoma.[29, 80] In unilateral cryptorchism the predisposition to develop carcinoma may also be present in the contralateral descended testicle.[12, 21, 41] In twenty-three out of 840 testicular neoplasms associated with unilateral cryptorchism the tumor developed in the contralateral scrotal testicle,[21] not the undescended testicle.

All the types of carcinoma common to the testicle may develop in the undescended testicle. Seminoma is relatively more common and teratoma relatively less common in the undescended testicle than in the scrotal testicle.[12, 21, 91]

Usually the presentation of the tumor occurs well into adult life, many years after orchiopexy. Altman and Malamont[2] reviewed cases of postorchiopexy testicular tumors to acquire some understanding of the relationship between age at the time of operation and the development of testicular tumor. Their findings suggest that the older the child at the time of orchiopexy, the greater the likelihood that testicular carcinoma will develop.

The undescended testicle is certainly more prone to develop carcinoma, but the risk is very small. These testicles should not be removed in all patients just to prevent tumor formation. Other functions of the testicle (hormonal activity, fertility) and psychologic effects have to be weighed before orchiectomy is considered.

PARATESTICULAR TUMORS

The paratesticular group includes all tumors enclosed within the external spermatic fascia from the internal inguinal ring to the testicle, as well as those arising from the testicular appendages, epididymis, testicular tunics, and spermatic cord. Seventy-five percent of extratesticular tumors occurring within the scrotum are found in the spermatic cord,[15] and 20% to 30% of these are malignant.[15, 32, 47] In a review of cases from the London Hospital, slightly less than 3% of all intrascrotal tumors were found to be sarcomatous and paratesticular in location.[94] The exact origin of sarcomatous lesions in the paratesticular area and spermatic cord is often difficult to ascertain because of the size of the tumor and the extent of invasion at the time of excision. Primary and metastatic epididymal tumors and adenocarcinoma of the appendix testis are extremely rare in the pediatric age group.[9, 94] Lymphoma may present in the scrotum first on one side and then on the other. In most instances this is associated with widespread disease.[60] One case of lymphosarcoma with deposits of tumor in the spermatic cord has been recorded in a 10-year-old patient with generalized disease.[94]

In an extensive review of the literature, El-Badawi and Al-Ghorab[16] listed 387 spermatic cord tumors, of which 222 were benign, 125 malignant, and 40 unclassified. The malignant tumors were primarily soft tissue sarcomas, but there were also lymphomas and other rare tumors. Sarcomas, especially rhabdomyosarcomas, are the most common malignancies and are often found in children or young adults.

Presentation and clinical features

Paratesticular tumors vary greatly in size. Often the sarcomas are 10 to 15 cm in diameter before diagnosis is made because of their rapid growth. They occur on either side with equal distribution and rarely, if ever, occur bilaterally.[94] The lesion is seldom found on routine examination. Usually the patient or his parent notices a lump, which is rarely associated with pain. The rhabdomyosarcomas generally present before 20 years of age.[94] The mean age varies with different reports (e.g., 42 months,[34] 15 years,[75] and 10 to 18 years[30]). In malignant lesions other than rhabdomyosarcoma the age at onset is usually over 40 years.

Malignant paratesticular lesions usually progress rapidly in size. The patient with rhabdomyosarcoma may have a symptomatic course measured in weeks. With fibrosarcoma and leiomyosarcoma the history tends to be longer. Benign lesions may date back years.

A hydrocele or a transilluminating mass may be seen on physical examination even in the presence of a malignant lesion.[76, 94] The tumor usually arises above the testicle and below the superficial inguinal ring. Benign lesions are well circumscribed and movable. Sarcomas extend upward toward the inguinal ring but are usually scrotal.[15, 44] They are lobulated, heavy, and usually nontender. They are attached to the structure of origin and may invade adjacent tissue so extensively that the site of origin cannot be determined. The differential diagnosis should include hematocele, tuberculosis, hydrocele, spermatocele, herniated fat, abscess, varicocele, and hernia.

Pathology

The origin of these sarcomatous tumors is not known.[30, 76] It has been suggested that embryonal rhabdomyosarcoma resembles the skeletal muscle tissue of the 7- to 10-week fetus.[64] Willis[95] states that this tumor may develop from embryonal mesenchymal tissue. Origin from cremasteric fibers is questionable.[23, 44]

Rhabdomyosarcoma is a large, unencapsulated, lobulated, rubbery tumor that frequently invades or compresses the testis. It is tan to reddish brown and often has foci of hemorrhage or degeneration. Microscopically, irregular multinucleated giant cells are seen, which may or may not have cross striations. Other tumor cells are markedly pleomorphic and anaplastic.

Treatment

The reported methods of treatment of these very malignant and relatively rare tumors differ greatly due to the general lack of experience with them. Most authors[44, 47, 75] suggest radical orchiectomy with early clamping and high ligation of the cord. The entire tumor and all invaded tissue should be removed; this may necessitate removing part of the scrotum or abdominal wall.[47] Some authors[4, 32] advocate retroperitoneal lymph node dissection; however, others[27, 44, 47] believe that this procedure is not indicated. Banowsky and Schultz[4] advocate node dissection because of the high incidence of lymphatic spread. In a good-risk patient with no demonstrable hematogenous metastasis a radical surgical approach may be indicated.[19, 27] Irradiation has been advocated by some authors.[26, 44, 47, 55, 75] A few successes have been reported with chemotherapy with methotrexate,[33] cyclophosphamide and vincristine,[75, 82] and actinomycin D, cyclophosphamide, and methotrexate.[30]

Prognosis

Unfortunately, few patients with sarcomatous lesions of the spermatic cord survive.[34, 38, 65, 75] Death due to widespread lymphatic and hematogenous metastasis to lymph nodes, lung, bone, and liver usually comes within a year. With more aggressive radical surgery, chemotherapy, and radiation, the prognosis appears to be improving.

REFERENCES

1. Abell, M. R., and Holtz, F.: Testicular neoplasms in infants and children. I. Tumors of germ cell origin, Cancer **16**:965-981, 1963.

2. Altman, B. L., and Malament, M.: Carcinoma of the testis following orchiopexy, J. Urol. **97**:498-504, 1967.
3. Aron, B. S., and Gross, M.: Renal adenocarcinoma in infancy and childhood: evaluation of therapy and prognosis, J. Urol. **102**:497-503, 1969.
4. Banowsky, L. H., and Shultz, G. N.: Sarcoma of the spermatic cord and tunics: review of the literature, case report and discussion of the role of retroperitoneal lymph node dissection, J. Urol. **103**:628-631, 1970.
5. Batsakis, J. G.: Urogenital rhabdomyosarcoma: histogenesis and classification, J. Urol. **90**:180-186, 1963.
6. Bjelke, E.: Malignant neoplasms of the kidney in children, Cancer **17**:318-321, 1964.
7. Bloom, H. J. G., and Wallace, D. M.: Hormones and the kidney. Possible therapeutic role of testosterone in a patient with regression of metastases from renal adenocarcinoma, Br. Med. J. **2**:476-480, 1964.
8. Boyd, W.: A textbook of pathology, ed. 8, Philadelphia, 1970, Lea & Febiger, pp. 679-680.
9. Broth, G., Bullock, W. K., and Morrow, J.: Epididymal tumors. 1. Report of 15 new cases including review of literature. 2. Histochemical study of the so-called adenomatoid tumor, J. Urol. **100**:530-536, 1960.
9a. Brown, J. H., and Kennedy, B. J.: Mithramycin in the treatment of disseminated testicular neoplasms, N. Engl. J. Med. **272**:111-118, 1965.
10. Campbell, H. E.: The incidence of malignant growth of the undescended testicle: a reply and re-evaluation, J. Urol. **81**:663-668, 1959.
11. Charny, C. W., and Wolgin, W.: Cryptorchism, New York, 1957, Paul B. Hoeber, Inc.
12. Collins, I. H., and Pugh, R. C. B.: Classification and frequency of testicular tumors, Br. J. Urol. **36**(Supp.):1-11, 1964.
13. Davis, L.: Christopher's textbook of surgery, ed. 6, Philadelphia, 1956, W. B. Saunders Co., p. 846.
14. Dehner, L. P., Leestma, J. E., and Price, E. B., Jr.: Renal cell carcinoma in children: a clinicopathologic study of 15 cases and review of the literature, J. Pediatr. **76**:358-368, 1970.
15. Dixon, F. J., and Moore, R. A.: Tumors of the male sex organs. In Atlas of tumor pathology, Section VIII, Fascicles 31b and 32, Washington, D. C., 1952, Armed Forces Institute of Pathology.
16. El-Badawi, A. A., and Al-Ghorab, M. M.: Tumors of the spermatic cord: a review of the literature and a report of a case of lymphangioma, J. Urol. **94**:445-450, 1965.
17. Engel, R. M., and Wilkinson, H. A.: Bladder exstrophy, J. Urol. **104**:699-704, 1970.
18. Fagan, W. T., Jr., and Clark, C. W.: Successful treatment of inoperable hypernephroma in childhood, J. Urol. **103**:652-659, 1970.
19. Fox, T. A., Jr., and Collier, R. L.: Rhabdomyosarcoma of the spermatic cord: a review and case presentation, Am. Surg. **33**:483-489, 1967.
20. Gangai, M. P.: Testicular neoplasms in an infant, Cancer **22**:658-662, 1968.
21. Gilbert, J. B., and Hamilton, J. B.: Incidence and nature of tumors in ectopic testes, Surg. Gynecol. Obstet. **71**:731-743, 1940.
22. Gittes, R. F., Smith, G., Conn, C. A., and Smith, F.: Local androgenic effect of interstitial cell tumor of the testis, J. Urol. **104**:774-777, 1970.
23. Goldstein, H. H., and Casilli, A. R.: Rhabdomyosarcoma of the cremasteric muscle and concomitant polyorchidism, J. Urol. **41**:583-591, 1939.
24. Goodwin, W. E.: Regression of hypernephromas, J.A.M.A. **204**:609, 1968.
25. Gordan, D. A.: The extrarenal manifestations of hypernephroma, Can. Med. Assoc. J. **88**:61-67, Jan., 1963.
26. Graf, R. A.: Malignant tumors of the spermatic cord: a brief review and presentation of a lipofibromyxosarcoma of the spermatic cord, J. Urol. **93**:74-76, 1965.
27. Gray, C. P., and Biorn, C. L.: Myosarcoma of the spermatic cord, J. Urol. **84**:562-564, 1960.
28. Grosfield, J. L., Clatworthy, H. W., Jr., and Newton, W. A., Jr.: Combined therapy in childhood rhabdomyosarcoma: an analysis of 42 cases, J. Pediatr. Surg. **4**:637-645, 1969.
29. Haines, J. S., and Grabstald, H.: Tumor formation in atrophic testes, Arch. Surg. **60**:857-860, 1950.

30. Hays, D. M., Mirabal, V. Q., Patel, H. R., Shore, N., and Woolley, M. M.: Rhabdomyosarcoma of the spermatic cord, Surgery **65**:845-849, 1969.

31. Herbst, A. L., and Scully, R. E.: Adenocarcinoma of the vagina in adolescence, Cancer **25**:745-751, 1970.

32. Hinman, F., and Gibson, T. E.: Tumors of the epididymis, spermatic cord and testicular tunics, Arch, Surg. **8**:100, 1924.

33. Hoffman, W. W., and Baird, S. S.: A rare tumor of the spermatic cord: rhabdomyosarcoma, J. Urol. **84**:376-381, 1960.

34. Holtz, F., and Abell, M. R.: Testicular neoplasms in infants and children. II. Tumor of non-germ cell origin, Cancer **16**:982-992, 1963.

35. Hopkins, B. G.: Interstitial cell tumor of the testis: case report and review of the literature, J. Urol. **103**:449-451, 1970.

36. Horn, R. C., Jr., and Enterline, N. T.: Rhabdomyosarcoma: a clinicopathological study and classification of 39 cases, Cancer **11**:181-199, 1958.

37. Houser, R., Izant, R. J., and Persky, L.: Testicular tumors in children, Am. J. Surg. **110**:876, 1965.

38. Irvine, E. W., Jr., Berg, O. C., and Nelson, R.: Rhabdomyosarcoma of paratesticular tissues; report of case, N. Engl. J. Med. **266**:994-995, 1962.

39. Joelson, J. J.: Primary sarcoma of the penis, Surg. Gynecol. Obstet. **38**:150, 1924.

40. Johnson, D. E., Keutter, C. R., and Guinn, G. A.: Testicular tumors in children, J. Urol. **104**:940, 1970.

41. Johnson, D. E., Woodhead, D. M., Pohl, D. R., and Robison, J. R.: Cryptorchism and testicular tumorigenesis, Surgery **63**:919-922, 1968.

42. Kaplan, G., and Roswit, B.: Bilateral testicular tumors following bilateral orchiopexy, J.A.M.A. **144**:1557-1558, 1950.

43. Kobayashi, A., Hoshino, H., Ohbe, Y., Sawaguchi, S., and Shimizu, K.: Bilateral renal cell carcinoma, Arch. Dis. Child. **45**:141-143, Feb., 1970.

44. Kyle, V. N.: Leiomyosarcoma of the spermatic cord: a review of the literature and report of an additional case, J. Urol. **96**:795-800, 1966.

45. Lockhart, H.: Cancer of uterus in childhood, Am. J. Obstet. Gynecol. **30**:76-80, 1935.

46. Lowry, E. C., Soanes, W. A., and Forbes, K. A.: Carcinoma of the bladder in children: case report, J. Urol. **73**:307-310, 1955.

47. Lundblad, R. R., Mellinger, G. T., and Gleason, D. F.: Spermatic cord malignancies, J. Urol. **98**:393-396, 1967.

48. MacKenzie, A. R., Whitmore, W. F., and Melamed, M. R.: Myosarcomas of the bladder and prostate, Cancer **22**:833-844, 1968.

49. Magner, D., Campbell, J. S., and Wiglesworth, F. W.: Testicular adenocarcinoma with clear cells, occurring in infancy, Cancer **9**:165-175, 1956.

50. Manson, A. D., Soule, E. H., Mills, S. D., and Deweerd, J. H.: Hypernephroma in childhood, J. Urol. **103**:336-340, 1970.

51. Marcus, R., and Watt, J.: Renal carcinoma in children, Br. J. Surg. **53**:351-353, 1966.

52. Matsumeto, K., Nakauchi, K., and Fugita, K.: Radiation therapy for the embryonal carcinoma of testis in childhood, J. Urol. **104**:778-780, 1970.

53. Mayers, M. M.: Interstitial cell tumors of the testicle: a report of three cases, J. Urol. **68**:834-844, 1952.

54. McFarland, J.: Dysontogenetic and mixed tumors of urogenital region, with report of new case of sarcoma botryoides vaginae in child, and comments upon probable nature of sarcoma, Surg. Gynecol. Obstet. **61**:42-57, 1935.

55. McNeer, G. P., Cantin, J., Chu, G., and Nickson, J. J.: Effectiveness of radiation therapy in management of sarcoma of the soft somatic tissues, Cancer **22**:391-397, 1968.

56. Melicow, M. M.: Classification of tumors of testis: a clinical and pathological study based on 105 primary and 13 secondary cases in adults, and 3 primary and 4 secondary cases in children, J. Urol. **73**:547-574, 1955.

57. Mostofi, F. K.: Infantile testicular tumors, Bull. N. Y. Acad. Med. **28**:684-687, 1952.

58. Mostofi, F. K., Theiss, E. A., and Ashley, D. J. B.: Tumors of specialized gonadal stroma in human male patients. Androblastoma, Steroli cell tumor, granulosa-theca cell tumor of the testis, and gonadal stromal tumor, Cancer **12**:944-957, 1959.

59. Nelson, A. J.: Embryonal rhabdomyosarcoma: report of 24 cases and study of the effectiveness of radiation treatment upon primary tumor, Cancer 22:64-68, 1968.

60. Nelson, W. E., Vaughan, V. C., III, and McKay, R. T. Textbook of pediatrics, Philadelphia, 1969, W. B. Saunders Co., p. 1458.

61. Norris, H. J., Bagley, G. P., and Taylor, H. B.: Carcinoma of the infant vagina. A distinctive tumor, Arch. Pathol. 90:473-479, 1970.

62. Palma, L. D., Kenny, G. M., and Murphy, G. M.: Childhood renal carcinoma, Cancer 26:1321-1324, 1970.

63. Palomino, S. J., Gilbert, E. F., and Jones, B.: Embryonal rhabdomyosarcoma of the perineum: a clinicopathologic report and survey of the literature, Clin. Pediatr. 6:425-432, 1967.

64. Patton, R. B., and Horn, R. C., Jr.: Rhabdomyosarcoma: Clinical and pathological features and comparison with human fetal and embryonal skeletal muscle, Surgery 52:572-583, 1962.

65. Phelan, J. T., Woolner, L. B., and Bayles, A. B.: Testicular tumors in infants and children, Surg. Gynecol. Obstet. 105:569-576, 1967.

66. Pierce, G. B., and Dixon, F. J., Jr.: Testicular teratoma: I. Demonstration of teratogenesis by metamorphosis of multipotential cells, Cancer 12:573-583, 1959.

67. Pochedly, C., Suwansirikul, S., and Penzer, P.: Renal-cell carcinoma with extrarenal manifestation in a 10-month-old child, Am. J. Dis. Child. 121:528-530, 1971.

68. Pollack, R. S., and Taylor, H. C.: Carcinoma of the cervix during the first two decades of life, Am. J. Obstet. Gynecol. 53:135-141, 1947.

69. Pomer, F. A., Stiles, R. E., and Graham, J. H.: Interstitial cell tumors of the testis in children. Report of a case and review of the literature, N. Engl. J. Med. 250:233-237, 1954.

70. Poole, C. A., and Viamonte, M., Jr.: Unusual renal masses in the pediatric age group, Am. J. Roentgenol. 109:368-379, 1970.

71. Ravich, L., Lerman, P. H., Drabkin, J. W., and Noya, J.: Embryonal carcinoma of the testicle in childhood: review of literature and presentation of 2 cases, J. Urol. 96:501-507, 1966.

72. ReMine, W. H., Woolner, L. B., Judd, E. S., and Hopkins, D. M.: Testicular teratoma in infancy: report of a case with a 10-year followup, Mayo Clin. Proc. 36:661-664, 1961.

73. Riches, E., Sir: The place of irradiation, J.A.M.A. 204:230-231, 1969.

74. Riches, E. W., Griffiths, I. H., and Thackray, A. C.: New growths of the kidney and ureter, Br. J. Urol. 23:297-356, 1951.

74a. Robson, C. J., Churchill, B. M., and Anderson, W.: The results of radical nephrectomy for renal cell carcinoma, Trans. Am. Assoc. Genitourin. Surg. 60:122-126, 1968.

75. Rosas-Uribe, A., Luna, M. A., and Guinn, G. A.: Paratesticular rhabdomyosarcoma: a clinicopathologic study of seven cases, Am. J. Surg. 120:787-791, 1970.

76. Ross, L. A. R.: Rhabdomyosarcoma of the spermatic cord, Pediatrics 43:890-892, 1969.

77. Rusche, C.: Twelve cases of testicular tumor occurring during infancy and childhood, J. Pediatr. 40:192-199, 1952.

78. Schoenberg, H. S., and Murphy, J. J.: Neurofibroma of the bladder, J. Urol. 85:899-901, 1961.

79. Shanberg, A. M., Srouji, M., and Leberman, P. R.: Hypernephroma in the pediatric age group, J. Urol. 104:189-192, 1970.

80. Sohval, A. R.: Testicular dysgenesis in relation to neoplasm of the testicle, J. Urol. 75:285-291, 1956.

81. Staubitz, W. J., Jewell, T. C., Jr., and Magoss, I. V.: Management of testicular tumors in children, J. Urol. 94:683-686, 1965.

82. Sutow, W. W.: Chemotherapy in childhood cancer (except leukemia). An appraisal, Cancer 18:1585-1589, 1965.

83. Sutow, W. W., Sullivan, M. P., Ried, H. L., Taylor, H. G., and Griffith, K. M.: Prognosis in childhood rhabdomyosarcoma, Cancer 25:1384-1390, 1970.

84. Talley, R. W., Moorhead, E. L., III, Tucker, W. G., San Diego, E. L., and Brennan, M. J.: Treatment of metastatic hypernephroma, J.A.M.A. 207:317-321, 1969.

85. Tefft, M., Vawter, G. F., and Mitus, A.: Radiotherapeutic management of testicular neoplasms in children, Radiology **88**:457-465, 1967.
86. Teilum, G.: Classification of testicular and ovarian androblastoma and Sertoli cell tumors; survey of comparative studies with consideration of histogenesis, endocrinology and embryological theories, Cancer **11**:769-782, 1958.
87. Teilum, G.: Endodermal sinus tumors of ovary and testis: comparative morphogenesis of so-called mesonephroma ovarii (Schiller) and extra-embryonic (yolk-sac-allantoic) structures of rat's placenta, Cancer **12**:1092-1105, 1959.
88. Teoh, T. B., Steward, J. K., and Willis, R. A.: The distinctive adenocarcinoma of the infant's testis: an account of 15 cases, J. Pathol. Bacteriol. **80**:147-156, July, 1960.
89. Walsh, P. N., and Kissane, J. M.: Nonmetastatic hypernephroma with reversible hepatic dysfunction, Arch. Intern. Med. **122**:214-282, 1968.
90. Wilbur, J. R., Sutow, W. W., Sullivan, M. P., Castro, J. R., and Taylor, H. A.: Successful treatment of rhabdomyosarcoma with combination chemotherapy and radiotherapy, American Society of Clinical Oncology, Chicago, April 7, 1971.
91. Williams, D. I., editor: Pediatric urology, London, 1968, Butterworth & Co., Ltd.
92. Williams, D. I., and Schistad, G.: Lower urinary tract tumors in children, Br. J. Urol. **36**:51-65, 1964.
93. Williams, D. L., and Young, D. G.: Malignant tumors of the genitourinary tract in childhood, Practitioner **200**:678-685, 1968.
94. Williams, G., and Banerjee, R.: Paratesticular tumors, Br. J. Urol. **41**:332-339, 1969.
95. Willis, R. A.: The pathology of the tumors of children, Chapter 6, Springfield, Ill., 1962, Charles C Thomas, Publisher.
96. Woodruff, M. W., Gailani, S. D., and Jones, R., Jr.: The current status of chemotherapy for advanced renal carcinoma in renal neoplasia. In King, J. S., Jr., editor: Renal neoplasia, Boston, 1967, Little, Brown & Co., pp. 573-592.
97. Young, P. G., Mount, B. M., Foote, F. W., and Whitmore, W. F., Jr.: Embryonal adenocarcinoma in the prepuberal testis. A clinicopathologic study of 18 cases, Cancer **26**:1065-1075, 1970.

CHAPTER 23

Malignant gynecologic tumors

JULIAN P. SMITH
FELIX RUTLEDGE

Since gynecologic cancer is infrequent in children, most of the available information about these tumors has been obtained from small series of patients or from collected case reports. The prognosis that has been reported in the past has been extremely poor. Because of the limited experience in treating these tumors, improvement in treatment for these patients has been slow. In the past 15 years, however, with better understanding of the behavior of the tumors and the availability of new and superradical surgery, radiotherapy, and chemotherapy, more aggressive treatment has been employed, and some success has been achieved.

Twenty-eight patients with gynecologic cancer (an incidence of 2%) were included among the 1372 pediatric cancer patients (under 14 years of age) at The University of Texas M. D. Anderson Hospital and Tumor Institute (MDAH) from 1944 through 1970. The ovary was the most common site; 19 of the 28 patients had ovarian cancer. The occurrence of gynecologic cancer in the other pelvic sites is shown in Table 23-1.

Since the M. D. Anderson Hospital is a cancer center, it is perhaps significant that the same predominance of ovarian tumors was also noted by Kaplan and Acosta[6] in a review of malignant gynecologic tumors at the Texas Children's Hospital; these investigators found 7 patients with ovarian tumors among 11 with gynecologic cancer.

OVARIAN TUMORS

Ovarian cancer in pediatric patients differs in several ways from that found in adults. For example, among 915 patients of all ages reported by Burns,[2] 85% had epithelial tumors. In children, however, the germ cell tumors—dysgerminoma, embryonal carcinoma, malignant teratoma, and choriocarcinoma*—

---

*See Chapter 24 for a discussion of choriocarcinoma.

Table 23-1. Malignant pelvic tumors in children (M. D. Anderson Hospital)

Site	Number of patients	Age range
Ovary	19	6-13 yr
Uterus	0	—
Vagina	4	6-34 mo
Bladder	3	2-6 yr
Vulva	2	13 yr

predominate, although these tumor types account for only about 6% of ovarian cancer in adults. Only one pediatric patient in the MDAH series and one in the report from Texas Children's Hospital had an epithelial cancer of the ovary. Malignant germ cell tumors, however, were present in 17 of the 19 patients in our series and in 5 of the 7 patients reported by Kaplan and Acosta.[6]

Burns[2] reported that 68% of patients of all ages with ovarian cancer had tumor extending beyond the pelvis when they were first examined. In our pediatric patients only 7 had tumors extending beyond the pelvis, although in most instances the tumors were rather large at the time of surgical intervention. In our experience most ovarian tumors of the germ cell type are already large at the time of discovery, although symptoms may have been present for only a short time. These symptoms are usually related to the enlargement of the tumor, which produces such complications as torsion, hemorrhage into or rupture of a cyst, and pain or discomfort from adhesions and pressure on surrounding structures. Ascites, a frequent presenting finding in adult ovarian cancer patients, was present in 5 of our patients.

The treatment of children with ovarian cancer depends on the extent of tumor at diagnosis and the predominant cell type. It is most important that the histologic diagnosis be correct. Embryonal carcinoma has been confused with such diagnoses as dysgerminoma, teratoma, or undifferentiated adenocarcinoma. Such errors are understandable in view of the rarity of these tumors, but every effort should be made to establish the histologic nature of the tumor because of the therapeutic and prognostic implications. Mixed ovarian germ cell tumors will usually follow the behavior pattern associated with the cell type that is the most malignant. Three patients in our series had dysgerminomas with embryonal carcinoma, and each of these tumors metastasized or recurred as pure embryonal carcinoma.

The Cancer Committee of the International Federation of Gynecology and Obstetrics has proposed a detailed staging scheme for carcinoma of the ovary.[1] Cancer limited to the ovaries is Stage I, cancer limited to the pelvis is Stage II, cancer spread to the abdomen is Stage III, and cancer spread beyond the abdominal cavity is Stage IV.

Dysgerminoma

Of the 6 patients with pure dysgerminoma in our series (Table 23-2), 2 had cancer limited to one ovary (Stage I), 2 had cancer extending beyond the ovary but limited to the pelvis (Stage II), and two had cancer extending beyond the pelvis into the abdomen (Stage III) (Table 23-3). These tumors are rarely bilateral.

Patients with unilateral tumors less than 10 cm in diameter who do not have any evidence of metastases may be treated by excision of the affected ovary and tube only. After surgery a lymphangiogram should be obtained; if there is no evidence of metastases, no further treatment is indicated, although the patient should be observed carefully.

Total abdominal hysterectomy and bilateral salpingo-oophorectomy is the initial treatment for (1) patients with unilateral tumor larger than 10 cm, (2) those with metastatic cancer in the pelvis, (3) those with affected abdominal or regional lymph nodes, (4) patients with bloody ascites, and (5) those with bilateral tumors.

Table 23-2. Malignant ovarian tumors in children (M. D. Anderson Hospital)

Histology	Number of patients	Age range
Dysgerminoma	6	7-12 yr
Dysgerminoma with embryonal carcinoma	3	12-13 yr
Embryonal carcinoma	3	7-13 yr
Teratoma	1	10 yr
Teratoma with embryonal carcinoma	3	10-11 yr
Teratoma with malignant neural tissue	1	11 yr
Undifferentiated arrhenoblastoma	1	10 yr
Undifferentiated adenocarcinoma	1	6 yr

Table 23-3. Results of treatment of ovarian cancer in children

	Number of patients	Number living[*]		Number dead	
Pure dysgerminoma	6	6	24-42 mo	0	
Stage I	2	2	42,42 mo	0	
Stage II	2	2	24,36 mo	0	
Stage III	2	2	24,24 mo	0	
Embryonal carcinoma, pure and mixed	9	5	6-36 mo	4	3-10 mo
Stage I	3	2	6,7 mo	1	3 mo
Stage II	4	2	7,36 mo	2	3,10 mo
Stage III	2	1	30 mo	1	4 mo
Teratoma	2	1	12 mo	1	3 mo
Others	2	0		2	4,7 mo

[*]As of November, 1971.

When the tumor is pure dysgerminoma, the patient receives 2000 rads to the entire abdomen with a cobalt 60 unit by the moving strip technique, plus 2000 rads to the pelvis or the para-aortic nodes or both with the 22 mev Betatron. If metastatic cancer is found in the para-aortic lymph nodes at surgery or by lymphangiogram after a 3- to 6-week rest, 2500 rads is given in a 3-week period to the mediastinum and the left supraclavicular nodes. Patients with mixed or poorly differentiated dysgerminoma receive 2600 rads to the entire abdomen and, if indicated, additional pelvic, para-aortic, mediastinal, and supraclavicular irradiation.

These 6 patients with pure dysgerminoma were without evidence of cancer 2 to 3½ years after treatment (Table 23-3). One of the 6 with cancer limited to one ovary (Stage I) did not receive prophylactic irradiation and developed metastatic cancer that could not be resected in the para-aortic nodes 15 months after initial surgical intervention. She was well 20 months after abdominal irradiation by the moving strip technique, followed by irradiation to the pelvis and para-aortic nodes, the mediastinum, and the left supraclavicular nodes.

Embryonal carcinoma

Three of the children in our series had pure embryonal (or endodermal sinus) carcinoma, 3 had mixed dysgerminoma and embryonal carcinoma, and 3 had malignant teratoma with embryonal carcinoma (Table 23-2). Three were Stage I, 4 were Stage II, and 2 were Stage III (Table 23-3).

Patients with embryonal cancer usually had more localized disease than those with other kinds of ovarian cancer, probably because these tumors are fast growing and cause symptoms earlier. Despite this apparently earlier disease, the prognosis associated with these tumors is poor, and postoperative treatment with chemotherapy is essential. Embryonal carcinoma is radioresistant, and postoperative irradiation should be used only when the greater part of the tumor is dysgerminoma or if the tumor has metastasized as dysgerminoma.

Initially the primary treatment is surgical removal of all visible tumor, if possible. Unlike adult patients with ovarian cancer, children with embryonal carcinoma seldom have bilateral disease; both ovaries are affected in only 5% to 10% of these patients, and it is doubtful whether removal of a normal ovary or uterus contributes anything to cure.

Chemotherapy, a combination of actinomycin D, 5-fluorouracil, and cyclophosphamide (ActFuCy) or a combination of vincristine, actinomycin D, and cyclophosphamide (VAC), should be given for a period of from 1 to 2 years, even though the tumor is believed to be completely excised. The dosage and the schedule for these two combinations are shown in Table 23-4. Based on a larger experience with this tumor in adults, we noted that embryonal carcinoma is resistant to a single-agent chemotherapy with the alkylating agents; however, more than 50% of patients will benefit from the combination chemotherapy.[12]

Of the 9 patients, 4 died within 10 months after surgery, and 4 were receiving chemotherapy 6 to 36 months after surgery (Table 23-3). The other patient was without evidence of cancers 3 years after surgery and after 2 years of postoperative treatment with chemotherapy.

Teratoma

Two patients had malignant teratoma in addition to the one who had mixed teratoma and embryonal carcinoma. Treatment for malignant teratoma is similar to that for embryonal carcinoma except that both ovaries and the uterus should be removed, since these tumors are frequently bilateral. Like the embryonal carcinoma, they are radioresistant, but they will frequently respond to a combination regimen of VAC or ActFuCy.

Teratomas with malignant neural tissue are reported to be less virulent than teratomas with other malignant elements.[8] At MDAH, however, two young adults treated for teratoma containing neural elements that were believed to be benign developed widespread intra-abdominal metastases early and died.

Table 23-4. Combination chemotherapy for ovarian cancer

ActFuCy—repeated every 3 wk	
Actinomycin D	0.015 mg/kg/day IV for 5 days (not to exceed 0.5 mg/day)
5-Fluorouracil	8-10 mg/kg/day IV for 5 days
Cyclophosphamide	6-8 mg/kg/day IV for 5 days
VAC	
Vincristine	2 mg/M^2 IV weekly for 8-12 wk (not to exceed 2 mg/wk)
Actinomycin D	0.075 mg/kg IV over 5-7 days, repeated every 6 wk for 1-2 yr
Cyclophosphamide	8-10 mg/kg/day IV over 5-7 days, repeated every 6 wk; given with actinomycin D for 1-2 yr

Stromal cell carcinoma or sex cord mesenchyme carcinoma

One patient in our series had a stromal cell carcinoma; this was an undifferentiated arrhenoblastoma. The stromal tumors such as granulosa cell carcinoma, theca cell cancer, and arrhenoblastoma are often described as hormone producing, but actually most are inactive hormonally, and precocious puberty is a rare occurrence.

The histology of the stromal cancers is often misleading, and it is difficult to predict which tumors will recur or metastasize when the tumor is confined to one ovary. Furthermore, late recurrences are common; granulosa cell carcinoma is reported to recur more frequently after than before the fifth anniversary of the original treatment.[7] These tumors are relatively sensitive to irradiation, but this modality should be used only when metastases are small and localized.

If a granulosa cell cancer or an arrhenoblastoma is present in only one ovary, unilateral salpingo-oophorectomy is probably adequate treatment, since the stromal cell carcinomas are usually unilateral. When the tumor is undifferentiated, there is evidence of pelvic or abdominal metastases, and the masses are less than 2 cm in diameter, total abdominal hysterectomy and bilateral salpingo-oophorectomy with postoperative irradiation is the indicated treatment. If the cancer has spread beyond the abdominal cavity or there are large residual tumor masses, combination treatment with ActFuCy or VAC is indicated.

Epithelial cancer

Only one child in this series had an epithelial cancer, and this diagnosis was made from the biopsy of a metastatic lesion. Children for whom this diagnosis is established should have a total abdominal hysterectomy and bilateral salpingo-oophorectomy. After this treatment the patient should receive irradiation to the entire abdomen if all the tumor is removed or if the residual masses are less than 2 cm in diameter. If the residual masses are larger than 2 cm or if there is tumor outside the peritoneal cavity, the child should receive an alkylating agent rather than irradiation.[10]

UTERINE TUMORS

In his review[5] Huffman was able to find reports of only four adenocarcinomas of the uterine corpus in children, although mixed mesodermal sarcoma of the uterus is occasionally reported. These latter tumors are probably identical to the sarcoma botryoides (embryonal rhabdomyosarcoma) of the vagina and cervix and are included in the same series. One child (34 months of age) in our series who had a sarcoma botryoides of the vagina had an apparent separate focus in the uterine wall.

Adenocarcinoma is the only epithelial cancer of the cervix that has been reported in children. Most of these tumors in children are probably mesonephric in origin.[3] These patients should be treated with a radical hysterectomy and pelvic lymphadenectomy. Although this adenocarcinoma is probably sensitive to irradiation, this type of treatment is impractical for children, since the vagina and uterus are too small for standard radium applicators. The use of external irradiation probably would be less effective than the combination of external irradiation and intracavitary radium used for adults and would cause loss of ovarian function.

VAGINAL TUMORS
Adenocarcinoma

There were no patients with adenocarcinoma of the vagina in our series, but several types of this kind of cancer have been described in pediatric patients. An extremely rare and very virulent endodermal sinus tumor is found in infants.[9] These latter tumors clinically resemble sarcoma botryoides but are histologically identical with embryonal carcinoma of the ovary. Children with these tumors have a poor prognosis; the only possibility for survival is afforded by radical removal of the uterus and the vagina or by exenteration.

The other adenocarcinomas of the vagina are found in older children, usually after menarche. Some are thought to be of mesonephric origin, and others are believed to be of mullerian origin.[4] These tumors are usually extensive, often filling the vagina when the patient is first examined; therefore complete surgical removal including radical hysterectomy, vaginectomy, and pelvic lymphadenectomy has been recommended.[11]

Although radical surgery is the favored treatment for adenocarcinoma of the vagina in pediatric patients, three young adults (under 25 years of age) at our institution have been successfully treated with irradiation. Two of these have had local excision of residual tumor after irradiation; both were free of disease for more than 3 years, and each has a functional vagina. The third patient, 18 years of age, was treated with external irradiation and subsequently by radium applicators.

Sarcoma botryoides

Sarcoma botryoides (embryonal rhabdomyosarcoma) is the most common malignant tumor of the lower genital tract in children. This tumor is also reported under such descriptive names as mixed mesodermal sarcoma or mesenchymal sarcoma. Histologically, the tumors frequently have a myxoid or loose stroma that may resemble embryonic mesenchyme. With proper staining and careful searching, rhabdomyoblasts or striated muscle can often be found.

The diagnosis is occasionally difficult. One 17-year-old patient with a polypoid lesion of the cervix was thought to have a benign cervical polyp because of both histologic and clinical appearances until the lower abdomen was filled with tumor. Another patient with a diagnosis of sarcoma botryoides that was confirmed by several well-known pathologists was found to have a bobby pin in the vagina. After the bobby pin was removed, biopsy specimens were interpreted as normal and have continued to be normal for several years.

Sarcoma botryoides arises in the walls of the vagina, the bladder (Fig. 23-1), the substance of the cervix, or occasionally in the uterine wall; some are multifocal in origin. Abnormal vaginal bleeding is the most common presenting complaint, but occasionally a child will present without bleeding with an edematous polypoid mass protruding through the introitus (Fig. 23-2). Sarcoma botryoides is associated with lymph node metastases. Three of the 8 patients (6 children and 2 young adults) who have been treated surgically at our institution either had lymph node metastases or later developed recurrence in the regional lymph nodes.

The prognosis for patients with sarcoma botryoides has been poor, but the situation has improved with the use of such superradical surgical procedures as pelvic exenteration (Fig. 23-3).[10] Any surgical procedure that divides the vagina or cervix from the bladder or rectum may cut through the tumor and leave microscopic foci behind. It is also necessary to remove the entire vagina or bladder, since sarcoma botryoides may be multifocal.

Among the 6 girls under 14 years of age with sarcoma botryoides in our series, 5 underwent exenteration, and 1 was treated with radical hysterectomy and vaginectomy (Table 23-5). Three who had pelvic exenteration were without evidence of recurrent cancer more than 3 years after the surgical procedure. One who underwent exenteration and pelvic lymphadenectomy had pelvic nodal metastases and died 23 months later, despite treatment with irradiation and chemotherapy. The other, who was treated by exenteration without pelvic lymphadenectomy, died after recurrence of cancer in the pelvic nodes. The child who underwent radical hysterectomy and vaginectomy developed recurrent cancer 4 months later and died 8 months after treatment.

Three children with sarcoma botryoides have received chemotherapy for recurrent cancer. One had a complete disappearance of a large pelvic mass after chemotherapy and survived for a total of 28 months after the recurrence was noted. She received vincristine weekly for 18 weeks with concomitant external pelvic irradiation for 5 weeks; VAC was given for 8 months when the tumor recurred a second time.

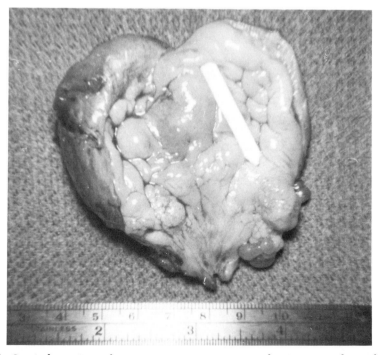

Fig. 23-1. Surgical specimen from an anterior exenteration showing an embryonal rhabdomyosarcoma in opened bladder. (Courtesy Medical Communications, The University of Texas at Houston, M. D. Anderson Hospital and Tumor Institute.)

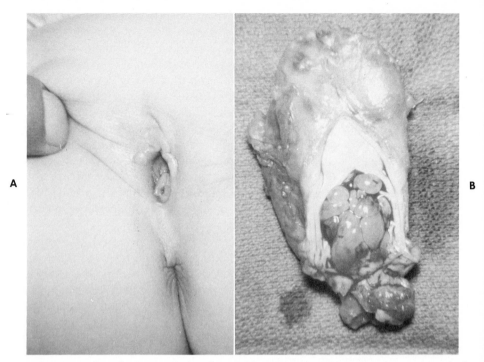

Fig. 23-2. A, Polypoid sarcoma botryoides of the vagina. **B,** Same patient as in **A,** with the anterior vagina opened. (Courtesy Medical Communications, The University of Texas at Houston, M. D. Anderson Hospital and Tumor Institute.)

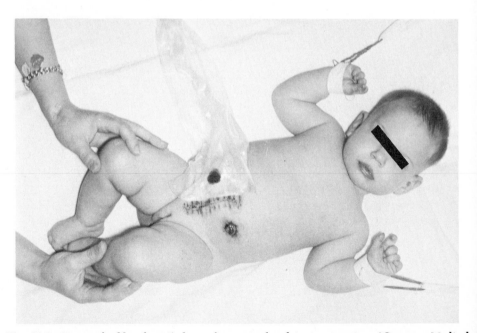

Fig. 23-3. Six-month-old infant 7 days after a total pelvic exenteration. (Courtesy Medical Communications, The University of Texas at Houston, M. D. Anderson Hospital and Tumor Institute.)

Table 23-5. Sarcoma botryoides of the pelvis

Age	Site	Histology	Primary treatment	Result
23 mo	Vagina	Embryonal rhabdo-myosarcoma	Total exenteration	Dead (34 mo)
34 mo	Vagina	Mixed mesodermal sarcoma	Radical hysterectomy	Dead (8 mo)
6 mo	Vagina	Sarcoma botryoides	Total exenteration	Living (75 mo)
27 mo	Vagina	Sarcoma botryoides	Total exenteration	Living (10½ yr)
4 yr	Bladder	Embryonal rhabdo-myosarcoma	Anterior exenteration	Living (30 mo)
6 yr	Bladder	Embryonal rhabdo-myosarcoma	Anterior exenteration	Dead (23 mo)

TUMORS OF THE VULVA AND PERINEUM

Huffman[5] reported only 7 cases of epithelial vulvar carcinoma in pediatric patients in his review. Sarcomas of the vulva are also uncommon but are more frequently reported than carcinomas. Our series of 28 patients contained 2 with sarcoma of the vulva.

The best treatment for these uncommon tumors is difficult to determine, but by utilizing knowledge of the natural history of sarcoma in older children and adults, some guidelines can be formulated. The fibrosarcomas, leiomyosarcomas, and probably most undifferentiated sarcomas should be widely excised with a clear margin of normal tissue, but regional lymphadenectomy is unnecessary unless the tumor is a rhabdomyosarcoma. Neither is it essential to remove all the vulva as is indicated in squamous cell carcinoma of the vulva in older women, since these tumors are seldom multifocal.

The rhabdomyosarcomas of the vulva and perineum are very virulent, and possibly the best treatment is a combination of irradiation and chemotherapy. Three older teen-agers with rhabdomyosarcoma of the pelvis have been treated with regional arterial infusions of vincristine plus external irradiation. All received vincristine, 0.015 to 0.02 mg/kg as a continuous intra-arterial infusion 5 to 7 days weekly for 5 weeks. They also received 5000 rads of external irradiation to the tumor area through anterior and posterior portals or through a perineal portal. All had severe neurologic toxicity, which included personality changes, severe pain, and severe but temporary motor loss in the legs. However, two are without evidence of recurrent disease at the present time; the third died of widespread distant metastasis shortly after treament was completed. There was no evidence of cancer in the perineal area.

SUMMARY

Although at one time malignant gynecologic tumors in pediatric patients were almost always lethal, today some success can be achieved with better understanding of the behavior of these tumors and the use of radical measures. Specifically, our experience with 28 patients has indicated the following:

1. Location and treatment with adequate irradiation of the sites of metastatic disease may afford the patient with dysgerminoma of the ovary a chance for cure.

2. Intensive chemotherapy in addition to the indicated surgical procedure may benefit children with embryonal carcinoma of the ovary.

3. Children with sarcoma botryoides, once a uniformly fatal disease, may be cured with pelvic exenteration in uncomplicated cases. When tumor size is unfavorable, preoperative chemotherapy or chemotherapy and irradiation may improve results.

4. The combination of chemotherapy and irradiation for patients with rhabdomyosarcoma of the pelvis may prove to be the most effective treatment.

REFERENCES

1. Annual report on the results of treatment in carcinoma of the uterus and vagina, vol. 14, published under the patronage of the International Federation of Gynecology and Obstetrics, Stockholm, 1967, AB P.A. Norstedt & Söner, p. 30.
2. Burns, B. D., Jr., Underwood, P. B., Jr., and Rutledge, F. N.: A review of carcinoma of the ovary at The University of Texas M. D. Anderson Hospital and Tumor Institute at Houston. In Cancer of the uterus and ovary, Chicago, 1969, Year Book Medical Publishers, Inc., pp. 123-147.
3. Fawcett, K. J., Dockerty, M. B., and Hunt, A. B.: Mesonephric carcinoma and adenocarcinoma of the cervix in children, J. Pediatr. **69:**104-110, 1966.
4. Herbst, A. L., and Scully, R. E.: Adenocarcinoma of the vagina in adolescence, Cancer **25:**745-757, 1970.
5. Huffman, J. W.: The gynecology of childhood and adolescence, Philadelphia, 1968, W. B. Saunders Co.
6. Kaplan, A., and Acosta, A.: Personal communication.
7. Kottmeier, H. L.: Carcinoma of the female genitalia, Baltimore, 1953, The Williams & Wilkins Co., pp. 174-192.
8. Mayberger, H. W., Carlson, A. S., and Lim, S.: Immature neural elements (neuroblastomatous change) in benign cystic teratoma: malignant or not? J. Obstet. Gynecol. **32:**114-117, 1969.
9. Norris, H. J., Bagley, G. P., and Taylor, H. E.: Carcinoma of the infant vagina, Arch. Pathol. **90:**473-479, 1970.
10. Rutledge, F., and Sullivan, M. P.: Sarcoma botryoides, Ann. N. Y. Acad. Sci. **142:**694-708, 1967.
11. Smith, F. R.: Primary carcinoma of the vagina, Am. J. Obstet. Gynecol. **69:**525-537, 1955.
12. Smith, J. P.: Unpublished data.

CHAPTER 24

Tumors of the endocrine glands

GEORGE W. CLAYTON

Malignant tumors of the endocrine glands are rare but constitute a diverse and highly interesting group of neoplasms. These tumors frequently secrete the native hormone, producing symptoms of hormone excess such as cortisol hypersecretion (Cushing's syndrome) in cancer of the adrenal cortex, or they may produce in excess intermediate products of hormone synthesis as seen in virilizing or feminizing tumors of the adrenal cortex. Of great interest have been those tumors that secrete substances that have the effect of pituitary trophic hormones. These are the choriocarcinomas, which produce a gonadotropin-like substance, and certain cancers of the lung, which secrete adrenocorticotropin-like substances.

Dysgenetic endocrine tissue tends to undergo malignant degenerations, and the etiologic factors are poorly understood. The risk of malignancy in the dysgenetic male gonad is high.

Cancer of the testes and ovaries in children is extensively covered in Chapters 22 and 23; hence this chapter will primarily be devoted to malignant tumors of the thyroid and adrenal cortex. In addition, discussions on cancer in the dysgenetic gonad and tumors producing substances with endocrine functions are included.

THYROID CARCINOMA

In a survey on the incidence of thyroid carcinoma in children in 1951, Winship[26] found reports of 93 cases in the literature and 95 cases from a survey of hospitals and medical centers. In the next 10 years, he was able to obtain reports of over 600 cases.[27] These reports demonstrate that the pathogenesis of the disease in children differs from that in adults primarily in that there is a high incidence in children with previous irradiation to the neck for such conditions as thymic enlargement, hemangioma, and cervical adenopathy. In addition, children exhibit a greater relative frequency of papillary carcinoma as compared to other types and a greater incidence of metastasis at the time of diagnosis. That thyroid carcinoma is only twice as common in females as in males is unique, since thyroid disease in general is much more common in females in a ratio of 7:1. Some investigators believe that there has been an increase in the incidence of reported cases of thyroid carcinoma in childhood in recent years, but since the incidence of irradiation to the region of the thyroid has markedly decreased, it is thought that the incidence of thyroid cancer should as well.

Pathology

Although there are great differences between types of thyroid neoplasms, it would seem that the best classification for those occurring in children is as follows: *differentiated forms,* papillary and follicular carcinomas, which are most commonly seen in children, and *undifferentiated forms,* solid and anaplastic tumors, which occur for the most part in adults.[18]

   Differentiated forms. Papillary carcinomas (Fig. 24-1) appear as pink or dark red, circumscribed, moderately soft masses that on cut surface are finely divided, soft, and friable. They may be single or multiple, and multiple microscopic foci may be present. Histologically, they are usually well differentiated. The cells are uniformly columnar with few mitoses and are supported by vascularized connective tissue stalks. Pink-staining material that resembles colloid but contains no iodine lies between the papillae. Psammoma bodies are common. These are concentrically layered calcium deposits that are characteristic of the tumor. These tumors tend to infiltrate the surrounding tissues by direct extension. Metastases occur in the regional lymph nodes and lungs. Invasion of the trachea and esophagus or systemic involvement occurs occasionally.

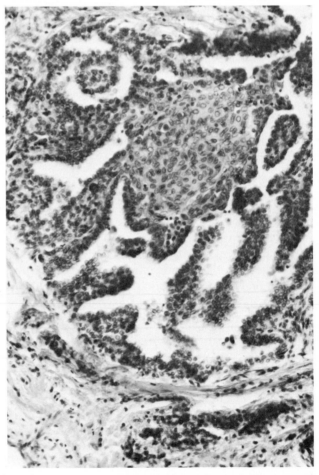

Fig. 24-1. Papillary carcinoma. (Courtesy Department of Visual Education, Baylor University College of Medicine.)

Follicular carcinoma (Fig. 24-2) is homogenous and yellow. Histologically, it consists of a microfollicular pattern in which the cells and nuclei have dense chromatin and heavy nuclear membranes and mitoses are common. Papillary and mixed papillary-follicular tumors are most commonly seen in children.

Undifferentiated forms. Undifferentiated, or anaplastic, carcinoma may be made up of a variety of cell types consisting of spindle, giant, or squamous cells. In these types metaplasia is common. These tumors grow and spread by local extension very rapidly. Prognosis is usually poor. In those series of carcinoma of the thyroid in children that report cell types, the incidence of anaplastic carcinoma is very low and in some completely absent.

Medullary carcinoma. Medullary carcinoma of the thyroid is a recently described tumor that occasionally occurs in children.[24] It probably arises from follicular cells and has distinctive clinical features. It may occur as an autosomal dominant trait in some families and is associated with pheochromocytomas and

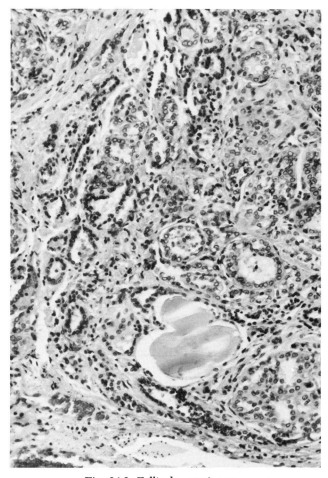

Fig. 24-2. Follicular carcinoma.

neuromas. Clinical symptoms due to secretion by the tumor of calcitonin, serotonin, and prostaglandins may occur. Metastases to lymph nodes may occur. Surgery seems to be the only effective therapy.

Pathogenesis

Experimental thyroid carcinoma has been produced in a number of ways, but its production has usually been based on an increased secretion of thyrotropin (TSH). Experimental neoplasms have been produced by the long-term administration of thiourea derivatives to rats.[16] Regression of these tumors was brought about by administering thyroid hormone. Thyrotropin-secreting pituitary tumors grafted into rats produced thyroid hyperplasia and adenomatous and malignant changes.[10] Radiation, both external and internal, has been used to produce experimental thyroid cancer. Doniach[4] produced thyroid cancer in rats, using a combination of ^{131}I and methylthiouracil. Goldberg and Chaikoff[9] reported the occurrence of thyroid carcinoma in rats receiving 400 μc of ^{131}I. However, Doniach[4] reported that similarly high doses of ^{131}I so damaged the thyroid epithelium that it was incapable of producing experimental thyroid carcinoma. External radiation also has a carcinogenic effect when combined with methylthiouracil administration.[5, 12] These studies suggest that radiation alone is incapable of carcinogenesis, unless there is prolonged thyrotropin stimulation of the thyroid. In addition, iodine deprivation and goitrogen ingestion act to stimulate thyrotropin secretion, which may in turn produce thyroid hyperplasia, adenoma, and carcinoma. Most studies indicate that experimental thyroid cancer is initially hormone dependent, but autonomy may eventually occur.

Duffy and Fitzgerald[6] were the first to report an association between irradiation therapy in infancy and the later occurrence of thyroid carcinoma. Of 28 patients reported with thyroid carcinoma, 10 had received thymic radiation during infancy. Many other investigators have confirmed this observation.* Many instances of x-ray therapy given during infancy and early childhood for thymic enlargement, tonsillar and adenoidal hypertrophy, hemangiomas, cystic hygroma of the neck, cervical adenitis, and mastoiditis have been reported with the later occurrence of thyroid carcinoma. It has been reported that radioactive fallout may be a causal factor in the development of thyroid cancer.[11, 20] Winship[27] reported that a history of prior irradiation was found in as high as 80% of patients with thyroid cancer in children. Although some have doubted the association, it seems certain that the thyroid gland in infancy and early childhood is highly susceptible to ionizing radiation. The incidence of deaths due to thyroid carcinoma in Switzerland decreased in the endemic goiter region with the introduction of iodized salt, but no such correlation has been found in this country.[14] The occurrence of cancer in patients with enzymatic defects in the synthesis of thyroxine has been reported.[7, 22] Wilkins and co-workers[23] reported a goitrous cretin who was inadequately treated for a long period. Histologically, the thyroid contained areas suggesting carcinoma, although no capsular or vascular invasion could be found. Other reports[19] have concluded that the changes represent hyper-

---

*References 2, 3, 8, 13, 17, 25.

plasia and nodule formation due to intense thyrotropin stimulation and are not true neoplastic changes.

The role of therapeutic or diagnostic doses of ^{131}I as a possible cause of carcinoma of the thyroid in infancy and childhood has not been established.

Clinical manifestations

The finding of a nodule in the thyroid of a child is very suggestive of carcinoma and should prompt immediate diagnosis and treatment. The nodule is usually very firm and irregular, but it may be smooth and circumscribed. Generalized enlargement of the thyroid may be present, since carcinoma and thyroiditis may occur concomitantly. Cervical metastases are frequent and may be unilateral or bilateral. Pulmonary metastases are said to be present in as high as 30% of patients at the time of diagnosis and are often mistaken for inflammatory conditions of the lung. Although the majority of children with thyroid carcinoma are euthyroid, instances of associated hyperthyroidism have been reported.[21] Hypothyroidism is extremely rare.

Most tests that measure the functional capacity of the thyroid such as the PBI, BEI, and radioiodine uptake are of little value. Scan studies usually reveal a decreased concentration of radioiodine in the nodule. Concentration of radioiodine in metastases is uncommon. Functional follicular adenomas, or those accumulating an increase of radioiodine, are rare in children. The uptake of radioactive phosphorus (^{32}P) by thyroid cancer has been used with some success in the diagnosis[1] but has not been evaluated in children. Psammoma bodies or calcific masses may be demonstrated on x-ray examination of the soft tissues of the neck.

Therapy

It is well known that carcinoma of the thyroid is compatible with long life and that the disease in many instances has a very slow progression. Long survival after the diagnosis has been made is not uncommon, and recurrence after as long as 20 years is not unusual. This is particularly true in childhood. Despite its benign nature in children, a fatal outcome occurs in a definite number of the patients afflicted. In Winship's[27] series of 602 cases, 63 died within 5 years of diagnosis, 19 within 10 years of diagnosis, and 25 10 years after diagnosis.

Total thyroidectomy is the treatment of choice, thus eliminating the possible presence of microscopic foci of tumor within apparently unaffected thyroid tissue as possible sites of recurrence. Surgery is indicated even if distal metastases are present. Radical neck dissection has no place in the therapy of carcinoma of the thyroid in children. Affected lymph nodes should be removed at the time of thyroidectomy and later if additional nodes appear.

The complications of surgical management are those that are attendant to thyroidectomy for any cause, and the more extensive the surgical procedure, the greater the incidence and severity of complications. It is thought by some that residual thyroid tissue remaining after surgery should be eliminated by administering therapeutic doses of radioiodine. In addition, radioiodine may be indicated if there is extensive local disease or metastases.

Stimulation of the tumor by thyrotropin before the therapeutic administration of radioiodine is mandatory. If the patient is receiving thyroid hormone, it should be discontinued.

There is an increased incidence of leukemia after radioiodine therapy for thyroid carcinoma.[15] Other complications of radioiodine therapy have been pulmonary fibrosis in patients with pulmonary metastases, sterility, and bone marrow depression with pancytopenia.

Thyroid hormone in doses somewhat greater than physiologic requirements should always be given after surgical and/or radioiodine therapy has been carried out. Many investigators believe that in those cancers that are hormone dependent, complete inhibition of thyrotropin secretion will eliminate the stimulus for further tumor growth. In such instances, metastases may regress or disappear when thyroid therapy is instituted. This may not be true in every instance, but it is now recognized that thyroid therapy is an important adjuvant in the therapy of thyroid cancer. It is particularly applicable to young patients in whom the administration of large doses of radioiodine is thought to be hazardous and when there is such extensive pulmonary involvement that radioiodine therapy might result in pulmonary fibrosis.

CANCER OF THE ADRENAL CORTEX

Cancer of the adrenal cortex in children is rare, and its incidence is relatively unknown. As in other functional endocrine tumors, the distinction between carcinoma and benign adenoma is frequently difficult insofar as clinical manifestations are concerned.

Tumors producing virilism are said to be the most common. In a series reported by Bierich,[28] there were 134 children, of whom 40 were boys and 94 girls. Virilizing tumors occurred in 76, whereas 52 demonstrated evidence of Cushing's syndrome, the majority with evidence of virilism. Feminizing tumors are rare, as are aldosterone-secreting tumors. There is a greater incidence of functional adrenal tumors in females than in males, and the reason is unexplained. Primary nonfunction adenocarcinoma of the adrenal does occur, but the incidence is unknown. The occurrence of Cushing's syndrome due to tumors of the adrenal in young infants in association with hemihypertrophy, urinary tract anomalies, and various other anomalies[29] suggests oncogenic factors occurring during embryonic development. Otherwise the cause of tumors of the adrenal cortex is unknown. (Further details may be found in articles and texts pertaining to adrenal cortical carcinomas listed in the general references, p. 539.)

Adrenal tumors causing virilism

These tumors may rarely occur in infants but most commonly occur after 2 years of age.[38, 41] They elaborate large quantities of dehydroepiandrosterone (DHIA), a naturally occurring 17-ketosteroid, and although this adrenal steriod is a weak androgen, it is probably responsible for the virilization. Conversion of DHIA into more potent androgens such as Δ 4-androstenedione and testosterone may occur. In addition, some tumors, produce excessive amounts of cortisol, resulting in symptoms of Cushing's disease as well as virilization.

The manifestations are those of excessive androgen production, with rapid growth, increased muscle mass, and accelerated epiphyseal development in the preadolescent child. In the boy the classic signs of puberty—enlargement of the penis, the appearance of pubic and axillary hair, wrinkling and stippling of the scrotum, and the appearance of acne and seborrhea—are seen. In the girl there is enlargement of the clitoris and labia majora, as well as the appearance of pubic and axillary hair, seborrhea, and acne. In children with excessive cortisol secretion the excess may be considerably less evident in the presence of excessive androgen production.

The differential diagnosis in the boy is that of constitutional sexual precocity, interstitial cell tumor of the testis, and the late appearance of signs of congenital adrenal hyperplasia. The testes of boys with virilizing adrenal tumors remain small, which may help differentiate this condition from sexual precocity and testicular tumors, but the signs may be undistinguishable from congenital hyperplasia and require precise laboratory studies. In the girl virilizing neoplasms of the adrenal must be differentiated from mild adrenal hyperplasia with late onset of virilism and rarely from acquired adrenal hyperplasia or arrhenoblastoma of the ovary. In both sexes the early appearance of pubic and axillary hair, which has been called *premature pubarche* by Wilkins,[36] may be indistinguishable from the early signs of adrenal tumor.

The diagnosis of a virilizing adrenal tumor may be made only by means of accurate endocrine laboratory studies. Usually the urinary 17-ketosteroids are markedly elevated, much more so than in other virilizing conditions, as are the levels of 17-ketosteroid sulfates in the plasma. In our laboratory we have had one sample with levels of over 1000 mcg/100 ml in the plasma. The most prominent steroid in the urine is usually 5-androstane, 3-β-ol, 17-one, dehydroepiandrosterone, and this compound may account for the preponderance of urinary ketosteroid excretion. Dehydroepiandrosterone may be assayed by a number of practical methods, the most prominent of which is the "Allen blue test."[37, 42] In children with cushingoid features, cortisol, its metabolites, and precursors may be excreted in large quantities. In addition, large quantities of adrenal estrogens may also be found. Administration of corticosteroids fails to cause a fall in 17-ketosteroid excretion and may be important in differentiating virilizing tumors from adrenal hyperplasia.[40] In sexual precocity and premature development of pubic and axillary hair the excretion of 17-ketosteroids is of normal pubertal levels or perhaps below pubertal levels. In very rare instances of interstitial cell tumor of the testis the urinary 17-ketosteroid excretion is as great as in adrenal tumors, but the principal excretory product is androsterone rather than dehydroepiandrosterone.

It is not possible to differentiate virilizing adenomas from carcinomas on the basis of laboratory studies, and frequently children with metastasis continue to grow excessively, gain weight, and generally appear well.

If a tumor is suspected, intravenous pyelography may demonstrate it. Very small tumors may be difficult to demonstrate by the usual means, and procedures such as presacral air insufflation are generally not helpful, although tomography may be. Bone x-ray films reveal a marked advance in osseous maturation.

The treatment is surgical. The tumor is usually unilateral but may be bilateral in approximately 10% of the cases. The majority are well encapsulated and histologically appear to be adenomas but may recur locally, whereas tumors showing capsular and blood vessel invasion when removed frequently never recur (Fig. 24-3). Metastasis at the time of surgery is evidence of malignancy, and there is

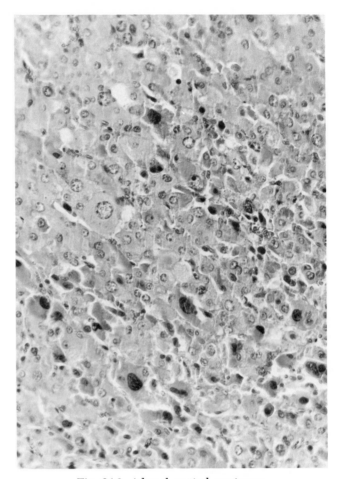

Fig. 24-3. Adrenal cortical carcinoma.

no satisfactory therapy. *o, p′*-DDD may reduce signs of virilism and, according to Hutter and Kayhoe,[39] may prolong life.

Case 1 (Fig. 24-4). R. J., a 3½-year-old boy, began having signs of virilism 2 months prior to admission. The pregnancy and delivery had been normal, and the child had had no serious illnesses or injuries. Two months prior to admission pubic hair was noted, and this increased. His penis became larger, and he developed acneform lesions on the face. His appetite was excellent.

Examination showed a height age of 6½ years. He was a muscular boy with a deep voice. The dental age was normal. Acne was present on the face and shoulders. The penis was enlarged (10 by 2 cm); the testes measured 2.8 by 1.5 cm bilaterally. The scrotum was wrinkled and stippled. Pubic and axillary hair was abundant. An ill-defined mass was palpable in the right upper quadrant.

Laboratory examination revealed a bone age of 9 years; a flat plate of the abdomen was normal. The 17-ketosteroid level was 40 mg/24 hr (normal: 1-2 mg/24 hr), the 17OH corticoid level was 1.7 mg/100 ml (normal: 0.5-1 mg/24 hr), 17-ketosteroid fractionation revealed 21 mg (normal: 0.5-1 mg/24 hr) DHIA. A dexamethasone test was carried out, and there was no suppression of the 17-ketosteroids.

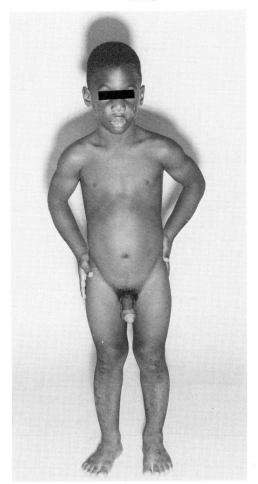

Fig. 24-4. Boy, 4½ years old, with virilizing tumor of the adrenal cortex.

An intravenous pyelogram showed depression of the right kidney.

At surgery a large, oval, well-encapsulated tumor was found. Histologic examination revealed capsular and blood vessel invasion; however, the patient is well 7 years after surgery.

Adrenal tumors causing Cushing's disease

Cushing's syndrome is due to the overproduction of cortisol by the adrenal cortex in children and may be caused by either cancer, adenoma, or adrenal hyperplasia. In general, adrenal hyperplasia occurs in older age groups, whereas cancer of the adrenal tends to occur in infants and young children.[45] Cushing's syndrome is extremely rare in pure form when due to tumor, since there is frequently an element of virilism and occasionally signs of feminization.

The pathogenesis of adrenal cortical neoplasms causing Cushing's syndrome is unknown. The manifestations of Cushing's syndrome are due to excessive cortisol secretion and result from its effect on carbohydrate and protein metabolism. Excessive cortisol secretions result in diversion of amino acids from protein synthesis to glucose and eventually to fat. The inhibition of protein synthesis causes muscle wasting, osteoporosis, and growth retardation, although there is evidence that excessive cortisal inhibits growth hormone secretion. Hypertension may be due to excessive cortisol or aldosterone secretion. Virilism is due either to androgen or cortisol excess.

Clinical manifestations. The major clinical manifestation in infants and children is obesity, which is progressive and may be extreme. Deposits of fat characteristically occur in the cheeks, causing a "fish-mouth" appearance and obscuring the ears, in the pectoral girdle, resulting in the well-known "buffalo hump," and over the trunk. In infants obesity may be generalized, whereas in older children the extremities may appear thin due to muscle wasting. Muscle weakness may be profound. The face appears plethoric with downy hair on the cheeks. Acne and seborrhea may be present. Retardation of growth is inevitably present. Striae, which progress from pink to violaceous, may appear on the abdomen and legs, although they are rarely seen in infants and very young children. Signs of virilism are frequently present. Hypertension may be extreme, and cardiomegaly may be present. Psychotic behavior, which is common in adults, is rare in children, although infants exhibit marked irritability and difficulty in sleeping. Infants may have enormous appetites.

Laboratory findings and diagnosis. Skeletal x-ray films may reveal osteoporosis and retardation of epiphyseal development. The vertebrae may be compressed, and fractures may occur, resulting in back pain in older children. Elevation of hemoglobin and hematocrit levels and neutrophilia, as well as lymphopenia and eosinopenia, are frequently found. Hypokalemia and hypokalemic alkalosis may be severe.[43] Changes in the electrocardiogram are frequent because of hypertension and occasionally hypokalemia.

In Cushing's disease due to carcinoma the levels of plasma cortisol and excretion of urinary corticosteroids are markedly increased above levels found in Cushing's disease due to adrenal hyperplasia, adenoma, and obesity. In addition, ACTH administration causes no change in plasma levels and excretory values in infants and children with cancer, whereas children with adrenal hyperplasia demonstrate hyperresponsiveness, exogenously obese children show a normal response, and children with benign adenomas demonstrate a subnormal response. The same responses are also obtained when metyrapone (Metopirone) is administered.

Dexamethasone suppression tests may also help differentiate adrenal neoplasia from hyperplasia.[47] Large doses (2 mg) will suppress corticosteroid excretion in the child with adrenal hyperplasia but not in those with adrenal tumors.[48]

Increased excretion of 17-ketosteroids, pregnanetriol, and estrogens is suggestive of adrenal carcinoma. Increased aldosterone excretion has been reported in some instances.[46]

Approximately 50% of the cases of Cushing's syndrome in childhood are due to carcinoma. Of the remaining, most are due to bilateral adrenal cortical hyperplasia and are in general found in older children and adolescents. Perhaps 15% are due to benign adenomas and a very small group due to ACTH-secreting tumors.

Treatment. The treatment of Cushing's syndrome due to adrenal neoplasm is surgical. An anterior transverse incision is believed to be the approach of choice because both adrenals may be affected. Intramuscular injections of corticosteroids before and intravenous infusions of corticosteroids during the procedure are mandatory. If one adrenal is involved, suppression of the hypothalamic-pituitary-adrenal axis will result in atrophy of the contralateral adrenal, necessitating the use of corticosteroids during convalescence with subsequent tapering of dose. The use of ACTH to stimulate the atrophic contralateral adrenal has been recommended by some.[44] If both adrenals are removed, mineralocorticoids such as desoxycorticosterone and 9 α-fluorohydrocortisone may be required. Prognosis after surgery is unpredictable unless there are definite signs of metastasis. Recurrence after many years has been reported. Metastatic disease may be manifested by a complete alteration of symptomatology and hormonal excretion. Instead of the cushingoid features returning predominantly, virilizing or feminizing processes may occur, and in some instances metastasis may occur without increased hormonal secretion. Treatment with aminoglutethimide or o, p'-DDD may control the progress of metastatic disease.

Case 2 (Fig. 24-5). N. M. K. was born on October 28, 1959, to a gravida I, Para 1, 25-year-old mother after a full-term, uncomplicated pregnancy. Her birth weight and length were 4313 gm and 49.5 cm, respectively. A 4 cm, soft, red-purple mass was present over the midline of the lumbar area. Diagnosis of hemangioma or lipoma was entertained at this time. The left side of the tongue was noted to be larger than the right side. During the first 5 days of life she lost approximately 450 gm. The mother felt that she was not a normal baby. But no clear reason was given for this except that "she did not sleep like a normal baby." At the age of 1 month her weight was 4313 gm. At 6 weeks of age she began to rapidly deposit fat on the face, the posterior aspect of the neck, and over the pubis. At 2 months, hirsutism on the face, forehead, and pubic area was noted, as was clitoral enlargement. She became irritable, and her blood pressure was noted to be "abnormally high."

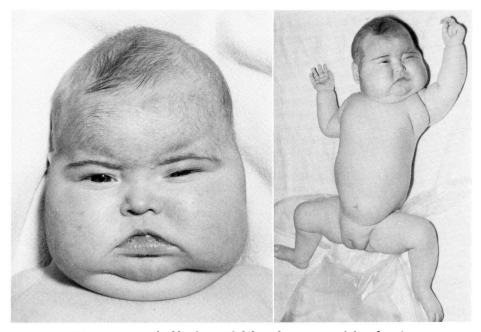

Fig. 24-5. Fourteen-week-old infant with bilateral carcinoma of the adrenal cortex.

She entered Texas Children's Hospital on December 4, 1959, at the age of 14 weeks. Physical examination revealed a weight of 6129 gm (approximately 60th percentile) and a length of 60 cm (the 3rd percentile). She appeared flabby, with a plethoric "moon" facies. There was a mild degree of acne and fine pubic and facial hair, more prominent on the forehead and cheeks. The left side of the tongue was larger than the right side and appeared to be deviated to the right. Her respirations were rapid and grunting. The blood pressure was 160/90. The labia majora were flabby and increased in size, and the clitoris was slightly enlarged. The muscular development of the extremities and spinal region appeared to be diminished. A movable 6 by 6 cm mass in the right lumbosacral area was present. Abdominal palpation revealed a 4 to 5 cm mass in the right upper quadrant. The left kidney was easily palpated. Laboratory examinations revealed 141 mEq/L of Na, 5.8 mEq/L of K, 104 mEq/L of Cl, and 22.5 mM/L of CO_2. The hemoglobin was 16.9 gm/100 ml, the hematocrit 51, and the white blood cell count 11,400. Electrocardiogram revealed left ventricular hypertrophy. X-ray examination of the skull, chest, and abdomen showed milk osteoporosis of the thoracic cage and shoulder girdle. The heart was slightly enlarged. Vaginal smear was negative for estrogenic effect. Urinary 17-ketosteroids (17-KS) and 17-hydroxycorticosteroids (17-OHCS) were 13.85 and 3.98 mg/24 hr, respectively. The plasma 17OH corticoids were 80 mg/100 ml before and after an infusion of ACTH.

Three days after admission the patient underwent surgery. Both adrenals and the left lobe of the liver contained tumor. A bilateral adrenalectomy and left hepaticolobectomy were carried out. The right adrenal gland was enlarged, measuring 4.5 by 2 by 1.2 cm and weighing 4.5 gm. At one pole of the gland the normal architecture was distorted by a subcapsular and somewhat rubbery nodule measuring 2 by 1.5 by 1 cm. Its sectioned surface was smooth and yellow-brown, with numerous golden yellow and red striations. The central part of the gland had a large hemorrhagic cyst with a necrotic center. The left adrenal appeared hemorrhagic; it measured 3.5 by 1.9 by 2 cm and weighed 2 gm. On the posterior edge of the left lobe of the liver there was a 4.5 cm subcapsular spheric neoplastic growth. Its sectioned surface was similar in appearance to that described in the adrenals. The rest of the liver was normal. Pathologic examination revealed carcinoma of both adrenals with metastasis to the liver.

The 17-ketosteroids returned to zero on the fourth postoperative day. The patient was discharged from the hospital 8 weeks after admission. She was maintained on a regimen of cortisone acetate and desoxycorticosterone. The blood pressure normalized, and the acne, hirsutism, excessive fat, and pubic hair generally regressed and disappeared over a period of several months.

She was observed in the outpatient clinic at regular intervals for control and implantation of desoxycorticosterone acetate (Doca) pellets. Bilateral bowing of the legs was noted at 9 months of age. The hypertrophy of the right side of the tongue persisted. She was readmitted to Texas Children's Hospital on June 5, 1962, at the age of 33 months for removal of a lipoma of the lumbar region. The lipoma was noted to extend intravertebrally and attached to the cauda equina. The lipoma was incompletely removed, but she was discharged a few days later in good condition.

Her development has been slow since the age of 14 months. At that time her weight was 8850 kg (approximately 18th percentile) and her length 69.8 cm (less than 3rd percentile). Thereafter her weight has always been in the 10th percentile or below and her length below the 3rd percentile. Ten years postoperatively she has no evidence of recurrence.

Feminizing tumors

Feminizing tumors are extremely rare in childhood, with less than a dozen reported in the last 50 years.[49-54] The majority have been reported in boys.

In addition to the appearance of breasts, there are inevitably signs of virilism such as pubic and axillary hair and acne. Enlargement of the penis or clitoris, however, does not occur. Menses have been reported in girls with this tumor, Although the height may be increased, ossesous development is usually accelerated to a greater degree. In some instances hypertension has been recorded.

The urinary 17-ketosteroid excretion is elevated, occasionally to high levels, the major portion being dehydroepiandrosterone. The 17-hydroxycorticoids may also be elevated. Estrogen excretion is moderately elevated, with the principal estrogens estrone and estradiol.

The tumors are usually unilateral, and approximately half the reported cases have been carcinomas.

Aldosterone-secreting tumors

Aldosterone-secreting tumors have been reported in children but are extremely rare.[55-58] They are usually benign and must be differentiated from primary aldosteronism due to adrenal hyperplasia.

NEOPLASIA IN UNDESCENDED TESTES AND IN TESTICULAR DYSGENESIS

Although frequently deemphasized, malignancy in undescended testes occurs with considerable frequency if true cryptorchidism is differentiated from retractile testes.[59, 60] It has been estimated that malignancies develop in 5% of abdominal testes and in 1% of inguinal testes. The relatively high incidence of malignancy in abdominal testes suggests that they are initially abnormal and position does not predispose them to malignant change. In addition, the risk is not changed by surgery; hence an effort to preserve the abdominal testes is not believed to be warranted. The tumors are frequently seminomas, which, as has been pointed out previously, are extremely rare in childhood.

There is a high incidence of neoplasia in a number of conditions in which the testis is dysgenetic. These include male pseudohermaphroditism, which may be due to a variety of causes, the syndrome of feminizing testes, and true hermaphroditism. Melicow and Unson[61] reviewed 140 cases of gonadal neoplasia in patients with ambiguous genitalia and added 5 patients. Seminoma and gonadoblastoma are the two neoplasms most often associated with dysgenetic gonads.

Table 24-1. Malignant tumors in children secreting hormone or hormonelike substances

Tumor	Hormone(s) produced	Syndrome
Thyroid carcinoma	Thyroxine	Hyperthyroidism
Medullary tumor of thyroid	5-Hydroxytryptophan	Carcinoid syndrome
Carcinoid	Serotonins ACTH-CRF?	Cushing's syndrome
Adrenal carcinoma	Cortisol	Cushing's syndrome
	Aldosterone	Conn syndrome
	Androgen	Precocity in male; virilism in female
	Estrogen	Feminizing tumors
Granulosa cell tumor of ovary	Estrogen	Feminization
Sertoli cell tumor of testis	Estrogen	Feminization
Sertoli-Leydig cell tumor of ovary	Androgens	Virilism
Leydig cell tumor of testis	Androgens	Virilism
Choriocarcinoma hepatoma	Gonadotropins	Sexual precocity

The occurrence of these tumors is rare in childhood, and the risk of tumor in dysgenetic gonad seems to increase with the occurrence of gonadotropin stimulation. Inasmuch as gonadotropin release frequently occurs early in many instances of testicular dysgenesis, it would seem highly indicated to remove these gonads at an early age. It is thought that the testis should be preserved only if testis biopsy appears normal and the testis is normally located, and even then there is probably an increased risk of malignancy.

TUMORS SECRETING HORMONE OR HORMONELIKE SUBSTANCES

Certain malignant tumors secrete hormone or hormonelike substances. They have been listed in Table 24-1, and the associated clinical syndromes have been indicated.

REFERENCES
Thyroid carcinoma

1. Ackerman, M. B., Shahon, D. B., and Marvin, J. F.: The diagnosis of thyroid cancer with radioactive phosphorus, Surgery **47**:615, 1960.
2. Clark, D. E.: Association of irradiation with cancer of thyroid in children and adolescents, J.A.M.A. **159**:1007-1009, 1955.
3. Crile, G. Jr.: Carcinoma of the thyroid in children, Ann. Surg. **150**:959, 1959.
4. Doniach, I.: Effect of radioactive iodine alone and in combination with methylthiouracil upon tumor production in the rat's thyroid gland, Br. J. Cancer **7**:181-202, June, 1953.
5. Doniach, I.: Comparison of the carcinogenic effect of x-irradiation with ratioactive iodine on the rat's thyroid, Br. J. Cancer **11**:67, March, 1957.
6. Duffy, B. J., Jr., and Fitzgerald, P. J.: Cancer of the thyroid in children: a report of 28 cases, J. Clin. Endocrinol. Metab. **10**:1296, 1950.
7. Elman, D. S.: Familial association of nerve deafness with nodular goiter and thyroid carcinoma, N. Engl. J. Med. **259**:219, 1958.
8. Fetterman, G. H.: Carcinoma of the thyroid in children: report of 10 cases, Am. J. Dis. Child. **92**:581, 1956.
9. Goldberg, R. C., and Chaikoff, I. L.: Induction of thyroid cancer in the rat by radioactive iodine, Arch. Pathol. **53**:22, 1952.
10. Haran-Ghera, N., Pullnar, P., and Further, J.: Induction of thyrotropin-dependent thyroid tumors by thyrotropes, Endocrinology **66**:694, 1960.
11. Hollingsworth, D. R., Hamilton, H. B., Tamagaki, H., and Beebe, G. W.: Thyroid disease: a study in Hiroshima, Japan, Medicine **42**:47-71, Jan., 1963.
12. Lindsay, S., Sheline, G. E., Potter, G. D., and Chaikoff, I. L.: Induction of neoplasms in the thyroid gland of the rat by x-irradiation of the gland, Cancer Res. **21**:9-16, Jan., 1961.
13. Majarakis, J. D., Slaughter, D. P., and Cole, W. H.: Thyroid cancer in childhood and adolescence, J. Clin. Endocrinol. Metab. **16**:1487, 1956.
14. Pendergrast, W. J., Milmore, B. K., and Marcus, S. C.: Thyroid cancer and thyrotoxicosis in the United States: their relation to endemic goiter, J. Chronic Dis. **13**:22-38, Jan., 1961.
15. Pochin, E. E.: The occurrence of leukemia following radioiodine therapy. In Advances in thyroid research, Elmsford, N. Y., 1961, Pergamon Press, Inc., pp. 392-397.
16. Purves, H. D., and Griesbach, W. E.: Studies on experimental goiter: thyroid carcinomata in rats treated with thiouria, Br. J. Exper. Pathol. **27**:294, 1947.
17. Rooney, D. R., and Powell, R. W.: Carcinoma of the thyroid after x-ray therapy in early childhood, J.A.M.A. **161**:1, 1959.
18. Root, A. W.: Cancer of the thyroid in childhood and adolescence, Am. J. Med. Sci. **246**:734, 1963.
19. Smith, J. F.: The pathology of the thyroid in the syndrome of sporadic and congenital deafness, Q. J. Med. **29**:297, 1960.
20. Socolaw, E. L., Hashizune, A., Neriishi, S., and Niitani, R.: Thyroid carcinoma in man after exposure to ionizing radiation. A summary of the findings in Hiroshima and Nagasaki, N. Engl. J. Med. **268**:406, 1963.

21. Sussman, L., Librik, L., and Clayton, G. W.: Hyperthyroidism attributable to a hyperfunctioning thyroid cancer, J. Pediatr. **72**:208, 1968.

22. Thieme, E. J.: A report of the recurrence of deafmutism and goiter in four of six siblings of a North American family, Ann. Surg. **146**:941, 1957.

23. Wilkins, L., Clayton, G. W., and Berthrong, M.: Development of goiters in cretins without iodine deficiency, hypothyroidism due to apparent inability of thyroid gland to synthesize hormone, Pediatrics **13**:235, 1954.

24. Williams, E. D., Brown, C. L., and Doniach, I.: Pathological and clinical findings in a series of 67 cases of medullary carcinoma of the thyroid, J. Clin. Pathol. **19**:103-113, March, 1966.

25. Wilson, E. H., and Asper, S. P., Jr.: The role of x-ray therapy to the neck region in the production of thyroid cancer in young people: a report of 37 cases, Arch. Intern. Med. **105**:244, 1960.

26. Winship, T.: Carcinoma of the thyroid in children, J. Am. Goiter Assoc. **3**:64, 1951.

27. Winship, T., and Rosvoll, R. V.: Childhood thyroid carcinoma, Cancer **14**:734, 1961.

Cancer of the adrenal cortex

28. Bierich, J. R.: Nebennierenrinden-Tumoren mit Wirkung auf die Sexualsphäre, Minerva Pediatr. **17**:725, 1965.

29. Fraumeni, J. F., and Miller, R. W.: Adrenal cortical neoplasms and hemihypertrophy, brain tumors and other disorders, J. Pediatr. **70**:129, 1967.

General references

30. Forsham, P. H. The adrenal cortex. In Williams, R. H., editor: Textbook of endocrinology, ed. 4, Philadelphia, 1968, W. B. Saunders Co.

31. Goldstein, A. E., Rubin, S. W., and Ashin, J. H.: Carcinoma of the adrenal with adrenogenital syndrome in children: a complete review of the literature and report of a case with recovery in a child eight months of age, Am. J. Dis. Child. **72**:563, 1946.

32. Grass, R. E.: Neoplasms producing endocrine disturbances in childhood, Am. J. Dis. Child. **59**:579, 1940.

33. Hovas, A. G.: Adrenal cortical carcinoma, clinical pathological study of 34 cases, Cancer **25**:354, 1970.

34. Lloyd, C. W., Labotsky, J., Jane, J., Fredericks, J., and Wyatt, L. C.: Hormone studies in a case of adrenogenitalism due to neoplasm of the adrenal cortex, J. Clin. Endocrinol. Metab. **11**:857, 1951.

35. Soffer, L. J.: Disease of the endocrine glands, ed. 2, Philadelphia, 1956, Lea & Febiger.

36. Wilkins, L.: The diagnosis and treatment of endocrine disorders in childhood and adolescence, ed. 3, Springfield, Ill., 1965, Charles C Thomas, Publisher.

Virilizing adrenal tumors

37. Allen, W. M., Hayward, S. J., and Pinto, A.: A color test for dehydroisoandrosterone and close related steroids of use in the diagnosis of adrenocortical tumor, J. Clin. Endocrinol. Metab. **10**:54, 1950.

38. Cahill, G. F., Melicow, M. M., and Darby, H. H.: Adrenal cortical tumors: the types of non-hormonal and hormonal tumors, Surg. Gynecol. Obstet. **74**:281, 1942.

39. Hutter, A. M., Jr., and Kayhoe, D. E.: Adrenol cortical carcinoma: results of treatment with O, P' DDD in 138 patients, Am. J. Med. **41**:581, 1966.

40. Garderner, L. I., and Migeon, C. J.: Urinary dehydroisoandrosterone in hyperadrenocorticism: influence of cortisone and hydrocortisone- A.C.T.H., J. Clin. Endocrinol. Metab. **12**:1117, 1952.

41. Garrett, R. A.: Adrenal cortical carcinoma in children, J. Urol. **66**:477, 1951.

42. Jensen, C. C.: Quantitative determination of dehydroisoandrosterone. II. Determination in urinary extracts, Acta Endocrinol. **4**:374, 1950.

Cushing's syndrome

43. Bagshaw, K. D.: Hypokalemia carcinoma and Cushing's syndrome, Lancet **2**:284, 1960.

44. Graber, A. L., Ney, R. L., Nicholson, W. E., Island, D. P., and Liddle, G. W.: Natural history of pituitary-adrenal recovery following long term suppression with corticosteroids, J. Clin. Endocrinol. **25**:11, 1965.

45. Guin, G. H., and Gilbert, E. F.: Cushing's syndrome in children associated with adrenal cortical carcinoma, Am. J. Dis. Child. **92**:297, 1956.
46. Jackson, W. P. U., Zilberg, B., Lewis, B., and McKenzie, D.: Cushing's syndrome in childhood: report of case of adrenocortical carcinoma with excessive aldosterone production, Br. Med. J. **2**:130, July 19, 1958.
47. Liddle, G. W.: Tests of pituitary-adrenal suppressibility in the diagnosis of Cushing's syndrome, Arch. Intern. Med. **111**:471, 1963.
48. Linn, J. E., Jr., Boudoin, B., Farmer, T. A., and Meador, C. K.: Observations and comments on failure of dexamethasone suppression, N. Engl. J. Med. **277**:403, 1967.

Feminizing tumors

49. Bacon, G. E., and Lowery, G. H.: Feminizing adrenal tumor in a six-year-old boy, J. Clin. Endocrinol. Metab. **25**:1403, 1965.
50. Higgins, G. H., Brownlee, W. E., and Monty, F. H., Jr.: Feminizing tumors of the adrenal cortex, Am. Surg. **22**:56, 1956.
51. Kepler, E. J., Walters, W., and Dixon, R. K.: Menstruation in a child aged 19 months as the result of tumor of the left adrenal cortex, successful surgical treatment, Mayo Clin. Proc. **13**:362, 1938.
52. Mosier, H. D., and Goodwin, W. E.: Feminizing adrenal adenoma in a seven year old boy, Pediatrics **27**:1016, 1961.
53. Snoithe, A. H. A.: A case of feminizing adrenal tumor in a girl, J. Clin. Endocrinol. Metab. **18**:318, 1958.
54. Wilkins, L. A.: Feminizing adrenal tumor causing gynecomastia in a boy of five years contrasted with a virilizing tumor in a 5 year old girl. Classification of 40 cases of adrenal tumor in children according to their hormonal manifestations and a review of eleven cases of feminizing tumor in adults, J. Clin. Endocrinol. Metab. **8**:111, 1948.

Aldosterone-secreting tumors

55. Cavell, B., Sandegard, E., and Hakfelt, B.: Primary aldosteronism due to an adrenal adenoma in a three year old child, Acta Pediatr. **53**:205, 1964.
56. Conn, J. W.: Aldosteronism and hypertension, Arch. Intern. Med. **107**:813, 1961.
57. Crane, M. G., Holloway, J. E., and Winsor, W. G.: Aldosterone secreting adenoma: report of a case in a juvenile, Ann. Inst. Med. **54**:280, 1961.
58. Orndahl, G., Hokfelt, B., Ljunggren, E., and Hood, B.: Two cases of primary aldosteronism: comments on differential diagnosis and difficulties in screening, Acta Med. Scand. **165**:445, 1959.

Neoplasia in undescended testes and in testicular dysgenesis

59. Campbell, H. E.: The incidences of malignant growth of the undescended testicle: a reply and re-evaluation, J. Urol. **81**:663, 1951.
60. Grass, R. E., and Jewett, L. C., Jr.: Surgical experiences from 1,222 operations for undescended testes, J.A.M.A. **160**:634, 1958.
61. Melicow, M. M., and Unson, A. C.: Dysgenetic gonadomas and other gonadal neoplasms in intersexes—report of 5 cases and review of literature, Cancer **12**:552, 1959.

CHAPTER 25

Carcinoma of the nasopharynx

JAMES B. SNOW, Jr.

Carcinoma of the nasopharynx occurs in children as well as in adults. In younger individuals the tumor is often composed of large epithelioid cells that display the usual characteristics of malignant cells such as pleomorphism, hyperchromatism, frequent mitosis, and normal appearing lymphocytes. Although this histologic picture is often designated as lymphoepithelioma, most authorities consider lymphoepitheliomas to be squamous cell carcinomas.

INCIDENCE

The incidence of carcinoma of the nasopharynx varies greatly among ethnic groups. It is unusually high among the Chinese and relatively low in white populations. In some reports from China, it accounts for 18% of all malignant neoplasms.[3] In white populations nasopharyngeal cancer comprises 0.25% of all malignancies and has an incidence of 2 per 100,000 population per year.[2] The tumor is more common in males than in females with a sex ratio of 2:1 in all races.[6]

Carcinoma of the nasopharynx occurs at relatively young ages. In white populations 6% occur before 30 years of age, and 30% occur before 50 years of age.[2] The youngest patient was a four-year-old girl reported by Lederman.[6]

PATHOLOGIC CHARACTERISTICS

Carcinoma of the nasopharynx arises in areas that bear respiratory epithelium and stratified squamous epithelium in close proximity. The nasopharynx normally is lined by pseudostratified, ciliated columnar epithelium and stratified squamous epithelium. In those areas where attrition from the movement of mucous membrane surfaces against each other is great, the epithelium is stratified squamous. This type of epithelium predominates on the posterior surface of the soft palate and the posterior wall of the nasopharynx.[1] Malignant tumors of the nasophrynx include squamous cell carcinomas, adenocarcinomas, adenoid cystic carcinomas, mucoepidermoid carcinomas, malignant mixed tumors, melanomas, chordomas, sarcomas (including fibrosarcomas, rhabdomyosarcomas, liposarcomas, and myxosarcomas), plasmacytomas, and lymphomas. Among children, the lymphomas and lymphosarcomas are the most common malignant tumors arising from and secondarily involving the nasopharynx. Among the carcinomas, lymphoepitheliomas or squamous cell carcinomas are by far the most common type.

The term *lymphoepithelioma* was introduced in 1921 by Regaud[9] to describe a highly radiosensitive tumor composed of a syncytium of anaplastic epithelial cells surrounded by lymphoid cells. In the same year, Schmincke[10] described a similar tumor in which the epithelial cells were scattered through lymphocytes.

541

Many have been unwilling to accept that the lymphocytes might be normal. The presence of the lymphocytes in metastases tends to support the concept of the mixed origin of the tumor. Today most pathologists interpret the presence of the lymphocytes in the primary site and in the metastases as possible evidence of a cellular immunologic response.

The nomenclature of carcinoma of the nasopharynx has been complicated in another way. In 1927 Quick and Cutler[8] used the term *transitional cell epidermoid carcinoma* to describe a carcinoma that lacks squamous cell features. The omission of "epidermoid" in the term has led to confusion. The term has been generally abandoned.

Squamous cell carcinomas are composed of sheets and strands of epithelioid cells with pleomorphic and hyperchromatic nuclei, prominent nucleoli, and a relatively large cytoplasmic to nuclear ratio. Intercellular bridges, individual cell keratinization, and epithelial pearls are characteristics. When the tumors lack these characteristics, the cells are large with pale-staining nuclei, prominent and multiple nucleoli, and poorly defined cytoplasm, and the stroma contains numerous lymphocytes as illustrated in Fig. 25-1, the term *lymphoepithelioma* is appropriate. This form of the tumor is particularly likely to be found in children and young adults.

Anatomic relationships do much to determine the clinical manifestations of carcinomas of the nasopharynx; an expanding neoplasm may infiltrate rapidly into the parapharyngeal space, cranial cavity, and orbit.

Roughly two thirds of carcinomas of the nasopharynx arise from the lateral wall (37%) and the roof of the nasopharynx (32%). Only 15% arise from the

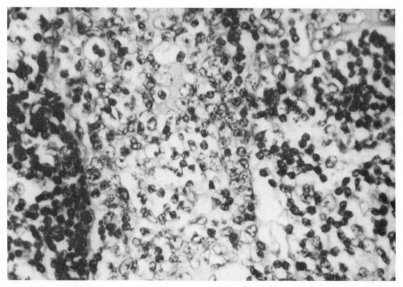

Fig. 25-1. Photomicrograph of a lymphoepithelioma showing large, pale-staining nuclei, prominent and multiple nucleoli, poorly defined cytoplasm, and numerous lymphocytes (×400).

posterior wall.[6] The site of origin in the lateral wall is usually the fossa of Rosenmüller. The fossa of Rosenmüller is a lateral extension of the nasopharynx posterior to the torus tubarius, or prominence of the cartilage of the eustachian tube. The fossa of Rosenmüller is frequently 1 cm in depth and usually contains lymphoid tissue.

CLINICAL MANIFESTATIONS
Symptoms and signs

The majority of patients with carcinoma of the nasopharynx have symptoms of aural or nasal obstruction. In Lederman's series, 17% presented with symptoms of eustachian tube obstruction.[6] Such obstruction may result in retraction of the tympanic membrane or in an effusion in the middle ear (serous otitis media), which may be recognized by the amber or dark gray color of the eardrum, the immobility of the tympanic membrane, and the conductive hearing loss. Obstruction of the eustachian tube may occur because of edema or infiltration of the mucous membrane or extrinsic pressure, but actual invasion of the lumen of the eustachian tube by tumor is rare. Nasal obstruction was the presenting symptom in 38% of Lederman's patients, and this symptom is often associated with rhinorrhea, particularly purulent, blood-tinged rhinorrhea, and frank epistaxis.

The more dramatic symptoms resulting from cranial nerve involvement and lymph node metastases are unfortunately common presenting complaints. Trotter's triad of unilateral hearing loss, fixation of the soft palate, and neuralgia or anesthesia of the third division of the trigeminal nerve is occasionally seen as the presenting symptom complex. These findings can be explained by invasion of the prestyloid compartment of the parapharyngeal space through the anterior inferior aspect of the fossa of Rosenmüller through the fascial space surrounding the levator muscle of the palatine velum.

Metastasis

Metastasis to the cervical lymph nodes occurs early in carcinoma of the nasopharynx. Enlargement of cervical lymph nodes was the presenting symptom in 18% of Lederman's series and is the next most common chief complaint after the symptoms of obstruction of the eustachian tube and nose.[6] Enlarged lymph nodes were present in 70% of his patients, bilaterally in 39%. Bilateral metastases are more likely in patients whose primary tumor arises from the roof of the nasopharynx. Males are more likely to present with lymph node enlargement than females, and children are more likely to have lymph node enlargement than are older patients.[6]

Distant metastases become clinically evident late. They may appear in the viscera, skeleton, lung, and central nervous system. Of 218 cases, Lederman demonstrated distant metastases in 26 cases at the time of initial evaluation: nine to the viscera, seven to the skeleton, five to the lung, two to the central nervous system, and three to other sites.

The natural history of carcinoma of the nasopharynx is characterized by early but subtle aural and nasal symptoms and dramatic symptoms and signs of cranial nerve paralysis and lymph node metastasis. Early cervical metastasis is common, whereas early generalized dissemination is uncommon.

DIAGNOSTIC FEATURES
Clinical evaluation

Diagnosis of carcinoma of the nasopharynx depends on awareness of its manifold presentations. It should be suspected in patients with serous otitis media, particularly in adults, nasal obstruction, rhinorrhea and epistaxis, cervical lymphadenopathy, particularly in the superior part of the posterior cervical triangle, and any cranial paralysis.

Physical diagnosis plays a most important role in the identification of the lesion. There may be clues in a conductive hearing loss and an otoscopic picture with the characteristics of serous otitis media. A granular mass or ulcer may be seen through the nasal cavity. The palate may be deformed by the bulk of the nasopharyngeal mass, or its mobility may be limited by paralysis of the levator muscle of the palatine velum. Of prime importance is visualization of the nasopharynx by either mirror or nasopharyngoscope. Characteristically carcinoma presents in the nasopharynx as a granular mass. Not infrequently the tumor extends deep to the mucous membrane, appears as only a slight fullness, and produces no abnormality of the mucous membrane. It is this feature of carcinoma of the nasopharynx that makes biopsy through apparently normal mucous membrane occasionally fruitful.

The diagnosis is made by biopsy of the primary tumor. Adequate access to the nasopharynx ordinarily requires general anesthesia. General anesthesia also allows the opportunity to judge the extent of the primary lesion by palpation. Carcinoma produces a firm mass in the nasopharynx that stands out from any remaining adenoid tissue. In the absence of a definite mass, removal of the adenoid tissue as in an adenoidectomy is most likely to provide the histologic diagnosis.

Roentgenographic evaluation

A lateral view of the nasopharynx and a submental-vertex view of the base of the skull are necessary for the evaluation of the patient. Laminograms of the orbits, sinuses, and petrous pyramids are frequently helpful.

The lateral view is of value in demonstrating soft tissue masses contrasted with the air column of the nasopharynx. In children the adenoid tissue normally produces a soft tissue density projecting from the posterior wall and the roof of the nasopharynx. A similar appearance in an adult should raise suspicion of a neoplasm. The air column of the nasopharynx is bilaterally concave in the submental-vertex view. In obese individuals the concavities may be lost. In nasopharyngeal tumors the two sides of the air column may become asymmetrical. In particular, the concavity of the air column may be lost on the side bearing the tumor.

Destruction of the base of the skull can be demonstrated in approximately 30% of the cases with the submental-vertex view.[6] Destruction of the base of the skull occurs mainly in four areas: foramen lacerum, carotid canal, greater wing of the sphenoid, and hypophyseosphenoidal area. Destruction of the greater wing of the sphenoid may be produced by tumor that gains access to it intracranially but extradurally through the carotid canal or by invasion of the prestyloid compartment of the parapharyngeal space. With destruction of the greater wing of the sphenoid the foramen ovale and foramen spinosum may become indistinct on the submental-vertex view. Destruction of the tip of the petrous pyramid can occur by the same intracranial but extradural route. Laminograms of the petrous pyramid are helpful in demonstrating the destruction.

Destruction of the base of the skull is seen five times more frequently in patients with cranial nerve paralysis.[4] Invasion of the base of the skull occurs more frequently with carcinomas than with lymphomas or sarcomas.[6]

DIFFERENTIAL DIAGNOSIS

The differential diagnosis of carcinoma of the nasopharynx includes other malignant tumors such as lymphomas and sarcomas, benign tumors such as the juvenile angiofibromas, cysts of the nasopharynx, and the infectious granulomas. In children the lymphoma is the lesion most likely to require differentiation.

The diagnosis of carcinoma of the nasopharynx is based on biopsy. It is preferable that the primary lesion be biopsied. Biopsy of the metastases in the neck should be avoided until the nasopharynx has been inspected and palpated and any suspicious lesion has been biopsied. Biopsy of the cervical metastases violates the integrity of the block of tissue that must be removed in a radical neck dissection. It may result in implantation of the tumor in the skin and subcutaneous tissue. The necessity for demonstrating the tumor in the nasopharynx prior to treatment remains even if a histologic diagnosis is obtained from biopsy of the cervical metastases.

TREATMENT
Irradiation therapy

The treatment of choice for carcinoma of the nasopharynx is irradiation. The irradiation should be delivered to the primary tumor-bearing area of the nasopharynx and to both sides of the neck whether there is clinically demonstrated metastasis or not. It is essential that the full extent of the primary lesion be determined as accurately as possible so that all tumor-bearing areas may be included in the treatment fields. Such determinations must include careful physical examination and radiographic studies. A supervoltage source should be used, with fractionated therapy at the rate of 150 to 200 rads per day for a total tumor dose of 7000 rads to the primary lesion and 5000 rads to each side of the neck.

Surgery

Surgery plays no role in the initial therapy of carcinoma of the nasopharynx. Those cervical metastases that remain clinically palpable after irradiation therapy or that subsequently become apparent should be eradicated by radical neck dissection. As a general rule, control of the secondary lesion should be attempted only after there is evidence that the primary lesion has been controlled. Although clinical evidence of control of the primary lesion is usually all that is appropriate, biopsy of the nasopharynx should be repeated prior to the radical neck dissection if the nasopharynx has a suspicious appearance.

Chemotherapy

The role of chemotherapy in the management of nasopharyngeal carcinoma is not defined at present, although responses to chemotherapeutic agents have been reported.[5, 7] The major problem in this area is the lack of a specific agent for the treatment of carcinomas such as are available for use in children with other hematologic and solid malignancies. There is little likelihood of a specific agent becoming available in the near future, and management must be based on the likelihood of cure by surgery and radiation therapy.

Two basic problems may benefit directly from the use of cancer chemotherapy in children with lymphoepithelioma. The first is the extensive lymphoid infiltration that is found in childhood nasopharyngeal carcinoma and that has led to its consideration as a lymphomatous malignancy. The extreme morbidity and debility, apparently from the host's response to the tumor, may be attenuated by drug therapy. My experience is limited (one patient) to the use of cyclophosphamide (30 mg/kg/day in three divided doses at weekly intervals), but the overall improvement in symptomatology was impressive. Prednisone, methotrexate, vincristine, and other chemotherapeutic agents probably function just as well for this purpose, but they have yet to be adequately evaluated, primarily because of the rarity of this tumor in children. Secondly, chemotherapy may also be useful as part of a total treatment regimen with drugs used to reduce the possibility of metastasis or local recurrence or both. Since surgery and radiation therapy markedly reduce the tumor mass without necessarily destroying all malignant cells, the size of the residual tumor may be small enough for adequate chemotherapy to destroy the remaining cells. Leone and co-workers[7] reported on the use of high-dose (60 mg/M^2 once weekly) methotrexate intravenously in the treatment of 35 patients with carcinoma of the head and neck, most of whom had received prior surgery and radiation. There were eleven complete remissions (mean duration of 160 days) and nine partial remissions, thereby demonstrating the activity of methotrexate in carcinoma despite its inability to effect cure. Methotrexate may have a role in a combined regimen of surgery-radiation-chemotherapy but requires further evaluation.

Cryosurgery

Occasionally the primary lesion in the nasopharynx persists after irradiation therapy without evidence of local extension beyond the nasopharynx and without evidence of uncontrolled local or distant metastases. Under these circumstances cryosurgery may be applied to the persisting tumor in the nasopharynx through a transpalatal approach. Useful palliation and an occasional cure may result from this rather aggressive approach. Careful selection of patients with tumor persisting only in the nasopharynx is essential to avoid subjecting patients to a futile procedure.

PROGNOSIS

The overall 5-year survival rate for carcinoma of the nasopharynx is approximately 35%. The survival rate for irradiation therapy ranges from 76% for Stage I lesions of the vault to 17% for Stage IV lesions of the lateral wall.[11] Lederman[6] reports an overall 5-year survival rate of 13%. The results were very similar for patients with cervical metastases and patients without cervical metastases probably because of the failure to eliminate the primary tumor in both groups. Females have a higher survival rate than males. Likewise, younger individuals have a higher survival rate than older individuals. In Lederman's series the 5-year survival rate of patients with posterior wall lesions was 26%, whereas the patients with lateral wall lesions had a 12% 5-year survival rate.[6] The statistics of the American Joint Committee also demonstrated a higher survival rate among the patients with posterosuperior wall lesions as compared to patients with lateral wall lesions.[11]

CASE REPORTS

In the last 10 years, 7 patients under 21 years of age have been treated at the University of Oklahoma Medical Center for carcinoma of the nasopharynx. There were 5 boys and 2 girls; four were white, and 3 were Negro. Their ages ranged from 9 to 17 years at the time of diagnosis. Five are living and free of disease, and 2 are dead. There are 3 5-year survivors. The following case reports illustrate important factors in the management of carcinoma of the nasopharynx.

Case 1. This 12-year-old white boy presented with a right cervical mass in September, 1963. A right radical neck dissection was performed, and the diagnosis of lymphoepithelioma was established histopathologically. The nasopharynx was subsequently biopsied, and the lymphoepithelioma was again demonstrated. He received irradiation therapy to the nasopharynx and both sides of the neck from September to November, 1963. He is now living and well 8 years after the diagnosis was made.

Comment. As a general rule in evaluating cervical masses, the primary lesion should be sought and biopsied first.

Case 2. This 15-year-old white boy was seen in September, 1966, with a large left cervical mass. The left cervical mass was biopsied, but no diagnosis was established. A mass in the nasopharynx was biopsied, and the diagnosis of lymphoepithelioma was established histologically. The patient received irradiation therapy to the nasopharynx and both sides of the neck from September to November, 1966. In January, 1967, a left radical neck dissection for a persistent left cervical mass was performed. No tumor could be demonstrated in the surgical specimen. In March, 1967, he had a resection of the proximal portion of the left fibula because of pain in the leg and a radiolucent defect in the fibula. The tissue removed was similar to the primary tumor in the nasopharynx. He is now living and well 5 years after the diagnosis was made.

Comment. This case demonstrates the exceptional situation in which surgical control of a distant metastasis proved to be beneficial.

Case 3. This 12-year-old Negro boy presented in November, 1963, with the complaints of headache, epistaxis, and frequent tonsillitis for 1 year and a 2 by 2 cm nontender node in the right posterior cervical triangle. In December, 1963, he had a tonsillectomy and adenoidectomy. In February, 1964, the right cervical mass had increased in size. Reexamination of the adenoid tissue demonstrated a lymphoepithelioma. Irradiation therapy to the nasopharynx and both sides of the neck was carried out from March to May, 1964. The patient is now living and well 7 years after the diagnosis was made.

Comment. This case demonstrates the importance of careful histopathologic study of all tonsillar and adenoid tissue.

Case 4. This 14-year-old Negro boy, the younger brother of the patient in Case 3, was noted to have bilateral, posterior cervical triangle lymphadenopathy and a mass in the nasopharynx in July, 1967. A biopsy of the nasopharyngeal mass established the diagnosis of lymphoepithelioma. From August to October, 1967, the patient received irradiation therapy to the nasopharynx and both sides of the neck. In December, 1967, a right radical neck dissection for a persistent right cervical mass was performed. No tumor could be demonstrated in the surgical specimen. The patient developed a staphylococcal wound infection and massive necrosis of the cervical skin flaps and died after carotid artery rupture.

Comment. The development of lymphoepithelioma in two siblings is of great interest from an environmental and genetic point of view. The older brother developed the clinical manifestations of the tumor at 12 years of age, and 4 years later the younger brother developed them at 14 years of age. None of the previously proposed environmental etiologic factors could be elicited in this family, and no new factors came to light.

The survival rate in this group of patients is very good. There were no cranial nerve palsies and no roentgenographic evidence of destruction of the base of the skull in this group of patients. Cranial nerve palsies and destruction of the base of the skull have an adverse effect on prognosis.

These patients illustrate that carcinoma of the nasopharynx should be managed as a regional disease rather than a systemic one. Because of the confusion attendant to the name *lymphoepithelioma,* systemic drug therapy is sometimes advocated rather than regional irradiation therapy on the assumption that these tumors are more related to lymphomas and lymphosarcomas than to carcinomas. It is very clear that lymphoepitheliomas should be managed as carcinomas.

The only deaths in this group of young patients were directly related to radical neck dissection. Five radical neck dissections were performed in 4 patients. One of these was performed prior to irradiation therapy; 2 of 4 who had radical neck dissections performed after irradiation therapy died. Each of these procedures was clearly indicated by the persistence of a cervical mass. Although failure to demonstrate tumor in a surgical specimen does not exclude its existence, no tumor could be demonstrated in any of the postirradiation dissection specimens. The value of radical neck dissection in this age group after irradiation therapy for carcinoma of the nasopharynx merits further critical review.

No serious complication of irradiation therapy has so far been encountered in this group of patients.

REFERENCES

1. Ali, N. Y.: Distribution and character of the squamous epithelium in the human nasopharynx. In Muir, C. S., and Shammugaratnam, K., editors: Cancer of the nasopharynx, Flushing, N. Y., 1967, Medical Examination Publishing Co.
2. Bailar, J. C.: Nasopharyngeal cancer in white populations—a worldwide survey. In Muir, C. S., and Shanmugaratnam, K., editors: Cancer of the nasopharynx, Flushing, N. Y., 1967, Medical Examination Publishing Co.
3. Digby, K. H., Fook, W. L., and Che, Y. T.: Nasopharyngeal carcinoma, Br. J. Surg. **28:** 517-537, 1941.
4. Godtfredsen, E.: Opthalmologic and neurologic symptoms of malignant nasopharyngeal tumours, Acta Psychiatrica et Neurologica Suppl. XXXIV, Copenhagen, 1944, Munksgaard, International Booksellers & Publishers, Ltd.
5. Lane, M., Moore, J. E., Levin, H., and Smith, F. E.: Methotrexate therapy for squamous cell carcinomas of the head and neck, J.A.M.A. **204:**561-564, 1968.
6. Lederman, M.: Cancer of the nasopharynx—its natural history and treatment, Springfield, Ill., 1961, Charles C Thomas, Publisher.
7. Leone, L. A., Albala, M. M., and Rege, V. B.: Treatment of carcinoma of the head and neck with intravenous methotrexate, Cancer **21:**828-837, 1968.
8. Quick, D., and Cutler, M.: Transitional cell epidermoid carcinoma, Surg. Gynecol. Obstet. **45:**320-331, 1927.
9. Regaud, C.: Discussion of paper by Reverchon, L., and Coutard, H.: Lymphoepitheliome de l'hypopharynx traite par le roentgentherapie, Bull. Soc. Franc. Oto-rhino-lar. **34:**209-214, 1921.
10. Schmincke, A.: Ueber lymphoepitheliale Geschwülste, Beitr. Pathol. Anat. **58:**161-170, 1921.
11. Smith, R. R., Frazell, E. L., Caulk, R., Holinger, P. H., and Russell, W. O.: The American Joint Committee's proposed method of stage classification and end-results reporting applied to 1,320 pharynx cancers, Cancer **16:**1505-1520, 1963.

CHAPTER 26

Tumors of the respiratory tract[*]

DANIEL M. LANE

The respiratory system is a very common site for cancer in adults, both for primary tumors and for metastatic tumors. In children and adolescents the incidence of primary tumors is much lower, but metastatic tumors very commonly spread to involve the respirtory tract.

THE LARYNX

Carcinoma of the larynx is most frequent in persons between 55 and 75 years of age with few cases in individuals less than 40 years of age. In a recent review of cases occurring in the first two decades of life, Jones and Gabriel[7] found 98 cases, to which they added their own case. The number of cases occurring in the second decade outnumbered those in the first decade approximately 3:1. The sex incidence revealed a male to female ratio of 5:3, a much higher representation of females than is found in adult cases. Hoarseness, cough, and weak voice are usually the first signs of difficulty, and their sudden appearance in a child should be as aggressively studied as in older age groups. Lesions are most often localized at the time of diagnosis, although metastasis to the regional lymph nodes can occur if the disease progresses. Treatment with radiation therapy alone has resulted in cures, although laryngectomy with regional node dissection has also been a successful approach. A comment should be made here about the frequency of carcinoma in juvenile papillomas. Twelve of the 99 cases reviewed by Jones and Gabriel arose from papillomas; consequently, juvenile papillomas should receive continuing, careful observation for possible malignant change.

Tumors of the supporting tissues of the larynx also occur in children, although again less frequently than in adults. Primary malignant tumors are exceedingly rare in the pediatric age group. Fibrosarcoma has been reported in a 15-year-old girl,[4] but most other cases reported in this age group have been questioned as to their authenticity as true fibrosarcomas. Rhabdomyosarcoma of the larynx does occur, and 4 cases have been reported in children, all in the first decade of life.[1] Initial symptoms resulted from respiratory obstruction and included a croupy coughing, audible breath sounds, and hoarseness. All 4 patients were treated by laryngectomy and were free of recurrence at last report. Rhabdomyosarcoma is important also because it has been confused in the past with two benign tumors, granular cell myoblastoma and rhabdomyoma. Careful differentiation should be made to separate these lesions from the highly malignant rhabdomyosarcomas. Neurogenous and vascular malignant tumors have not been reported to occur in the larynx.[2]

*This manuscript was completed during the tenure of a National Institutes of Health Special Research Fellowship (5 FO3 HE43135-03) from the National Heart and Lung Institute.

THE LUNGS AND MEDIASTINUM
Metastatic tumors

More tumors of the lung and mediastinum in children originate from sites outside the thorax than from inside. Malignancies can reach the lungs through three major routes: the blood, the lymphatics, and direct extension.

1. Hematogenous (bloodborne)
   a. Wilms' tumor
   b. Osteogenic sarcoma
   c. Rhabdomyosarcoma
   d. Carcinomas
   e. Ewing's tumor
2. Lymphogenous (lymphatic extension)
   a. Neuroblastoma
   b. Hodgkin's disease
   c. Lymphosarcoma
   d. Testicular tumors
   e. Carcinomas
3. Direct spread
   a. Hepatomas
   b. Rhabdomyosarcoma
   c. Ewing's tumor

One of the most common sources of metastatic tumors to the lungs, Wilms' tumor (nephroblastoma), disseminates from the abdominal cavity by way of the blood. Osteogenic sarcoma, Ewing's tumor, and rhabdomyosarcoma also metastasize in this manner to pulmonary tissues. Neuroblastoma and ganglioneuroblastoma are major malignancies that spread by the lymphatics to the lungs, although mediastinal rather than pulmonary involvement is more characteristic. Lymphomas also may involve the mediastinal lymph nodes, but it may be difficult to determine whether the tumor is primary or metastatic. Testicular lesions usually progress up through the abdominal lymphatics to the thoracic cavity. Finally, the lungs or mediastinum can be involved by direct extension of a tumor. Hepatomas can force their way through the diaphragm. Chest wall tumors such as rhabdomyosarcoma or Ewing's sarcoma may extend to involve the pleura, lungs, and mediastinum.

Treatment for metastatic tumors is somewhat controversial at this time. Aggressive surgical resection has been advocated, even if repeated operations are necessary, particularly in patients with metastatic Wilms' tumor.[9] Radiation therapy, when the ports are small, is an excellent modality, but its effectiveness decreases as the size of the tumor increases. Chemotherapy can produce regression of masses in the lung and mediastinum, depending on the tumor sensitivity, but its most important use is as adjuvant therapy. More specific information about management of metastatic tumors is available in the chapters on each tumor type.

Primary tumors

Carcinoma of the lung occurs in childhood, although it is extremely rare. Only 15 cases could be found in children 14 years of age or younger up to 1951.[3] Additional cases have been reported, including one 16-year-old patient in whom smoking may have been a cause.[12] Of special note is the association of carcinoma with congenital malformations of the lung, especially cystic changes. The most frequent initial symptom is pain, either from the primary lesions or from a metastatic lesion. Dyspnea and coughing are fairly frequent, whereas pallor, fever, and weight loss are less common symptoms. Chest roentgenograms almost invariably show a mass, and the diagnosis is confirmed by tissue studies. Treatment has been primarily surgical resection with other modalities contributing palliative help. Prognosis is extremely poor, except when early diagnosis has made complete resection possible before metastasis.

Bronchial adenomas, which are often thought to be benign tumors because of their name, have been reported in children.[13] These slow-growing tumors usually arise in the primary or secondary bronchi and invade into the bronchial wall and surrounding tissues. Histologically, 80% to 85% of the tumors are carcinoids, resembling intestinal carcinoids, with the remainder cylindroid or mucoepidermoid. Presenting symptoms include persistent cough and hemoptysis with atelectasis and pneumonia late manifestations as bronchial obstruction progresses. Fortunately, cures can be obtained by adequate surgical resection. Endoscopic removal is not adequate, and the effectiveness of radiation or chemotherapy or both has yet to be proved.[5]

Primary sarcomas of the lung and mediastinum occur in children, but again less commonly than in adults. Lymphosarcoma and Hodgkin's disease are found most often, usually arising in the lymphoid tissues of the mediastinum. Neurogenic tumors can arise in the chest, with neuroblastoma and ganglioneuroblastoma the major malignant varieties. Soft tissue sarcomas are extremely rare but have included angiosarcoma and rhabdomyosarcoma.[6, 10]

PLEURA, CHEST WALL, AND DIAPHRAGM

Primary tumors of the pleura are limited almost exclusively to mesotheliomas. These tumors arise as solitary lesions of the visceral pleura (including the pericardium) and are usually fibrous mesotheliomas histologically.[8] The onset of symptoms is most often sudden with pain and a pleural effusion found initially. Therapy has been surgical resection with little or no success. Although only limited experience is available, radiation or chemotherapy, including intrapleural administration, may offer hope for the future.

The chest wall consists of several different tissues from which malignant tumors may arise.[14] Chondrosarcomas have been reported in individuals under 20 years of age, usually presenting as a mass or as an incidental finding on x-ray examination of the chest.[11] Ewing's sarcoma and osteogenic sarcoma may both originate in the chest wall. Lymphoid tissues have been the source of both lymphosarcomas and reticulum cell sarcomas. Finally, the skeletal muscles between the ribs are tissues from which rhabdomyosarcomas can arise.

The diaphragm is an extremely rare site for primary tumors both in children and adults. However, both a malignant hemangiopericytoma and a rhabdomyosarcoma have been reported in children less than 15 years of age.[15]

REFERENCES

1. Batsakis, J. G., and Fox, J. E.: Rhabdomyosarcoma of the larynx, Arch. Otolaryngol. **91:** 136-140, 1970.
2. Batsakis, J. G., and Fox, J. E.: Supporting tissue neoplasms of the larynx, Surg. Gynecol. Obstet. **131:**989-997, 1970.

3. Cayley, C. K., Caez, H. J., and Mersheimer, W.: Primary bronchogenic carcinoma of the lung in children, Am. J. Dis. Child. **82**:49-60, 1951.
4. Davies, D. G.: Fibrosarcoma and pseudosarcoma of the larynx, J. Laryngol. Otol. **83**:423-434, 1969.
5. Donahue, J. K., Weichert, R. F., and Ochsner, J. L.: Bronchial adenoma, Ann. Surg. **167**:873-884, 1968.
6. Heimburger, J. L., and Battersby, J. S.: Primary mediastinal tumors in childhood, J. Thorac. Cardiovasc. Surg. **50**:92-103, 1965.
7. Jones, D. G., and Gabriel, C. E.: The incidence of carcinoma of the larynx in persons under twenty years of age, Laryngoscope **79**:251-255, 1969.
8. Kauffman, S. L., and Stout, A. P.: Mesothelioma in children, Cancer **17**:539-544, 1964.
9. Kilman, J. W., Kronenberg, M. W., O'Neill, J. A., and Klassen, K. P.: Surgical resection for pulmonary metastases in children, Arch. Surg. **99**:158-165, 1969.
10. Martini, N., Hajdu, S. I., and Beattie, E. J., Jr.: Primary sarcoma of the lung, J. Thorac. Cardiovasc. Surg. **61**:33-38, 1971.
11. Salvador, A. H., Beabout, J. W., and Dahlin, D. C.: Mesenchymal chondrosarcoma-observations on 30 new cases, Cancer **28**:605-615, 1971.
12. Sawyer, K. C., Sawyer, R. B., Lubchenco, A. E., McKinnon, D. A., and Hill, K. A.: Fatal primary cancer of the lung in a teen-age smoker, Cancer **20**:451-457, 1967.
13. Verska, J. J., and Connolly, J. E.: Bronchial adenomas in children, J. Thorac. Cardiovasc. Surg. **55**:411-417, 1968.
14. Walkins, E., Jr., and Gerard, F. P.: Malignant tumors involving the chest wall, J. Thorac. Cardiovasc. Surg. **39**:117-129, 1960.
15. Wiener, M. F., and Chou, W. H.: Primary tumors of the diaphragm, Arch. Surg. **90**:143-152, 1965.

CHAPTER 27

Tumors of the gastrointestinal tract

DANIEL M. LANE*
DERRICK LONSDALE

Tumors of the gastrointestinal tract are infrequent in children, especially when compared to adults. Hepatomas and tumors of the colon are the two major malignancies covered in this section with a more limited discussion about other sites and types of gastrointestinal cancer. No discussion of lymphomas and lymphosarcomas will be included here, since those disorders are dealt with in Chapters 13 and 14. Nevertheless, before considering the gastrointestinal tumors, a few brief comments should be made about the lymphomatous disorders. They are the most common tumors involving the gastrointestinal tract in infants and children. The diagnosis of lymphoma should always be considered in the differential diagnosis in any child with possible cancer of the gastrointestinal tract. A very important feature of the lymphomatous disorders is their tendency to disseminate widely, and no lymphoma involving the bowel should be considered a local lesion until an intensive search for other sites of involvement has been completed.

The gastrointestinal tract malignancies are peculiar in that several are related to genetic defects and still others are capable of hormone production. Their relationship to genetic disorders is discussed in Chapter 2. The functioning gastrointestinal tumors are considered in Chapter 24.

SALIVARY GLANDS

Primary tumors of the salivary glands are uncommon in children, not only when compared to their frequency in adults, but also when compared to the occurrence of other tumors in the pediatric age group. Histologically, the malignant tumors include mixed tumors (because both epithelial and mesenchymal constituents are present), mucoepidermoid carcinomas, adenocystic carcinomas, and undifferentiated carcinomas.[10] Adenocarcinoma is the least common type, and undifferentiated carcinoma is probably the anaplastic form of the mucoepidermoid variety.

Although their appearance on histologic review is benign, mixed tumors of the parotid should be considered malignant because of their location and capacity to infiltrate.[2] They tend to recur locally, and the extent of the recurrence may produce as much difficulty as if the tumor were malignant. This is especially true when the facial nerve becomes involved as the tumor infiltrates.

If mixed tumors, which are considered to be somewhere between benign and malignant, are excluded from consideration, the most common type of malignant tumor of the salivary gland is mucoepidermoid carcinoma.[2] Histologically, these

*This manuscript was completed during the tenure of a National Institutes of Health Special Research Fellowship (5 FO3 HE43135-03) from the National Heart and Lung Institute.

tumors contain both epidermoid and mucoid cells; the degree of differentiation ranges from low-grade lesions, with predominately mucoid elements, to high-grade lesions, with predominately epidermoid cells. The parotid gland is by far the most common site with the palatal and submaxillary glands next most frequent. [7]

Patients with parotid gland tumors usually seek medical attention because a mass has been found. A good correlation exists between the degree of malignancy of the tumor and the duration that the mass has been present. The more benign types may be present for years before the problem is presented to a physician, whereas the more anaplastic forms are seen earlier. Pain is variable as well and is most intense with the more malignant varieties. Inflammation around the tumor is usually found only with the highly anaplastic carcinomas. Facial paralysis is infrequent but can occur if the facial nerve is extensively involved.

Therapy of primary tumors is by total surgical removal, with the degree of malignancy of the tumor dictating whether or not a radical neck dissection is performed. Mixed tumors should be resected by total parotid lobectomy with removal of all the previous biopsy tract. The temptation to "shell-out" these encapsulated tumors should be ignored. Mucoepidermoid carcinomas require complete removal of the affected gland (or the involved lobe if in the parotid) with examination of regional nodes by frozen section. If the nodes contain malignant cells, then radical neck dissection should follow resection. This is also appropriate management for adenocarcinomas. The highly anaplastic type does not respond well to surgical resection. However, a wide radical excision with prophylactic radical neck dissection should be performed, followed by adequate radiation therapy. Chemotherapy plays no role in the management of these tumors at the present time.

The success of therapy will depend on the adequacy of surgical removal and the degree of differentiation of the tumor.[12] Five-year survival rates have been reported to be as high as 90% in adults, but probably are lower in children because of the more rapid growth of the tumor in this age group.

Other malignancies such as lymphoma and rhabdomyosarcoma may involve the salivary gland but are also uncommon. In addition, the parotid gland may be the initial site of involvement with histiocytosis. As with any tumor involving uncommon sites in children, a high degree of suspicion and aggressive therapy are critical to the management of this group of tumors.

THE ESOPHAGUS

Primary esophageal malignancy is extremely rare in children, whereas metastatic involvement from tumors outside the esophagus is more common. In a review by Moore[19] only one definite case of childhood squamous cell carcinoma of the esophagus could be found. In the absence of more extensive experience, the management of esophageal cancer would be assumed to be essentially the same as in adults.

THE STOMACH

The stomach, in contrast to the esophagus, is a more common site of carcinomas and is second only to the colon as a site for cancer involving the gastrointestinal tract. In order of decreasing frequency, polypoid, ulcerating, and scirrhous carcinomas of the stomach are all found in children and young adults. The frequency, however, is very low. Only 19 patients less than 15 years of age were found in a total literature survey of 501 patients with gastric carcinoma.[18] Except for more extensive involvement of the mucosal surface, the disease is basically the same as in adults.

Presenting complaints of gastric carcinoma are usually those of pain, vomiting, and weight loss. The duration of the disease from symptoms to diagnosis is about 12 months and is referable primarily to delay in diagnosis. Physical examination reveals that almost three fourths of the patients have a palpable abdominal mass in addition to evidence of weight loss. Overall survival is very poor, with a 6% 3-year survival reported for patients under 30 years old.[18] Because of the rarity of the tumor in children, no specific recommendation for management can be made. However, surgical resection would appear to be as appropriate in the child as it is in the adult. Perhaps the most critical fact about carcinoma of the stomach in children is simply to remember that it does occur and that an aggressive diagnostic evaluation should not be delayed because of the patient's age whenever symptoms appear.

SMALL INTESTINES

The discussion of the small intestines will include the appendix, since both organs are uncommon sites for primary tumors and share most of the same tumors. If adenocarcinomas of the small bowel do exist in children less than 15 years of age, they are exceedingly rare. Carcinoid tumors are found almost exclusively in the appendix in individuals under 20 years old.[1] They are of low-grade malignancy, and it has not been proved that they produce metastatic disease in the pediatric age group. They rarely present with the full-blown malignant carcinoid syndrome as seen in the adult, but an occasional patient may show some of the manifestations. The peculiar patchy cyanosis, transient vasodilatation of the skin, tachycardia, hyperperistalsis, and diarrhea may occur, but presentation as acute appendicitis is most likely. Carcinoid tumors are functioning endocrine tumors, producing serotonin, which is excreted in the urine as 5-hydroxyindole acetic acid (5-HIAA). Normally, 2 to 9 mg of 5-HIAA is excreted daily, but in the presence of a carcinoid the levels are at least two to three times greater, which can be useful for diagnosis.[4] Histologic examination of the tumor is still necessary for definitive diagnosis. Leiomyosarcomas of the small intestine are very rare. Surgical resection would be the treatment of choice for all the tumors discussed.

THE PANCREAS

Pancreatic malignancy is a rare malignancy in children and is much less common than in adults. Up to 1970, only 25 cases of malignant pancreatic tumors have been reported in children.[11] Except for one rhabdomyosarcoma arising in the wall of a cystadenoma, all have been carcinomas.

Carcinomas of the pancreas can be divided into nonfunctioning and functioning types. The nonfunctioning variety can be further subdivided into cystic and solid groups. The cystic adenocarcinoma is extremely rare in children and involves primarily the tail of the pancreas. The solid carcinomas can arise from any of the pancreatic tissues, occur more frequently (with peaks in the preschool and early adolescent age groups), and involve primarily the head of the pancreas.

The functioning carcinomas of the pancreas can also be subdivided into two groups, beta type islet cell and nonbeta type islet cell carcinomas. The malignant beta type tumors are usually discovered at laparotomy for hypoglycemia, a problem most commonly caused by benign adenomas. The nonbeta carcinomas are associated with the Zollinger-Ellison syndrome, a disorder in which malignant change ordinarily is unusual. However, in one series of 8 children, 7 were found to have carcinomas with metastasis.[26]

The symptoms and signs of pancreatic carcinoma have been summarized by Welch.[25] Abdominal pain and the presence of an abdominal mass were by far the most common findings. Less common were icterus, anorexia, and vomiting. Diarrhea was also seen but was assumed to be associated with the Zollinger-Ellison syndrome. Additional findings such as anemia and weight loss, which are common to many malignancies, were infrequent.

Therapy is based on an aggressive surgical attack on the tumor, a procedure more successful in children than in adults.[11, 25] Nonfunctioning carcinomas involving the head of the pancreas should be treated by pancreatoduodenectomy. If only the body or tail is involved, then distal pancreatectomy may be possible, although there is little evidence to support this approach in children. For beta type islet cell carcinomas, resection of the tumor is probably adequate, since malignant change is so uncommon. The nonbeta type islet cell carcinomas associated with the Zollinger-Ellison syndrome require total gastric resection, but removal of the pancreatic neoplasm itself is dependent on its location and extent. If the tumor is in the body or tail and is not widespread, resection should probably be performed. Other therapeutic modalities such as radiation therapy and chemotherapy do not appear to play a role in the management of these tumors at the present time.

THE LIVER
Hepatoma

The liver is an uncommon site for primary neoplasms in infants and children when compared to other organs and tissues. However, they are frequent enough to be considered a major diagnostic problem in any child with an abdominal swelling. The age of onset of hepatomas in children is related to the histologic classification of the tumor.[15] Hepatoblastomas are almost always found in patients under 2 years of age, whereas hepatocarcinomas are usually seen in children over 5 years of age. Both types of hepatomas occur more frequently in males by a wide margin. In addition, hepatomas have a peculiar geographic distribution with a greater incidence both in children and in adults in Asia and Africa as compared to the United States and Europe.[6] No satisfactory explanation for this pattern has yet been proposed. Hepatomas are much less frequent than other childhood solid tumors such as Wilms' tumor or neuroblastoma, except in the newborn period, when they are found with a frequency higher than at any other time in childhood.[9]

Several systems for pathologic classification have been proposed, such as the one by Ishak and Glunz.[13] These workers subdivide the hepatomas of childhood into two major types. The first type is hepatoblastoma, which occurs both in a relatively pure form consisting predominately of epithelial cells and in a mixed form in which mesenchymal tissues are present in addition to the epithelial tissue. The mesenchymal tissue most commonly present is osteoid tissue, but its frequency is variable both as to site and extent. The other type of hepatoma is hepatocellular carcinoma, which is morphologically indistinguishable from adult carcinoma of the liver. Several morphologic features are differentiated between the two types, and the reader should refer to the Ishak and Glunz article[13] for further information.

The presenting symptoms and signs of hepatoma in infants and children are fairly consistent. The most common complaint is one of progressive enlargement of the abdomen, which may or may not be associated with a mass. If a mass is present, it is usually felt to be freely movable and not attached to surrounding tissues. Pallor, frequently associated with an anemia, is the second most common finding. Abdominal complaints, especially of pain or discomfort, are not a constant feature, although they do appear to be more frequent in hepatocarcinomas than in hepatoblastomas. Weight loss or underdevelopment appears to be infrequent but becomes more common with progression of the disease. Acute symptoms also appear to be more frequent as the disease progresses, when jaundice, hepatic coma, and other evidence of extensive liver involvement develop.

Diagnostic evaluation follows the discovery of abdominal enlargement or a mass or both. Careful physical examination usually localizes the mass to the liver. Splenomegaly may be present but is infrequent. The presence of jaundice is rarely of any diagnostic significance because of its infrequency. Laboratory studies of liver function are rarely helpful. A recent review has suggested that the presence of α_1-fetoglobulin may be both characteristic of and a specific test for hepatoma.[23] Although frequently absent in patients with hepatomas, a positive test for this abnormal protein has been diagnostic of a hepatoma with few exceptions, most of which were teratoblastomas. However, the usual determination of the presence of the hepatoma depends on radiologic or radioisotope procedures. A flat plate of the abdomen will usually reveal enlargement of the liver with occasional evidence of impingement on adjacent structures. The most useful procedure with which to demonstrate a liver mass is a radioisotope scan. Liver scans can demonstrate the presence of a mass but do not usually differentiate one type of mass from another. Hepatic arteriography may be the critical tool in differentiating hepatomas from other causes of liver masses when an abdominal mass is demonstrated by isotope scan. When hepatic arteriography and isotope scanning have been used together, excellent correlation with the diagnosis of hepatoma has been achieved.[17, 24]

Once a mass in the liver has been demonstrated, the diagnosis of hepatoma still depends on tissue studies. Needle biopsies of the hepatic mass are not satisfactory for this purpose. The procedure of choice to obtain a satisfactory specimen is a laparotomy with open biopsy. It offers the advantage not only of a satisfactory specimen but also an opportunity to evaluate the extent of the patient's disease. The decision to combine biopsy with resection depends on the judgment of the surgeon at the time of surgery.

Additional studies should be performed either before or after tissue confirmation to determine if the tumor has metastasized. This should include at least a chest film and skeletal survey to rule out metastasis to the lungs and bones. Bone marrow aspiration or biopsy may be useful to verify the presence of metastatic tumor. Isotope scanning procedures of other organs are becoming increasingly effective for demonstrating metastatic lesions and should be considered. Inferior venacavograms may also be used to determine if the tumor has spread into this vessel. Metastasis is most commonly regional, and studies on organs adjacent to the liver may be additional aids in evaluation of tumor spread.

The liver is a complex organ perfused with a large volume of blood, thereby making it a target for many different types of disorders. Consequently, the differential diagnosis of hepatomas in infants and children is complicated. Congenital hepatic cysts are fairly frequent, occurring either as solitary or multiple lesions; it is critical to differentiate this lesion from hepatoma because of its presentation as a hepatic mass by isotope scan. Areas of necrosis may also be a differential point to consider, especially when the necrosis is due to an amebic abscess or systemic mycotic infection. Cirrhosis with areas of cellular proliferation present between areas of fibrosis may be confused with a hepatoma. Trauma to the liver can lead to an intrahepatic hematoma and is especially difficult to deal with, since it may occur in the presence of a hepatoma. Two benign tumors of the liver should be considered in the differential diagnosis when a mass is found. Hamartomas are most likely to be confused because of their large size and increased frequency in males. Hemangiomas do occur but are relatively infrequent. Metastatic tumors will be discussed later in this section but should always be a major feature in the differential diagnosis of hepatomas.

Treatment of primary hepatomas of the liver in children is surgical at the present time. The specific techniques for surgical management will not be discussed, and the reader desiring more information should refer to the excellent review by Raffucci and Ramirez-Schon.[21] These authors beautifully describe the anatomic structures of the liver and the use of this information in determining the appropriate operation for resection of primary tumors. As discussed by Foster,[8] the success of resection of primary hepatomas depends less on the specific surgical procedure chosen for resection than it does on the adequacy of the tumor removal. The most important factor in surgical treatment is whether all the visible tumor and a margin of normal liver tissue can be removed at the time of operation. Hepatomas in children tend to metastasize later than in adults, making surgical resection more likely to be successful. When surgical removal is performed, it should be as aggressive as possible, since the liver in a young child has a tremendous capacity to regenerate. Despite an operative death rate of almost 25%, a 5-year cure rate of 33% justifies an aggressive surgical approach.

Cancer chemotherapy and radiation therapy play no definite role at the present time in the management of childhood hepatomas for cure. Both modalities have produced tumor regression when used alone and therefore can be used for palliation. The control of ascites and the relief of pain are two uses in which their effectiveness has been demonstrated. Until new drugs or more sophisticated uses of currently available drugs are developed, chemotherapy will continue to have an insignificant role. Since radiation therapy has been uniformly unsuccessful, nothing short of a major advance in methodology will add that technique to the treatment. The most hopeful procedure for the future for primary hepatomas in children is complete hepatic transplantation. Experience to date has been unrewarding, but progressively improving surgical and immunologic techniques may lead to this procedure ultimately becoming the treatment of choice.

Prognosis at the present time is difficult to define, except when complete surgical removal of the tumor has been possible. Approximately 1 out of 3 pediatric patients with primary hepatoma will survive. The cure rate for children under 2 years of age with hepatoblastoma is much better than that for the child over 5 years of age with hepatocarcinoma.[14]

Biliary system

Carcinomas of the bile duct and gallbladder are exceedingly rare in infants and children. The most common tumor of the biliary system is rhabdomyosarcoma, which has been reported in several patients.[16] Details on the diagnosis and treatment of rhabdomyosarcoma are presented in Chapter 20.

Metastatic tumors

The liver is a common site for metastases from other tumors. The most common metastatic tumor in children is neuroblastoma, which spreads by direct extension from the adrenal gland. Metastatic Wilms' tumor is almost as frequent and usually involves the liver by direct extension. Hematogenous metastases from both of these tumors do occur but are less common. Lymphomas and lymphosarcomas frequently involve the lymphatic tissues around the liver and can spread into hepatic tissue. Any carcinoma or other tumor arising from intra-abdominal organs may metastasize to the liver, which should always be studied for possible metastatic disease in such patients.

THE COLON AND RECTUM

A discussion of cancer of the colon and rectum could not be begun without first considering the problem of polyposis. There are three types of polyposis that involve infants and children: (1) juvenile polyps, (2) the Peutz-Jeghers syndrome, and (3) familial polyposis. Juvenile polyps are actually congenital cystic hamartomas that occur in the colon or rectum, producing variable abdominal symptoms, and are not associated with carcinomas. The Peutz-Jeghers syndrome is also associated with polyps that are hamartomas. The polyps involve the small intestine and stomach more commonly than the colon and are not associated with malignant disease, although changes suggesting malignancy have been noted in polyps from individuals with the Peutz-Jeghers syndrome. The final form of polyposis, familial multiple polyposis, is transmitted as a mendelian dominant trait with incomplete penetrance. Affected individuals with this disorder are at great risk for developing carcinomatous changes within the polyp.[22]

Treatment for the first two types of polyps is surgical removal of the polyp when it becomes symptomatic. Treatment of familial polyposis is total colectomy with removal of the rectal stump at the earliest possible age. If total colectomy cannot be performed because of possible complications, a subtotal colectomy may be performed, but only if frequent and regular follow-up examinations are made.

Another disorder associated with a high risk of the development of carcinoma is chronic ulcerative colitis in children. The frequency of carcinoma in these patients has been reported as ranging from 3% up to 33%. In one series the risk of developing carcinoma increased by 20% per decade after the first decade of disease.[3] Consequently, an aggressive approach must be taken in the management of ulcerative colitis if carcinoma is to be avoided. The operation of choice is total colectomy and proctectomy with ileostomy, although the time of surgery must be related to the patient's course.

In addition, carcinoma of the colon and rectum occurs without any association with the two disorders just discussed. Its greatest frequency is in children between 10 and 16 years of age, but it has been reported in children less than 5 years old. The male to female ratio is approximately 2:1. The site is much more commonly in the rectum than in other areas of the large bowel, and no difference is found between the right and left side of the colon. The patients usually have abdominal pain and vomiting, although weight loss, change of bowel habits, and rectal bleeding are also seen. Rectal bleeding is the most frequent symptom in lesions of the rectum with abdominal pain next most common. A palpable mass is usually found only in tumors of the transverse colon. About half the tumors are mucoid adenocarcinomas, which contrasts with an adult frequency of only 5%.[20] Therapy is based on adequate surgical resection, to which "second-look" surgery should probably be added to search for recurrences.[5] Chemotherapy using 5-fluorouracil has been effective and may play a role in management of this tumor. Even with improved methods the prognosis is poor, and major advances are still to come.

REFERENCES

1. Barclay, G. P. T., and Robb, W. A. T.: A clinicopathologic study of carcinoid tumors, Surg. Gynecol. Obstet. **126**:483-496, 1968.
2. Baum, R. K., and Perzik, S. L.: Tumors of the parotid gland in children, Am. Surg. **31**:719-722, 1965.
3. Devroede, G. J., Taylor, W. F., Saver, W. G., Jackman, R. J., and Stickler, G. B.: Cancer risk and life expectancy of children with ulcerative colitis, N. Engl. J. Med. **285**:17-21, 1971.
4. Dollinger, M. R., and Gardner, B.: Newer aspects of the carcinoid spectrum, Surg. Gynecol. Obstet. **122**:1335-1347, 1966.
5. Donaldson, M. H., Taylor, P., Rawitscher, R., and Sewell, J. B.: Colon carcinoma in childhood, Pediatrics **48**:307-312, 1971.
6. El-Domeiri, A. A., Huvos, A. G., Goldsmith, H. S., and Foote, F. W., Jr.: Primary malignant tumors of the liver, Cancer **27**:7-11, 1971.
7. Eversole, L. R.: Mucoepidermoid carcinoma: review of 815 reported cases, J. Oral Surg. **28**:490-494, 1970.
8. Foster, J. H.: Survival after liver resection for cancer, Cancer **26**:493-502, 1970.
9. Fraumeni, J. F., Miller, R. W., and Hill, J. F.: Primary carcinoma of the liver in childhood: An epidemiologic study, J. Natl. Cancer Inst. **40**:1087-1099, 1968.
10. Galich, R.: Salivary gland neoplasms in childhood, Arch. Otolaryngol. **89**:878-882, 1969.
11. Grosfeld, J. L., Clatworthy, H. W., Jr., and Hamoudi, A. B.: Pancreatic malignancy in childhood, Arch. Surg. **101**:370-375, 1970.
12. Healey, W. V., Perzin, K. H., and Smith, L.: Mucoepidermoid carcinoma of salivary gland origin, Cancer **26**:368-388, 1970.
13. Ishak, K. G., and Glunz, P. R.: Hepatoblastoma and hepatocarcinoma in infancy and childhood, Cancer **20**:396-422, 1967.
14. Kasai, M., and Watanabe, I.: Histologic classification of liver-cell carcinoma in infancy and childhood and its clinical evaluation, Cancer **25**:551-563, 1970.
15. Keeling, J. W.: Liver tumours in infancy and childhood, J. Pathol. **103**:69-85, Feb., 1971.
16. Kissane, J. M., and Smith, M. G.: Pathology of infancy and childhood, St. Louis, 1967, The C. V. Mosby Co.
17. Kreel, L., Jones, E. A., and Tavil, A. S.: A comparative study of arteriography and scintillation scanning in space-occupying lesions of the liver, Br. J. Radiol. **41**:401-411, 1968.

18. McNeer, G.: Cancer of the stomach in the young, Am. J. Roentgenol. **45**:537-550, 1941.
19. Moore, G.: Visceral squamous cancer in children, Pediatrics **21**:573-581, 1958.
20. O'Brien, S. E.: Carcinoma of the colon in childhood and adolescence, Can. Med. Assoc. J. **96**:1217-1222, 1967.
21. Raffucci, F. L., and Ramirez-Schon, G.: Management of tumors of the liver, Surg. Gynecol. Obstet. **130**:371-385, 1970.
22. Sachatello, C. R.: Familial polyposis of the colon. A four-decade follow-up, Cancer **28**: 581-587, 1971.
23. Stillman, A., and Zamcheck, H.: Recent advances in immunologic diagnosis of digestive tract cancer, Am. J. Dig. Dis. **15**:1003-1018, 1970.
24. Wang, I., Wood, D. E., Colapinto, R. F., and Langer, B.: Scintigraphy and arteriography in the diagnosis of diseases of the liver, Can. Med. Assoc. J. **104**:989-993, 1971.
25. Welch, K. J.: Pancreatic neoplasms. In Mustard, W. T., Ravitch, M. M., Snyder, W. H., Jr., Welch, K. J., and Benson, C. D., editors: Pediatric surgery, vol. I, ed. 2, Chicago, 1969, Yearbook Medical Publishers, Inc., pp. 758-761.
26. Wilson, S. D., and Ellison, E. H.: Total gastric resection in children with the Zollinger-Ellison syndrome, Arch. Surg. **91**:165-173, 1965.

Review references

1. Janower, M. L., Dreyfuss, J. R., and Weber, A. L.: Cancer of the gastrointestinal tract in young people, Radiol. Clin. North Am. **7**:121-130, 1969.
2. Kissane, J. M., and Smith, M. G.: Pathology of infancy and childhood, St. Louis, 1967, The C. V. Mosby Co.
3. Landing, B. H., and Martin, J. W.: Tumors of the gastrointestinal tract and pancreas, Pediatr. Clin. North Am. **6**:413-426, 1959.
4. Pickett, L. K., and Briggs, H. C.: Cancer of the gastrointestinal tract in childhood, Pediatr. Clin. North Am. **14**:223-234, 1967.
5. Synder, W. H., Chaffin, L., and Synder, M. H.: Neoplasms of the colon and rectum in infants and children, Pediatr. Clin. North Am. **3**:93-111, 1956.

CHAPTER 28

Miscellaneous childhood tumors

MARY ELLEN HAGGARD

A variety of miscellaneous tumors occurring in childhood remain to be considered. Some of these are common and truly benign. Others, although benign microscopically, are potentially malignant because of location or mode of growth. Other very rare malignant tumors should be considered early in the differential diagnosis. In all these cases adequate consultation must be obtained and optimum treatment and support given.

TERATOMA

Histologically, teratomas contain a variety of different types of tissues arising from all three embryonic layers, that is, endodermal tissue such as respiratory or intestinal, mesodermal such as connective or vascular, and ectodermal such as skin, teeth, or nerves. Teratomas occur at a variety of sites but mainly in the midline of the body or in the gonads. They are predominantly benign but may be malignant. In many series, incuding those cited by Gross and co-workers[3] and Woolley,[6] the most common site is the sacrococcygeal region. Other sites include the retroperitoneum, mediastinum, cerebrum, base of the skull, and palate.

Sacrococcygeal teratoma is particularly important because it is the most common solid tumor of the newborn. Even so, its rarity is emphasized by Gelb's[2] estimate that it occurs once in every 40,000 live births. Histologically, these tumors may be classified as mature teratomas, immature teratomas, embryonal teratomas, and mixed germ neoplasms (teratocarcinomas).[1] In Conklin and Abell's series,[1] 75% of the tumors were either benign mature or immature teratomas, whereas 25% were of the more malignant types. Fig. 28-1 illustrates the latter variety.

Clinically, the tumor must be differentiated from meningomyelocele, pilonidal cyst, hemangioma, chordoma, or a neurogenic pelvic tumor. The size of the teratoma may be impressive. In the fetus it may contribute to difficult labor and delivery. Other consequences of the tumor are infection, bleeding, pain, and a tendency to undergo malignant transformation. The tumor is usually resectable in the newborn but is likely to undergo malignant change if not removed early in life. On the basis of their own experience and that reflected in a survey of the literature, Hunt and associates,[5] state that the likelihood of malignancy is time dependent. Before the age of 4 months the incidence of malignancy is about 6%. Tumors resected in the newborn period, although containing microscopic evidence of malignant cells, have resulted in surgical cure. Between the age of 4 months and 5 years the incidence of malignancy is 50% to 60%. The importance of early identification and surgical resection is further emphasized by the fact that these tumors are not sensitive to irradiation and are only sporadically and temporarily responsive to chemical agents.[4]

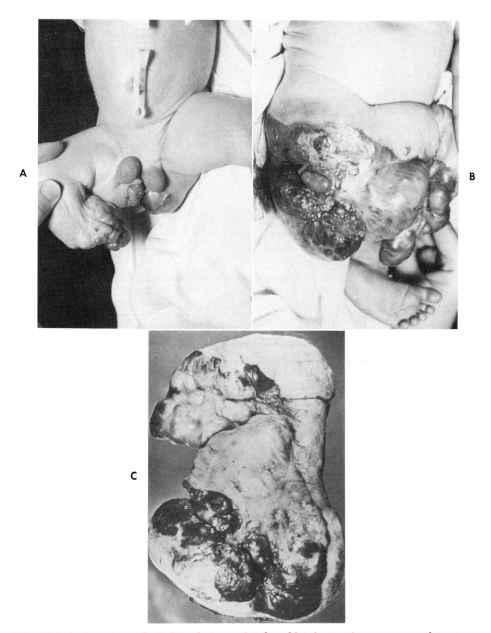

Fig. 28-1. A, Anterior and, **B,** lateral views of 2-day-old infant with sacrococcygeal teratoma involving right lower extremity, perineum, and buttock. **C,** Surgical specimen removed by hemipelvectomy. When the infant died from infection at 26 days, malignant cells were identified at the margins of the surgical wound. (Courtesy J. Ternberg, M.D.)

Teratomas in the mediastinal region usually occur in the anterior compartment. Although they are said to arise in the midline, the majority (80%) extend either principally or partially into one of the thoracic cavities. In the cervical region teratomas must be differentiated from cystic hygromas. Cystic hygroma usually occurs in the posterior cervical triangle and can be transilluminated. Teratomas of the testis and ovary are discussed in Chapters 22 and 23.

NEOPLASMS INVOLVING THE SKIN
Malignant melanoma

Malignant melanoma is an extremely rare neoplasm, particularly in children, accounting for only 0.6% of cancer deaths among all ages. About 50% to 75% of malignant melanomas arise in pigmented nevi, most commonly during the fourth decade of life. In 1971 Lerman and Murray,[9] adding 5 previously unreported cases, were able to find only 73 cases of malignant melanoma capable of metastases occurring in children.

Congenital malignant melanoma may occur as a result of transplacental passage of tumor cells from the mother or malignant transformation within a giant pigmented nevus that, unlike most other pigmented nevi, is present at birth. Leptomeningeal melanocytosis, the presence of nevus cells in the leptomeninges, is most likely to occur with giant nevi involving dermatomes of the cranial or cervical nerves. Associated features may include mental retardation, seizures, hydrocephalus, spina bifida, and meningomyelocele. Malignant melanoma may occur at any site of melanocytosis.[12]

Melanoma occurring before puberty other than congenitally is most likely to arise in a junctional nevus or the junctional component of a compound nevus. The likelihood of junctional nevi occurring on the soles, palms, genitalia, anorectal mucosa, nailbeds, and lower extremities is such that pigmented nevi in these areas should be removed prophylactically.

A junctional nevus undergoing malignant change may reveal certain sequential changes during a 3- to 4-month period of observation. It may become darker in color, gradually spread horizontally, then show roughness and scaliness, followed by vertical growth with the surface becoming smooth and bulging. Inflammation of the surrounding skin may also be observed with malignant change. Observation during adolescence is particularly important because of an increased incidence of malignant transformation compared with other childhood age groups. However, it must be borne in mind that with adolescence benign pigmented nevi tend to become more prominent and may also show some of these changes.[14]

Wide surgical excision in suspected malignant lesions is indicated. Metastatic disease is difficult to control, but chemotherapy may have palliative effects.[10] Immunologic studies of the tumor and immunotherapy are under active investigation.[11]

Nevoid basal cell carcinoma

A syndrome with this tumor, usually involving multiple sites, has been observed in a number of individuals.[8] The syndrome is characterized by cutaneous tumors, skeletal anomalies (rib defects, spina bifida, kyphosis, and scoliosis), cysts of the mandible or maxilla, pitting of the skin of the hands or feet, central nervous system anomalies, and occasionally medulloblastoma. The skin lesions tend to occur in crops. In childhood they may seem to be benign unless the associated defects are identified and the microscopic malignant nature of the lesions is observed.

Xeroderma pigmentosum

This recessive hereditable disorder of childhood is also characterized by a high incidence of squamous cell and basal cell carcinoma of the skin.[13] An abnormal sensitivity to sunlight with the development of skin changes resembling those of senility may be noted early in life with malignant lesions terminating in childhood or late adolescence. Recent observations suggest that the basic defect in this disorder is one of impaired DNA synthesis in cells of the skin on exposure to irradiation[7] (Figs. 28-2 and 28-3).

Basal cell carcinoma may also occur in children without associated anomalies.[15]

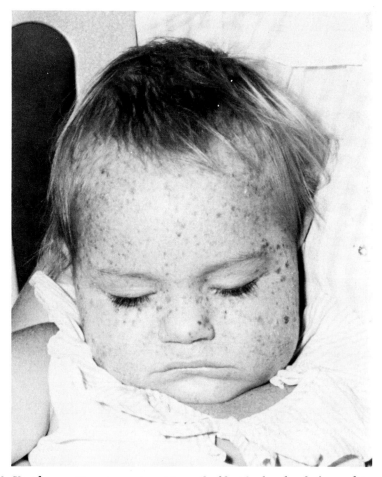

Fig. 28-2. Xeroderma pigmentosum in a 16-month-old girl who already has malignant lesions.

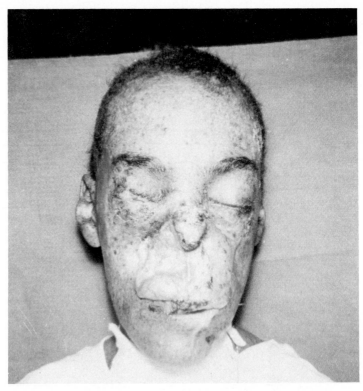

Fig. 28-3. Xeroderma pigmentosum in an 11-year-old boy showing progressive, extensive involvement of the face with squamous and basal cell carcinoma.

JUVENILE NASOPHARYNGEAL ANGIOFIBROMA

Juvenile nasopharyngeal angiofibroma is a rare but interesting tumor that, as its name implies, occurs in the nasopharynx and microscopically has vascular and fibrous components. Its characteristics have been reviewed and defined by Apostol and Frazell.[16] The tumor is characterized by its predilection for prepubertal and older boys, so much so that when the diagnosis is made in a girl it should be suspect, and chromosomal sex should probably be determined in the patient. Of the 230 cases cited by Apostol and Frazell, less than 15 were in girls, and some of these had no histologic verification.

These tumors arise in submucous connective tissue. The younger tumors tend to be cellular with fibrocytes and numerous thin-walled, endothelial-lined blood and lymph vessels. Cellularity diminishes with age.

Common presenting symptoms are epistaxis, which occurs in over a third of the patients, and nasal obstruction, which is seen in over half. Ultimately 90% develop nasal obstruction, and 80% have epistaxis. Other findings in addition to a nasopharyngeal mass include bulging of the cheek or palate or both, exophthalmos, headache, and deafness.

The tumor characteristically is unilateral in its growth and spares the contralateral antrum. The mass tends to ulcerate; subsequent infection was a cause of

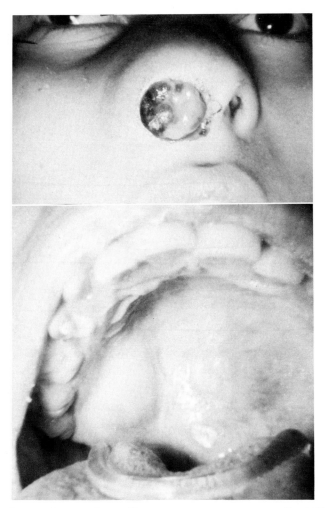

Fig. 28-4. Juvenile nasopharyngeal angiofibroma presenting as an externally visible mass. Tumor has destroyed walls of the nares, posterior walls of the right maxillary antrum, pterygoid, clinoids, and floor of the sella turcica. In spite of surgery, hormones, and chemotherapy, the child died of recurrent tumor 18 months after initial therapy.

some deaths attributed to the tumor prior to the advent of antibiotics. Malignant transformation, if it occurs at all, is extremely rare, and no instances of metastasis have been reported. The tumor grows slowly and in some instances regresses spontaneously.[16] Regression has been observed as early as 1 year and as late as 22 years after diagnosis. Prior to regression, however, the tumor may produce erosion of bone or life-threatening nasopharyngeal obstruction and hemorrhage.

Diagnosis is based on histologic appearance of the tumor and age and sex of the patient. It must be differentiated from other tumors arising in this area. Local resection is considered the treatment of choice, although temporary regression can be achieved by radiotherapy.[17, 18] Antibiotics may be necessary to control superimposed infection. The potential seriousness of epistaxis must be appreciated, and at times ligation of the external carotid artery may be necessary to control bleeding. Since these tumors often regress with completion of puberty, testosterone has been a form of treatment, but beneficial results have not been convincing. Stilbestrol has also been used but has been abandoned because of undesirable side effects.

Prognosis is generally good; complete cure is usual even in those tumors that are incompletely resected, but deaths have occurred (Fig. 28-4).

LYMPHANGIOMA

Lymphangiomas, congenital in origin, originate from lymphatic tissue sequestered during embryonic development.[28] They comprise 5% to 6% of benign tumors of infancy and childhood.[20] In some series girls predominate over boys,[21, 29] but in others the distribution is about equal.[24, 26] Classification includes three principal types. *Simple lymphangioma,* consisting of dilatations of lymph channels in the skin, subcutaneous tissue, or mucous membrane, is very rare. A specific entity usually included as part of this group has been called *lymphangioma cutis circumscriptum.* Lesions of this type develop in the superficial corium, most commonly as a single circumscribed lesion. *Cavernous lymphangioma* commonly involves the trunk or structures about the oral cavity. It may be large enough to cause dystocia or to be incompatible with life. The term *systemic lymphangiomatosis* has been applied[19] when the lymphangioma involves an entire extremity, producing a markedly deformed and enlarged organ.

Cystic hygroma is the term applied to lymphangiomas characterized by proximity to major lymph channels and by multiloculated cystic structure. Combined varieties of two or more of the three major types are also observed, but attempts are usually made to classify the tumor by its predominant features. Some observers add a fourth category of *lymphangiohemangioma* for tumors that seem to have both vascular and lymphatic components. This type is extremely rare and seen almost exclusively in adults. Ariel and Pack [19] were able to cite only one instance of sarcomatous degeneration in a cystic hygroma.

Clinical manifestations depend on the size of the tumor and the anatomic area involved. Simple lymphangioma, because of its often superficial location, may have an insignificant wartlike appearance.[24] Worthy of mention are the special problems associated with involvement of the tongue.[25, 26] The tongue alone may be involved, or the floor of the mouth, lips, cheeks, and epiglottis may also be involved. There may be associated macroglossia and overgrowth of the mandible. The lymphangiomas appear on the dorsum of the tongue as small vesicles filled with clear fluid; many of them disappear spontaneously, but some develop into papillomatous lesions that are painful and bleed easily. Glossitis with swelling of the tongue, often following an upper respiratory infection, may be a further complication.

The neck is the most common site of involvement of cystic hygroma (64%[21] to 93%[29]). Other sites include the axilla, popliteal fossa, groin, and retroperitoneal region. In the neck the tumor must be differentiated from thyroglossal duct cyst, branchogenic cyst, dermoid cyst, lipoma, or diseases of lymph nodes such as tuberculosis or malignant lymphoma. Cystic hygroma may fluctuate markedly in size; it is usually compressible and not attached to the skin. It frequently involves deeper structures.

Cavernous lymphangioma may also involve the neck and is likely to be noted at birth or within the first year of life. It is more invasive than the cystic variety.[24] These tumors tend to be multiple. The interesting association of chylopericardium[23] or chylomediastinum with lymphangioma of the posterior mediastinum and with anomalies of the skeletal system is worthy of note.[27]

The histologic finding of lymph-filled cysts and dilated vessels lined by endothelial cells is common to all these tumors. The simple or capillary variety has a very thin stroma, and dilatation is of lesser degree than with other varieties. Cavernous lymphangioma differs from the cystic variety in the smaller size of the cystic dilatations and the presence of thicker stroma.

Treatment depends on location and extent of involvement. Early surgical resection of cystic hygroma of the neck is recommended because of the likelihood of progressive growth leading to more extensive disease and respiratory obstruction. Resection is likely to require more extensive surgery than is initially thought because of the tumor's extension about deeper structures.

Extensive tumors not considered resectable may at times benefit from partial resection, especially where ulceration has occurred. Lymphangiomas are not radiosensitive, and the use of sclerosing solutions has few proponents.

PRIMARY TUMORS OF THE SPLEEN

Splenic tumors at any age are extremely rare. They may arise from any tissue represented in the spleen, that is, lymphoid, vascular, or fibrous tissue that makes up the capsular and trabecular framework.[31] The possibility also exists that primary splenic tumors could arise from embryonic rests such as dermoid cysts and teratomas. Of the reported cases, lymphosarcoma and reticulum cell sarcoma are by far the most common,[30] although hemangioendothelioma would appear to be the most common type observed in children.[32, 33] The rapidity with which progressive disease is observed after splenectomy in many of the reported cases of lymphoma of the spleen suggests the possibility of occult systemic disease at the time of surgery.

BREAST TUMORS

The rarity of *carcinoma* of the breast among the young has long been appreciated. deCholnoky's[36] review found 2% of all breast cancer occurring in patients under 30 years of age and less than 0.1% in those under 20 years of age. Only sixteen instances of primary carcinoma of the breast have been found in children 15 years of age or younger, the youngest of whom was 3 years of age.[39-41, 43-48] It has been observed that the rarity of the condition, as well as an understandable reluctance to undertake disfiguring surgery in a child, particularly a girl, makes the physician's decision regarding management all the more difficult. Although some authors suggest that this tumor is less likely to spread in children than in adults,[43] there are case reports of dissemination. Therefore children with malignancy should probably be managed the same as adults with carcinoma of the breast.

Certain benign tumors are much more common than malignant breast tumors.[35, 38, 42] This is especially true in prepubertal and adolescent 10- to

20-year-old girls. In a series of 237 girls with breast lesions, which Farrow and Ashikari[38] accumulated over a 10-year period, 76.4% proved microscopically to have *fibroadenomas*. In another series, 94% had fibroadenomas.[35] These lesions may be bilateral and assume massive proportions, making them difficult to distinguish from virginal hypertrophy.[42] Some observers consider the term *cystosarcoma phylloides* appropriate for tumors in this group that have a characteristic stromal pattern. They further subdivide this latter group into benign and malignant forms. Cystosarcoma phylloides of the malignant variety is extremely rare, and no cases have been reported in children.[38] Most masses in the breast can be treated by simple excision.

Other breast lesions occurring in the adolescent age group include *intraductal papillomatosis, lipoma, cysts,* and *inflammatory lesions*.[34, 35, 37, 38] Certain metastatic tumors may also involve the breast. Farrow and Ashikari[38] observed two instances of metastatic rhabdomyosarcoma involving the breast and only one primary neoplasm. We have observed one 15-year-old girl with massive bilateral breast enlargement developing over 4 weeks that proved to be due to infiltrates associated with acute leukemia.

HEMANGIOMA

A variety of classifications have been applied to vascular nevi.[51, 61, 62, 64] Many observers consider these as vascular malformations or hamartomas rather than neoplasms. Hemangiomas are composed of endothelial-lined vascular spaces of varying size and extent. Much of the rapid growth observed in these lesions shortly after birth is related to their becoming distended by blood and not to cellular proliferation. It is important to recognize that lesions already present at birth and showing little tendency to increase in size after birth are most likely to contain mature vascular channels with little tendency toward subsequent involution, whereas those that grow rapidly in the first few months of life are the more likely to involute.[60]

The natural history of the common strawberry hemangioma, cavernous or mixed hemangioma, and hemangioendothelioma is one of increasing size during the first 6 months of life and a period of slower growth when size increases parallel to the infant's growth, followed by involution, which may not reach its maximum for 4 to 5 years. Management should therefore be as conservative as possible. Surgery for removal or cosmetic revision should await maximal involution. Some investigators claim that involution has been hastened by adrenocortical hormone administration[53, 54, 66, 67]; therefore this approach might be considered for those lesions of such size, extent, or anatomic location that surgical resection is not possible and for those associated with thrombocytopenia. Radiation should be avoided if at all possible because of the high incidence of complications, which include interference with growth of underlying bone, malignancy arising in the radiation scar, and possible brain damage when administered to an area involving the skull.[56] Cutaneous hemangioma may be irradiated by electron beam, thereby avoiding the deep complications of radiotherapy.

Complications during the period of involution, whether induced or spontaneous, include ulceration with or without hemorrhage (usually slight) and infection. These can usually be easily managed. One complication requiring

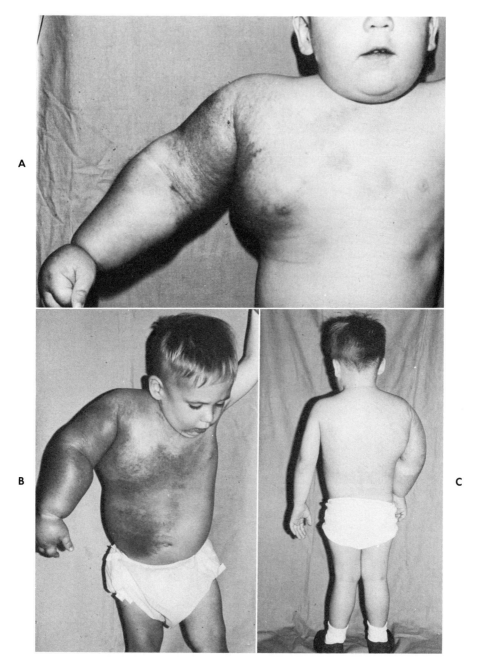

Fig. 28-5. A, Giant mixed hemangioma in a 22-month-old boy. Several small hemangiomas present at birth had been noted to grow rapidly in the ensuing 5 months. Thrombocytopenia with sequestration of ^{51}Cr-tagged platelets within the tumor failed to respond to electron beam irradiation. Heparin administration resulted in a return of platelet count to normal and amelioration of concurrent hemolytic anemia. **B,** Discontinuance of anticoagulants was followed by marked enlargement of the tumor. The administration of anticoagulants, diuretics, and digitoxin for associated oliguria and congestive heart failure was followed by gradual weight loss and regression in tumor size. **C,** With the patient on a regimen of crystalline sodium warfarin (Coumadin) for 4 years, there has been gradual regression in tumor size with maintenance of full use of the right arm and hand.

special attention is the syndrome first described by Kasabach and Merritt.[58] This entity is most commonly observed in the first year of life among those infants with rapidly growing giant cavernous hemangioma, but it also occurs as a chronic and sustained problem among older children with multiple hemangiomas that do not involute. Studies subsequent to Kasabach and Merritt's observation have shown that platelets are sequestered within the tumor and clotting factors depleted, leading to the development of consumption coagulopathy. Accompanying this phenomenon may be massive hemorrhage. In addition to adrenal cortical hormones, platelet transfusion, replacement of clotting factors, and use of anticoagulants[55] have been beneficial (Fig. 28-5).

Several clinical syndromes associated with hemangiomas have been observed. Diffuse neonatal hemangiomatosis, that is, nonmalignant hemangioma involving viscera and three or more organ systems, may result in early death.[57] Encephalotrigeminal angiomatosis (Sturge-Weber syndrome) with hemangioma involving skin, mucous membranes, choroid, and pia mater may be associated with mental retardation and visual defects. Syndromes associated with bone involvement include developmental hypertrophy of bone and extremity with hemangioma and venous varicosity, referred to as the *Weber-Klippel-Trenaunay syndrome*. When the associated bony defect is one of dyschondroplasia, the term *Maffucci's syndrome* is used. Gorham's disease is characterized by osteolysis of bone with replacement by hemangioma.[61]

Hemangiopericytoma[49] is differentiated from other vascular tumors by the presence of peculiar elongated and contractile cells proliferating and com-

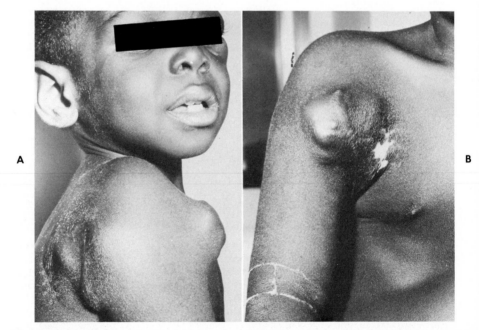

Fig. 28-6. A, Lateral and, **B,** anterior views of malignant hemangiopericytoma diagnosed in a 9-month-old infant. Attempts at surgical resection and chemotherapy were unsuccessful. The infant expired with pulmonary metastases at 19 months of age.

pressing capillaries. Attempts to distinguish a benign and malignant variety are difficult microscopically, but behavior of the tumor suggests an overall recurrence rate of 52% after surgical resection. In the central nervous system recurrence may be as high as 80% and in the lung and mediastinum 36%. The tumor is relatively radioresistant but may respond to chemotherapy[63] (Fig. 28-6).

Two malignant varieties of vascular tumors merit consideration. Angiosarcoma may develop in a hemangioma or hemangioendothelioma but does so extremely rarely.[50, 59] Local excision is usually possible, but extensive lesions may respond to chemotherapy such as vincristine. Endovascular papillary angioendothelioma[52] is a term assigned to a rare tumor of the skin characterized by plugs of endothelium extending into lumina of vascular channels. Although the tumor rarely may show lymph node invasion, prognosis after local excision is good.

REFERENCES

Teratoma

1. Conklin, J., and Abell, M. R.: Germ cell neoplasms of sacrococcygeal region, Cancer **20:** 2105, 1967.
2. Gelb, A., Rosenblum, H., Jaurigue, V. G., Liboro, C., and Francisco, P.: Sacrococcygeal teratoma, Del. Med. J. **36:**119, June, 1964.
3. Gross, R. E., Clatworthy, H. W., and Meeker, J. A.: Sacrococcygeal teratomas in infants and children, Surg. Gynecol. Obstet. **92:**341, 1951.
4. Hickey, R. C., and Schwindt, W. D.: Sacrococcygeal teratoma—surgical ground rounds, Wis. Med. J. **65:**91, 1966.
5. Hunt, P., Van Leeuwen, G., Bingham, H., and Sights, W.: Sacrococcygeal teratomas, Clin. Pediatr. **7:**165, March, 1968.
6. Woolley, M. M.: Teratomas in infancy and childhood, Z. Kinderheilkd. **4:**289, 1967.

Neoplasms involving the skin

7. Epstein, J. H., Fukuyama, K., Reed, W. B., and Epstein, W. L.: Defect in DNA synthesis in skin of patients with xeroderma pigmentosum demonstrated in vivo, Science **168:**1477, 1970.
8. Howell, J. B., Anderson, D. E., and McClendon, J. L.: Multiple cutaneous cancers in children; the nevoid basal cell carcinoma syndrome, J. Pediatr. **69:**97, 1966.
9. Lerman, R. T., and Murray, D.: Malignant melanoma of childhood, Cancer **25:**436, 1971.
10. Livingston, R. B., and Carter, S. K.: Single agents in cancer chemotherapy, New York, 1970, IFI/Plenum Data Corp.
11. Morton, D. L., Eibler, F. R., Joseph, W. L., Wood, W. C., Trahan, A., and Ketcham, A. S.: Immunological factors in human sarcomas and melanomas: A rational basis for immunotherapy, Ann. Surg. **172:**740, 1970.
12. Reed, W. B., Becker, S. W., Sr., Becker, S. W., Jr., and Nickel, W. R.: Giant pigmented nevi, melanoma and leptomeningeal melanocytosis, Arch. Dermatol. **91:**100, 1965.
13. Siegelman, M. H., and Sutow, W. W.: Xeroderma pigmentosum, J. Pediatr. **67:**625, 1965.
14. Walton, R. G.: Pigmented nevi, Symposium on Pediatric Dermatology, Pediatr. Clin. North Am. **18:**897, 1971.
15. Weitzner, S., and Harville, D. D.: Basal cell carcinoma of the cheek in a 12 year old girl, Am. J. Dis. Child. **116:**678, 1968.

Juvenile nasopharyngeal angiofibroma

16. Apostol, J. V., and Frazell, E. L.: Juvenile nasopharyngeal angiofibroma, Cancer **18:**869, 1965.
17. Briant, T. D. R., Fitzpatrick, P. J., and Book, H.: The radiological treatment of juvenile nasopharyngeal angiofibroma, Ann. Otol. Rhinol. Laryngol. **79:**1108, 1970.
18. Jereb, B., Anggard, A., and Baryd, I.: Juvenile nasopharyngeal angiofibroma, Acta Radiol. **9:**302, 1970.

Lymphangioma

19. Ariel, I. M., and Pack, G. T.: Cancer and allied diseases of infancy and childhood, Boston, 1960, Little, Brown & Co., p. 417.
20. Dargeon, H. W.: Tumors of childhood, a clinical treatise, New York, 1960, Hoeber Medical Division, Harper & Row, Publishers, p. 29.
21. Fuller, W.: Cystic hygroma, Surg. Gynecol. Obstet. **108**:457, 1959.
22. Goetsch, E.: Hygroma collicysticum and hygroma axillare, Arch. Surg. **36**:394, 1938.
23. Goldstein, M. R., Benchimol, A., Cornell, W., and Long, D. R.: Chylopericardium with multiple lymphangioma of bone, N. Engl. J. Med. **280**:1034, 1969.
24. Harkins, G. A., and Sabiston, D. C.: Lymphangioma in infancy and childhood, Surgery **47**:811, 1960.
25. Koop, C. E., and Moschakis, E. A.: Capillary lymphangioma of the tongue complicated by glossitis, Pediatrics **27**:800, 1961.
26. Litzow, T. J., and Lash, H.: Lymphangiomas of the tongue, Mayo Clin. Proc. **36**:229, 1961.
27. Morphis, L. G., Arcinue, E. L., and Kraus, J. R.: Generalized lymphangioma in infancy with chylothorax, Pediatrics **46**:556, 1970.
28. Sabin, F. R.: The origin and development of the lymphatic system, Johns Hopkins Hosp. Rep. **17**:347, 1916.
29. Ward, G. E., Hendrick, J. W., and Chambers, R. G.: Cystic hygroma of the neck, West. J. Surg. **58**:41, Feb., 1950.

Primary tumors of the spleen

30. Das Gupta, T., Coombes, B., and Brasfield, R. D.: Primary malignant neoplasms of the spleen, Surg. Gynecol. Obstet. **120**:947, 1965.
31. Hausmann, P. F., and Gaarde, F. W.: Malignant neoplasms of spleen, Surgery **14**:246, 1943.
32. Lazarus, J. A., and Marks, M. S.: Primary malignant tumor of the spleen, Am. J. Surg. **71**:479, 1946.
33. Stowens, D.: Pediatric pathology, Baltimore, 1966, The Williams & Wilkins Co., p. 546.

Breast tumors

34. Battle, W. H., and Maybury, B. C.: Primary epithelioma of the nipple in a girl aged 11 years, Lancet **1**:1521, 1913.
35. Daniel, W. A., Jr., and Matthews, M. D.: Tumors of the breast in adolescent females, Pediatrics **41**:743, 1968.
36. deCholnoky, T.: Mammary cancer in youth, Surg. Gynecol. Obstet. **77**:55, 1943.
37. Diethrich, E. G., Hammond, W. W., Jr., and Holtz, F.: Intraductal papillomatosis of the breast. Report of a case in a ten-year-old girl, Am. J. Surg. **112**:80, 1966.
38. Farrow, J. H., and Ashikari, H.: Breast lesions in young girls. Surg. Clin. North Am. **49**:261, 1969.
39. Festenstein, H.: Adenocarcinoma of the breast in a South African Bantu boy aged fourteen, S. Afr. Med. J. **34**:517, 1960.
40. Hartman, A. W., and Margrish, P.: Carcinoma of the breast in children: Case report: Six-year-old boy with adenocarcinoma, Ann. Surg. **141**:792, 1955.
41. Levings, A. H.: Carcinoma of the mammary gland in a 12-year-old girl: Report of a case, N. Engl. J. Med. **223**:760, 1940.
42. Lewis, D., and Gieschickter, C. F.: Gynecomastia, virginal hypertrophy and fibroadenomas of breast, Ann. Surg. **100**:779, 1934.
43. McDivitt, R. W., and Stewart, F. W.: Breast carcinoma in children, J.A.M.A. **195**:338, 1966.
44. Puente Duany, N., and Garciga Ramirez, C. E.: Cancer of the breast in children: observation in a patient aged 11, Arch. Cubanos Cancerol. **10**:36, Jan.-March, 1951.
45. Rameriz, G., and Ansfield, F. J.: Breast carcinoma in children, Arch. Surg. **96**:222, 1968.
46. Sears, J. B., and Schlesinger, M. J.: Carcinoma of the breast in a 12-year-old girl, N. Engl. J. Med. **223**:760, 1940.
47. Simmons, R. R.: Adenocarcinoma of the breast occurring in a boy of 13, J.A.M.A. **68**:1899, 1917.

48. Widmann, B. P., and Howell, J. C.: Carcinoma of the breast in a 14-year-old girl, Surg. Clin. North Am. **12**:1363, 1932.

Hemangioma

49. Backwinkel, K. D., and Diddamus, J. A.: Hemangiopericytoma: Case report and comprehensive review of the literature, Cancer **25**:896, 1970.
50. Burgoon, C. F., Jr., and Soderberg, M.: Angiosarcoma, Arch. Dermatol. **99**:773, 1969.
51. Dargeon, H. W.: Tumors in childhood, New York, 1960, Harper Brothers.
52. Debska, M.: Malignant endovascular papillary angioendothelioma of skin in childhood: Clinicopathologic study in six cases, Cancer **24**:503, 1969.
53. Fost, N. C., and Esterly, N. B.: Successful treatment of juvenile hemangiomas with prednisone, J. Pediatr. **72**:351, 1968.
54. Goldberg, S. J.: Successful treatment of hepatic hemangioma with corticosteroids, J.A.M.A. **208**:2473, 1969.
55. Hillman, R. S., and Phillips, L. L.: Clotting-fibrinolysis in a cavernous hemangioma, Am. J. Dis. Child. **113**:649, 1967.
56. Hliniak, A., Czownicki, Z., and Medyńska, A.: Long-term results and complications after the irradiation of haemangiomas in children, Radiobiol. Radiother. **7**(2):141, 1966.
57. Holden, K. R., and Alexander, F.: Diffuse neonatal hemangiomatosis, Pediatrics **46**:411, 1970.
58. Kasabach, H. H., and Merritt, K. K.: Capillary hemangioma with extensive purpura, Am. J. Dis. Child. **59**:1063, 1940.
59. Kauffman, S. L., and Stout, A. P.: Malignant hemangioendothelioma in infants and children, Cancer **14**:1186, 1961.
60. Lampe, I., and Latourette, H. B.: Management of cavernous hemangiomas in infants, Pediatr. Clin. North Am. **6**:511, 1959.
61. Margileth, A. M.: Developmental vascular abnormalities. Symposium on Pediatric Dermatology, Pediatr. Clin. North Am. **18**:773, 1971.
62. Michael, P.: Tumors of infancy and childhood, Philadelphia, 1964, J. B. Lippincott Co.
63. Ortega, J. A., Finkelstein, J. Z., Issacs, H., Hittle, R., and Hastings, N.: Chemotherapy of malignant hemangiopericytoma of childhood, Cancer **27**:730, 1971.
64. Rook, A., Wilkinson, D. S., and Ebling, F. J. B.: Textbook of dermatology, Philadelphia, 1968, F. A. Davis Co.
65. Thatcher, L. G., Clatanoff, D. B., and Steihm, E. R.: Splenic hemangioma with thrombocytopenia and afibrinogenemia, J. Pediatr. **73**:345, 1968.
66. Touloukian, R. J.: Hepatic hemangioendothelioma during infancy. Pathology, diagnosis, and treatment with prednisone, Pediatrics **45**:71, 1970.
67. Zarem, H. A., and Edgerton, M. T.: Induced resolution of cavernous hemangiomas following prednisolone therapy, Plast. Reconstr. Surg. **39**:76, Jan., 1967.

Index